Volume

II

ROENTGENOLOGIC DIAGNOSIS

A Complement in Radiology to the
Beeson and McDermott Textbook of Medicine

J. GEORGE TEPLICK, M.D., F.A.C.R.

Professor and Director of General Diagnosis, Department of Diagnostic Radiology,
Hahnemann Medical College and Hospital

MARVIN E. HASKIN, M.D., F.A.C.P.

Professor and Chairman, Department of Diagnostic Radiology,
Hahnemann Medical College and Hospital

Third Edition

1976
W. B. SAUNDERS COMPANY • Philadelphia • London • Toronto

W. B. Saunders Company: West Washington Square
Philadelphia, PA. 19105

1 St. Anne's Road
Eastbourne, East Sussex BN21 3UN, England

833 Oxford Street
Toronto, Ontario M8Z 5T9, Canada

Listed here is the latest translated edition of this book together with the language of the translation and the publisher.

Japanese *(1st Edition)* (Volumes I and II) – Igaku Shoin, Ltd., Tokyo, Japan

Spanish *(2nd Edition)* (Volumes I and II) – NEISA, Mexico, D.F., Mexico

Roentgenologic Diagnosis

ISBN Vol I: 0-7216-8789-X
ISBN Vol II: 0-7216-8790-3

Last digit is the print number: 9   8   7   6   5   4   3   2   1

CONTENTS

CONTENTS

SECTION 7   PROTOZOAN AND HELMINTHIC DISEASES

SECTION 8   DISORDERS OF THE NERVOUS SYSTEM

CONTENTS

VOLUME II

SECTION 11   RENAL DISEASES

SECTION 12   DISEASES OF THE DIGESTIVE SYSTEM

SECTION 18 CERTAIN CUTANEOUS DISEASES WITH SIGNIFICANT SYSTEMIC MANIFESTATIONS

SECTION 19 MISCELLANEOUS HEREDITARY DISORDERS AFFECTING MULTIPLE ORGAN SYSTEMS

RENAL DISEASES

PHYSIOLOGIC CONSIDERATIONS OF INTRAVENOUS PYELOGRAPHY

The intravenous contrast media currently employed are removed from the blood almost exclusively by glomerular filtration. Renal disease that impairs glomerular clearance affects the rate of contrast removal from the blood. In the absence of glomerular disease, the rate of clearance depends on pressure relationships in the glomerular tuft. Only after the dilute filtrate is concentrated by tubular reabsorption of water will opacification occur. Glomerular filtration and tubular concentration of the contrast material occur extremely rapidly. Within a minute or so after the intravenous injection, the presence of concentrated contrast material in the tubules produces opacification of the renal parenchyma; this opacification is termed the *nephrogram.* The more rapid the injection, the sooner and more intense the nephrogram. Normally the nephrographic density decreases rapidly as the opaque medium leaves the tubules and enters the calices and pelvis. Within 10 or 15 minutes after the usual intravenous injection, the nephrogram becomes less dense, and opacification of the calices, pelvis, and ureters occurs. The pyelogram is now well established.

Impairment of glomerular filtration or tubular reabsorption, or both, will decrease the intensity of both the nephrogram and the subsequent pyelogram. In a nonfunctioning kidney, neither nephrogram nor pyelogram will appear.

If ureteral obstruction prevents steady emptying of the collecting system, and if the increased pressure in this system has not yet completely blocked glomerular filtration, the nephrogram may appear more slowly, but will persist for abnormally long periods. Gradual diffusion of the contrast material into the distended calices and pelvis will produce a pyelogram, although a few minutes to over 24 hours can lapse between the onset of the nephrogram and the appearance of a pyelogram. Once a nephrogram has developed, a pyelogram will eventually appear; however, delayed films are usually required.

If the obstruction is sufficiently severe or chronic, the obstructive pressure may approach or exceed the glomerular filtration pressure, so that glomerular filtration will be greatly diminished or absent. The tubules are then able to excrete the contrast material, and this may continue as long as tubular function persists. With cessation of tubular excretion, there will be no nephrogram, and, of course, no pyelographic opacification will occur. If a nephrogram never develops, delayed films are useless, since no pyelogram can develop.

Prolonged bilateral nephrograms with delayed opacification of the collecting systems can occur not only in bilateral obstructive uropathy but also during a hypotensive episode and when the renal tubules are blocked by precipitated mucoproteins.

Unilateral renal artery narrowing in an otherwise normal kidney will decrease renal blood flow. Consequently, after a rapid intravenous injection, the nephrogram will be delayed and will usually be less dense than that of the normal kidney. There is subsequent delay in caliceal opacification of the affected side. If a segmental artery is the site of narrowing, a segmental change in nephrographic density may be observed. The diminished volume of filtrate passes more slowly through the tubules, allowing a longer period for reabsorption and concentration. Often, therefore, the density of the subsequent pyelogram may be greater than that of the opposite normal kidney. Furthermore, because of slower filling of the collecting system, the calices may appear smaller and thinner, especially in the earlier stages of the pyelogram. The chronic ischemic kidney is often measurably smaller than its normal fellow.

While the pyelographic density often parallels renal function, the intravenous urogram is at best only a crude yardstick of renal function. Unilateral decreased pyelographic density usually indicates unilateral diminished function. Bilateral diminished but equal pyelographic densities, however, are often difficult or impossible to correlate with true renal function, since many physiologic extrarenal factors and technical errors may be responsible. Conversely, it is not unusual to obtain good pyelographic densities in spite of mild to moderate bilateral renal disease.

The introduction of high dose pyelography has greatly increased the scope of the intravenous pyelogram. Diagnostic opacification of the collecting systems can often be obtained even in the presence of greatly increased blood urea nitrogen and plasma creatinine levels. An excellent pyelogram is usually obtained in a nonazotemic patient whose conventional intravenous pyelogram was faint or poor. The entire ureter is frequently outlined, which is uncommon in conventional pyelography. High dose pyelography will obviate the need for a retrograde study in most cases.

Other diagnostic studies that may be needed to supplement the findings of intravenous urography include retrograde pyelography, nephrotomography, renal isotope scans, ultrasound, and renal arteriography.[1-5]

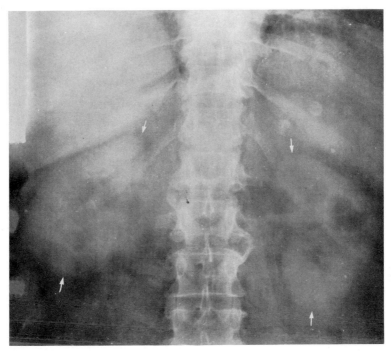

Figure 11-1 **Nephrogram Following Intravenous Pyelogram.** Serial films obtained immediately after rapid intravenous injection show bilaterally equal renal parenchymal opacification (*arrows*) (nephrogram). Nephrograms obtained by the intravenous method are less dense than those following an abdominal aortogram, because less contrast material reaches the kidney per unit of time. However, the ordinary intravenous nephrogram is usually adequate for delineating the size and shape of the kidney.

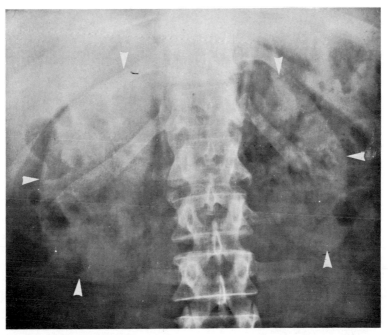

Figure 11-2 **Differential Nephrogram: Hypertension.** The nephrogram of the right kidney is denser than that of the left kidney (*arrowheads*). The left nephrogram was delayed, and the kidney on this side is smaller. These findings suggest stenosis of the left renal artery.

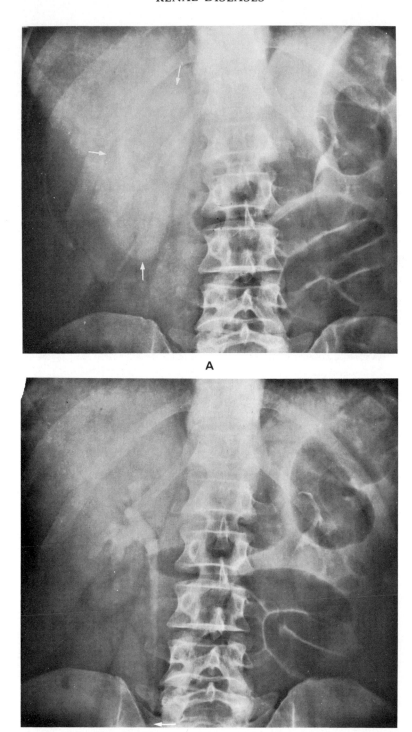

Figure 11–3   **Delayed Nephrogram: Obstructive Uropathy.**

A, There is a prolonged nephrogram and absence of caliceal opacification on the right (*arrows*); a normal pyelogram is seen on the left. Nephrographic opacification is prolonged in the acutely obstructed right kidney because the concentrated opaque medium in the renal tubules cannot rapidly enter the urine-filled calices.

B, Several hours later the tubular contrast material has diffused into the collecting system; the ensuing right pyelogram reveals the point of obstruction (*arrow*) to be a calculus in the right ureter. The ureter and collecting system above the point of obstruction are dilated. Occasionally in acute obstruction with a prolonged nephrogram, 24 hours may elapse before a pyelogram is seen.

RENAL FAILURE

Chronic Renal Failure and Uremia

In chronic renal failure due to advanced nephrosclerosis, chronic glomerulonephritis, chronic bilateral pyelonephritis, or interstitial nephritis, the plain film reveals small kidney shadows. In renal failure secondary to bilateral obstructive uropathy, the kidney shadows may be large and may contain calculi. In many other progressive bilateral renal conditions, such as polycystic disease, amyloidosis, tuberculosis, lymphosarcoma, and nephrocalcinosis, the kidney size is variable. (See text under these headings.)

Routine intravenous pyelography will frequently produce no opacification if the BUN or creatinine is elevated. However, high dose pyelography can often give satisfactory opacification even in uremia, especially if combined with tomography. When the kidneys are small, the cortices will be thinned, but the collecting systems will often be normal in nonpyelonephritic end-stage kidneys (see Figs. 11–31, 11–32, and 11–33); if pyelonephritis is the underlying cause, the calices will be blunted, and the cortices will be thin and irregular due to scarring (see Fig. 11–48).

In bilateral obstructive uropathy with large kidneys, the high dose pyelogram or retrograde studies are necessary to pinpoint the sites of obstruction for possible surgical correction.

Renal angiography in patients with uremia and small kidneys usually shows a tapered decrease in size of the main renal arteries, attenuated intrarenal arteries, decreased or absent vascularity in the periphery, and prolonged arterial opacification. The nephrographic density is moderately to severely diminished. Angiographic distinction between chronic glomerulonephritis and advanced nephrosclerosis is generally impossible. In chronic pyelonephritis the kidneys often are not symmetric in size, and the renal outline usually shows irregularities from focal scarring; the early nephrogram may be quite nonhomogeneous. However, in end-stage pyelonephritis and in diffuse noninfectious interstitial pyelonephritis (interstitial nephritis) the kidneys are often symmetric and smoothly outlined, making angiographic distinction from chronic glomerulonephritis or nephrosclerosis difficult or impossible.

In uremic patients with gastrointestinal complaints, there is often radiographic evidence of gastric atonicity and delayed gastric emptying. The mucosal folds in the stomach, the duodenal bulb, and the postbulbar area are often prominent, thickened, and somewhat stiffened. A greater than normal incidence of peptic ulcer and pancreatitis is associated with chronic uremia.[6-11]

The radiographic changes in bones, soft tissues, and chest are described on pages 780 and 786.

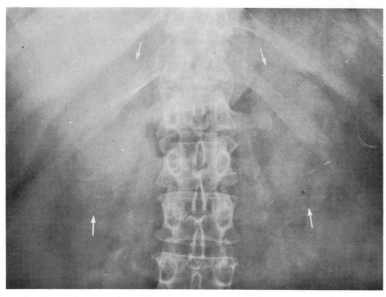

Figure 11-4 **Chronic Renal Insufficiency and Uremia.**   The kidneys are small (*arrows*). The patient had longstanding chronic pyelonephritis. There was nonvisualization of the urinary tracts by routine intravenous urography. Renal biopsy was necessary to establish the diagnosis.

Renal Osteodystrophy

Skeletal changes can occur in chronic renal failure and in the renal tubular dystrophies without renal failure. In the latter group, osteomalacia is the major finding, while in the much more common chronic renal failure, osteomalacia and secondary hyperparathyroidism are the underlying factors.

In the renal tubular dystrophies, which include renal tubular acidosis, the Fanconi syndrome, and the various aminoacidurias, the skeletal changes of osteomalacia in adults or rickets in children often develop. Adult osteomalacia is characterized by bone demineralization, coarsened trabeculations, and occasionally pseudofractures. Renal rickets is radiographically identical to ordinary rickets, with frayed, irregular, and cupped metaphyses, a widened epiphyseal line due to increased uncalcified osteoid tissue, flared rib ends, and bone demineralization. (See *Osteomalacia*, p. 1324, and *Rickets*, p. 1129). If chronic renal failure complicates the tubular dystrophy, the bone changes of secondary hyperparathyroidism will be superimposed.

In chronic renal failure, biochemical changes of secondary hyperparathyroidism develop in nearly every patient. Prolonged survival through maintenance dialysis eventually leads to radiographic evidence of osteodystrophy in about 80 per cent of patients. The bone changes are quite similar to those of primary hyperparathyroidism (see p. 1304). Subperiosteal resorption of the phalanges is usually the earliest finding but may require magnification techniques for early detection. Resorption of the outer and less often inner ends of the clavicles is a striking and relatively early finding. Later, subperiosteal erosions may appear in the proximal femora, humeri, and other bones. The tufts of the phalanges often show resorptive changes. Skull and skeletal demineralization is common. Brown tumors are encountered less frequently than in primary hyperparathyroidism. However, osteosclerosis is much more common in secondary hyperparathyroidism, occurring in about 20 per cent of cases. The vertebral bodies are most often involved, and thick sclerotic bands adjacent to the superior and inferior margins (rugger jersey spine) are almost pathognomonic. Vascular and periarticular soft tissue calcifications, sometimes massive, are frequently seen in advanced secondary hyperparathyroidism. Chondrocalcinosis occurs but is relatively infrequent. Following restoration of renal function by successful transplant, the skeletal and biochemical changes of secondary hyperparathyroidism usually slowly regress. Sometimes, however, persistence or progression of these changes occurs, necessitating parathyroid surgery (tertiary hyperparathyroidism?).

Osteomalacia or renal rickets is generally the earliest manifestation of azotemic osteodystrophy, since vitamin D resistance (absorptive failure?) constantly occurs in chronic uremia. These bone changes will coexist with the later changes of hyperparathyroidism.

In advanced azotemic osteodystrophy, rib fractures and epiphyseal dislocations are not uncommon.

Erosive periarticular changes may occur in the hands or wrists and may simulate rheumatoid arthritis. These are probably extensions of the subperiosteal resorption into the periarticular area. However, a true synovitis may also be present, perhaps related to the hyperuricemia of chronic renal disease.[12-24]

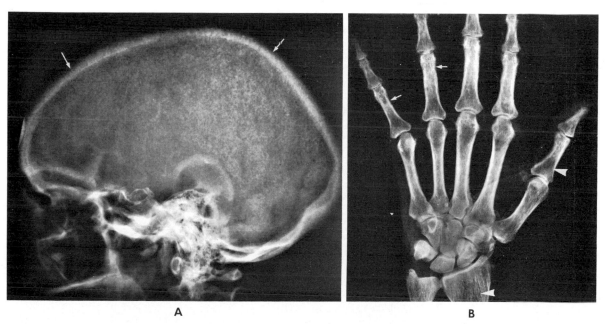

A   B

Figure 11–5   **Azotemic Osteodystrophy: Secondary Hyperparathyroidism.**

A, Characteristic sandy stippling of the bones of the cranial vault is due to demineralization. The outer table is demineralized and indistinct (*arrows*).

B, There is subperiosteal bone resorption of the phalanges (*arrows*), which is characteristic of hyperparathyroidism. Demineralization (*arrowheads*) of the remaining bones is frequently associated. The patient was a 56 year old woman with chronic glomerulonephritis and azotemia.

Subperiosteal bone resorption with demineralization of the skeleton is characteristic of advanced primary and secondary hyperparathyroidism. The larger cystic bony changes seen in primary hyperparathyroidism are less common in the secondary form.

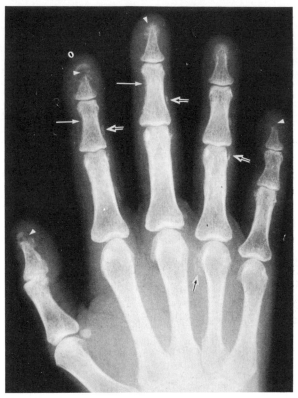

Figure 11–6 **Chronic Uremia: Secondary Hyperparathyroidism: Hand Changes.** A film of the hand reveals subperiosteal bone resorption on the radial side of several phalanges (*white arrows*), resorptive changes in the tufts (*arrowheads*), and soft tissue calcifications (*black-white arrows*). There was no apparent osteoporosis.

The resorptive changes in the tufts resemble the findings in Raynaud's phenomenon; however, soft tissue atrophy of the finger tips, which accompanies the tuft changes in Raynaud's disease, are not seen in secondary hyperparathyroidism. This patient also had resorption of the outer clavicles.

Roentgen evidence of secondary hyperparathyroidism, especially resorptive bone changes and soft tissue calcification, is being encountered more frequently because of longer survival of chronic uremic patients on dialysis therapy.

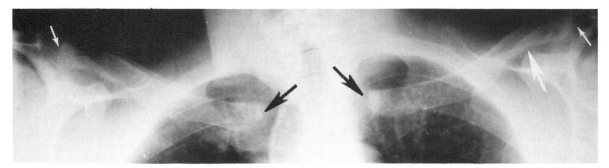

Figure 11–7 **Renal Osteodystrophy: Clavicular Changes.** There are marked erosive changes of the inner ends of the clavicles (*black arrows*), causing narrowed irregular articular margins.

The outer ends are also eroded (*small white arrows*), with loss of the articular white line and increased distance from the acromial articulation.

A concave erosive deformity is also seen (*large white arrow*) in the inferior margin of the outer third of the left clavicle.

The outer ends of the clavicles are the second most frequent site of erosions in osteodystrophy (the phalanges are the most common site). Inner clavicular erosions are less frequent but may be the only finding of osteodystrophy to be recognized on the chest film.

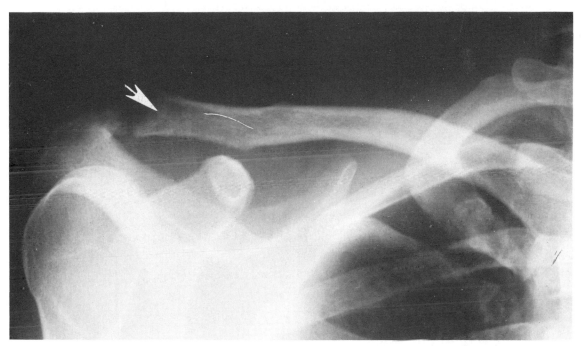

Figure 11–8 **Renal Osteodystrophy: Erosion of Outer Ends of Clavicles.** The outer end of the right clavicle is eroded and irregular (*arrow*), increasing the acromoclavicular space. The other clavicle was similarly affected. The inner ends were normal.

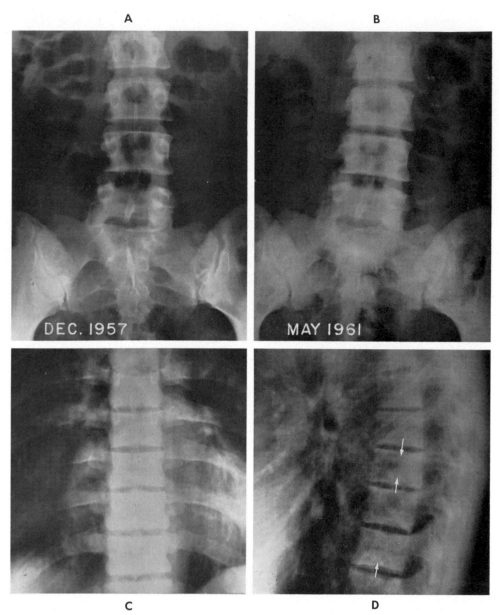

A

B

C

D

Figure 11-9 **Azotemic Osteodystrophy: Osteosclerosis with Secondary Hyperparathyroidism.**

A, Normal lumbar spine, 1957.

B, Sclerotic lumbar spine, 1961.

C and *D,* Enlarged anteroposterior and lateral views of the thoracic spine show sclerotic changes in the end plates of the thoracic vertebrae (*arrows*) due to secondary hyperparathyroidism.

The patient was a 36 year old woman with chronic pyelonephritis; sclerosis of the spine was associated with other bony changes typical of secondary hyperparathyroidism. These sclerotic changes occur in about 20 per cent of cases of secondary hyperparathyroidism; they are generally seen most clearly in the thoracolumbar spine and are most pronounced at the borders of the vertebral bodies. (Courtesy Dr. Harold B. Zimmerman, University of Rochester School of Medicine, Rochester, New York.)

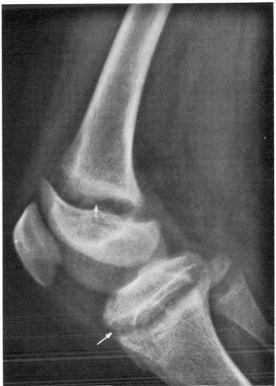

Figure 11–10 **Renal Rickets: Renal Tubular Acidosis.**
The typical rachitic alterations of the cuffed, widened, and frayed metaphysis are due to an irregular overgrowth of noncalcified osteoid tissue. This osteoid tissue also produces an increased width of the epiphyseal line *(arrows)*. These changes are seen only before epiphyseal closure; after closure, the picture is that of osteomalacia. The patient was a 14 year old girl who had renal tubular acidosis. The blood urea nitrogen was normal; serum phosphorus and calcium were decreased.

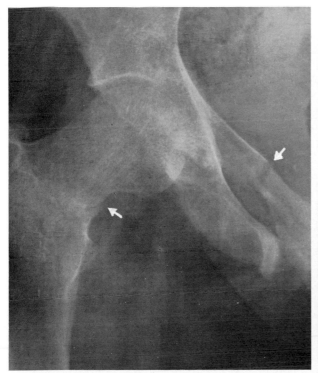

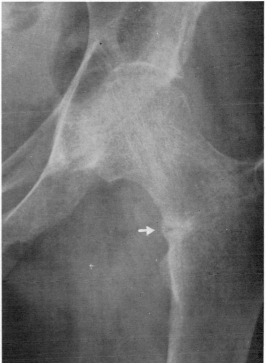

Figure 11–11 **Osteomalacia: Renal Tubular Acidosis.**   There are bilateral and symmetric lucent lines in the femoral neck; there is another lucent line in the superior ramus of the pubis on the right *(arrows)*. These are typical pseudofractures and are diagnostic of osteomalacia. The primary trabeculae of the femoral neck appear prominent because of the demineralization of the secondary trabeculae. (Courtesy Dr. R. C. Powell, Indiana University Medical School, Indianapolis, Indiana.)

The Chest In Uremia

Many of the significant metabolic alterations and complications of chronic uremia are mirrored in the findings on chest radiographs of patients surviving through maintenance dialysis. (See also *Maintenance Dialysis: Radiologic Considerations,* p. 795).

Episodes of pulmonary edema are not uncommon in the uremic patient and may be due to congestive failure, uremic toxicity to the pulmonary capillaries (uremic lung), or overhydration. Combinations of these factors may be the cause. When pulmonary edema is cardiac in origin, there will be cardiomegaly and other changes of congestive failure. When due to uremic toxicity or overhydration, there may be little or no cardiac enlargement. The pulmonary edema most often presents with characteristic perihilar alveolar densities (batwing appearance), but more random distributions of the fluffy alveolar densities can occur. Uremic pulmonary edema may persist for prolonged periods unless dialysis is instituted, and it may simulate a pneumonia.

Numerous other conditions can cause pulmonary edema without cardiomegaly (see *Pulmonary Edema,* p. 499), but distinction is readily made on clinical grounds.

Enlargement of the cardiac silhouette is extremely common in uremia and is most often due to hypertension or congestive failure. Pericardial effusions, sometimes massive, are frequently encountered, and it may be difficult to distinguish the swollen silhouette from true cardiomegaly on plain films. (See *Pericarditis with Effusion,* p. 706). Cardiac tamponade requiring pericardiectomy or a pericardial window occasionally occurs.

Pleural effusion from uncomplicated uremia can occur but is infrequent. More often pleural fluid is due to congestive failure or a metabolic or infectious complication. A higher than normal incidence of pulmonary infections occurs during chronic uremia and at times it may be difficult to distinguish a bilateral alevolar pneumonia from patchy pulmonary edema.

The changes of azotemic osteodystrophy are often first recognized on chest films. Erosive changes of the outer and/or inner ends of the clavicles and unsuspected rib fractures (pseudofractures) are not infrequently encountered. Rarely, diffuse punctate parenchymal calcifications are noted and are probably due to secondary hyperparathyroidism.[25-29]

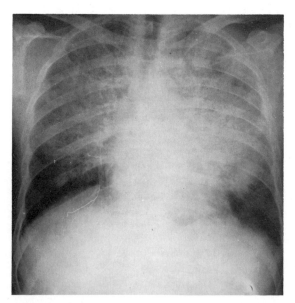

Figure 11–12 **Uremia: Pulmonary Edema.** Fan-shaped alveolar densities extend from both hilar regions but tend to spare the periphery. This batwing appearance is frequently associated with uremia. The heart is not enlarged.

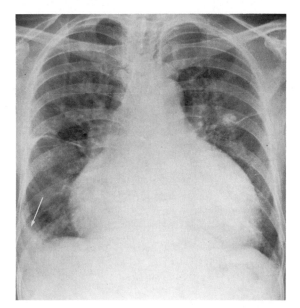

Figure 11–13 **Uremia: Congestive Failure and Pericardial Effusion.** The heart is huge and symmetrically enlarged, the superior pulmonary veins are prominent, and there is a right pleural effusion (*arrow*). The findings were due to congestive failure and uremic pericarditis with effusion. The bulging of the right heart border was due to the pericardial effusion, but it is difficult to distinguish cardiac enlargement from pericardial effusion on plain films.

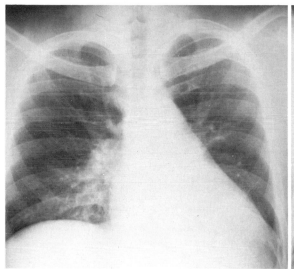

A

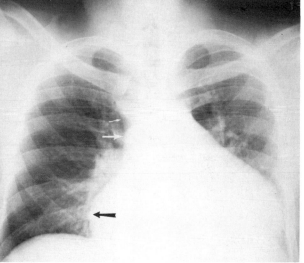

B

Figure 11–14 **Chronic Uremia: Cardiac Tamponade.**

A, Chest film of a 37 year old man on chronic maintenance dialysis shows a moderately enlarged heart shadow with a straightened left border. A pericardial effusion was present. The lungs are clear.

B, Two weeks later, there was a rather sudden onset of tachycardia, hypotension, and distended neck veins. The cardiac silhouette has become much larger, with a marked bulge (*black arrow*) of the right atrial border. The superior vena caval shadow (*small white arrow*) and the azygos vein (*large white arrow*) have become prominent. The lung fields remain clear. These changes are strongly suggestive of cardiac tamponade.

C, An immediate right heart angiocardiogram discloses a greatly increased pericardial space (*double-headed arrow*) and a concavity of the opacified right atrial border (*white arrows*). These findings are pathognomonic of cardiac tamponade (of right atrium). An immediate pericardial window was surgically made, providing prompt clinical improvement.

Cardiac tamponade is an infrequent but life-threatening complication of uremic pericarditis.

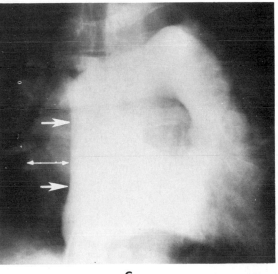

C

Acute Renal Failure

Acute renal failure can occur from various causes, including chemical and drug nephrotoxicity, shock, and mismatched transfusion.

Radiographic findings are generally noncontributory. Abdominal films may show progressive increase in kidney size due to parenchymal edema. Small kidneys or nephrocalcinosis indicates pre-existing renal disease. Retrograde studies cautiously performed rule out ureteral obstruction. Excretory pyelography will not opacify the kidneys and is therefore not employed.

Renal angiography will show similar findings in acute renal failure whether from nephrotoxins, shock, or hemolysis. The cortical vessels are absent and no cortical nephrogram develops. Transit time of the contrast medium is prolonged. These changes are apparently due to preglomerular vasoconstriction.[10, 11, 30, 31]

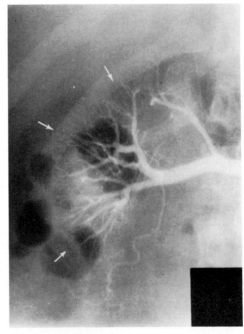

Figure 11–15 **Acute Renal Failure from Carbon Tetrachloride Poisoning: Selective Renal Angiogram.** There is a smooth, rapid attenuation of the interlobar and arcuate renal arteries. Cortical vessels are entirely absent *(arrows)*, and no cortical nephrogram appeared. The arterial transit time was prolonged.

These are the characteristic angiographic changes seen in acute renal failure from shock, mismatched transfusions, or nephrotoxins. (Courtesy Dr. D. Adams: N. Engl. J. Med., *282*:1329, 1970.)

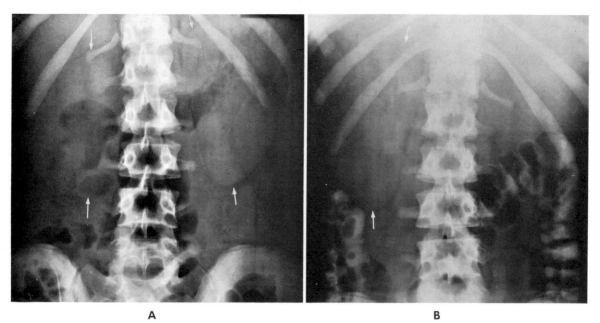

A   **B**

Figure 11–16   **Acute Renal Failure: Intravenous Urogram.**

A, The patient was a 15 year old girl who had renal tubular necrosis. There is no opacification of the kidneys or collecting system. The kidneys are slightly enlarged *(arrows).*

B, Twenty-four hours later, with persisting anuria, the kidneys appear larger *(arrows).* The colon is opacified by the intravenous contrast medium, which probably is excreted by the small intestine because of failure of renal excretion.

Progressive increase in kidney size may be noted during acute renal failure, but after diuresis and recovery the kidneys decrease in size.

Hypotension

Hypotension can occur from many causes, including shock, anaphylaxis, and vagal syncope. If it is present or develops during the course of excretory urography, there will be a marked prolongation of the nephrographic phase, but delayed opacification of the collecting system.

In some cases, the hypotension is due to a reaction to the injected contrast medium. The prolonged nephrogram will promptly disappear and the collecting system will become opacified as the blood pressure is raised during the radiographic study. The prolonged nephrogram in hypotension apparently is due to continued but slow filtration of the contrast material into static columns of tubular fluid.

Prolonged nephrograms and delayed filling of the calices and pelvis can also occur in bilateral obstructive uropathy and when the renal tubules are blocked by precipitated mucoproteins—for example, in multiple myeloma.[32, 33]

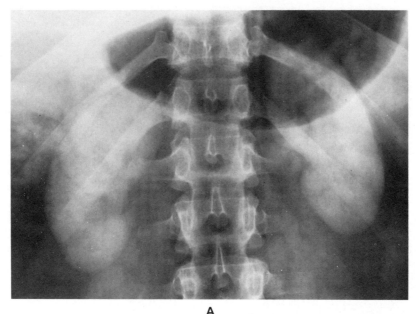

A

B

Figure 11–17 **Prolonged Bilateral Nephrograms in Hypotension.** *A* and *B* reveal persistent nephrograms without opacification of the collecting system at 30 and 60 minutes, respectively, after injection of contrast material.

The patient had a ruptured gallbladder and unrecognized hypotension.

A prolonged bilateral nephrogram during intravenous pyelography should be a signal for immediate blood pressure reading. (Courtesy Dr. M. T. Korobkin, San Francisco, California.)

Bilateral Renal Cortical Necrosis

This condition is one of the recognized causes of acute renal failure and apparently results from acute bilateral cortical ischemia. Its cause is uncertain; a variety of agents have been implicated. (See *Acute Renal Failure*, p. 788.)

During the acute episode there is a marked radiographic impairment of excretory function. However, the pelves and calices appear normal on retrograde studies. The kidneys are often edematous and somewhat enlarged.

In surviving patients, within one or two months a characteristic calcification of the cortex develops, sometimes as a thin double line (tramway calcification). The kidney gradually diminishes in size, and its outline may show some irregularities.

Clinically, cortical necrosis is indistinguishable from acute tubular necrosis, but cortical calcification does not occur in the latter. Radiographically, the predominantly cortical location of the calcifications differentiates renal cortical necrosis from other forms of nephrocalcinosis. The rare cortical calcifications of chronic glomerulonephritis (Fig. 11–33) may be indistinguishable from those of cortical necrosis, but differentiation of these two conditions can usually be made clinically.[34, 35]

A

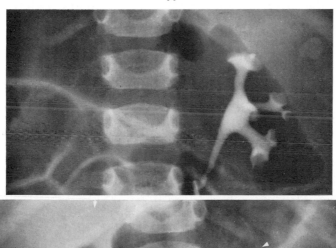

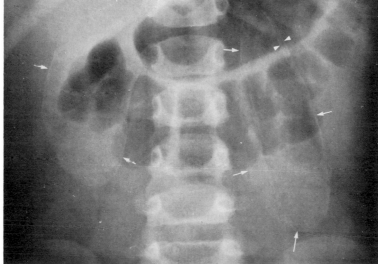

B

Figure 11–18 **Bilateral Cortical Necrosis: Cortical Calcification.**

A, A left retrograde pyelogram of a 16 month old child with acute anuria and elevated BUN (121 mg. per 100 ml.) shows a normal pelvis and calices. Biopsy disclosed acute renal cortical necrosis.

Acute arterial ischemia of the kidney prevents opacification on intravenous pyelography, but, characteristically, the retrograde study is normal.

B, Abdominal film made one month after the acute episode shows cortical calcification of both kidneys (*arrows*). A double-line (tramway) calcification (*arrowheads*) is seen on the left. This double-line calcification is considered characteristic and pathognomonic. Cortical calcification develops rapidly after acute cortical necrosis. (Courtesy Dr. J. G. Whelan, Louisville, Kentucky.)

Renal Transplantation: Radiologic Considerations

After renal transplantation, significant radiologic information can be obtained about the changing size and function of the transplanted kidney, impending rejection, postoperative urinary tract complications, and pulmonary infections.

Radiographic estimation of renal size is facilitated if metallic clips are attached to the poles of the transplanted kidney. Some increase in kidney size usually occurs shortly after transplantation. A successful transplant has a fairly normal pyelographic and arteriographic appearance, although in some cases adequate kidney function may not appear for several weeks.

Acute rejection of the transplant can occur within a few days after surgery; more chronic rejection may develop after several weeks. Both forms are accompanied by pyelographic and arteriographic changes. The kidney undergoing acute rejection may enlarge up to 20 per cent of its original size because of medullary edema. Pyelographic opacification is diminished or absent. Arteriography shows poor filling of the peripheral renal arteries, and the arterial phase is prolonged to more than 4 seconds (2.5 to 3 seconds is normal). The major intrarenal branches are stretched by the parenchymal edema. Nephrographic density is diminished. Severe or chronic rejection is characterized by narrowing of the main renal artery and its branches, and by nonvisualization of the peripheral vessels; the nephrogram is absent.

Postsurgical complications can cause oliguria or anuria and will clinically simulate rejection. Obstruction at the ureteral anastamosis can be detected by intravenous or retrograde pyelography. Arteriography demonstrates thrombosis of the renal artery, a not uncommon complication. Renal vein thrombosis can cause arteriographic changes similar to those of rejection: namely, stretching of the intrarenal branches, poor filling of peripheral arteries, a prolonged arterial phase, and the absence of a nephrogram. Retrograde venography of the renal vein may be necessary for distinction from rejection.

A postoperative lymphocele develops in from 1 to 6 per cent of cases. This appears radiographically as a soft tissue mass compressing the bladder and often displacing and sometimes obstructing the transplant ureter.

Pulmonary infections by common and uncommon microorganisms are frequent during prolonged periods of immunosuppressive therapy. These infections are a major cause of death. The causative organisms include fungi (Candida, Aspergillus, Nocardia), *Pneumocystis carinii,* cytomegalovirus, Klebsiella, and Staphylococcus. Nodular lesions are usually of fungal origin, whereas localized or diffuse alveolar infiltrates are usually due to Pneumocystis, Klebsiella, or Staphylococcus organisms. The diffuse alveolar densities of pneumocystis infections may be mistaken for pulmonary edema of cardiac or renal origin.

Prolonged steroid therapy may cause widening of the mediastinum due to fat deposition in the mediastinum and probably also causes the high incidence of bleeding peptic ulcer in post-transplant patients.

In all transplant recipients receiving immunosuppressive therapy, there is an increased incidence of malignancy, most often lymphomatous.[36, 37]

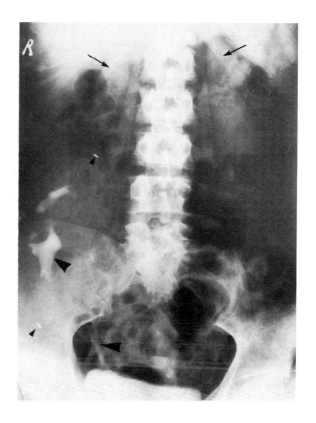

Figure 11–19 **Functioning Renal Transplant.** High close pyelogram shows excellent opacification of the collecting system of the transplanted kidney (*large arrowheads*) in the right iliac fossa. Metal clips (*small arrowheads*) at the upper and lower borders indicate considerable enlargement of this kidney. Incidentally, the patient's small, diseased kidneys show some function, evidenced by nephrographic opacification (*arrows*).

Every transplanted kidney undergoes some degree of enlargement.

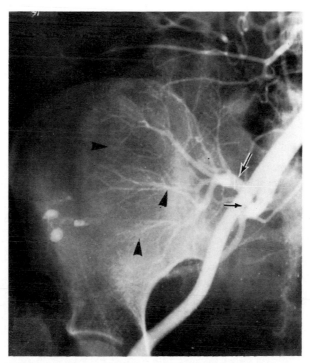

Figure 11–20 **Chronic Rejection of Renal Transplant: Angiogram.** All the intrarenal branches are narrow and sparse (*arrowheads*), especially at the periphery. Arterial filling was prolonged, and the nephrographic phase was absent. These changes are characteristic of chronic rejection.

The main renal artery and its anastomosis to the deep iliac artery (*arrows*) appear intact.

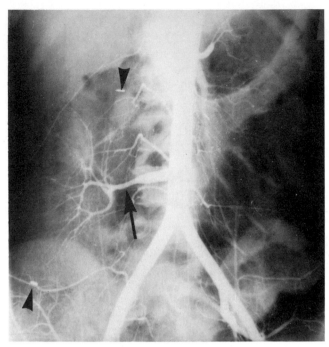

Figure 11–21 **Severe Rejection of Renal Transplant: Arteriogram.**   The artery of the transplanted kidney is anastomosed directly to the aorta. The kidney is greatly enlarged (*arrowheads*). There is marked tapering of the renal artery (*arrow*), and the intrarenal branches are narrow and somewhat stretched. There is virtually a complete absence of peripheral arteries.

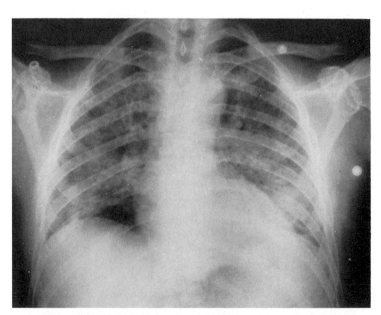

Figure 11–22 **Pneumocystis carinii Pneumonia Complicating Immunosuppressive Therapy Following Renal Transplant.**   Alveolar densities are scattered diffusely throughout both lungs, with coalescence at the left base. The infiltrates developed rather rapidly and were associated with fever and dyspnea. The patient was on intense immunosuppressive therapy because of threatened rejection of a renal transplant.

The bilateral alveolar involvement under these circumstances suggested a pneumocystis infection; this was verified histologically. The radiographic appearance of diffuse *Pneumocystis carinii* pneumonia can sometimes mimic pulmonary edema.

Maintenance Dialysis: Radiologic Considerations

Radiologic information of various types is necessary for proper management of patients on maintenance dialysis. Reversal or disappearance of the chest findings that can occur in chronic uremia is dramatic evidence of successful maintenance dialysis. The cardiac silhouette, if greatly enlarged from pericardial effusion, may rapidly decrease in size. Persistent alveolar infiltrates of the uremic lung may disappear dramatically. The cardiac and pulmonary changes of congestive failure frequently respond to the treatment. It is interesting to note that infusion pyelography, if performed shortly after a dialysis session, may sometimes opacify urinary tracts that could not be visualized previously.

The pulmonary complications of peritoneal dialysis include basal plate-like lobular atelectasis, occasional pleural effusions, and basal pneumonia; the latter may be superimposed upon an atelectatic area.

In patients on maintenance hemodialysis, angiographic studies of the shunt (shuntogram) or fistula must be performed periodically to evaluate its patency and efficacy. Complications that may require revision of the shunt include arterial or venous thrombosis, arteritis, thrombophlebitis, abnormal cannula angulation, and leakage around the shunt.

Other radiographic findings that may be encountered in the patient on maintenance dialysis include peptic ulcer, periarticular calcinosis, arterial calcifications, and azotemic osteodystrophy. Occasionally, cerebral dural calcification occurs.

A small percentage of patients regularly undergoing dialysis develop a subdural hematoma. Diagnosis and localization can be made by cerebral angiography or a CT scan.[48-54]

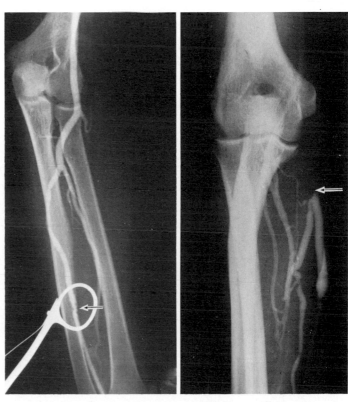

Figure 11–23 **Shunt Complications: Shuntograms.**

A, Irregularity and small lucent defects (*arrow*) in the artery just above the cannula are due to several small clots.

B, Shuntogram in another patient reveals an occluding venous thrombus (*arrow*) a few inches above the cannula insertion. Collateral veins are filled, but total flow is diminished.

A

B

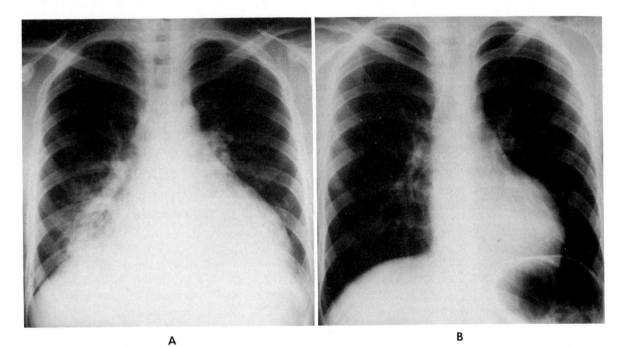

A   B

Figure 11-24   **Pneumonia and Cardiac Changes Following Peritoneal Dialysis.**

A, A pneumonic infiltrate has appeared at the right base two days after peritoneal dialysis. The greatly enlarged cardiac silhouette was due to pericardial effusion.

B, After repeated dialysis, the heart size has dramatically decreased. The pneumonia has cleared following antibiotic therapy.

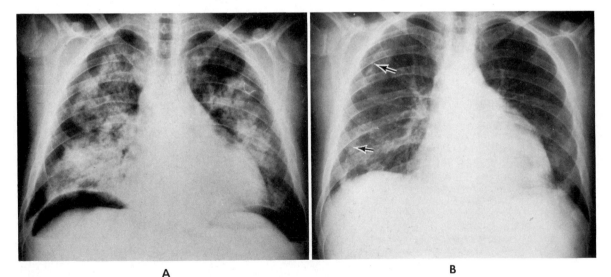

A   B

Figure 11-25   **Peritoneal Dialysis: Clearing of Uremic Pulmonary Edema.**

A, Bilateral, diffuse, fluffy, alveolar infiltrates were due to uremic pulmonary edema and not to cardiac failure. The free air under the diaphragms is from peritoneal dialysis.

B, After two weeks of dialysis, the infiltrates have almost completely disappeared except for some peripheral densities (*arrows*). The heart size is unchanged.

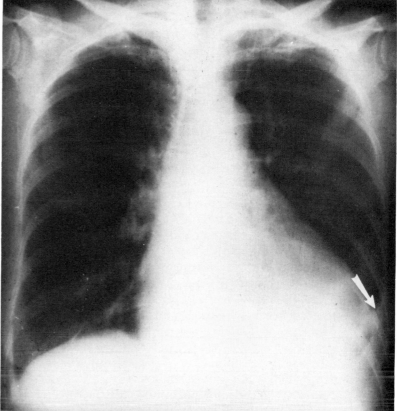

Figure 11–26 **Peritoneal Dialysis: Pleural Effusion and Basal Atelectasis.** There is a small pleural effusion in the left costophrenic angle (*arrow*) and atelectatic densities behind the heart, obliterating the left diaphragm. These were caused by peritoneal dialysis.

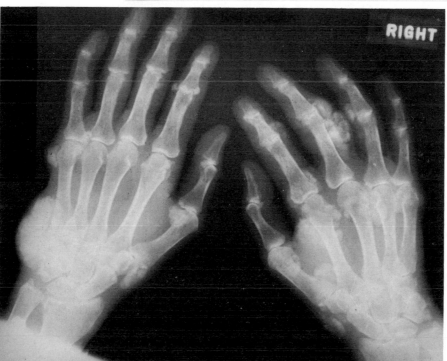

Figure 11–27 **Chronic Uremia and Maintenance Dialysis: Periarticular Calcifications.** Extensive collections of soft tissue calcification are seen in both hands and wrists. The bones are greatly demineralized, with extensive subperiosteal resorptive changes.

Although the periarticular soft tissue calcifications are generally part of the changes due to secondary hyperparathyroidism, these changes sometimes occur after prolonged dialysis without other bone changes of renal osteodystrophy.

GLOMERULAR DISEASE

Acute and Chronic Glomerulonephritis

Intravenous pyelography gives little or no diagnostic information in acute glomerulonephritis, since the kidneys appear normal. Occasionally, cortical swelling increases the distance between the calices and the kidney border, but this is very difficult to evaluate.

Cardiomegaly of nonspecific appearance develops in over half of the acute cases in children and is associated with some degree of hypertension, but the exact cause is uncertain.

In 50 to 75 per cent of cases, pulmonary changes are noted. Increased size of the hilar vessels and indistinct borders of the more prominent intrapulmonary vessels are the most common and often the early findings. Pleural fluid (sometimes interlobar or infrapulmonic) or pulmonary edema, or both, are also frequently seen. Occasionally the findings are unilateral. The lung changes promptly disappear after the peripheral edema clears. The mechanism is unclear, but fluid retention and circulatory failure are probably the etiologic factors. Pulmonary inflammatory or atelectatic consolidation may complicate the lung picture.

In chronic glomerulonephritis the kidneys are small as a result of loss of parenchymal cortical tissue. Before renal function is severely impaired, opacification by regular or high dose pyelography discloses relatively normal collecting systems in small kidneys with thin cortices.

Rarely, there may be diffuse calcification of the cortices of the kidneys. Histologically, the calcifications are not in the glomeruli but, rather, primarily in the lumina of the tubules. Small kidneys with extensive cortical calcification produce a pathognomonic picture of chronic glomerulonephritis.

Advanced bilateral chronic pyelonephritis can produce a clinical and biochemical picture indistinguishable from chronic glomerulonephritis. However, the small pyelonephritic kidneys are generally irregular in outline and their calices, if opacified, are usually blunted.

In well-advanced chronic glomerulonephritis, renal angiography discloses small renal and intrarenal arteries with a sparse peripheral vasculature. Arterial filling is prolonged. The nephrographic density is greatly diminished but homogeneous. The cortices are thin and relatively lucent compared to the medullary density. The angiographic appearance, however, is often indistinguishable from that of other forms of bilateral diffuse parenchymal chronic renal disease.[55-62]

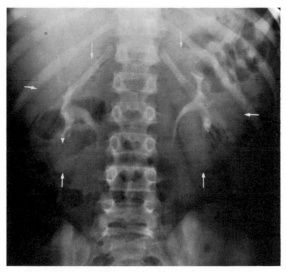

Figure 11–28 **Acute Glomerulonephritis: Intravenous Urogram.** The kidneys are slightly enlarged, and the cortices are swollen, as shown by the increased distance from the calix *(arrowhead)* to the outer border of the kidney *(arrows).* The urogram is otherwise normal. Intravenous urography is generally unrevealing and rarely indicated in acute glomerulonephritis.

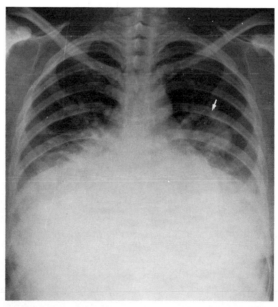

Figure 11–29 **Acute Glomerulonephritis: Pulmonary and Cardiac Changes.** In posteroanterior view there is evidence of bilateral vascular congestion, pulmonary edema *(arrow),* and bilateral pleural effusions. The cardiomegaly is obscured by the pleural effusions. The nonspecific findings of pulmonary edema and congestive failure were caused in this case by acute glomerulonephritis.

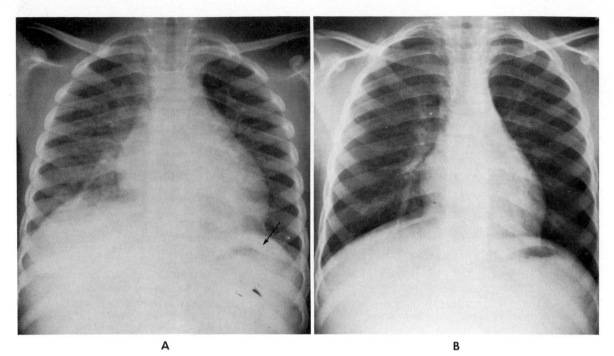

A   B

Figure 11–30 **Acute Glomerulonephritis: Cardiac Changes.**

   A, The heart is considerably enlarged, and there is some vascular congestion; this film was taken during the acute process. There is an increased distance between the lung and the stomach air bubble due to an infrapulmonic effusion (*arrow*). This is frequently seen in acute glomerulonephritis.

   B, Three weeks later, clinical recovery is paralleled by return of the heart and lungs to normal. The stomach bubble is now close to the lung field, due to resorption of the infrapulmonic effusion.

   Often the extent of cardiac dilatation can be appreciated only by changes seen on serial films.

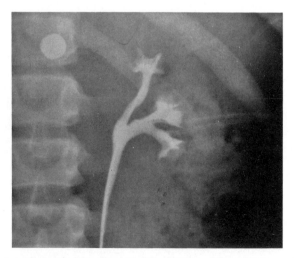

Figure 11–31 **Chronic Glomerulonephritis: Retrograde Study.** The pelvis and calices of the kidney are normal, while the renal parenchyma is markedly reduced and extremely thin. Even with planigraphy, it was difficult to visualize the outline of the kidney because of the loss of perirenal fat.

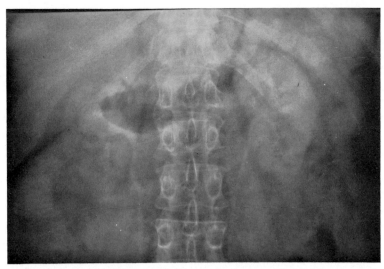

Figure 11–32 **Chronic Glomerulonephritis: Intravenous Urogram.** Both kidneys are functioning, although the pyelographic density is diminished. No significant alterations of the pelves or calices are apparent, but both kidneys are abnormally small. As the disease progresses, opacification by conventional intravenous urogram becomes increasingly fainter and finally unobtainable.

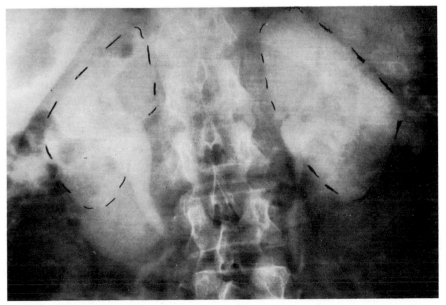

Figure 11–33 **Chronic Glomerulonephritis: High Dose Pyelogram.** There was no opacification by routine pyelography of the small kidneys of this patient, who was a chronic hypertensive with a BUN of 70 mg. per 100 ml.

High dose pyelogram shows nephrographic opacification of the small kidneys (*borders outlined with ink*) and relatively normal collecting systems. The calices extend to the kidney borders, indicating marked cortical atrophy.

Advanced nephrosclerosis can produce an identical radiographic picture; in the small kidneys of chronic pyelonephritis, the calices would be blunted and dilated.

In some cases of azotemia, high dose pyelography is extremely useful for obtaining satisfactory opacification of poorly functioning kidneys without resorting to retrograde studies.

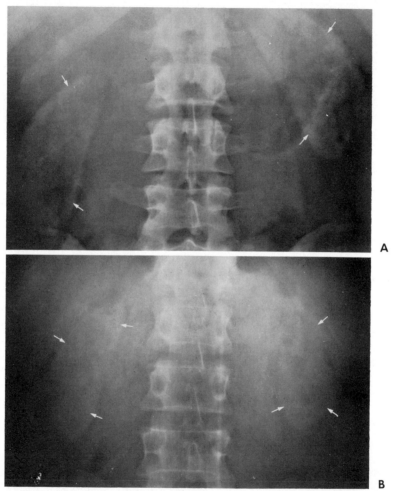

Figure 11–34 **Chronic Glomerulonephritis: Nephrocalcinosis in Two Patients.**   Both patients (*A,* age 32; *B,* age 47) had a greatly elevated BUN. Abdominal film of each reveals small kidney shadows with diffuse granular calcifications of the cortical areas (*arrow*s) clearly outlining each kidney. The diagnosis of chronic glomerulonephritis was confirmed in each patient at autopsy. (Courtesy Dr. W. J. Esposito, Summit, New Jersey.)

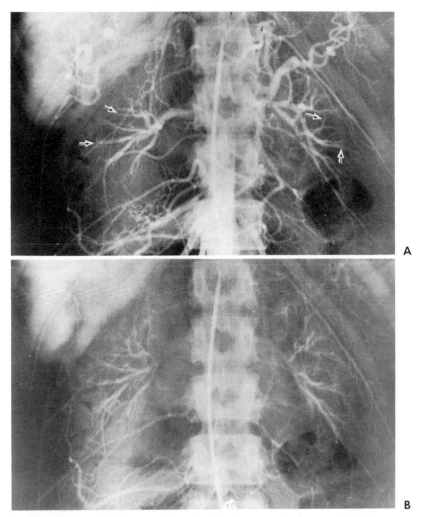

Figure 11–35 **Moderately Advanced Glomerulonephritis: Angiogram.**

A, The more peripheral arteries of both kidneys are attenuated and sparse (*arrows*), and the cortical arteries are not opacified. Both kidneys are small.

B, A later film made five seconds after injection shows persisting opacification of the renal arterial trees; the nephrogram is very faint. Normally, renal arterial opacification lasts two to four seconds.

These changes are the salient angiographic features of chronic glomerulonephritis. In far-advanced cases the lumina of the main renal arteries and their intrarenal branches are quite narrowed. However, advanced malignant nephrosclerosis and chronic interstitial nephritis produce virtually identical nephrographic findings.

Goodpasture's Syndrome

This progressive and fatal disease of unknown origin is characterized by repeated episodes of pulmonary alveolar hemorrhage associated with glomerulonephritis. In some cases, exposure to hydrocarbons is a possible etiologic factor.

The radiographic findings are limited to the chest. During an active bleeding episode there are irregular, rapidly changing areas of confluent alveolar infiltrates. Between episodes there is usually a fine reticular or nodular lung pattern, representing hemosiderin deposits from former hemorrhages. The roentgen findings are identical to those of idiopathic pulmonary hemosiderosis (see p. 505); the associated clinical renal findings in Goodpasture's syndrome differentiate these diseases.

The renal involvement causes hematuria and albuminuria, often associated with hypertension and anemia, but there are often no significant urographic findings. Impaired excretory function may occur in more advanced disease. It should be remembered that episodes of pulmonary hemorrhage can occur from pulmonary complications of chronic renal failure of any cause.[63-75]

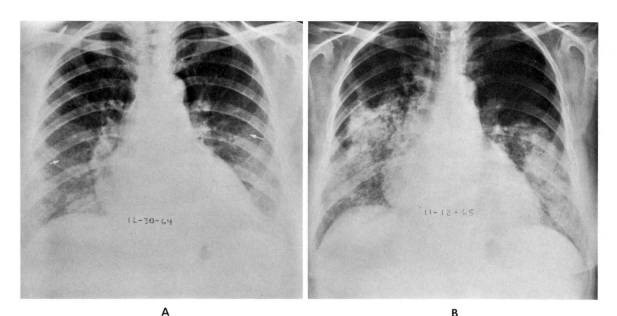

A   B

Figure 11–36 **Goodpasture's Syndrome: Chest Findings.**

A, This 40 year old female had a history of recurrent hemoptysis. There is a fine reticular and tiny nodular pattern (*arrows*) (difficult to see in this reproduction) in both lower lung fields. The heart is considerably enlarged, probably owing to chronic anemia. There were many red cells in the urine.

B, Chest film made almost a year later during an episode of severe hemoptysis reveals extensive irregular confluent densities due to intra-alveolar hemorrhage in both lower lung fields. The densities rapidly increased, and in a few days both lung fields were completely involved. At autopsy, glomerulonephritis was found.

Hereditary Nephritis (Alport's Syndrome)

This syndrome is characterized by progressive glomerulonephritis, usually fatal in the second or third decade. About 15 per cent of patients have associated deafness, and about 7 to 8 per cent show various ocular lesions. The condition is more severe in men, in whom deafness is often the earliest clinical symptom, although microscopic hematuria and albuminuria will be found. In women, the nephropathy may be asymptomatic indefinitely.

The urographic and angiographic findings are generally indistinguishable from those in ordinary glomerulonephritis. With progressive renal failure, the kidneys become small and angiographically show a faint or absent nephrogram, small major arteries, thinned avascular cortices, some tortuosities of smaller vessels, and increased transit time of the contrast material — findings quite similar to those of chronic glomerulonephritis or other end stage kidneys.[66, 67]

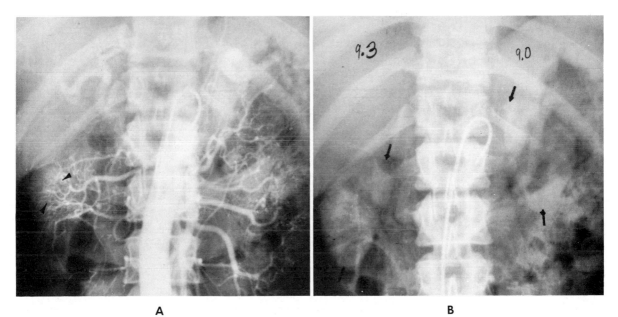

A   B

Figure 11–37 **Alport's Syndrome: Arteriogram.** A 37 year old man in chronic renal failure had bilateral deafness and proteinuria for 14 years. His father and brother had died from renal failure.

A, Arteriogram shows small and somewhat tortuous intrarenal vessels (*arrowheads*), with sparsity of small peripheral vessels and prolonged transit time.

B, The kidneys show poor nephrographic density following the arterial phase, and both kidneys are small (9.0 and 9.3 cm. respectively) (*arrows*).

The arteriographic appearance is indistinguishable from that of chronic glomerulonephritis.

Nephrotic Syndrome: Renal Vein Thrombosis

The nephrotic syndrome refers to chronic proteinuria due to increased permeability of the glomerular membrane. The majority of the cases are idiopathic (idiopathic lipoid nephrosis) and occur in children and young adults. The syndrome may occasionally appear during many other kidney diseases such as poststreptococcal glomerulonephritis, membranous glomerulonephritis, Kimmelstiel-Wilson syndrome, renal amyloidosis, and the nephritis of lupus erythematosus. Chronic renal venous congestion from renal vein thrombosis and, more rarely, from constrictive pericarditis can also cause the syndrome. Renal biopsy is usually necessary to determine the underlying renal disorder.

In the well-developed nephrotic syndrome there may be radiographic evidence of either pleural effusion or ascites, or both. The pleural fluid may appear as an infrapulmonic effusion. Pyelographic changes are minimal or absent except in some cases of renal vein thrombosis. In idiopathic lipoid nephrosis the kidneys may be enlarged but are otherwise normal.

Renal vein thrombosis, unilaterally or bilaterally, may cause a nephrotic syndrome. In adults, renal vein thrombosis may result from a variety of disorders, especially peripheral thromboembolic disease. In children, dehydration is a frequent cause. A nephrotic syndrome associated with episodes of pulmonary embolism should suggest renal vein thrombosis.

Radiographically, in acute or subacute renal vein thrombosis the involved kidney is enlarged; opacification by excretory urography is poor or absent. The renal pelvis and calices are distorted and often compressed by the congested and edematous parenchyma. The upper ureter may be notched or scalloped by distended collateral vessels. Retrograde contrast material can diffuse into the congested parenchyma. In more chronic cases, excretory urography may be normal, but ureteral notching due to distended collateral veins is sometimes seen.

Renal arteriography can be normal, or it may show narrowed and stretched intrarenal arteries. The arterial phase is prolonged, and later venous filling is absent. Cavography occasionally demonstrates a clot in the vena cava. However, precise diagnosis requires selective renal venography, which will disclose the occlusion or clot. Better opacification of the venous bed is obtained if renal blood flow is temporarily diminished by injection of epinephrine into the renal artery immediately prior to the venous study.[68–73]

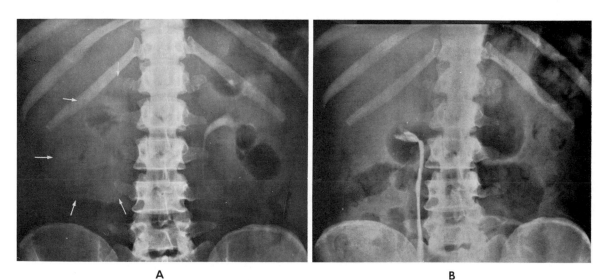

A   **B**

Figure 11–38 **Nephrotic Syndrome: Acute Renal Vein Thrombosis.**

A, The right kidney is enlarged (*arrows*) and does not function on intravenous pyelography. The left kidney is normal radiographically.

B, Retrograde study demonstrates compression and deformity of the pelvis caused by the edematous kidney substance. No caliceal or infundibular filling is seen.

The presence of an enlarged nonfunctioning kidney on intravenous urogram with pelvic or caliceal compression and distortion on the retrograde pyelogram is characteristic of renal vein thrombosis. In the above patient, nephrectomy led to complete clinical recovery.

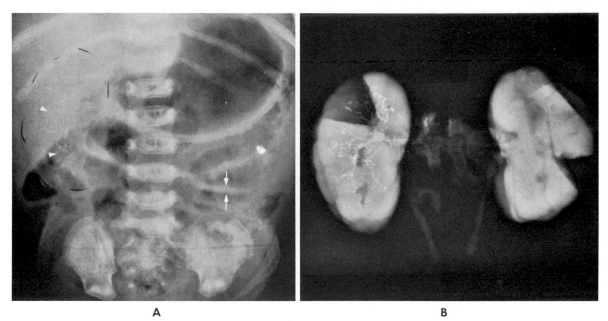

A   B

Figure 11–39   **Nephrotic Syndrome: Chronic Renal Vein Thrombosis in a 9 Month Old Boy.**

A, The distance between the bowel loops (*arrows*) is increased because of edema and ascites. The flanks bulge. Calcifications in the region of the right kidney (*arrowheads*) were in areas of necrosis of the kidney substance, a late result of renal vein thrombosis.

B, On a postmortem radiograph the renal calcification in the right kidney is more clearly seen.

In children, renal vein thrombosis is generally secondary to infection and dehydration, with subsequent thrombophlebitis of the renal vein.

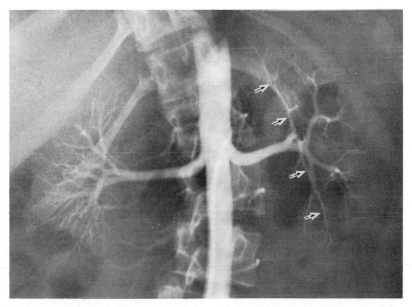

Figure 11–40   **Nephrotic Syndrome: Left Renal Vein Thrombosis: Arteriogram.**   In contrast with the normal right renal arteriogram, on the left there is no nephrogram; the kidney is enlarged; the arteries are stretched, somewhat thinner, and spread apart (*arrows*) by the swollen renal parenchyma; and there is poor opacification of the peripheral arterioles. On later films, only the right renal vein was opacified. (Courtesy Dr. G. P. Wegner, Madison, Wisconsin.)

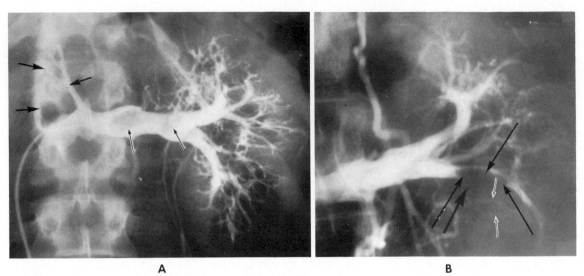

A   B

Figure 11–41 **Nephrotic Syndrome and Renal Vein Thrombosis in Two Adolescent Males: Selective Renal Venogram after Injection of Epinephrine into Renal Artery.**

A, Two large clots (*black-white arrows*) are seen as filling defects in the left renal vein. There is also a large triangular thrombus (*black arrows*) in the vena cava. The right renal venogram was normal.

B, In the second boy, a long oval clot (*black arrows*) is apparent in the inferior renal vein. There is a distinct sparsity of venous channels in the lower pole of the kidney. Several collateral venous pathways (*black-white arrows*) are opacified.

Selective renal vein angiography after renal blood flow is diminished by intra-arterial epinephrine is the definitive procedure for conclusive demonstration of thrombosis of a major renal vein. (Courtesy Dr. M. T. Gyepes, Los Angeles, California.)

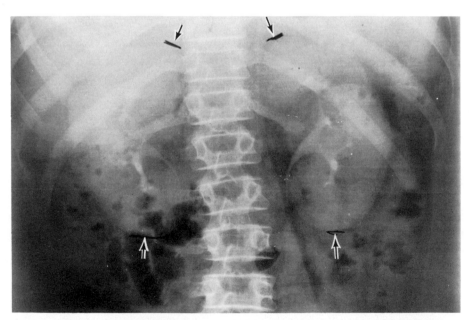

Figure 11–42 **Membranous Glomerulonephritis with Nephrotic Syndrome (Lipoid Nephrosis): Intravenous Pyelogram.**   Both kidneys are considerably enlarged (*arrows*), measuring over 16 cm. Excretion of contrast material is good, and the pelvicaliceal structures appear normal.

This somewhat stunted 20 year old boy had nephrotic syndrome for 12 years. Prolonged steroid therapy is responsible for the osteoporosis of the vertebrae. Renal biopsy taken shortly after this pyelogram disclosed membranous glomerulonephritis.

Large kidneys with normal collecting systems are typical radiographic findings in lipoid nephrosis, whether the disease be idiopathic or due to membranous glomerulonephritis.

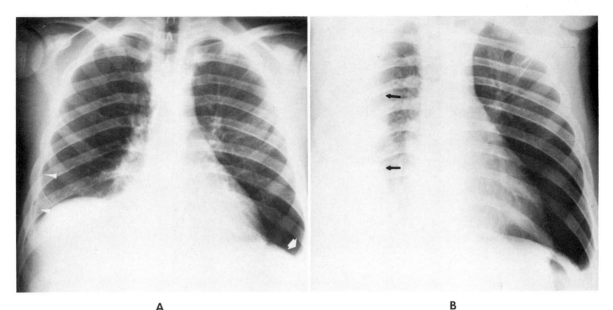

A   B

Figure 11–43 **Nephrotic Syndrome: Infrapulmonic Effusion.**

A, Chest film of an 18 year old girl with albuminuria shows a mild blunting of the left costophrenic angle (*arrow*). The right "diaphragm" is elevated, and although the right costophrenic angle is clear, there is a linear pleural density in the lower chest (*arrowheads*). An infrapulmonic effusion was suspected.

B, A right decubitus film confirms that the "elevated right diaphragm" was indeed an infrapulmonic collection that has layered along the right chest wall (*arrows*).

It is interesting that pleural effusion in nephrotic patients is frequently infrapulmonic.

THE KIDNEY DURING PREGNANCY

Beginning in the early stages of a normal pregnancy, there is a progressive dilatation of the upper ureters, pelves, and calices. Earlier and greater dilatation is seen on the right side in about 95 per cent of pregnant women. Ureteral pressure from the enlarging uterine mass and hormonal physiologic changes are responsible factors. On the right side the iliac artery and right ovarian vein cause additional pressure on the ureter at the level of the upper sacrum, resulting in greater dilatation.

This bilateral hydronephrosis may become suprisingly large, but the urinary tracts return to normal within a few weeks after delivery. Infrequently, moderate dilatation, especially of the right side, may continue to exist for prolonged periods post partum owing to pressure by a persistently engorged ovarian vein.

Radiation exposure from urography is prudently avoided during pregnancy. Moreover, the dilatation of the urinary tracts may make radiologic evaluation of other suspected renal pathologic conditions difficult or impossible. No distinctive urographic changes related to the toxemia of pregnancy have been reported.[74-77]

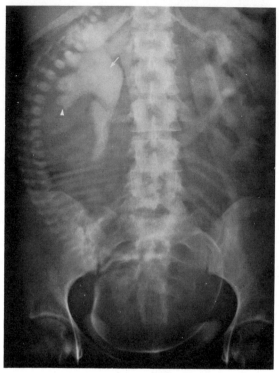

Figure 11-44   **Pregnancy: Physiologic Bilateral Hydronephrosis: Intravenous Pyelogram.**   There is a single intrauterine fetus near term. The renal pelvis (*arrow*) and calices (*arrowhead*) of both kidneys are dilated. The pelvis and ureter on the right are more dilated than those on the left—a common situation during pregnancy.

URINARY TRACT INFECTIONS AND PYELONEPHRITIS

Acute and Chronic Pyelonephritis

In acute pyelonephritis there are usually no significant urographic findings. In severe cases the renal cortex may be widened and swollen; if the entire renal parenchyma is involved, function may be impaired. Occasionally the calices and infundibula are narrowed from edema or spasm, although this finding is difficult to evaluate. Cortical or medullary abscesses may complicate acute pyelonephritis, especially in diabetics, but may produce no radiographic changes unless they displace an adjacent calix or communicate and become opacified. In diabetics, *Escherichia coli* infection may lead to gas formation within the pyelocaliceal system or even within the parenchyma (emphysematous pyelonephritis).

In chronic or healed pyelonephritis, fibrosis and scarring can produce focal or generalized cortical thinning, which is recognized by a decreased distance between the tip of a calix and the kidney border. The calices become blunted, and the infundibula are narrowed. These relatively late changes may be the first detectable radiographic abnormalities. With continuing disease the calices become rounded or clubbed, the cortex becomes thinner and irregular from scarring, and the kidneys shrink in size. Excretory urographic function may progressively diminish. Chronic pyelonephritis is probably the commonest cause of chronic renal insufficiency and is associated with small, often irregular end-stage kidneys. Hypertension usually develops. Chronic pyelonephritis is usually bilateral, although one side is often more severely affected.

In a significant percentage of cases, vesicoureteral reflux, often with ureteral dilatation, occurs during micturition. Whether this is a cause or a consequence of pyelonephritis is uncertain, although in some children reflux is undoubtedly an inherited abnormality.

Renal arteriography usually reveals a decrease in the size of the main renal artery and its major branches. The smaller intrarenal vessels appear tortuous, and localized areas of decreased vasculature are seen. Stenoses and occlusions of the intrarenal arteries are frequent. The nephrographic density is diminished and is not uniform, but it clearly demonstrates the cortical thinning and irregularity. In focal chronic pyelonephritis, nephrographic density may be absent focally, and the intralobar vessels in the involved area are sparse and thin.[78-86]

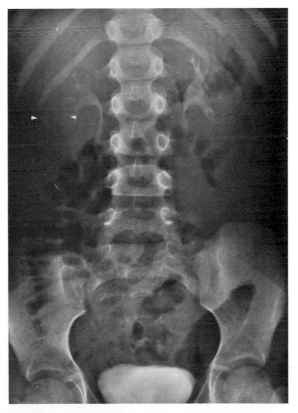

Figure 11–45 **Acute Pyelonephritis.** The density of the contrast material in the right kidney is decreased due to functional impairment; the cortex is swollen and widened (*arrowheads*). These changes are unusual, since generally there are no urographic findings in acute pyelonephritis. Occasionally there is irritability and spasm of the calices, but this is difficult to evaluate and is not diagnostic in itself.

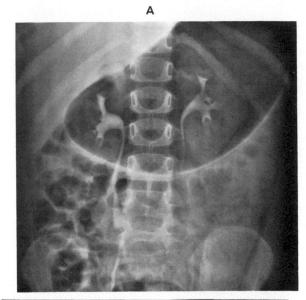

A

Figure 11–46 **Pyelonephritis: Progressive Changes.**

A, The urogram is essentially normal during an episode of acute right-sided pyelonephritis.

B, Two years later, following several other episodes of focal pyelonephritis, there is localized elongation and blunting of the right upper calix, with thinning and indentation of the cortex in this area (*arrow*).

C, Four years later, the right upper calix is blunted and dilated. The adjacent cortex is greatly thinned and scarred, so that one observes a puckered indentation toward the involved calices (*arrows*).

This series of films illustrates the progressive changes in focal pyelonephritis.

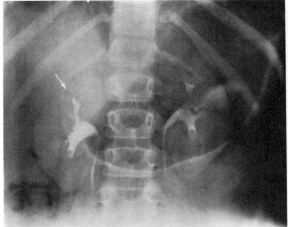

B

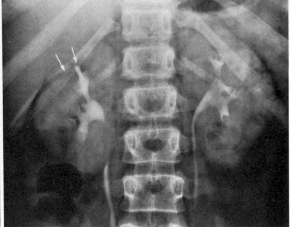

C

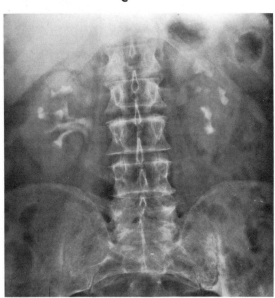

Figure 11–47 **Chronic Pyelonephritis.** There is bilateral marked irregularity, scarring, and thinning of the renal cortices. The calices are blunted and distorted by fibrous scars. The picture is typical of advanced bilateral chronic pyelonephritis.

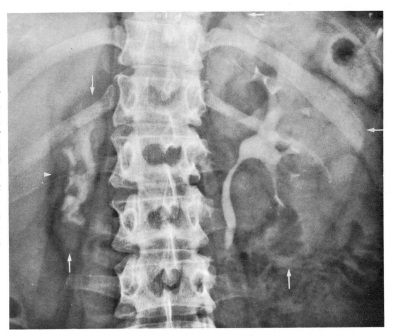

Figure 11–48 **Chronic Pyelonephritis.** The right kidney is much smaller than the left (*arrows*). The calices are dilated and distorted. Little cortical tissue remains. The cortex is irregular and scarred (*arrowhead*). These changes are the end result of chronic pyelonephritis. Pyelographic distinction between a shrunken chronic pyelonephritic kidney and a congenital hypoplastic kidney with distorted architecture may be impossible. Arteriographic distinction can sometimes be made (see Fig. 11–49).

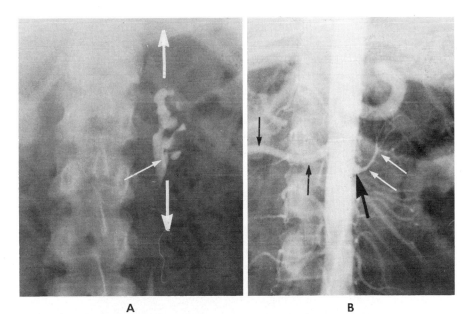

A   B

Figure 11–49 **Unilateral Chronic Atrophic Pyelonephritis: Arteriogram.**

A, Left retrograde pyelogram discloses a small kidney with blunted calices and a thin cortex, consistent with longstanding chronic pyelonephritis. However, the extreme medial position of this kidney, its abnormal vertical long axis (*large arrows*), and the low position of its pelvis (*small arrow*) are more in keeping with a congenital hypoplastic kidney.

B, Midstream aortogram demonstrates a normal-sized right renal artery (*small black arrows*) and a small narrow left renal artery (*white arrows*). However, at its aortic origin the artery is of normal width (*large black arrow*), indicating that the left kidney originally was of normal size. In a congenital hypoplastic kidney, the artery is small even at its point of origin from the aorta. The size of the aortic orifice of a renal artery can help distinguish acquired atrophic kidney from congenital hypoplastic kidney.

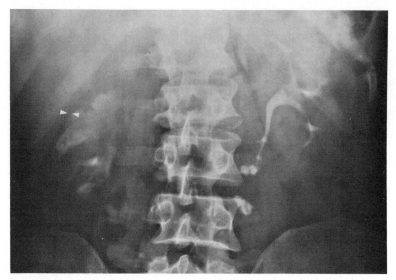

Figure 11–50 **Unilateral Chronic Pyelonephritis: Intravenous Urogram.**   There is a pronounced difference in density of the contrast medium in the calices. The decreased density on the right signifies impaired function of this kidney; the calices and infundibulum on the right, especially in the upper pole, are dilated and irregular; there is definite narrowing of the renal cortex (*arrowheads*). These changes indicate chronic pyelonephritis.

The calcifications on the left side of the abdomen represent unrelated calcified mesenteric lymph nodes, although the presence of calcified abdominal lymph nodes along with evidence of chronic pyelonephritis should raise the possibility of tuberculous pyelonephritis.

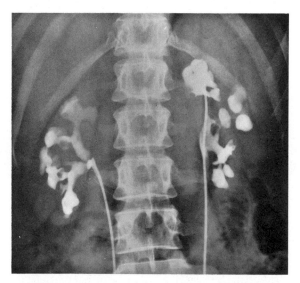

Figure 11–51 **Chronic Pyelonephritis with Azotemia.**   A bilateral retrograde pyelogram demonstrates the features characteristically found in chronic bilateral pyelonephritis. The calices have become blunted and dilated and extend almost to the periphery of the kidneys; this is indicative of marked thinning and atrophy of the cortex. The kidneys are small despite the dilatation of the collecting system.

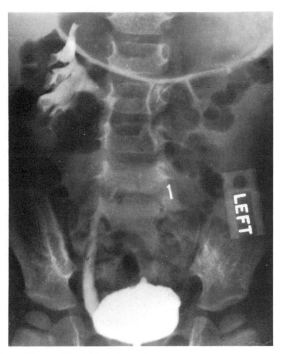

Figure 11-52 **Pyelonephritis with Reflux: Voiding Cystogram.** The patient was a 7 year old girl with pyelonephritis. The contrast material instilled into the bladder has refluxed into the dilated right ureter and the right kidney. Normally there is no such reflux.

Segmental or total ureteral dilatation is often associated with pyelonephritis, and in many cases there is also vesicoureteral reflux.

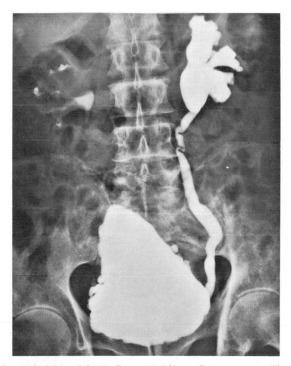

Figure 11-53 **Chronic Pyelonephritis with Reflux: Voiding Cystogram.** There are multiple diverticula and coarse trabeculations in the bladder. There is reflux of contrast material into both kidneys. The left pelvis and ureter are dilated, and the calices are blunted.

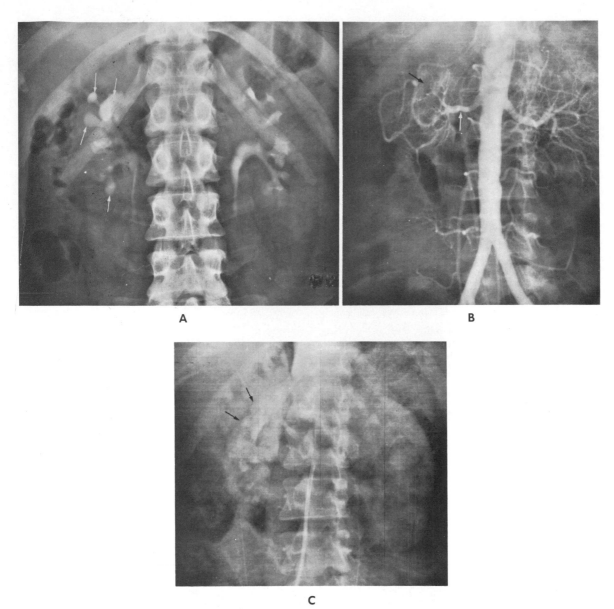

C

Figure 11–54   **Chronic Pyelonephritis with Hypertension: Aortogram.**

A, Intravenous urogram demonstrates a small right kidney. Pronounced caliceal clubbing and dilatation (*arrows*) indicate chronic pyelonephritis. Similar changes, although less severe, are seen in the middle and inferior caliceal system of the left kidney. Chronic pyelonephritis is most often bilateral, but one side may be more severely involved.

B, On the abdominal aortogram there is a normal vascular pattern in the left kidney, but there is distortion and tortuosity of the peripheral (cortical) vessels on the right (*black arrow*) owing to chronic pyelonephritis. The right main renal artery (*white arrow*) is smaller than the left; this is often seen in chronic inflammatory disease with renal atrophy.

C, On the nephrogram following the vascular phase of arteriography the right kidney is small, and the cortex is irregular and thin because of scarring (*arrows*). The left kidney is normal in size and shape, and the cortical tissue is normal.

Xanthogranulomatous Pyelonephritis

This rare unilateral disorder, usually seen in adults, is characterized by inflammatory necrosis and lipid degeneration (foam cell) of a kidney and is generally due to a gram-negative bacillus (Proteus, *E. coli*, Pseudomonas). Antecedent obstruction, calculi, and infection are almost always present. Occasionally, a solitary renal abscess is the underlying cause.

Radiographic findings are nonspecific; the correct roentgen diagnosis is rarely made. There is usually an enlarged nonfunctioning kidney containing calculi, suggesting calculus pyonephrosis. Occasionally focal dystrophic calcifications are seen in the parenchyma, suggesting tuberculosis. Retrograde studies will show the obstruction and usually are not helpful for diagnosis. If xanthogranulomatous changes develop from a primary renal abscess, the kidney may be functioning and urography may show a space-occupying mass, suggesting cyst, tumor, or abscess.

Angiographic findings usually reflect merely the obstructive and inflammatory nature of the condition. When a large xanthogranulomatous mass is present, the vascular changes suggest cyst, abscess, or even necrotic renal carcinoma.[87-89]

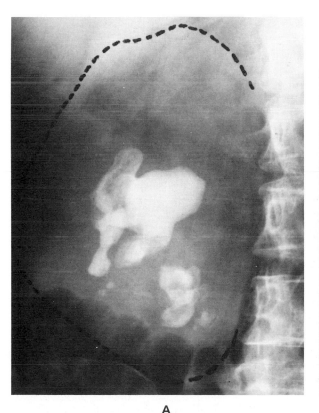
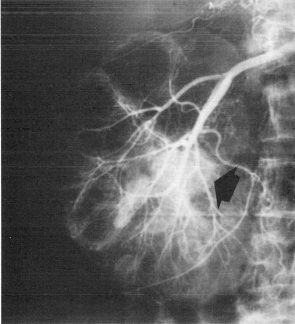

A

B

Figure 11-55 **Xanthogranulomatous Pyelonephritis.**

A, The kidney (*outlined in ink*) is enlarged and nonfunctioning and contains a large staghorn calculus and lower pole calculi.

B, Angiography shows crowded hypervascular small arteries draped around the lucent pyonephrotic sacs. Arrow points to the staghorn calculus.

The radiographic findings in xanthogranulomatous pyelonephritis are nonspecific and usually are merely those of chronic infection and renal calculi. (Courtesy Dr. A. J. Palubinskas, San Francisco, California.)

Renal Carbuncle

A renal carbuncle (abscess) is difficult to recognize clinically or radiographically. Most often urinary symptoms are lacking and urinalysis is negative, although occasionally flank pain with chills and fever will suggest renal involvement. The inflammation may be blood borne or may result from extension of a pyelonephritis.

In the acute phase, decreased opacification of all or part of the kidney will often occur. Multiple abscesses usually produce a swollen kidney with no opacification, similar to severe acute pyelonephritis. A single large abscess may cause a localized bulge on the renal outline and may distort the adjacent calices, suggesting a mass lesion. Uncommonly, the abscess extends into the collecting system and the pyelogram will show caliceal destruction and contrast material extending into the abscess area, a more definitive finding.

Nephrotomography may show a poorly demarcated lucent area in the kidney, simulating a cyst but with a less regular outline and often a thickened wall. More chronic lesions closely resemble a necrotic neoplasm.

Renal angiography will detect the lesion but usually fails to distinguish the abscess from a poorly vascularized neoplasm or granuloma. Sometimes the vascular displacement and draping is surprisingly minimal in contrast to the size of the nephrographic defect, a suggestive finding. In the nephrographic phase, loss of the normal corticomedullary junction and a relatively homogeneous blush may be suggestive findings.

If the parenchymal abscess involves the perinephric space, the angiographic findings are more definitive. (See *Perinephric Abscess,* p. 819.)

Definitive diagnosis of renal carbuncle is infrequently made prior to surgery.[90, 91]

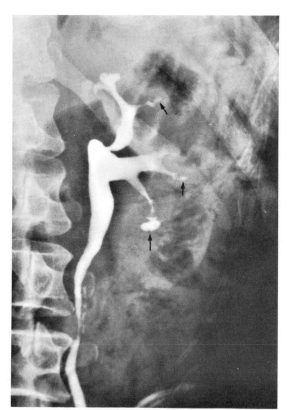

Figure 11–56 **Renal Carbuncles: Diabetes.** Multiple abscesses (*arrows*) filled with contrast material are separated from the calices. Contrast material has accumulated in an abscess just below the distorted lower calix (*lowest arrow*). These abscesses may have resulted from a previous episode of acute pyelonephritis. Pericaliceal edema is probably the cause of narrowing and shortening of some calices. In the absence of infection these cavities are indistinguishable from congenital caliceal diverticula.

Calcium may occasionally be deposited in chronic renal abscesses. Medullary abscesses produce no roentgenologic changes until they become large enough to displace adjacent calices or to communicate with the collecting system. In the present case the abscesses were caused by infection with *Aerobacter aerogenes.*

Perinephric Abscess

Perinephric abscess is generally caused by extension of a cortical inflammatory lesion to the renal capsule and perinephric tissues. A renal carbuncle or suppurative pyelonephritis is the most common underlying lesion. Renal trauma and extravasation can also initiate perinephric inflammation.

Abdominal and urographic films show an indistinct renal border or pole; the psoas shadow is also indistinct or obliterated. A localized lumbar scoliosis is often seen. The collecting system may be normal or may show localized caliceal distortion from the pre-existing renal inflammation. The most significant findings are some displacement of the involved kidney, and immobility with postural changes and respiration.

Angiography during the subacute or chronic phase may show localized, diminished or absent nephrographic density and an indistinct renal border adjacent to the perinephric mass. The capsular artery is prominent, displaced from the kidney and stretched over the inflammatory mass. It may send some branches into the mass, the bulk of which is avascular. There are often areas of vascular blush at the edges of the abscess. Though there are no "tumor" vessels, sometimes the angiographic picture is not easily distinguished from that of a necrotic neoplasm.[91-94]

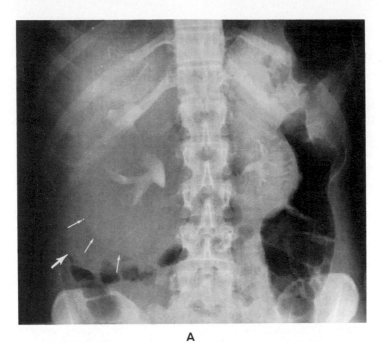

A

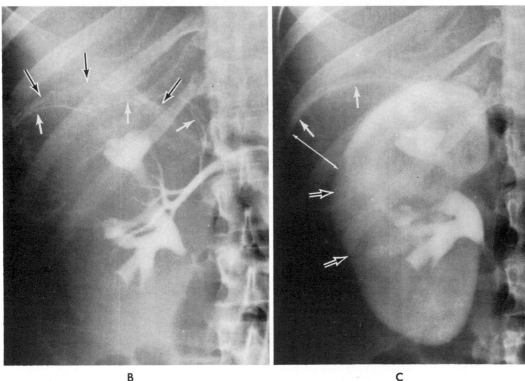

B   C

Figure 11–57 **Chronic Subcapsular Perinephric Abscess.**

A, Excretory urography was done because of postpartum fever and right flank pain. The left kidney is hypoplastic but has a regular pelvis and calices. The right kidney and its collecting system are somewhat enlarged, probably due to compensatory hypertrophy. Its lower border is visible (*small arrows*), but there appears to be another soft tissue mass (*large arrow*) below the border. The lateral and upper margins of the right kidney cannot be identified.

B, Selective right renal arteriography shows early filling of the capsular artery (*white arrows*), which courses far laterally, indicative of a displaced renal capsule. A band of opacification (*black-white arrows*) has appeared just above the capsular artery.

C, Nephrographic phase discloses an undistorted kidney. The opacified band (*white arrows*) was the thick wall of a subcapsular perinephric abscess (*double-headed arrow*). Inflammatory involvement of the lateral kidney border is evidenced by the focal absence of cortical opacification (*black-white arrows*).

OTHER SPECIFIC RENAL DISEASES

Hypercalcemic Nephropathy

Hypercalcemic nephropathy refers to calcification of the kidney parenchyma secondary to any condition associated with excessive calcium mobilization and excretion. Calcification generally begins in the distal tubules and collecting ducts and may progress to involve the renal pyramids, although any portion of the parenchyma may be affected. Renal calculi frequently develop. Eventually, renal insufficiency may supervene, and the kidneys may decrease in size. Among the causes are primary hyperparathyroidism, multiple myeloma, sarcoid, idiopathic hypercalcemia, vitamin D intoxication, hyperchloremic acidosis, Cushing's disease, and milk alkali syndrome. Hypercalcemic nephropathy is a relatively rare cause of renal failure.

Other diseases may also lead to precipitation of calcium within the kidney. Among these diseases are chronic pyelonephritis, medullary sponge kidney, tuberculosis, and chronic glomerulonephritis. Radiographically, these conditions may simulate hypercalcemic nephropathy, but studies of blood and urinary calcium will help differentiate the cause.[95-98]

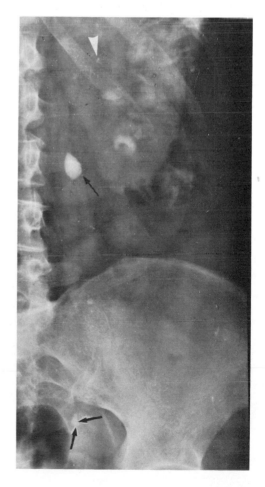

Figure 11–58 **Hypercalcemic Nephropathy: Hyperparathyroidism.** Urogram demonstrates medullary calcification in the upper pole *(arrowhead),* with calculi in the upper and lower ureter *(arrows).* The calices appear dilated.

Renal parenchymal calcifications and renal calculi are common complications of hyperparathyroidism.

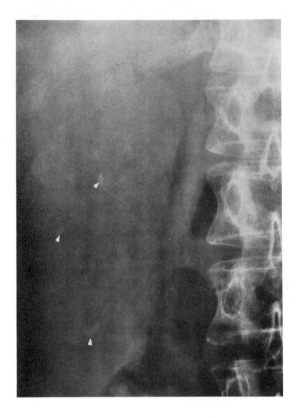

Figure 11–59 **Hypercalcemic Nephropathy Secondary to Cortisone Administration.** An enlarged view of the right kidney reveals extensive medullary calcification (*arrowheads*) similar to the nephrocalcinosis seen in Cushing's disease and hyperparathyroidism. The calcification is probably within the distal tubules and collecting ducts. The patient had received high doses of cortisone over a long period.

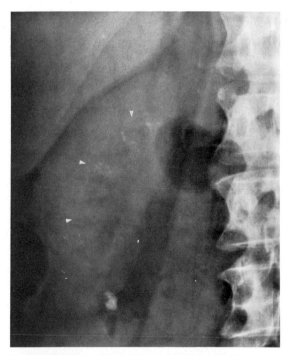

Figure 11–60 **Arteriosclerotic Calcification Simulating Nephrocalcinosis.** Multiple medullary calcifications (*arrowheads*) are indistinguishable from the calcification of nephrocalcinosis. However, these proved to be calcifications in arteriosclerotic plaques in the small renal arteries adjacent to the pyramids, which is a rare occurrence.

Renal Tubular Acidosis

This condition is due to a tubular defect that interferes with normal urinary acidification and leads to hyperchloremic acidosis. This is commonly an isolated defect, but it can occur as one of the multiple and complex tubular defects of Fanconi syndrome.

Hypercalcinuria is an almost constant feature and can result in diffuse nephrocalcinosis and renal calculi. In children, diffuse nephrocalcinosis is striking and often suggestive of the diagnosis. In adults, recurrent renal and urinary calculi with little or no parenchymal calcification are seen.

Renal function is generally normal or slightly impaired, but calculous obstructions, extensive nephrocalcinosis, and infection may lead to renal failure.

The other common radiographic findings are renal rickets in children and osteomalacia in adults. These conditions are apparently due to the hypophosphatemia from increased phosphate excretion.

Although nephrocalcinosis occurs in other conditions, including sarcoidosis, primary hyperparathyroidism, idiopathic hypercalcinuria, and medullary sponge kidney (see text under these headings), when accompanied by renal rickets or by pseudofractures of osteomalacia in the absence of renal failure, the diagnosis of renal tubular acidosis is probable.

Early nephrocalcinosis in renal tubular acidosis may show considerable resolution under proper treatment.[98-100]

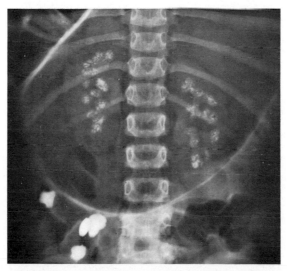

Figure 11–61 **Renal Tubular Acidosis in a Child: Urogram.** Areas of fine calcification are shown in the medullary portions of both kidneys, adjacent to the calices. This type of nephrocalcinosis is found, in various degrees, in about one fifth of children with renal tubular acidosis. When fragments of calcium become detached, renal colic may occur. Calculus formation is very common in adults with mild renal tubular acidosis.

Hypophosphatemia often develops in this condition and may cause renal rickets in children and osteomalacia in adults.

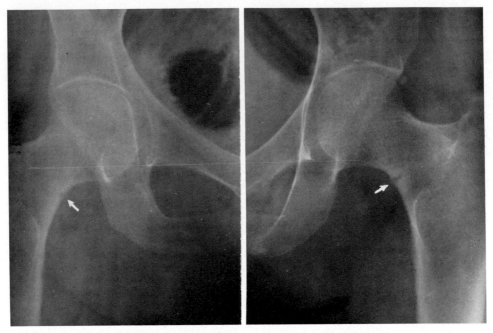

Figure 11–62 **Renal Tubular Acidosis: Osteomalacia.** There are bilateral symmetric pseudofractures (*lucent lines*) in both femoral necks (*arrows*). There is also bone demineralization.

Generally, pseudofractures are symmetric and occur at points of entry of the blood vessels into the bone. They are diagnostic of osteomalacia.

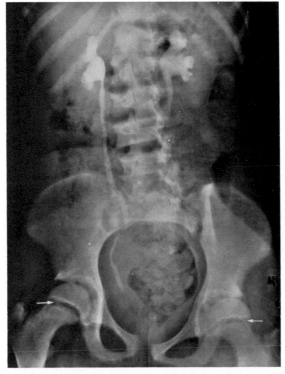

Figure 11–63 **Renal Tubular Acidosis: Renal Rickets: Intravenous Urogram.** Except for some fullness of the caliceal system on the left, the kidneys are not remarkable. Widening of the epiphyseal lines (*arrows*) is characteristic of rickets. In renal tubular dystrophies the pyelogram is usually normal unless nephrocalcinosis or calculi develop.

Renal Papillary Necrosis

The predisposing factors to development of renal papillary necrosis (ischemic necrosis of renal papilla) are urinary obstruction and infection, diabetes, sickle cell trait or disease, and chronic phenacetin or aspirin ingestion. Acute or chronic pyelonephritis is associated in most cases.

The radiographic changes are due to necrosis and later detachment of the papilla. Central necrosis may lead to an extension of contrast material from the center of the calix into the papilla (medullary type). Necrosis of the entire papilla causes extension of contrast material from the caliceal edges around the papilla. With sloughing, the papilla may present as a lucent defect within a pool of dye — a ring shadow (papillary type). Occasionally the sloughed papilla may calcify. There is usually evidence of pyelonephritis, even in cases associated with phenacetin abuse. Intravenous urography is generally adequate for diagnosis, since kidney function is usually unimpaired. The extent and distribution of the focal areas of destruction are best demonstrated by nephrotomography.[101-104]

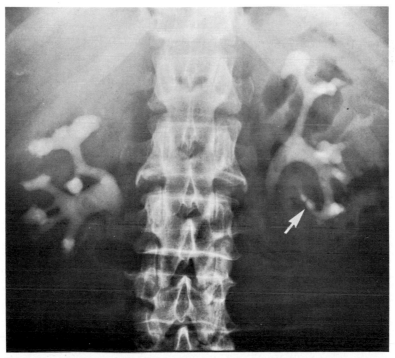

Figure 11–64 **Early Renal Papillary Necrosis: Intravenous Pyelogram.** In a 52 year old man who had hematuria, dysuria, and left flank pain, there are changes of early papillary necrosis: caliceal blunting caused by bilateral chronic pyelonephritis, and extension, into the parenchyma, of contrast material from the inferior left calix adjacent to a necrotic papilla (*arrow*).

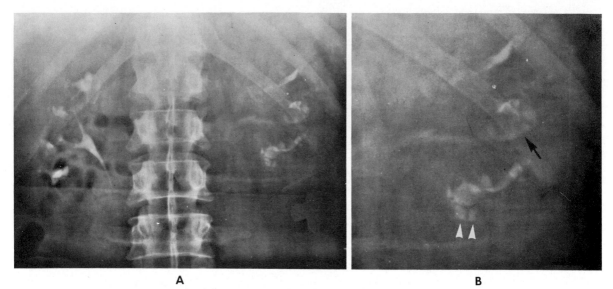

A   B

Figure 11–65   **Advanced Papillary Necrosis: Intravenous Urogram.**

A, Caliceal changes caused by chronic pyelonephritis are seen on the right, and on the left there is greater caliceal destruction with marked distortion and cortical thinning due to scarring. The left upper calix appears relatively normal.

B, Enlarged view of the left kidney shows the characteristic ring shadow (*black arrow*) of the detached papillae in the caliceal pool; contrast medium flowing into the parenchyma forms sinus tracts (*arrowheads*). The involved kidney is usually abnormally small.

Pyeloureteritis Cystica

This condition is generally a complication of chronic urinary tract infection, especially pyelonephritis. Multiple small cysts develop in the wall of the upper ureter, sometimes in the bladder, and occasionally in the renal pelvis. Although pyeloureteritis cystica is rare, the roentgenographic picture is characteristic: multiple small radiolucent filling defects due to the cysts are seen in the contrast-filled ureter or pelvis. These filling defects may be confused with air bubbles on a retrograde study.[105, 106]

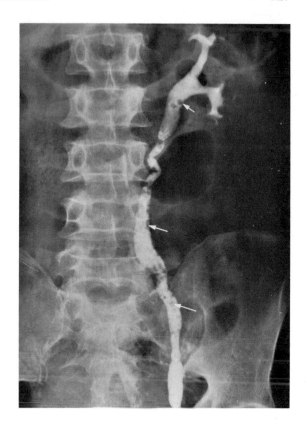

Figure 11–66 **Pyeloureteritis Cystica.** A retrograde study demonstrates multiple small round lucent defects (*arrows*) throughout the upper two thirds of the ureter and in the renal pelvis. Prior intravenous pyelogram indicated that both ureters were involved.

OBSTRUCTIVE NEPHROPATHY

Unilateral obstruction can result from lesions in the renal pelvis, the ureter, or the ureteropelvic junction. Lesions of the bladder neck or the urethra can produce bilateral obstructive uropathy.

The most common cause of ureteral obstruction is a calculus. It can lodge at any point but it is most frequently at the ureterovesical junction since this is the narrowest part of the ureter. Other intrinsic causes of ureteral obstruction include narrowing by a ureteral tumor, blood clot, inflammatory spasm, stricture, and ureterocele. Extrinsic causes include pressure or invasion by extrinsic tumor, inflammatory masses, an anomalous blood vessel such as a retrocaval ureter, and periureteral fibrosis.

The ovarian vein syndrome is a hydronephrosis in postgravid women caused by ureteral compression at L3–L4 from a dilated ovarian vein. While usually right sided, it may be bilateral.

Obstruction of the bladder outlet in the male adult results most often from prostatic hypertrophy and, less frequently, from prostatic or bladder tumor.

In children, obstruction is generally caused by congenital malformations, the most common of which are ureterocele, a posterior urethral valve, and ureteropelvic narrowing, which may be bilateral. The latter two conditions can cause bilateral hydronephrosis and chronic renal failure.

The significant roentgenographic finding is dilatation of the urinary tract proximal to the obstruction. The renal calices first become flattened and broadened and then progressively dilated. With prolonged obstruction they continue to enlarge and eventually destroy the surrounding parenchyma. The renal pelvis also becomes dilated and enlarged; an extrarenal pelvis dilates earlier and to a greater degree. Calculi often form in the chronically obstructed pelvis and calices. The proximal ureter becomes dilated and may also become tortuous, elongated, and eventually atonic. Films taken with the patient in erect position usually demonstrate most clearly the dilatation and point of obstruction.

In acute ureteral obstruction there may be delay or absence of excretion on the obstructed side. If function is present the nephrogram persists without caliceal filling because of distention and elevated pressure in the collecting system. However, after a variable time lapse, sufficient opaque medium diffuses from the tubules into the collecting system and allows visualization up to the point of obstruction. Rarely, more than 24 hours may be required for sufficient opacification, but if a nephrogram is initially present, opacification can be expected. The kidney is generally enlarged, and the calices are dilated.

In chronic persistent obstruction, kidney function may be greatly diminished, and neither a nephrogram nor a delayed pyelogram will be obtained. In these cases a successful retrograde pyelogram may show the site of obstruction and the extent of dilatation. Hydronephrosis can also be recognized on angiographic studies. The hydronephrotic sacs will cause characteristic stretching of the vessels and will appear as "holes" in the nephrogram. After selective renal arteriography, later films will usually show some contrast material in the hydronephrotic sacs, even when the kidney appeared totally nonfunctioning on pyelographic studies.

Occasionally, prolonged incomplete obstruction can cause renal atrophy, with reduction of the cortical and medullary substance, but with some preservation of the caliceal papillae. Function may be reduced; ischemia from pressure of the dilated infundibula and calices is a probable cause.[107, 112]

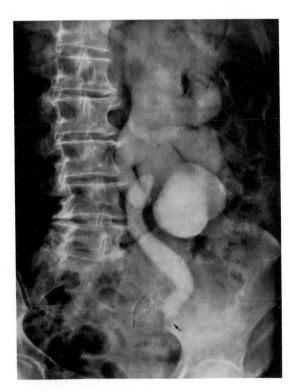

Figure 11–67 **Obstructive Nephropathy: Ureteral Calculus: Retrograde Pyelogram.** The pronounced hydronephrosis and hydroureter are proximal to an obstructing nonopaque calculus (*arrow*). The ureter is tortuous and redundant, thus indicating the chronicity of the obstruction. Dilatation of the collecting system has led to destruction of the adjacent kidney parenchyma. Almost no functioning urinary tissue remains, and there was nonvisualization on the intravenous study.

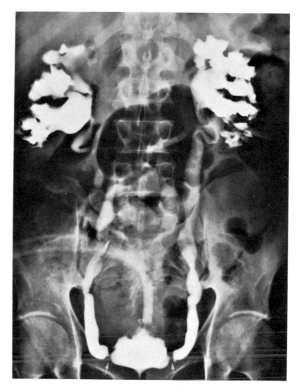

Figure 11–68 **Obstructive Nephropathy: Chronic Prostatic Enlargement.** The kidneys and pelves are extremely dilated. Blunting of the caliceal system suggests pyelonephritis. Both ureters are dilated and redundant. There is bilateral narrowing of the lower intramural end of the ureters, due to thickening of the bladder wall (*arrows*). Notice the curvature of the distal ureters—fish-hooking—the result of chronic obstruction and elevation of the bladder. The bladder wall is thickened and irregular. A cystotomy tube is in place.

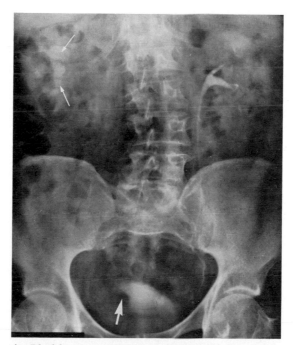

Figure 11–69 **Hydronephrosis: Bladder Tumor with Secondary Obstruction.** There is a radiolucent filling defect in the bladder and irregularity of the right lateral bladder wall due to a tumor mass (*large arrow*). Decreased opacification and hydronephrosis of the right kidney (*small arrows*) are secondary to ureteral obstruction by the tumor at the ureterovesical junction.

Although bladder tumors may usually be demonstrated by intravenous pyelogram, a cystogram is generally more accurate for diagnosis. Most bladder tumors do not involve the urethral orifice or cause obstruction.

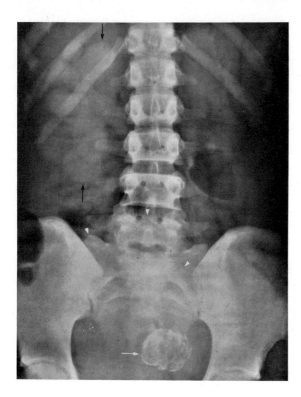

Figure 11–70 **Obstructive Nephropathy: Uterine Fibroids.** A three-hour intravenous urogram taken after the normal left kidney has emptied reveals marked dilatation of the right renal calices and pelvis, which are faintly opacified (*black arrows*). Obstruction of the right ureter is due to a large uterine fibroid (*arrowheads*). One of the fibroids is calcified (*white arrow*). After hysterectomy the kidney and ureter rapidly returned to normal size.

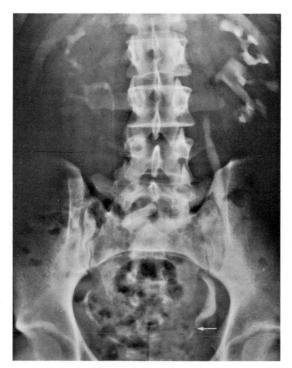

Figure 11–71 **Congenital Ureteral Stricture: Intravenous Pyelogram.** The distal ureter tapers to an area of stricture (*arrow*), and the ureter and kidney proximal to the stricture are dilated. The stricture was congenital. Following passage of a ureteral calculus, spasm and edema of the lower ureter may produce a similar appearance, but only temporarily.

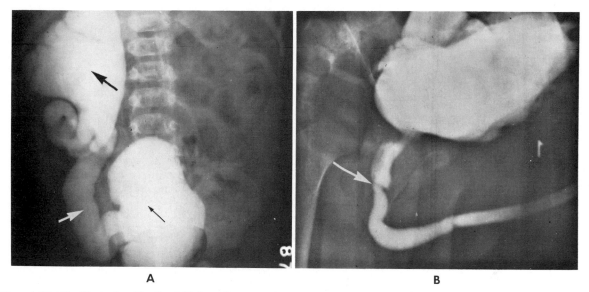

Figure 11–72 **Posterior Urethral Valve: Retrograde Cystourethrogram.**

A, Contrast material refluxes from the greatly dilated bladder (*small black arrow*), filling the distended ureter (*white arrow*) and hydronephrotic kidney (*large black arrow*) on the right side.

B, Voiding cystourethrogram demonstrates a defect in the opacified urethra. The defect was due to a posterior urethral valve (*arrow*), which has caused obstructive dilatation of the bladder, kidney, and ureter.

The value can be demonstrated only by voiding cystourethrography. If untreated, such a valve can cause renal failure and death.

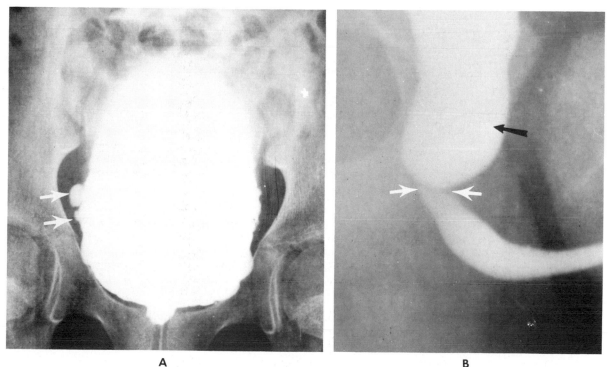

Figure 11–73 **Posterior Urethral Valve: Hydronephrosis and Chronic Renal Insufficiency in 4 Year Old Boy.**

A, Cystogram shows a large trabeculated bladder with cellules (*arrows*), characteristic findings of chronic bladder outlet obstruction.

B, Voiding cystourethrogram reveals a dilated prostatic urethra (*black arrow*) and a linear defect of the obstructing posterior urethral valve (*white arrows*).

Both hydronephrotic kidneys were nonfunctioning on excretory pyelography.

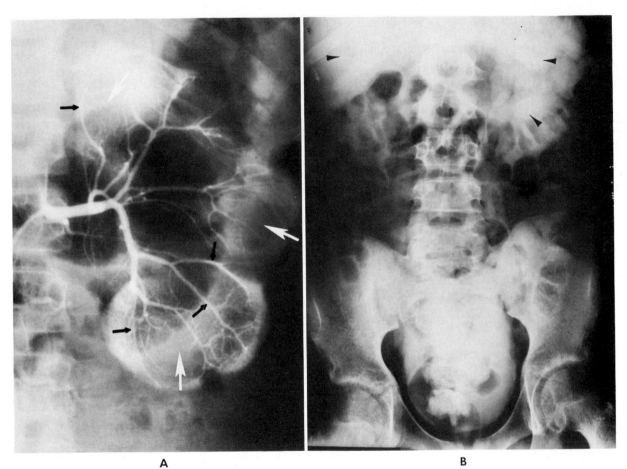

A   B

Figure 11–74 **Hydronephrosis: Selective Renal Angiography.**   This 12 year old boy was uremic from unsuspected bilateral obstructive uropathy due to a posterior urethral valve.

   A, The left intrarenal vessels are stretched (*black arrows*) around "holes" in the nephrogram (*white
arrows*). These characteristic findings of hydronephrosis were also present in the right kidney.

   B, A film taken 12 hours later shows some contrast material in the dilated hydronephrotic sacs (*arrowheads*).

TOXIC NEPHROPATHY

Radiation Nephritis

If the kidney is included in the fields of radiation, a diffuse renal vasculitis can occur after a latent period of six months to a year. This leads to diminished or absent function. Some degree of recovery may ensue, but most often the kidney remains nonfunctional. On retrograde study, however, the renal collecting system appears normal, findings similar to those of arterial renal infarction. Systemic hypertension may occur in the acute or chronic phase. The nonfunctioning kidney eventually decreases in size.[113-115]

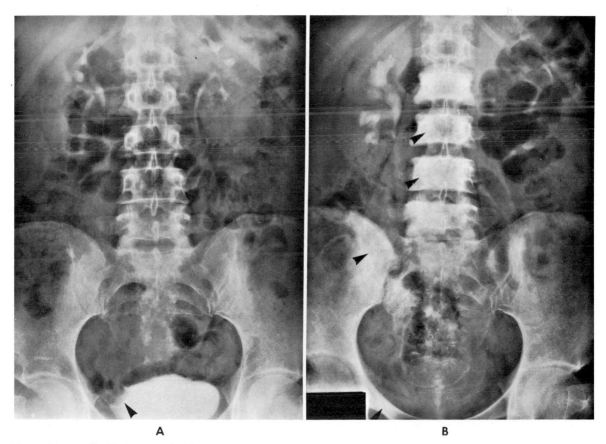

A   B

Figure 11–75 **Radiation Nephritis.**

A, A tumor of the bladder produces a filling defect (*arrowhead*). Both upper urinary tracts appear normal.

B, A few months after intensive radiotherapy for metastases, the left kidney is nonfunctioning. The size is unchanged. Slight compensatory dilatation of the right collecting system has occurred. Osteoblastic metastases (*arrowheads*) have developed in the pelvis and lumbar bodies.

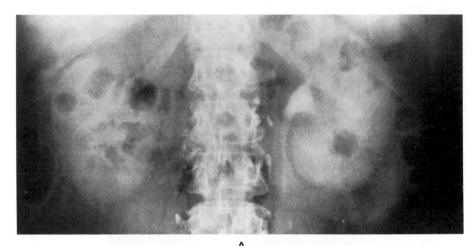

A

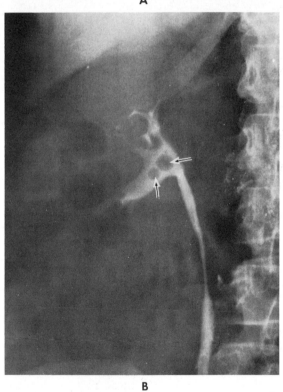

B

Figure 11–76 **Radiation Nephritis.**

A, Intravenous pyelogram reveals a normal left pyelogram, but no excretion from the right kidney. Both kidneys are identical in size. The patient had received intensive radiation a year previously for a retroperitoneal malignancy. The densities along the spine are residual opaque material from a prior lymphangiogram.

B, A right retrograde pyelogram shows a normal collecting system. The lucencies in the renal pelvis *(arrows)* are air bubbles.

Both arterial renal infarction and radiation nephritis cause avascularity of the kidney without affecting the collecting system. Characteristically, both conditions show a nonfunctioning kidney on excretory pyelography and a normal collecting system on retrograde pyelography.

Analgesic Nephropathy

Excessive and prolonged ingestion of phenacetin and other analgesics has been implicated in the development of chronic pyelonephritis and subsequent papillary necrosis. The changes are usually bilateral. The roentgenographic picture is indistinguishable from that of chronic pyelonephritis and papillary necrosis from other causes (diabetes, urinary tract obstruction; see p. 810). Symptoms of renal insufficiency may eventually develop. (See *Renal Papillary Necrosis*, p. 825.)[116, 117]

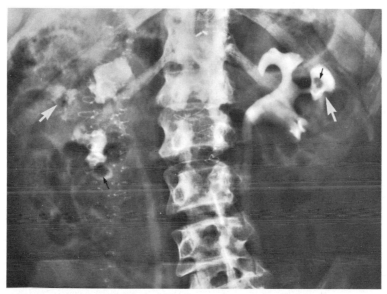

Figure 11–77 **Bilateral Phenacetin Nephritis.** This 40 year old woman had a history of heavy phenacetin ingestion for six years. An intravenous urogram done seven years earlier had been normal.

The urogram illustrated shows rounded lucencies (*black arrows*) in multiple areas of caliceal destruction (*white arrows*), characteristic of papillary necrosis. The lucencies represent the sloughed papillae within the contrast-filled calices. The caliceal blunting is indicative of chronic pyelonephritis.

Lithiasis

Nephrolithiasis—stones or calculi within the calices or pelvis of the kidney—should be distinguished from nephrocalcinosis, in which calcium deposits occur within the renal parenchyma. Nephrolithiasis is not a single entity but is a manifestation of various disease processes; however, the underlying metabolic abnormality is often unknown. Frequently, mechanical stasis is a predisposing factor. In nephrocalcinosis, calcium deposits in the papillae may break into the calices and become calculi. Radiologic examination is important not only to demonstrate the calculi but also to disclose a possible underlying renal abnormality.

Over 90 per cent of symptomatic renal calculi are radiopaque and detectable on a plain film examination of the abdomen. Most calculi contain either calcium phosphate or calcium oxalate. These calculi are smooth and uniformly dense. The less common magnesium ammonium phosphate stones have a lower degree of opacity; they frequently appear as casts of the renal pelvis and are generally secondary to renal infection. Uric acid and urate stones are radiolucent and account for only about 4 per cent of calculi. One per cent of calculi are cystine stones, which have a uniform ground-glass density.

Intravenous pyelogram confirms the presence and location of calculi and usually discloses the degree of obstruction and dilatation. It may also indicate mechanical causes of urinary stasis, such as ureteropelvic bands and vessel narrowing, which predispose to infection and stone formation.

Roentgenograms may occasionally furnish clues to the presence of predisposing endocrine diseases such as hyperparathyroidism and Cushing's disease, and there may be evidence of osteolytic metastases, myeloma, sarcoid, Paget's disease, and other diseases that cause hypercalcemia and subsequent nephrolithiasis.

Renal colic usually ensues when a pelvic or caliceal calculus descends into the ureter. Intravenous pyelogram very often demonstrates the stone in the ureter as well as dilatation of the proximal ureter and, usually, dilatation of the pelvis and calices. It is not uncommon, however, for caliceal filling to be delayed on the involved side. If a nephrogram develops, eventual filling of the collecting system can be expected, although it may not occur for 24 hours. If the kidney is not functioning, retrograde pyelography may be needed to confirm the diagnosis.

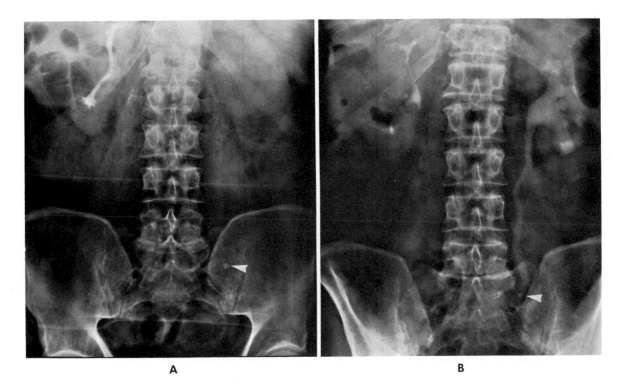

A   B

Figure 11–78 **Ureteral Calculus with Obstruction: Delayed Films.**

A, Ten-minute urogram shows good excretion on the right but only a nephrogram on the left. An opaque ureteral calculus overlies the left side of the sacrum (*arrowhead*).

B, Delayed film (two hours) demonstrates opacification of the left urinary tract, which is dilated down to the obstructing calculus (*arrowhead*). If a nephrogram develops during pyelography, delayed films will eventually show opacification of the collecting system down to the site of obstruction.

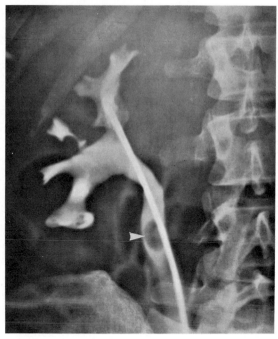

Figure 11–79 **Nonopaque Ureteral Calculus: Retrograde Pyelogram.** There is a round lucent filling defect in the upper ureter (*arrowhead*), and the ureter above the stone is dilated. Lucent calculi can be demonstrated only by contrast studies, in which the calculi appear as defects in the contrast material. Lucent calculi must be differentiated from blood clot and tumor masses. Only a small percentage of renal calculi are nonopaque.

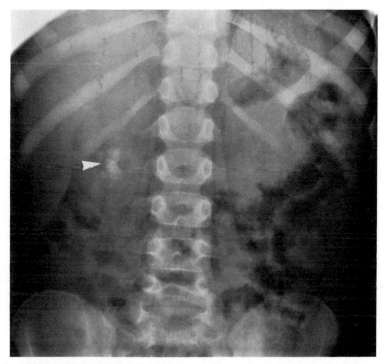

Figure 11–80 **Cystine Stone: Right Kidney.** There is a large, homogeneously dense calculus in the right kidney (*arrowhead*). It is pure cystine, uniformly dense, and nonlobulated, with a ground-glass appearance. Calcium salts are usually deposited as the calculus increases in size.

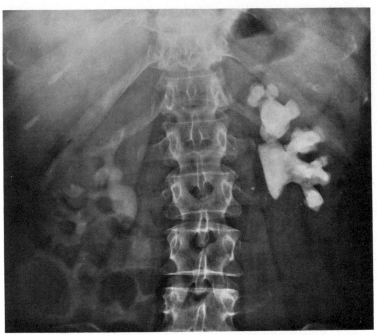

Figure 11–81 **Staghorn Calculus: Intravenous Pyelogram.** A huge staghorn calculus fills the left renal pelvis and calices. The left side appears to be nonfunctioning, while the right kidney is excreting normally. This type of calculus is almost always radiopaque. It forms a cast of the pelvis and calices, but the kidneys may remain functional over a surprisingly long period of time. Portions of a staghorn calculus may break off and enter the ureter, causing acute renal colic. In many cases, congenital ureteropelvic narrowing is thought to be an underlying cause.

During urography a staghorn calculus may be mistaken for contrast material. A preliminary film must always be made.

Nephrocalcinosis

In nephrocalcinosis, the visualized calcium deposits are diffusely scattered in the renal parenchyma and in the lumina of the collecting and distal convoluted tubules. The most common causes are hyperparathyroidism, renal tubular acidosis, idiopathic hypercalcinuria, medullary sponge kidney, and sarcoidosis. Less common causes include Cushing's disease, multiple myeloma, chronic glomerulonephritis, and steroid therapy.

Distinction between various nephrocalcinoses by the roentgenologic appearance of the calcifications is usually impossible. However, nephrocalcinosis associated with stag-horn calculi is most often due to renal tubular acidosis. When the calcifications are limited to the papillary portion of the pyramids, medullary sponge kidney is a likely diagnosis, and this is readily confirmed by the pyelographic findings.[117]

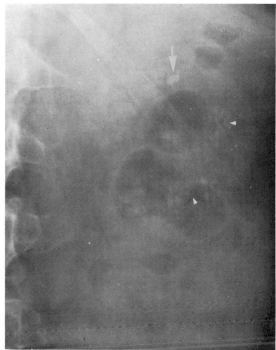

Figure 11–82 **Nephrocalcinosis: Hyperoxaluria.** An enlarged film of the left kidney shows widespread medullary calcifications *(arrowheads).* A larger calcification has formed in the upper pole *(arrow).* The calcific deposits are within the medullary portion of the kidney. In nephrocalcinosis, the scattered small calcific densities are in the medullary portion of the kidney. In the illustrated kidney the deposits were due to primary hyperoxaluria, a rare congenital metabolic disturbance. (See also Section 15.)

CYSTS OF THE KIDNEY

Adult Polycystic Disease

Polycystic kidney disease is progressive and often familial. In about one third of cases it is associated with liver cysts; intracranial berry-type aneurysms are found in up to 10 per cent of cases. Hypertension is often present. Progressive renal impairment and eventual chronic renal failure occur in most cases. An intracranial aneurysm occasionally ruptures, sometimes before renal disease is suspected.

When the cysts are large, the urographic findings are quite characteristic. Both kidneys are enlarged, often with some asymmetry and irregularity. The infundibula are thin and elongated, and often the calices are widened. The collecting system shows a distorted architecture. Individual large cysts may produce characteristic compression and bowing of calices; sometimes a peripelvic cyst displaces the upper ureter laterally.

If the cysts are small, renal enlargement is less marked or even absent and the collecting systems appear normal. Infusion nephrotomography will disclose the smaller lucent cysts and should be performed in any suspected case, even if the standard pyelogram is negative. Definitive diagnosis can be made by selective renal arteriography, which will show stretched and draped vessels and multiple scattered lucencies in the nephrogram. Hepatic arteriography will disclose lucencies in the opacified liver (hepatogram) if hepatic cysts are present.

In the younger hypertensive patient with suspected polycystic disease, cerebral arteriography is indicated to rule out asymptomatic intracranial aneurysm.

The urographic differential diagnosis includes diffuse renal enlargement from lymphomatous or leukemic disease and from bilateral multiple retention cysts.[119–122]

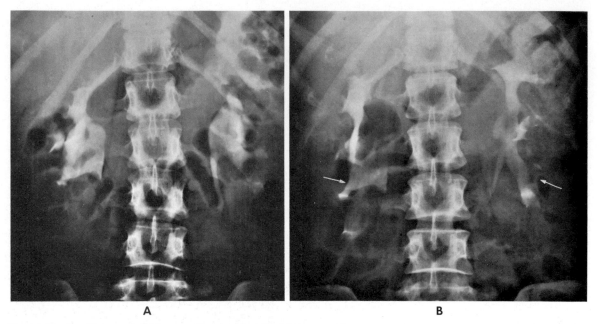

Figure 11–83   **Polycystic Disease: Unusually Rapid Progression.**

A, In intravenous urogram performed in 1959, the kidneys are large but there is little alteration of the caliceal contour.

B, Urogram three years later demonstrates considerable elongation and spreading of the caliceal system (*arrows*), with a characteristic polycystic appearance. Progressive enlargement of the cysts does occur in polycystic disease, but such rapid growth is unusual.

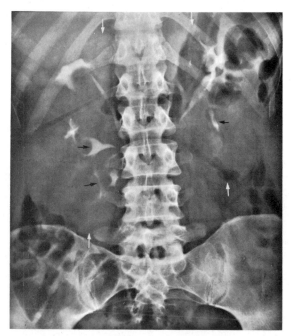

Figure 11–84   **Advanced Polycystic Kidney: Intravenous Pyelogram.**   Both kidneys are greatly enlarged (*white arrows*), and each has a double collecting system. The numerous cysts have produced pressure deformities on the calices (*black arrows*), which are irregular and bizarre due to the random location of the cysts. The infundibula are elongated. The picture is typical of polycystic kidneys.

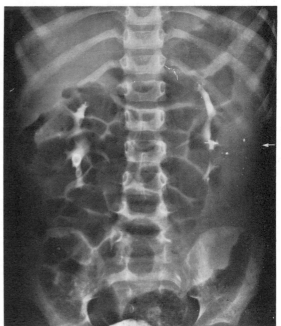

Figure 11–85 **Leukemic Infiltration of Kidney Simulating Polycystic Disease.**   The urogram demonstrates enlarged kidneys, with elongation and compression of the caliceal system similar to the changes seen in polycystic disease. The renal cortex is considerably widened *(arrows)* due to the infiltration with leukemic cells. This feature may help differentiate between infiltrating kidney disease and polycystic disease.

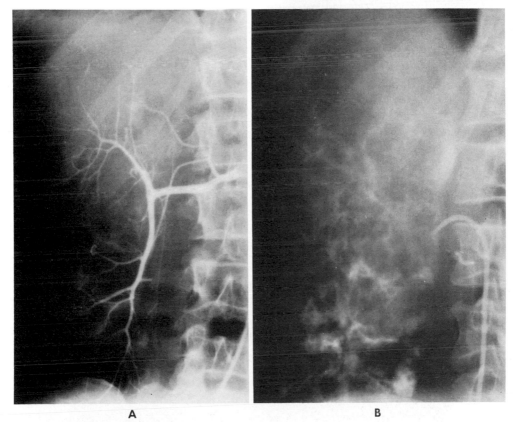

A   B

Figure 11–86 **Polycystic Kidney: Selective Angiogram.**

A, Virtually all the major and minor intrarenal arteries are elongated, stretched, and curved around the cysts. The kidney is greatly enlarged.

B, Nephrographic stage discloses rounded and oval filling defects throughout the entire kidney; these are due to the widely dispersed cysts. This swiss-cheese appearance of the nephrogram in an enlarged kidney is characteristic of polycystic disease.

Renal Cyst

Simple cysts are usually solitary but can be multiple and bilateral. They are somewhat more frequent in the lower pole. When near the periphery, a cyst will cause a local smooth bulge or enlargement. Calcification of the cyst wall is uncommon.

Urography demonstrates nondestructive displacement and stretching of the adjacent infundibula and calices; this is in contradistinction to the invasion and amputation of these structures by malignant tumors. However, distinction between cyst and malignant tumor is often impossible by urography alone, and nephrotomography, ultrasonography, or renal arteriography is necessary.

On the nephrotomograms made during high dose pyelography, the cyst appears as a nonopacified, thin-walled, smooth, circumscribed area within the nephrogram. The sharp, pointed appearance of the opacified renal border abutting the cyst is a characteristic finding (claw sign). Arteriography shows displacement of renal vessels around the cyst; the lesion is avascular and shows no abnormal vessels or tumor stain. A necrotic and avascular malignant tumor may produce identical angiographic findings, but usually its wall is thicker. Sometimes diagnosis can be made by means of direct transabdominal needle of the cyst and instillation of contrast material, which outlines the smooth cyst cavity.

Pyelogenic cysts (renal diverticula) communicate with the pelvis or calices and are opacified during pyelography.

In children, a rare multicystic disease of one kidney can result from a form of renal dysplasia; it has been called unilateral polycystic disease. The kidney is huge, irregular, and nonfunctioning. A few cases in adults have also been reported. (See *Congenital Multicystic Kidney*, p. 847.)[123–126]

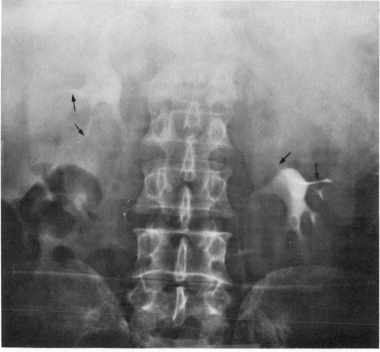

Figure 11–87 **Bilateral Renal Cysts: Intravenous Pyelogram.**   Intravenous urogram reveals downward displacement, compression, elongation, and spreading of the superior calices *(arrows)* of the enlarged left kidney. On the right, the smoothly stretched middle and lower caliceal system defines the cystic lesion *(arrows)*. There is no caliceal destruction. Bilateral renal cysts were found at surgery.

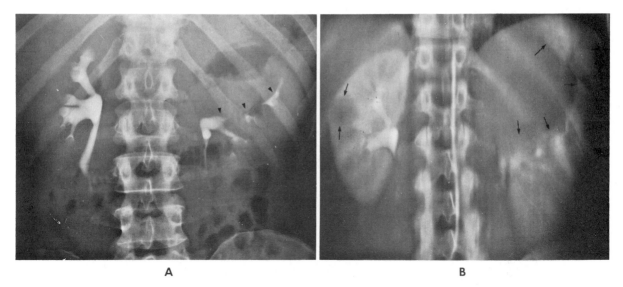

A   B

Figure 11–88   **Bilateral Renal Cysts: Nephrotomogram.**

A, Mass in the upper pole of the left kidney causes depression and stretching of the upper calices *(arrowheads).* There is no evidence of caliceal or infundibular destruction, and the right kidney appears to be normal.

B, Nephrotomogram following aortography demonstrates a characteristic large smooth defect of the left upper pole *(arrows).* An unexpected finding was the smooth defect *(arrows)* in the middle of the right renal cortex. The clearly circumscribed margins of the defects are characteristic of a benign cyst.

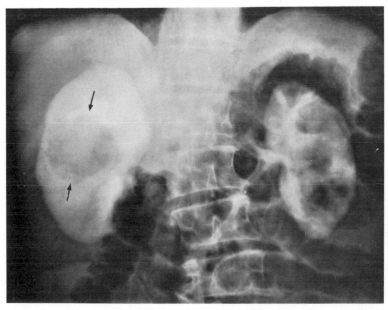

Figure 11–89   **Atypical Renal Cyst: Nephrogram.**   The large filling defect *(arrows)* in the opacified right kidney has an irregular margin, so that differentiation between cyst and necrotic tumor is impossible. Generally, a benign cyst has a smooth, well-demarcated border. At surgery a benign cyst was found.

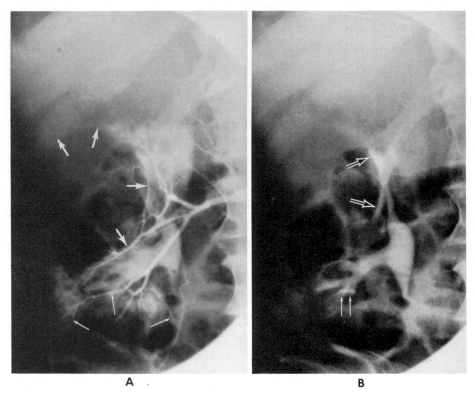

A   B

Figure 11–90   **Benign Renal Cysts: Angiogram.**

   A, Vascular opacification and nephrogram show a large, sharply demarcated defect, with vessels stretched and displaced around the cyst *(large arrows)*. The defect is avascular, and the findings are characteristic of a benign cyst. A smaller cyst has produced similar changes in the lower pole *(small arrows)*. The pyelographic opacification is from a prior injection.

   B, Pyelogram shows the smooth pressure deformity and stretching of the upper calices *(black-white arrows)*. The cyst in the lower pole is causing a slight pressure deformity of a lower calix *(white arrows)*.

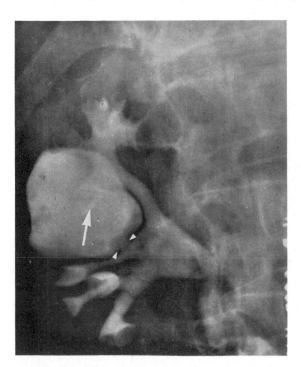

Figure 11–91   **Pyelogenic Cyst.** A large cyst filled with contrast material *(arrow)* communicates with the pelvis *(arrowheads)*. This is a congenital pyelogenic cyst. Urinary stasis can cause infection and calculi in these cavities.

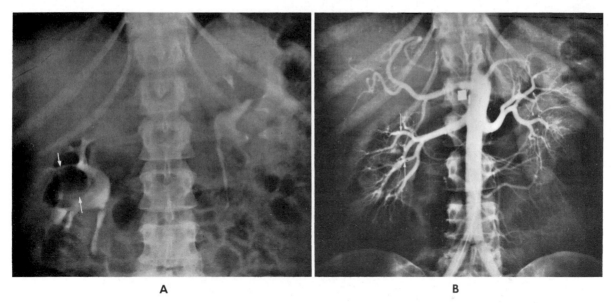

A   B

Figure 11-92   **Vascular Pressure on Calices Simulating a Cyst.**

A, Intravenous urogram reveals displacement and curvature of the infundibulum in the superior caliceal system, and spreading of the middle caliceal system of the right kidney *(arrows)*. These changes suggest pressure from a cyst.

B, Aortogram demonstrates a normal right kidney. Apparent displacement of the calices was due to pressure from the large intrarenal arterial branches *(arrows)*. Such vascular pressure and, sometimes, congenital variations in the calices can simulate the changes due to cyst. In either case, however, angiography will help to avoid erroneous diagnoses.

Medullary Cystic Disease

In this rare hereditary disease, sometimes called salt-losing nephritis, numerous medullary cysts of varying size develop in both kidneys. The cysts arise at the medullocortical junction and are associated with progressive fibrosis, leading to renal failure most often in the second and third decades. There are few or no cortical cysts. Chronic anemia, azotemia, and urine of low specific gravity are sometimes accompanied by severe urinary sodium loss, causing an addisonian-like syndrome.

Radiographically, in the fully developed disease the kidneys are small and do not visualize on intravenous pyelography. On retrograde studies the larger cysts may produce pressure deformities of the calices. Occasionally a medullary cyst may communicate with the pelvis and become opacified. Calcification of the cysts or parenchyma apparently does not occur. During infancy, before advanced renal failure, intravenous pyelography may reveal enlarged kidneys with caliceal distortion due to the numerous medullary cysts. Progressive pericystic fibrosis of the parenchyma causes decrease of kidney size and increasing azotemia.

Angiographic findings are sometimes characteristic and diagnostic. Although the vascular changes and thinned, poorly vascularized cortex are nonspecific changes of end-stage kidneys, stretching of interlobar and arcuate arteries may be seen if the cysts are large. In small or normal sized kidneys, the appearance of various sized cystic lucencies in the nephrogram, with some cortical tissue seen around the most peripheral cysts, is more specific. A cortical border is seen because the cysts do not involve the outer cortex, in contrast to the lesions of polycystic disease.[127-130]

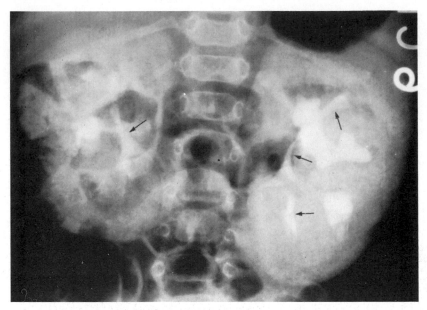

Figure 11–93 **Medullary Cystic Disease in an Infant.** Intravenous pyelogram shows greatly enlarged kidneys with caliceal distortion and stretching *(arrows)* from the multiple cysts, an appearance indistinguishable from that of ordinary polycystic disease.

Progressive azotemia over the following year was treated by bilateral nephrectomy and renal transplantation. (Courtesy Dr. Milton Elkin, New York City, New York.)

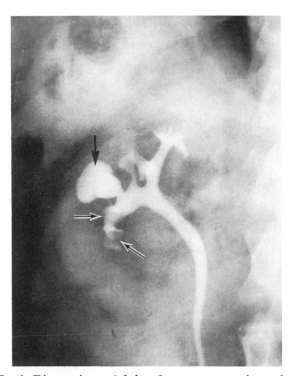

Figure 11–94 **Medullary Cystic Disease in an Adult.** Intravenous pyelography in a 30 year old man with anemia and renal failure showed no function from somewhat small kidneys. A right retrograde pyelogram shows elevation and pressure deformity of the lower calices *(black-white arrows)* and contrast filling of a large medullary cyst *(black arrow).* (Courtesy Dr. H. Grossman, New York City, New York.)

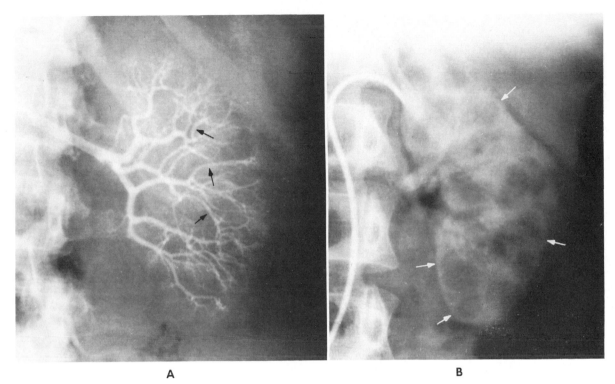

A   B

Figure 11-95 **Medullary Cystic Disease in an Adult with Chronic Renal Failure: Angiograms.**

A, The kidney is smaller than normal, and the interlobar arteries show some stretching and draping *(arrows)*. Tortuosity and tapering are also apparent.

B, The nephrogram discloses numerous cystic lucencies, but the thin cortex *(arrows)* is continuous and uninterrupted, suggesting that the cysts are of subcortical (medullary) origin.

In a younger patient with renal failure, angiographic demonstration of multiple cysts in a small or normal sized kidney is highly suggestive of medullary cystic disease.

Congenital Multicystic Kidney (Unilateral Renal Dysplasia)

This is the most common cystic renal disorder in children, and the most frequent cause of an abdominal mass in the newborn. Since the other kidney is normal, the patient is usually asymptomatic and the enlarged multicystic kidney may not be discovered until adulthood.

The dysplastic kidney is usually quite large, and a palpable mass may be the only clinical finding. On urography, the enlarged kidney may appear lobulated and is almost always nonfunctioning. Rarely, calcification of a cyst is identified. High dose urography in children may opacify the cyst walls. Retrograde studies will reveal an atretic ureter, ending blindly proximally. Often, small pseudosacculations give the ureter a beaded appearance.

Angiography will show an absent or atretic renal artery, with insignificant or disorganized internal vasculature.

Positive radiographic identification of the renal dysplasia by its atretic blind ureter and the angiographic findings can obviate nephrectomy in the adult.[131, 132]

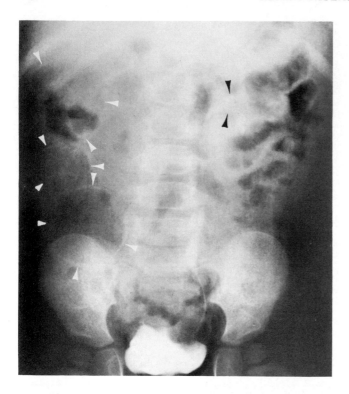

Figure 11–96 **Congenital Multicystic Kidney.** High dose (total body) excretory urography in an asymptomatic infant with a large right-sided abdominal mass shows a normal left renal pelvis and calices *(black arrowheads).*

The right kidney is nonfunctioning, but the walls of three large cysts *(white arrowheads)* have become faintly opacified by the high dose of contrast material. The multicystic kidney is huge. (Courtesy Dr. W. H. McAlister, St. Louis, Missouri.)

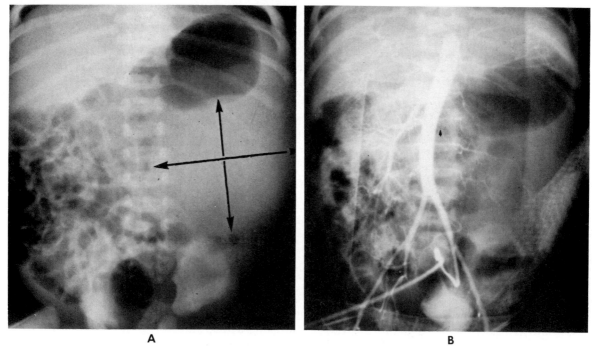

A   B

Figure 11–97 **Congenital Multicystic Kidney.**

A, Intravenous pyelogram in a neonate with an abdominal mass reveals a large mass filling the left flank *(arrows),* with no excretion from this side. The right pyelogram is normal.

B, Aortogram shows a hypoplastic left renal artery *(arrow).* The large mass is displacing the aorta. The ureter at surgery was atretic.

A unilateral nonfunctioning enlarged kidney and a hypoplastic renal artery and ureter are the characteristic triad of congenital multicystic kidney. Urinary findings are generally negative; a palpable asymptomatic mass is usually the only clinical finding.

Medullary Sponge Kidney (Renal Tubular Ectasia)

In this probably congenital disorder there are linear or cystic dilatations of the collecting tubules in the pyramids. Stasis predisposes to calculus formation and pyelonephritis. The ectatic changes may be confined to a single pyramid but are more often widespread and bilateral. Renal function remains unaltered. The condition is asymptomatic and is often uncovered only after one of the medullary calculi becomes dislodged and produces renal colic or hematuria.

Radiographically the kidneys are normal or slightly enlarged and may show collections of small medullary calculi. Urography reveals normal or slightly blunted calices, associated with opacified clusters of linear or oval cavities, extending from the calices into the kidney substance. The cavities are 1 to 6 mm. long. The calculi, if present, lie in clusters within these cavities. Papillary necrosis and caliceal diverticula may sometimes simulate tubular ectasia. Often, the pyramidal tubules of a normal kidney are opacified as a homogeneous smudge, especially if large amounts of contrast material are injected. These tubules should not be considered abnormal unless dilated.

Some cases of medullary sponge kidney are associated with hepatic fibrosis and dilated bile ducts.[133-138]

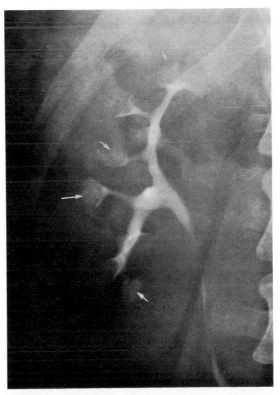

Figure 11–98 **Medullary Sponge Kidney: Intravenous Pyelogram.** The pelvis and calices are clearly outlined, and the kidney is of normal size. Numerous brush-like densities (*arrows*) extending from the calices into the parenchyma represent contrast medium within dilated tubules in the renal pyramids; they are diagnostic of medullary sponge kidney. Both kidneys are always involved.

In cases in which the pyramidal tubules are more dilated, the streaks of contrast medium extending from the calices are wider and coarser and may even appear cyst-like; calcium deposits may develop.

Diagnosis of medullary sponge kidney can almost always be made by intravenous pyelography.

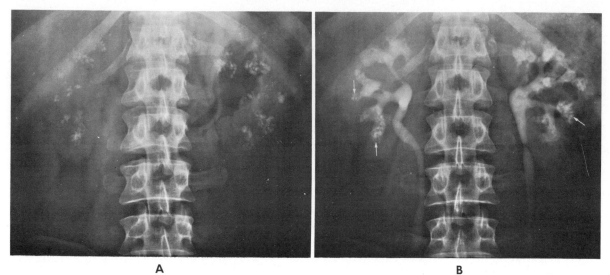

A   B

Figure 11–99 **Medullary Sponge Kidney.**

A, Plain film of the abdomen shows clusters of small calcifications throughout both kidneys.

B, Urogram shows that all calcifications are adjacent to the calices. These contrast-filled areas (*arrows*) are ectatic cystic dilatations of the pyramidal collecting tubules.

TUMORS OF THE KIDNEY

Benign Tumors

The majority of benign tumors of the parenchyma are small, insignificant lesions, incidentally found at autopsy. Clinically significant benign tumors are rare. They include the larger adenomas, hamartomas, and fibromas.

Radiographically the larger benign parenchymal tumors have few distinguishing characteristics. Most often they closely simulate the more common cyst, presenting as a renal mass and producing caliceal displacements and deformity. However, the hamartoma (angiomyolipoma) may contain sufficient fatty tissue to produce characteristic radiolucent shadows. Hamartomas often occur in tuberous sclerosis (see p. 395) as multiple and bilateral lesions, and they may simulate polycystic disease.

Renal adenomas are benign and arise as single or multiple nodules within the renal cortex. As a rule they are small and are found accidentally. Adenomas grow slowly and cause atrophy of the adjacent tissue and bulging of the cortex. Although most often asymptomatic, they occasionally cause hemorrhage and pain. Usually they cause displacement and elongation of the caliceal system indistinguishable from that caused by cysts. Nephrotomography demonstrates a smooth lucent mass without lobulation. If a thick capsular wall can be identified, it may help differentiate the adenoma from a cyst; however, thick-walled cyst-like masses are more likely to represent necrotic carcinoma. Renal angiography will usually distinguish adenoma from cyst. A rare but clinically significant parenchymal tumor is the small juxtaglomerular adenoma that secretes renin and causes hypertension (see p. 695).

The benign tumors of the renal pelvis or calices are usually papillomas or hemangiomas. The papilloma will produce a circumscribed defect in the opacified pelvis and may simulate a nonopaque calculus. Hemangioma of the renal pelvis gives rise to persistent hematuria and produces a filling defect in the opacified renal pelvis that cannot be distinguished from a papillary carcinoma.[74, 139–142]

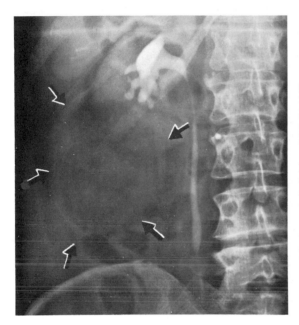

Figure 11–100 **Angiomyolipoma: Intravenous Pyelogram.** There is a large mass in the lower pole of the right kidney *(arrows)*. A rather thick capsule surrounding a more or less homogeneous lucency suggests a fatty mass. The kidney is rotated, and the calices of the lower pole are crowded.

Hamartomas of the kidney (such as angiomyolipoma) are uncommon and are rarely diagnosed preoperatively. There may be signs that suggest a mass compressing and displacing the collecting system, but this is not a specific finding. Fatty tissue may be suggested by defined areas of lucency, which occasionally are large enough to indicate the correct diagnosis. Multiple and bilateral hamartomas occur frequently in tuberous sclerosis.

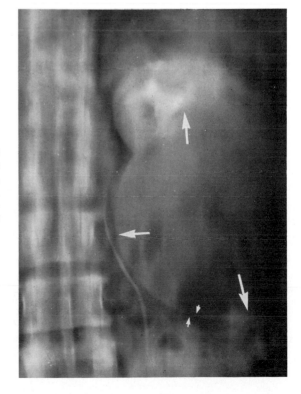

Figure 11–101 **Benign Renal Adenoma: Nephrogram.** There is a nonopacified mass in the lower pole of the left kidney *(large arrows)* whose wall *(small arrows)* is clearly defined and thicker than is generally seen in a simple cyst. Histologic examination disclosed a benign medullary adenoma with areas of hemorrhagic necrosis. (Courtesy Dr. Jack G. Rabinowitz, The Mount Sinai Hospital, New York.)

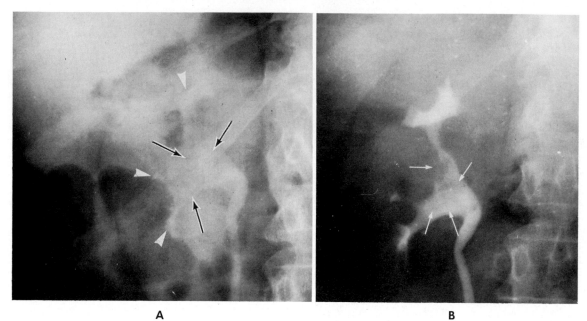

A   B

Figure 11–102 **Hemangioma of Renal Pelvis.**

A, Intravenous urogram of an elderly woman with a history of recurrent painless hematuria reveals a functioning right kidney with normal appearing calices *(arrowheads)* but with poor opacification of the distal infundibula and proximal pelvis *(arrows)*. The left kidney was completely normal.

B, Right retrograde pyelogram reveals an irregular filling defect located in the pelvis and extending into the infundibula *(arrows)*. This was an irregular but benign hemangioma. The roentgen appearance is indistinguishable from that of papillary carcinoma of the renal pelvis.

Malignant Tumors

In the adult, renal cell carcinoma (hypernephroma) is the most common malignant tumor of the kidney; transitional cell carcinoma of the renal collecting system develops much less often. In the child, Wilms' tumor is the most frequent renal tumor.

A small hypernephroma or renal cell carcinoma may produce little or no change on the urogram, and arteriography may be necessary for diagnosis. Large tumors may produce asymmetric enlargement. In about 15 per cent of cases, calcification may be found within the tumor. Metastases occur to the lung, liver, bone, adrenal gland, and lymph nodes.

Urography may show displacement and destruction of the collecting system by the tumor; the calices are often distorted, elongated, and amputated, and a portion of the collecting system may be obliterated. Sometimes the involved kidney may not function during excretory pyelography, which usually indicates invasion of the renal vein.

Renal arteriography may reveal enlargement of the main renal artery and displacement of its branches by the tumor. Within the tumor there are disordered fine tortuous vessels. These contain microaneurysms and small arteriovenous shunts, which cause small areas of puddling or pooling of the contrast medium. Abnormal vessels may be seen in both the arterial and capillary phase.

Early venous filling may occur. The instillation of epinephrine during arteriography permits better localization of tumor vessels and helps visualization of the tumor vein (since epinephrine causes constriction of only the normal vessels). The tumor area may be relatively lucent in the early nephrogram, but in later films persistent tumor stain often renders all or part of the lesion denser than the surrounding tissue. Distinction from a cyst, which is avascular and radiolucent in the nephrographic stage, is usually readily made. In some chronic inflammatory masses, however, there may be a network of fine vessels, a homogeneous blush, and early venous filling, making distinction from neoplasm difficult. An occasional avascular tumor may show no detectable pathologic vessels, but the nephrographic phase shows an irregularly lucent mass, frequently with a thick or irregular wall. Cyst and tumor can coexist in approximately one per cent of cases.

Neoplasms of the pelves and calices are usually epithelial. Because of their location within a pelvis or calix, these lesions lead to early hematuria and are generally discovered when small. On the pyelogram there is usually a slightly irregular filling defect in the calix or pelvis; occasionally the defect may appear smooth and regular. This appearance is simulated by radiolucent calculi and blood clots; calcification of the tumor is rare. Ureteral and bladder metastases are not infrequent consequences. Transitional cell carcinoma usually does not produce marked caliceal distortion.

Wilms' tumor is second only to neuroblastoma as the cause of a malignant abdominal mass in children. The child is usually asymptomatic, and the mass is discovered by accident. Plain films reveal a soft tissue density, usually without calcification, and the urogram generally reveals marked distortion of the collecting system by an intrarenal lesion.

Leukemia and lymphosarcoma may diffusely infiltrate the kidney and simulate polycystic disease, although caliceal destruction may sometimes occur. Generally the width of cortical tissue is markedly increased by the diffuse neoplastic infiltration. Angiography may show stretching of the intrarenal arteries by masses that contain a few clusters of pathologic vessels. The findings are not specific.

Tumors of the ureters are uncommon; most are carcinomas. The lesion radiographically simulates the defect of a calculus. Sometimes, there is dilatation distal to the defect, a more suggestive finding.

Occasionally one or both kidneys are involved by metastatic carcinoma, especially from the breast or lung. The metastatic masses may cause focal or diffuse enlargement of one or both kidneys. Caliceal irregularity and distortion usually occur. Renal function may be reduced.[121, 126, 143–152]

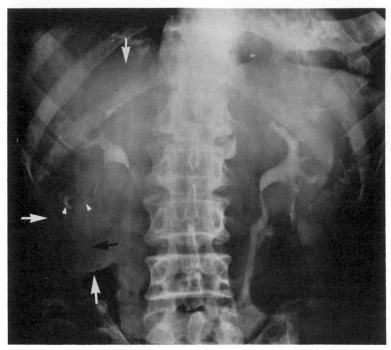

Figure 11–103 **Hypernephroma: Intravenous Urogram.**   The lower pole *(black arrow)* of the enlarged right kidney *(white arrows)* is greatly enlarged, with destruction and distortion of the lower calices *(arrowheads)*. This combination of a mass with distorted and destroyed calices is indicative of a malignant renal neoplasm.

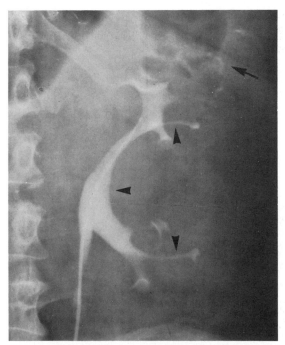

Figure 11–104 **Hypernephroma with Calcification: Intravenous Urogram.**   Amorphous calcification within a mass in the upper pole of the left kidney *(arrow)* has produced little change in the adjacent calices; however, extension of tumor to the middle of the kidney has resulted in elongation and spreading of the calices *(arrowheads)*. Without the calcification, the mass would be indistinguishable from a cyst. Calcification occurs in about 15 per cent of renal tumors. When amorphous, it strongly suggests a malignant neoplasm.

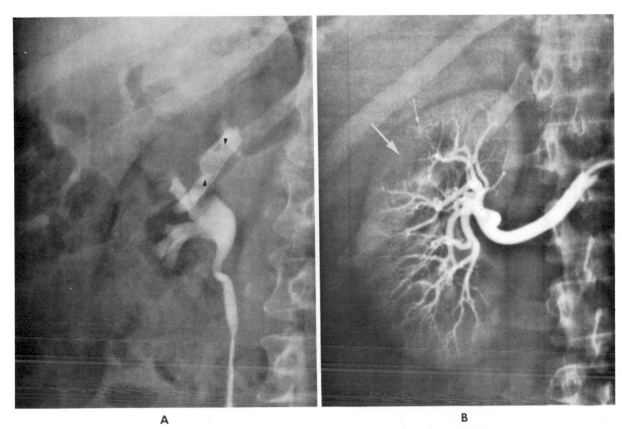

A   B

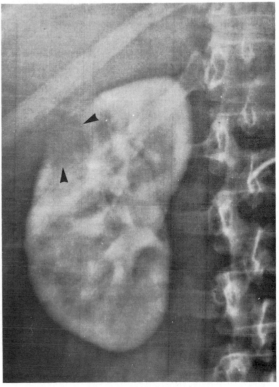

C

Figure 11–105 **Hypernephroma: Retrograde Pyelogram and Selective Renal Arteriogram.**

A, Right retrograde pyelogram demonstrates a filling defect in the superior calix *(arrowheads).* It was caused by blood clots. No clear-cut mass or caliceal displacement was observed. The patient had a history of repeated episodes of hematuria.

B, Selective arteriogram reveals an irregular area in which opacification and vascularity are decreased *(large arrow).* There are abnormally small tortuous vessels with some puddling *(small arrow);* these are characteristic of tumor. In contrast to the abnormal vascularity of a neoplasm, a benign cyst is avascular.

C, A few seconds later the nephrogram discloses a somewhat irregular area in the upper outer cortical region *(arrowheads).* It is not opacified and it corresponded exactly to the tumor found at surgery.

Smaller cortical neoplasms may be undetectable on pyelography yet readily demonstrated on arteriography. The technique also helps distinguish a solid mass from a cystic lesion, the latter having sharp borders, no internal vascular structure, and no tumor stain.

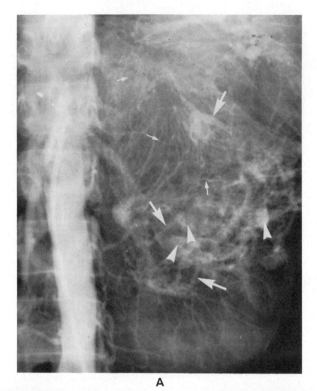

A

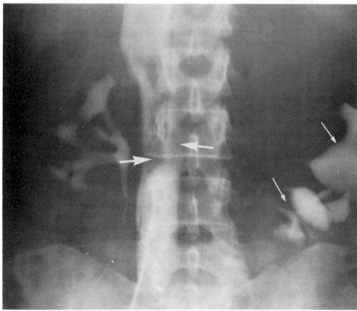

B

Figure 11–106   **Large Hypernephroma: Arteriogram and Vena Cavagram.**

A, Aortogram reveals extensive vascular abnormalities in a huge mass occupying the upper half of the left kidney. The smaller arteries are disorderly and abnormal *(small arrows).* Numerous collections of pooled dye *(arrowheads)* are seen throughout, particularly in the lower half of the mass. Early opacification of veins *(large arrows)* is indicative of multiple arteriovenous shunts.

These vascular changes are characteristic of a malignant tumor.

B, Opacification of the inferior vena cava through a catheter discloses filling defects *(large arrows)* in the vicinity of the kidney tumor. These defects represent extension of tumor masses into the vena cava. The distorted and displaced calices of the left kidney *(small arrows)* are striking.

Demonstration of malignant extension into the vena cava is extremely important for surgical decisions and for prognosis.

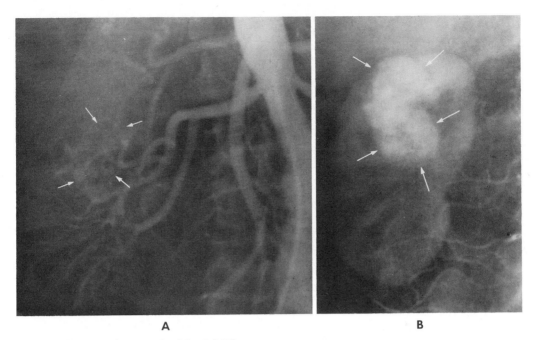

A   B

Figure 11–107 **Hypernephroma: Accidental Discovery.**

A midstream aortogram was performed on this elderly woman because of severe ischemic symptoms in the lower extremities. There were no renal symptoms.

A, Early film during aortography discloses a somewhat rounded, circumscribed collection of abnormal vessels *(within arrows).*

B, Later film discloses intense tumor staining of an irregular mass in the upper half of the kidney *(arrows).* The staining persisted for a considerable period of time. Note the absence of kidney enlargement. Later, pyelography disclosed distortion and compression of the upper calices.

A malignant kidney tumor may show extensive staining and density during arteriography, or may present as a relatively lucent area in the nephrogram. Abnormal vessels are generally seen in either case.

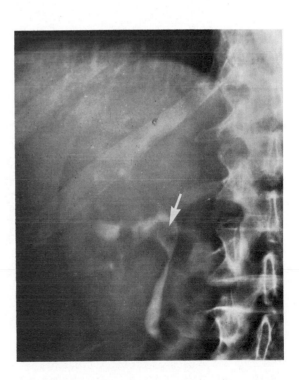

Figure 11–108 **Transitional Cell Carcinoma of Renal Pelvis: Intravenous Pyelogram.** Defect within the right renal pelvis *(arrow)* was a transitional cell carcinoma. The upper pole of the right kidney is hydronephrotic and poorly filled. The middle calix is also dilated.

Because of its location in the pelvis and calices, the carcinoma causes hematuria early in the disease. As a rule it presents as a somewhat irregular intraluminal lucency, which occasionally cannot be differentiated from a blood clot or nonopaque calculi. A small tumor of the renal collecting system may cause hydronephrosis and nonfunctioning of the kidney.

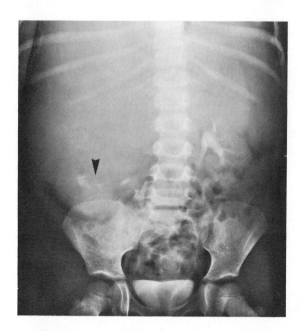

Figure 11–109 **Wilms' Tumor: Intravenous Urogram.** There is a huge mass filling the entire right side and extending into the left side of the abdomen. The calices of the right kidney are depressed, distorted, and partially destroyed *(arrowhead).* In a child these findings are characteristic of a huge Wilms' tumor.

The extension of the mass into the left side has depressed the left kidney.

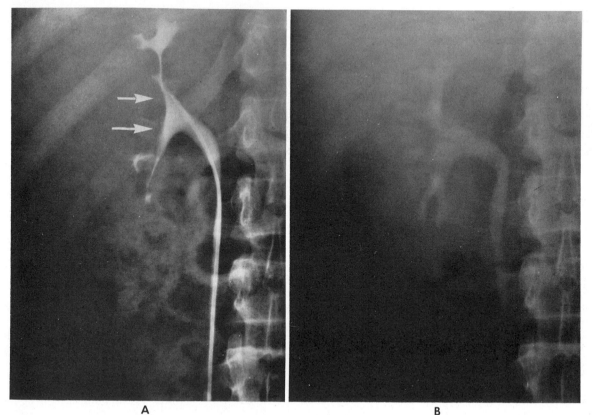

A   B

Figure 11–110 **Intrarenal Hemorrhage Simulating a Tumor.**

The patient was a 35 year old male who developed anemia and flank pain subsequent to receiving anticoagulants.

A, Right retrograde pyelogram shows a mass lesion in the right kidney, with medial displacement and compression of the calices, particularly the middle group *(arrows).* The findings are indistinguishable from those of cyst or tumor.

B, Intravenous urogram done one month later indicates a normal collecting system and a kidney of normal size. The mass was probably intrarenal hemorrhage secondary to anticoagulant therapy. (Courtesy Dr. Arlyne Shockman, Veterans Administration Hospital, Philadelphia, Pennsylvania.)

MISCELLANEOUS RENAL DISORDERS

Renal Arterial Infarction

Characteristic roentgenographic findings follow arterial occlusion of a major or main renal artery. Intravenous pyelography will always show complete nonvisualization of the involved kidney if the main artery has been occluded. In segmental occlusion, the collecting system in the affected portion may be only faintly opacified. Retrograde studies, however, show an anatomically normal collecting system. This combination of a nonfunctioning kidney and a normal retrograde pyelogram is practically specific for recent arterial obstruction of the kidney. Occasionally, similar findings develop after severe radiation nephritis; distinction is readily made by the history.

Occlusion of the renal artery or of one of its major branches can be confirmed by renal arteriography. The actual embolus or thrombus, however, is rarely demonstrated. In segmental infarction there will be a focal area of diminished or absent nephrographic density and a paucity of vessels. Midstream aortography is usually done prior to selective renal opacification, since the latter technique may fail to fill an accessory renal artery, thereby producing a nephrographic defect that simulates an area of infarction.

The totally infarcted kidney usually fails to recover function and may show progressive shrinkage and even eventual parenchymal calcification. Segmentally infarcted kidneys usually recover function, but there may be local shrinkage and caliceal distortion.[153-155]

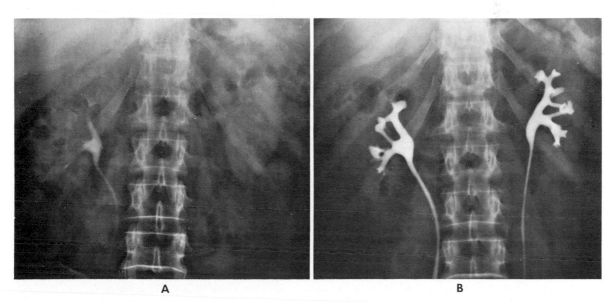

A **B**

Figure 11-111 **Left Renal Infarction.**

A, A 52 year old male experienced sudden left flank pain. Intravenous pyelogram demonstrates that functioning of the left kidney is greatly decreased, while the right kidney is within normal limits.

B, The retrograde pyelogram shows an anatomically normal left kidney. At surgery it was found to be segmentally infarcted.

Decreased or absent functioning associated with an anatomically normal retrograde pyelogram is characteristic of renal arterial infarction. Arteriography is essential for diagnosis.

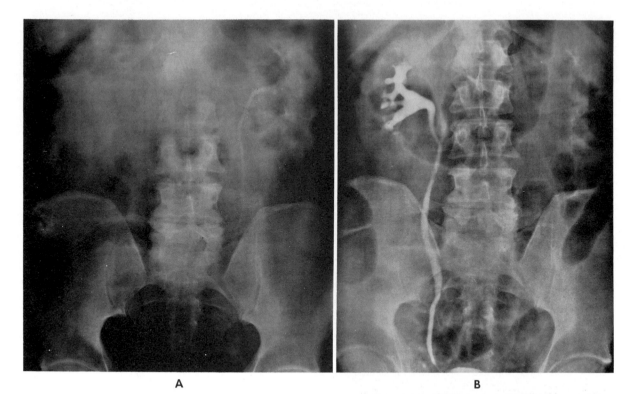

A   B

Figure 11–112   **Right Renal Arterial Occlusion: Diagnostic Pyelographic Findings.**

A, A 50 year old male developed severe right flank pain. Intravenous pyelogram made two days later demonstrates a nonfunctioning right kidney of normal size and shape. The left urinary tract was normal. A ureteral stone was suspected, especially since there was hematuria.

B, Right retrograde pyelogram made the following day reveals a normal right urinary tract. The calices are blunted due to overdistention. Another intravenous pyelogram made two days later again demonstrated a nonfunctioning right kidney.

C, Two months after clinical recovery, an intravenous pyelogram demonstrates that both kidneys are functioning normally.

A nonfunctioning kidney with a normal retrograde pyelogram is practically pathognomonic of renal arterial infarction, and this may be confirmed by demonstrating the arterial block on renal arteriography (renal arteriography was not done in the present case). Severe irradiation nephritis may produce similar pyelographic findings, but the history of radiation facilitates differentiation.

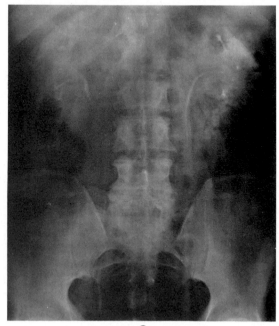

C

In many cases of arterial renal infarction, function in the affected kidney is not restored. Although arteriosclerotic occlusion is the most common cause of acute renal ischemia, emboli, trauma, and vasospastic vascular disease may be responsible.

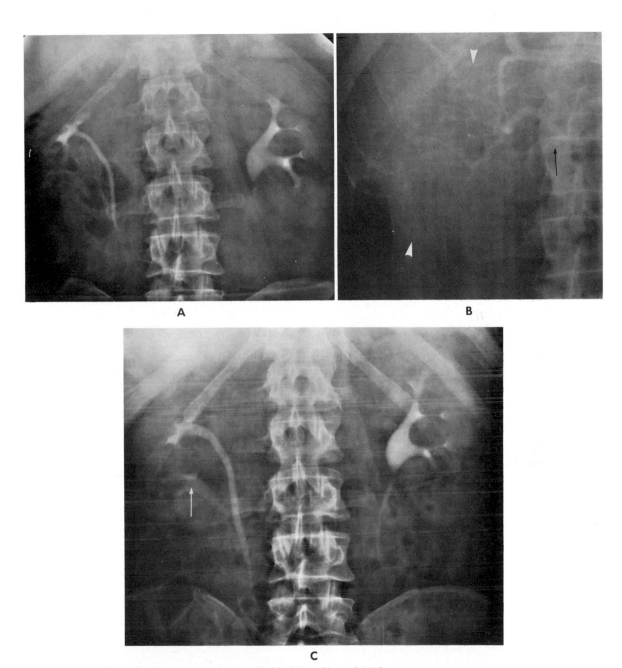

A

B

C

Figure 11–113 **Renal Infarction in Lower Half of Duplicated Kidney.**

A, The patient was a 59 year old male. Intravenous pyelogram made shortly after the onset of acute right flank pain demonstrates nonvisualization of the lower half of the duplicated right kidney. Only the upper portion of the double kidney is opacified. The left kidney is normal. Retrograde pyelogram *(not shown)* revealed a normal double pelvis and calices.

B, Renal arteriogram shows vascular filling of only the renal artery supplying the upper half of the duplicated kidney. The renal outline is shown by the arrowheads. The renal vessel supplying the lower half of the double kidney is completely occluded *(arrow).*

C, Excretory urogram done two months later indicates that the lower half of the duplicated right kidney is now functioning *(arrow).*

A

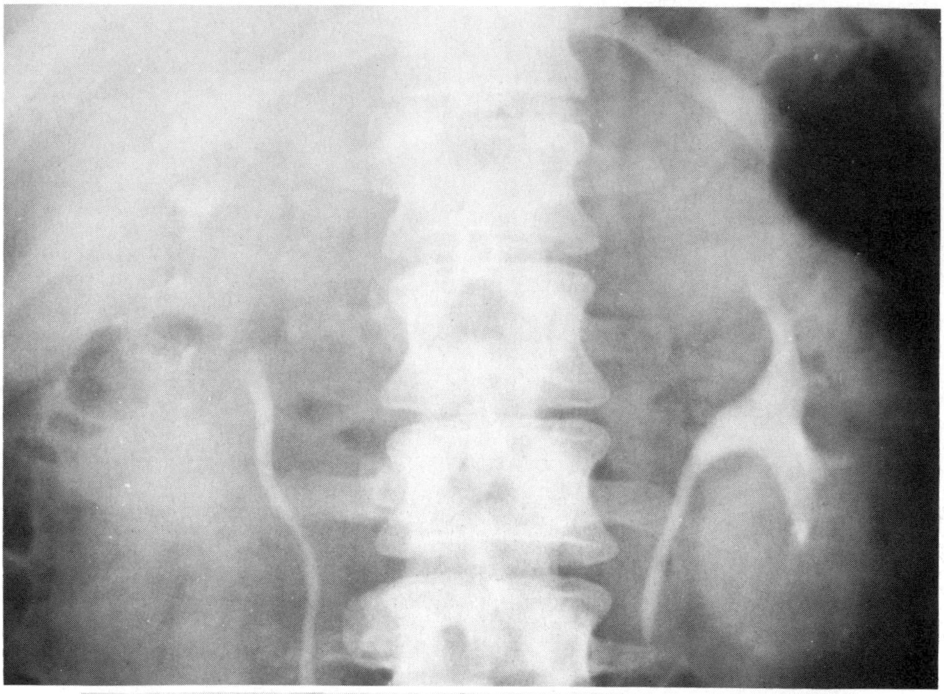

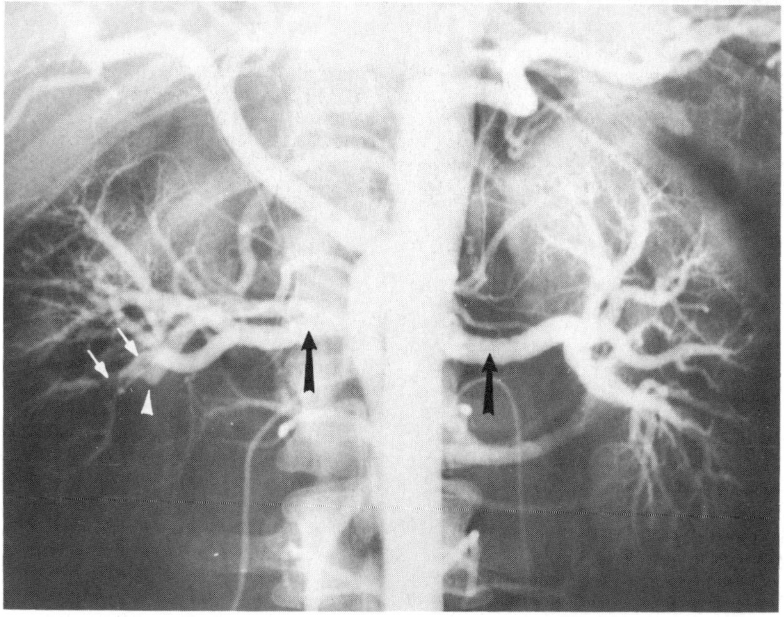

B

Figure 11–114 **Segmental Renal Infarction: Pyelogram and Arteriography.**

A, Excretory pyelogram made after onset of right flank pain and hematuria shows delayed and poor contrast filling of the right kidney, especially the middle and lower calices. The left kidney is normal.

B, Aortogram shows opacification of the main renal arteries on both sides *(black arrows)*, with normal vasculature on the left. The lower half of the right kidney is almost avascular and shows no nephrographic effect. Small lucent thrombi are seen in an interlobar artery *(white arrows)*, and an adjacent artery is abruptly occluded *(arrowhead).*

Pneumaturia

Pneumaturia is the passage of gas in the urine. It may be the result of a fistula, or it may be due to infection with a gas-producing organism. The fistulas may be congenital or acquired and are either vesicovaginal or vesicoenteric. Anaerobic gas-producing agents, such as *Escherichia coli, Aerobacter aerogenes,* or a yeast organism, may occasionally be the cause; they are most frequently found in the diabetic.

In many cases the bladder is partially or completely outlined by gas, and erect views demonstrate an air-fluid level. Fistulous tracts may be demonstrated by contrast cystography or barium studies of the gastrointestinal tract.[156, 157]

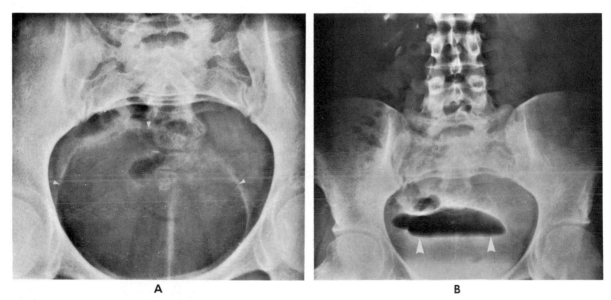

A   B

Figure 11–115 **Pneumaturia.**

A, The bladder is distended with gas. The dense stripe *(arrowheads)* surrounding the bladder represents the bladder wall.

B, Erect view during intravenous pyelography demonstrates an air-fluid level *(arrowheads)* in the contrast-filled bladder.

The patient was a young diabetic female with a severe bladder infection caused by *E. coli.*

Nephroptosis

Nephroptosis is an abnormal downward displacement of one or both kidneys. It is usually found in thin females who have a dearth of perirenal fat or poor tone of the abdominal muscles; it occurs most often on the right side.

An erect pyelographic film will show abnormal descent of the kidney. There is an associated rotation on the anteroposterior axis, placing the upper pole of the kidney more laterally than usual. Rotation on the longitudinal axis may also occur, and this can distort the caliceal appearance. The kidney often shows decreased postural drainage, but true stasis and clinical symptoms are infrequent. Dietl's crisis, which refers to colic in the erect posture from acute kinking of the upper ureter, is a rarity.[158]

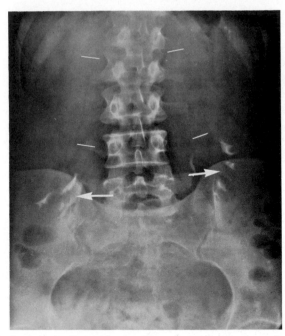

Figure 11–116 **Bilateral Nephroptosis: Intravenous Urogram.** Erect view shows the lower poles of each kidney *(arrows)* well below the iliac crest. With the patient recumbent, the kidneys were situated between the white lines. Downward rotation and angulation of the calices usually occurs in the severely ptotic kidney. No dilatation or obstruction of the collecting system is seen.

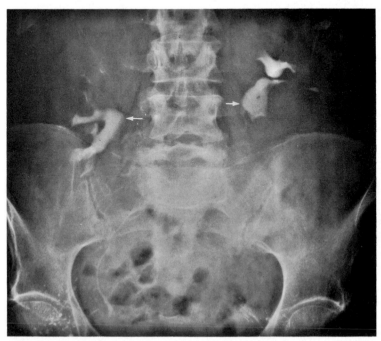

Figure 11–117 **Bilateral Nephroptosis.** In erect view both renal pelves *(arrows)* are seen opposite the body of L5; in the supine view they were at the level of L2. On the erect view, a descent equal to the height of two or more vertebral bodies is considered to be ptosis.

Renal Sinus Lipomatosis

The accumulation of excessive fatty tissue around the pelvicaliceal system occurs most often in obese individuals or in a person whose kidney has lost renal parenchyma as a result of ischemia or infection. In about 20 per cent of cases it may appear without evident cause.

The condition is asymptomatic and without clinical significance. However, on routine excretory urography, the fat deposits may cause pelvicaliceal deformities suggestive of solitary or multiple cysts or tumors, especially if the fat lucencies are ill defined or not well appreciated. Some enlargement of kidney shadows is common, simulating polycystic disease. High dose pyelography, especially with nephrotomography, will permit ready recognition of the lucent fat surrounding the pelvicaliceal system and will suggest the correct diagnosis.[159, 160]

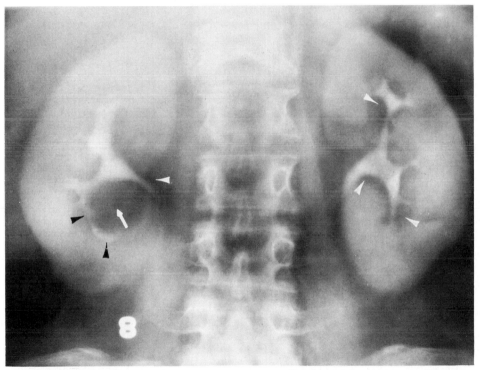

Figure 11–118 **Renal Sinus Lipomatosis.** Tomogram of high dose pyelogram shows unusual amounts of peripelvic and pericaliceal fat lucencies *(white arrowheads)*. A large collection of sinus fat *(arrow)* on the right has displaced the inferior calix and infundibulum *(black arrowheads)*.
On the regular pyelogram, a right peripelvic mass was suspected. The patient had no renal symptoms.

Malacoplakia of the Urinary Tract

In this infrequent condition, which most often affects women, granulomatous plaques or nodules involve the lower ureter and trigone. The entire ureter and bladder may be affected, and rarely the pelvicaliceal system is involved. The ureter becomes dilated, and hydronephrosis often results. Dysuria and occasionally hematuria are the usual symptoms.

Radiographically the involved ureter shows rounded and flat shallow irregularities of the wall with some dilatation. The bladder demonstrates smooth nodular filling defects, up to 2.5 cm. in diameter, suggesting multiple tumors or a bullous cystitis. The ureteral involvement simulates ureteritis cystica and even tuberculous ureteritis, but defects in malacoplakia are not as rounded and discrete as those in ureteritis cystica and rarely produce strictures as in tuberculous ureteritis.[161, 162]

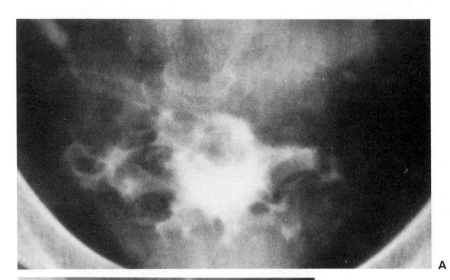

A

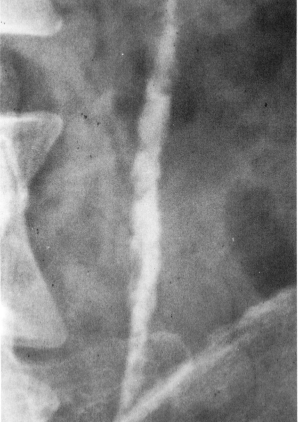

B

Figure 11–119 **Malacoplakia: Two Patients.**

A, The bladder on postvoiding film is deformed by multiple smooth nodular filling defects. The appearance resembles a severe cystitis with greatly swollen edematous mucosa.

B, In another patient, the ureter shows a feathery nodular irregularity. The kidney was hydronephrotic, with caliceal nodular defects. (Courtesy Dr. J. G. Clement, Vancouver, British Columbia, Canada.)

Anomalies of the Genitourinary Tract

A large number of anomalies of size, form, number, position, and structure of the kidneys, ureters, bladder, and urethra are encountered radiologically. Many are rare; most are of no great clinical importance. The more severe anomalies may cause symptoms in infancy or childhood, and are usually recognized and treated early. Anomalies discovered in adults are usually incidental and unimportant.

Anomalies of the Kidney

Unilateral agenesis and *supernumerary kidney* are rare anomalies. *Fetal lobulation* is of no clinical significance but may be mistaken for a renal mass.

A small *hypoplastic kidney* may be a perfect anatomic miniature of a normal kidney, or may show bizarre and distorted calices extending to the renal border. It may be difficult to distinguish the latter from the kidney of atrophic pyelonephritis. On arteriogram, the aortic orifice of the renal artery is small in the hypoplastic kidney but of normal size in the atrophic kidney.

Malrotation of various degrees is commonly seen in one or both kidneys. The calices are more medial, and the pelvis and upper ureter are more lateral, than normal.

In *horseshoe kidneys,* both kidneys are malrotated, and their lower poles are joined either by fibrous tissue or by functioning renal tissue. Urographically, the mass joining the lower poles can be seen extending across the spine. The mass will be opacified if it consists of renal tissue. The pelves and proximal ureters are lateral and anterior to the medial calices. The longitudinal axes are reversed, with the upper poles tilted away from the spine. The joined kidneys maintain a constant spatial relationship to each other in all postures. A complicating obstructive uropathy may result from compression of the abnormally located upper ureters.

An *ectopic kidney* is most often small and is usually located in the pelvis. Although the kidney generally functions, the contrast material may be faint or obscured by bone or fecal contents. Careful search for ectopic kidney should be made if only one kidney is seen on urography, or if there is a clinically palpable pelvic mass. *Crossed ectopia,* a condition in which an ectopic kidney lies on the same side as the normal kidney, can sometimes occur.[158, 163, 164]

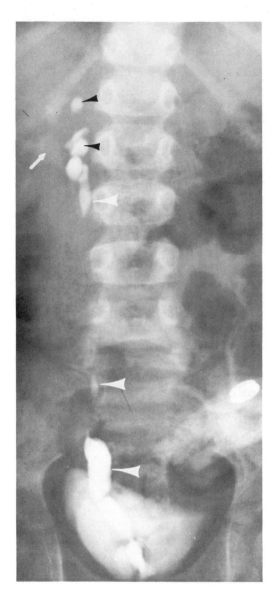

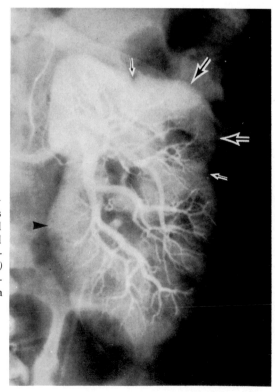

Figure 11–120 **Supernumerary (Third) Kidney.** Intravenous pyelogram of a child with recurrent urinary infections showed normal kidneys bilaterally.

Cystogram performed immediately afterward reveals a third ureter *(white arrowheads)* and blunted calices of a third kidney *(black arrowheads)* lying medial to the still faintly opacified *(arrow)* normal right kidney.

Chronic pyelonephritis of this supernumerary kidney was causing the urinary problem.

Figure 11–121 **Fetal Lobulation: Angiogram.** Nephrographic opacification during arteriography discloses a large lateral bulge *(large arrows)* and a smaller medial bulge *(arrowhead)*. These areas contain no abnormal vessels and exhibit a regular nephrographic density, characteristic of fetal lobules. The indentations *(small arrows)* resemble cortical scars. Without arteriographic clarification, a fetal lobule often cannot be distinguished from a cyst or tumor.

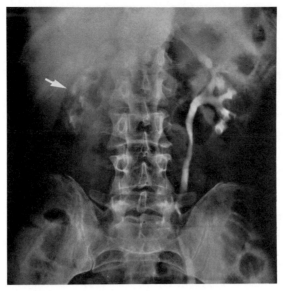

Figure 11–122 **Congenital Hypoplastic Kidney.** Intravenous urogram in a 55 year old hypertensive patient demonstrates a functioning hypoplastic right kidney *(arrow)*. The cortex is thin, and the calices are clubbed and irregular. This very small kidney is more nearly vertical than the normal one, and it is closer to the spine, characteristic of congenital hypoplasia.

There are two distinct types of congenital hypoplastic kidney: One type has a bizarre caliceal architecture extending to the periphery, as in the present example. Intercurrent pyelonephritis is difficult to evaluate in this type. The second type has small but otherwise normal calices, pelvis, and ureter, and appears to be well proportioned although miniature.

Congenital hypoplasia is associated with hypertension in about half the cases. Renal function may be normal, diminished, or absent. On the arteriogram the kidney appears small but with normal vessels. Differentiation of a congenital hypoplastic kidney from the small kidney that is seen in renal artery insufficiency or chronic pyelonephritis is difficult by means of urography alone. The size of the renal artery orifice at its origin may be a distinguishing feature (see Fig. 11–49).

Figure 11–123 **Malrotation and Chronic Pyelonephritis.** Intravenous pyelogram in a 34 year old hypertensive male reveals a malrotated left kidney, with the calices rotated anteriorly and medially. Intercurrent pyelonephritis is responsible for caliceal blunting and cortical thinning. The right kidney is low and also malrotated. The upper calices are also dilated from pyelonephritis. The lower caliceal system appears normal. In a malrotated kidney the calices are generally more medial than normal, and the pelvis and ureter are more lateral. Malrotation may be unilateral or bilateral.

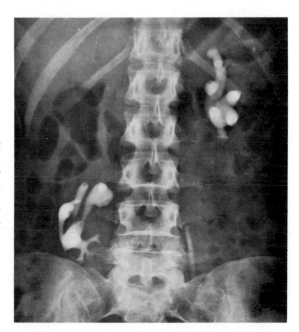

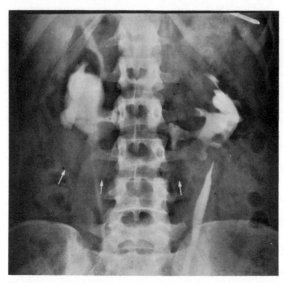

Figure 11–124 **Horseshoe Kidney.** The patient was a 25 year old woman. Intravenous pyelogram discloses the characteristic medial location of the calices; the pelves and ureters are more lateral. The kidneys are closer to the midline than normal. The lower poles are closer to each other than are the upper poles, which is the reverse of normal.

The lower poles are connected by functioning renal tissue or by a fibrous mass or band; in the case illustrated, the poles are connected by functioning renal tissue *(white arrows)*, which increases in density during pyelography.

The ureters arise laterally and anteriorly, and this abnormal course frequently leads to obstructive uropathy and subsequent pyelonephritis.

The horseshoe kidney is always rotated, so that the relationships of the pelvis, calices, and ureter are changed. The degree of rotation varies. When the connecting band between the two lower poles cannot be visualized, it may be difficult to distinguish between horseshoe kidney and bilateral malrotated kidneys. If the kidneys retain an identical spatial relationship in erect and recumbent views, one can assume that they are connected.

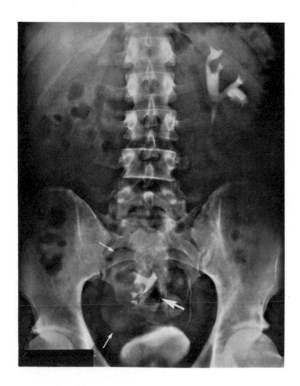

Figure 11–125 **Ectopic Kidney: Intravenous Pyelogram.** The left kidney appears normal. The right kidney *(small arrows)* is in the pelvis overlying the sacrum and has a more or less normal collecting system. The ureter *(large arrow)* is extremely short. An intravenous pyelogram should be performed on every patient who has a pelvic mass, both to assess the effect of the mass on the ureters and to rule out an ectopic pelvic kidney.

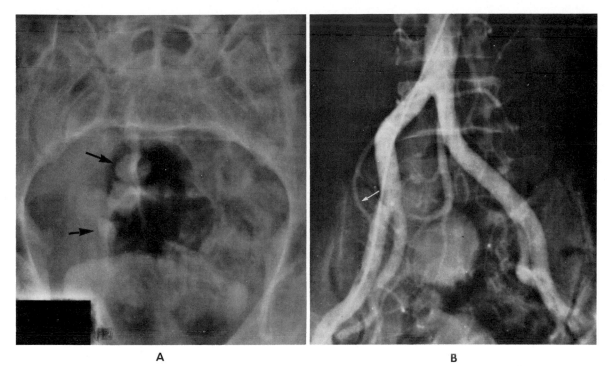

A   **B**

Figure 11–126 **Ectopic Kidney: Aortogram.**

A, Intravenous pyelogram discloses opacification in an ectopic right kidney overlying the sacrum *(arrows).* The calices are dilated due to chronic pyelonephritis, which is a frequent complication.

B, Aortogram demonstrates an anomalous arterial supply *(arrow)* to the ectopic kidney.

Every case of an obscure pelvic mass should be studied preoperatively by intravenous pyelography to avoid resecting a normally functioning pelvic kidney. If one kidney is not visualized, a careful search should be made for a pelvic kidney. Kidneys in abnormal positions are frequently difficult to visualize even by intravenous pyelography, since they are partially obscured by overlying bowel gas and bone shadows and since their functioning is often impaired.

Figure 11–127 **Crossed Ectopia: Retrograde Pyelogram.** Both kidneys are on the left side. The upper kidney is rotated along its longitudinal axis, so that the renal pelvis drains laterally instead of medially. The right kidney *(arrow)* is located in the left abdomen just above the sacrum. The collecting system is dilated because of infection and inadequate drainage—a frequent complication of ectopia. The ureter of the ectopic kidney crosses the midline and inserts in a normal location within the bladder.

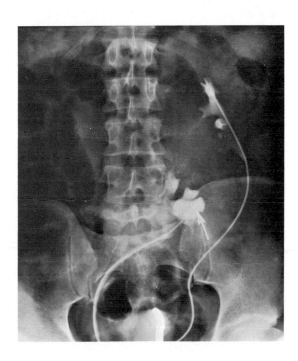

Anomalies of the Renal Pelvis and the Ureter

Duplication can vary from a simple bifid pelvis to a complete double pelvis, ureter, and ureteropelvic orifice. Some degree of duplication is seen in about 4 per cent of urograms. Obstructive hydronephrosis of one of the double collecting systems can simulate a mass lesion of one pole of the kidney.

Congenital strictures can cause hydronephrosis. The ureteropelvic junction is the most common site of structure.

Retrocaval ureter occurs only on the right side. The upper ureter has an abnormal medial and posterior curve around the vena cava, and it may become partially obstructed. Diagnosis is corroborated by a simultaneous cavagram and urogram.

Ureterocele is a cystic dilatation of the lower end of a ureter. It is either congenital or acquired. Urographically, this dilated segment may appear as a round or oval lucent shadow in the bladder density; or, if opacified, it is surrounded by a lucent zone (the ureteral wall), producing the characteristic cobra-head appearance.

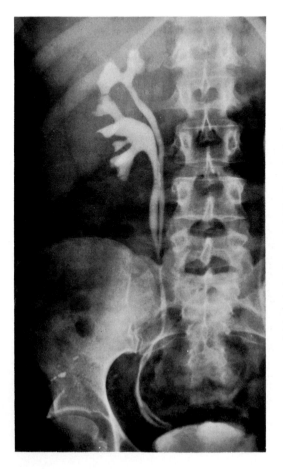

Figure 11–128 **Double Kidney: Intravenous Urogram.** There is complete duplication of the right urinary tract, with a double pelvis and complete double ureter to the bladder. Note the close resemblance of the collecting system of the lower kidney to the architecture of a single normal kidney. Characteristically, the upper collecting system has only one major calix, and if this system fails to opacify, the large superior pole can readily be mistaken for a mass.

Duplication of the urinary tract can be unilateral or bilateral and can vary from a mere bifid pelvis to a double tract. If there are two complete ureters, the ureter from the upper kidney characteristically enters the bladder below the normally situated ureter from the lower kidney. Duplicated ureters, however, often join well above the bladder to form a single lower ureter.

Figure 11–129 **Ureteropelvic Narrowing: Intravenous Pyelogram.** An enlarged film of the right kidney reveals tapering of the renal pelvis at the ureteropelvic junction *(arrow)* associated with infundibular and caliceal dilatation of the upper pole. The kidney drained poorly even when the subject was erect. The patient had right flank discomfort.

Although ureteropelvic narrowing may be an isolated asymptomatic finding, it can cause variable degrees of obstructive uropathy in which pelvic calculi and infection often develop. Drainage is usually delayed on erect view. As a rule the obstruction is due to a congenital narrowing, but it may also result from an aberrant vessel or fibrous band crossing the ureteropelvic junction. Rare causes include valves, abnormalities of nervous innervation affecting peristalsis, and acquired or congenital hypertrophy of the ureteral wall. A large extrarenal pelvis may simulate dilatation caused by ureteropelvic narrowing, but there is normal emptying of an extrarenal pelvis in erect views.

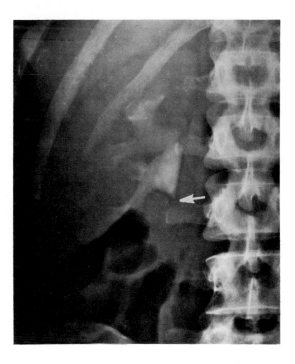

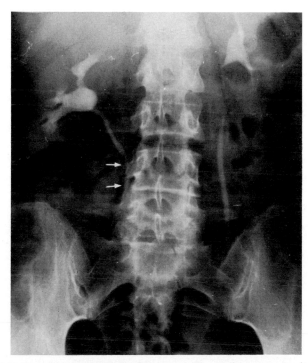

Figure 11–130 **Retrocaval Ureter: Intravenous Pyelogram.** The right ureter is displaced medially *(arrows)* at the level of the upper border of L4. Note the normal course of the left ureter. The lower pole of the right kidney is abnormally lateral, a developmental anomaly.

A retrocaval ureter may sometimes show a sharp upward course at its point of deviation, as it swings up and behind the vena cava. Obstructive hydronephrosis may ensue.

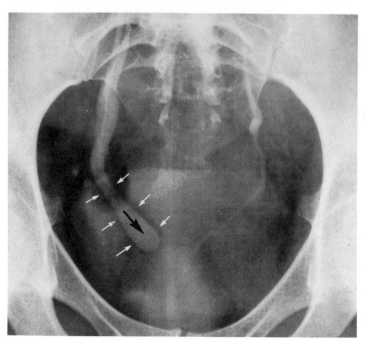

Figure 11–131 **Ureterocele.** The intravesical portion of the right ureter has a characteristic cobra-head dilatation *(black arrow)*. The contrast material is surrounded by a lucent layer *(white arrows)*, which is the wall of the ureterocele.

There is a double right kidney and ureter on the right; the ureter is dilated proximal to the ureterocele (compare with left ureter).

Anomalies of the Bladder and Urethra

A *persistent urachus* is identified on retrograde cystogram as a contrast-filled cyst-like blind pouch extending from the upper bladder in the direction of the umbilicus. Discovery of this anomaly is usually accidental.

In *exstrophy* of the bladder, there is characteristic separation of the pubic bones.

Other anomalies include *duplication* of the bladder and urethra, midline *müllerian duct cyst,* unilateral *cyst of the seminal vesicle, urethral diverticula, stricture,* and persistent *posterior urethral valve* (see Fig. 11–72).

Anomalies of the Renal Arteries

Anomalies of the renal arteries include congenital stricture and aneurysm, although often these are secondary to arterial disease. Fibromuscular hyperplasia of the renal arteries is a developmental and possibly familial disorder occurring most often in females. (See *Renovascular Hypertension*, p. 686.)

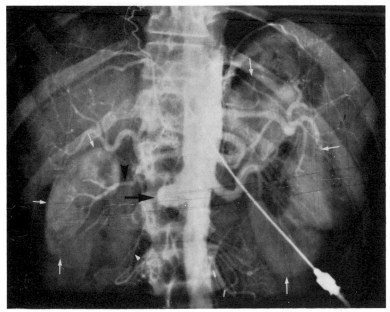

Figure 11–132 **Renal Artery Aneurysm.** Translumbar aortogram in a 36 year old hypertensive male demonstrates two renal arteries supplying the right kidney. The upper renal artery *(black arrowhead)* is patent; the lower one is obstructed by an aneurysm *(black arrow)*. The right kidney is much smaller than the normal left kidney *(white arrows)*. There are collateral vessels to the lower portion of the right kidney *(white arrowhead)*; on pyelography this may produce notching of the upper ureter and pelvis. (Courtesy Dr. Arlyne Shockman, Veterans Administration Hospital, Philadelphia, Pennsylvania.)

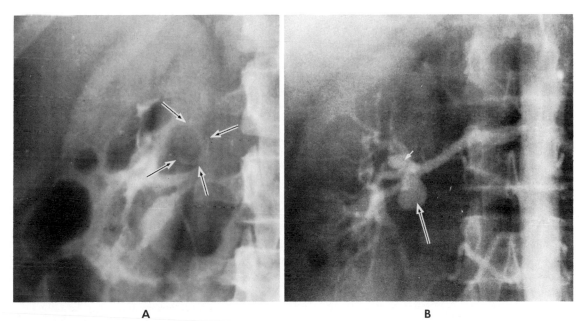

A   B

Figure 11–133 **Calcified Renal Artery Aneurysm.**

A, A faint ring calcification *(arrows)* is seen medial to the right renal pelvis. The right kidney is of normal size, and its collecting system is normal. The location and appearance of the calcification is characteristic of a renal artery aneurysm.

B, During aortography the aneurysm is opacified *(black-white arrow),* and a second aneurysm *(white arrow)* is seen arising from the same segment of the renal artery. The aorta and its branches showed no atherosclerotic changes.

Only a minority of renal artery aneurysms develop visible wall calcification.

REFERENCES

1. Meschan, I.: Background physiology of the urinary tract for the radiologist. Radiol. Clin. North Am., 3:13, 1965.
2. Leinbach, L. B.: The utilization of the intravenous pyelogram in a study of renal function. Radiol. Clin. North Am., 3:41, 1965.
3. Hoffman, W. W., and Grayhack, J. T.: The limitations of the intravenous pyelogram as a test of renal function. Surg. Gynecol. Obstet., 110:503, 1960.
4. Schreiber, M. H., et al.: The pyelogram-urea washout test: its value in the diagnosis of renovascular hypertension. N. Engl. J. Med., 270:1223, 1964.
5. Korobkin, M. T., and Kirkwood, R.: Nephrogram of hypotension. Radiology, 98:129, 1971.
6. Schwartz, W. B., Hurwit, A., and Ettinger, A.: Intravenous urography in the patient with renal insufficiency. N. Engl. J. Med., 269:277, 1963.
7. MacEwan, D. W., Dunbar, J. S., and Nogrady, M. B.: Intravenous pyelography in children with renal insufficiency. Radiology, 78:893, 1962.
8. Weiner, S. N., Vertes, V., and Shapiro, H.: The upper gastrointestinal tract in patients undergoing chronic dialysis. Radiology, 92:110, 1969.
9. Friedenberg, M. J., Eisen, S., and Kissane, J.: Renal angiography in pyelonephritis, glomerulonephritis, and arteriolar nephrosclerosis. Am. J. Roentgenol. Radium Ther. Nucl. Med., 95:349, 1965.
10. Bosniak, N. A., and Schweizer, R. D.: Urographic findings in patients with renal failure. Radiol. Clin. North Am., 10:433, 1972.
11. Halpern, M.: Angiography in chronic renal disease and renal failure. Radiol. Clin. North Am., 10:467, 1972.
12. Braband, H.: Metaphyseal and epiphyseal changes due to disturbances of kidney function. Fortschr. Roentgenstr., 94:693, 1961.
13. Valvassori, G. E., and Pierce, R. H.: Osteosclerosis in chronic uremia. Radiology, 82:385, 1964.
14. Zimmerman, H. B.: Osteosclerosis in chronic renal disease. Am. J. Roentgenol. Radium Ther. Nucl. Med., 88:1152, 1962.
15. Powell, R. C., and Deiss, W. P., Jr.: Symptomatic osteomalacia secondary to clinically occult causes. Ann. Intern. Med., 54:1280, 1961.
16. Craven, J. D.: Renal glomerular osteodystrophy. Clin. Radiol., 15:210, 1964.
17. Valvassori, G. E., and Pierce, R. H.: Osteosclerosis in chronic uremia. Radiology, 82:385, 1964.
18. Kirkwood, J. R., Ozonoff, M. D., and Steinbach, H. L.: Epiphyseal displacement after metaphyseal fracture and renal osteodystrophy. Am. J. Roentgenol. Radium Ther. Nucl. Med., 115:547, 1972.
19. Meena, H. E., Rabinovich, S., et al.: Improved radiographic diagnosis of azotemic osteodystrophy. Radiology, 102:1, 1972.
20. Calenoff, L., and Norfray, J.: Am. J. Roentgenol. Radium Ther. Nucl. Med., 118:283, 1973.
21. Resnick, D. L.: Erosive arthritis of hand and wrist in hyperparathyroidism. Radiology, 110:263, 1974.
22. Shapiro, R.: Radiologic aspects of renal osteodystrophy. Radiol. Clin. North Am., 10:557, 1972.
23. Agus, Z. S., and Goldberg, M.: Pathogenesis of uremic osteodystrophy. Radiol. Clin. North Am., 10:545, 1972.
24. Teplick, J. G., Eftekhari, F., and Haskin, M. E.: Erosions of the sternal ends of the clavicles: A new sign of primary and secondary hyperparathyroidism. Radiology, 113:323, 1974.
25. Nemir, R. L., and Beranbaum, S. L.: Pulmonary edema occurring during course of renal azotemia: its differential radiologic diagnosis. J. Dis. Child., 95:516, 1959.
26. Emmrich, J., Quellhorst, E., and Scheler, F.: Fluid-retention lung in course of renal diseases. Röntgenblätter, 20:357, 1967.
27. Schwartz, E. E., and Onesti, G.: The cardiopulmonary manifestations of uremia and renal transplantation. Radiol. Clin. North Am., 10:569, 1972.
28. Mootz, J. R., Sagel, S. S., and Roberts, T. H.: Roentgenographic manifestations of pulmonary calcifications. Radiology, 107:55, 1973.
29. Singh, S., et al.: Pericardiectomy in uremia. J.A.M.A., 228:1132, 1974.
30. Moëll, H.: Kidney size and its deviation from normal in acute renal failure. A roentgen diagnostic study. Acta Radiol. (supplement): 206, 1961.
31. Hollenberg, N. K., Adams, D. F., et al.: Acute renal failure due to nephrotoxins. N. Engl. J. Med., 282:1329, 1970.
32. Korobkin, M., Kirkwood, R., and Minagi, H.: The nephrogram of hypotension. Radiology, 98:129, 1969.
33. Korobkin, M.: The nephrogram of hemorrhagic hypotension. Am. J. Roentgenol. Radium Ther. Nucl. Med., 114:673, 1972.
34. Whelan, J. G.: Antemortem roentgen manifestations of bilateral renal cortical necrosis. Radiology, 89:682, 1967.
35. Palmer, F. J.: Renal cortical calcification. Clin. Radiol., 21:175, 1970.
36. Samuel, E.: Radiology in the diagnosis of renal rejection. Clin. Radiol., 21:109, 1970.
37. Kaftori, J. K., Munk, J., et al.: The pyelographic appearance of the transplanted cadaver kidney. Clin. Radiol., 21:119, 1970.

38. Rosenberger, A., Munk, J., et al.: Angiographic signs of rejection in cadaver kidney transplants. Clin. Radiol., *21*:135, 1970.
39. Fletcher, E. W. L., Lecky, J. W., and Gonick, H. C.: Selective phlebography of transplanted kidneys. Clin. Radiol., *21*:144, 1970.
40. Goodman, N., Daves, M. L., and Rifkind, D.: Pulmonary roentgen findings following renal transplantation. Radiology, *89*:621, 1967.
41. Navani, S., Christos, A., et al.: Renal homotransplantation: spectrum of angiographic findings of the kidney. Am. J. Roentgenol. Radium Ther. Nucl. Med., *113*:433, 1971.
42. White, R. I., Najarian, J., et al.: Arteriovenous complications associated with renal transplantation. Radiology, *102*:29, 1973.
43. Lewicki, A. M., Saito, S., and Merrill, J. P.: Gastrointestinal bleeding in renal transplant patients. Radiology, *102*:533, 1972.
44. Pierce, J. C., Madge, G. E., et al.: Lymphoma – a complication of renal allotransplantation in man. J.A.M.A., *219*:1593, 1972.
45. Gedgaudas, E., White, R. I., and Loken, M. K.: Radiology in renal transplantation. Radiol. Clin. North Am., *10*:529, 1972.
46. Mott, C., and Schreiber, M. H.:Lymphoceles following renal transplantation. Am. J. Roentgenol. Radium Ther. Nucl. Med., *122*:821, 1975.
47. Price, J. E., and Rigler, L. G.: Widening of the mediastinum resulting from fat accumulation. Radiology, *96*:497, 1970.
48. Berlyne, G. M., Lee, H. A., et al.: Pulmonary complications of peritoneal dialysis. Lancet, *2*:75, 1966.
49. Sinclair, D. J.: Radiological management of renal shunts. Clin. Radiol., *19*:287, 1968.
50. Moskowitz, H., et al.: Angiographic study of the arteriovenous shunt in hemodialysis patients. Am. J. Roentgenol. Radium Ther. Nucl. Med., *93*:72, 1969.
51. Schwartz, C., and Teplick, J. G.: Radiologic consideration in maintenance dialysis. Radiol. Clin. North Am., *10*:511, 1972.
52. Mirahmandi, K. S., Coburn, J. W., and Bluestone, R.: Calcific periarthritis and hemodialysis. J.A.M.A., *223*:548, 1973.
53. Ritchie, W. G. M., and Davison, A. M.: Dural calcification: a complication of prolonged periodic hemodialysis. Clin. Radiol., *25*:349, 1974.
54. Leonard, A., and Shapiro, F. L.: Subdural hematoma in regularly hemodialyzed patients. Ann. Intern. Med., *82*:650, 1975.
55. Holzel, A., and Fawcett, J.: Pulmonary changes in acute glomerulonephritis in childhood. J. Pediatr., *57*:695, 1960.
56. Caffey, J.: Cardiac dilatation in nephritis. In *Pediatric X-ray Diagnosis,* 6th ed. Chicago, Year Book Medical Publishers, Inc., 1972.
57. Foster, R. D., Shuford, W. H., and Weens, H. S.: Selective renal arteriography in medical diseases of the kidney. Am. J. Roentgenol. Radium Ther. Nucl. Med., *95*:291, 1965.
58. Esposito, W. J.: Specific nephrocalcinosis of chronic glomerulonephritis. Am. J. Roentgenol. Radium Ther. Nucl. Med., *101*:688, 1967.
59. Kirkpatrick, J. A., and Fleisher, D. S.: Roentgen appearance of the chest in acute glomerulonephritis in children. J. Pediatr., *64*:492, 1964.
60. Gill, W. M., Jr., and Pudvan, W. R.: The arteriographic diagnosis of renal parenchymal diseases. Radiology, *96*:81, 1970.
61. Mena, E., Bookstein, J. J., and Gikas, P. W.: Angiographic diagnosis of renal parenchymal disease. Radiology, *108*:523, 1973.
62. MacPherson, R. I., and Banerjee, A. K.: Acute glomerulonephritis; a chest film diagnosis? J. Can. Assoc. Radiol., *25*:58, 1974.
63. Brannun, H. M., McCaughey, W. T. E., and Good, C. A.: The roentgen appearance of pulmonary hemorrhage associated with glomerulonephritis. Am. J. Roentgenol. Radium Ther. Nucl. Med., *90*:83, 1963.
64. Wilde, W. T.: Goodpasture syndrome. Am. Rev. Resp. Dis., *94*:773, 1966.
65. Beirne, G. C.: Goodpasture's syndrome and exposure to solvents. (Editorial.) J.A.M.A., *222*:1555, 1972.
66. Purriel, P., Drets, M., et al.: Familial hereditary nephropathy (Alport's syndrome). Am. J. Med. *49*:753, 1970.
67. Chuang, V. P., and Reuter, S. R.: Angiographic features of Alport's syndrome. Am. J. Roentgenol. Radium Ther. Nucl. Med., *121*:539, 1974.
68. Scanlon, G. T.: The radiographic changes in renal vein thrombosis. Radiology, *80*:208, 1963.
69. Janower, M. L.: Nephrotic syndrome secondary to renal vein thrombosis. The value of inferior venography. Am. J. Roentgenol. Radium Ther. Nucl. Med., *95*:330, 1965.
70. Dunbar, J. S., and Favieau, M.: Infrapulmonary pleural effusion with particular reference to its occurrence in nephrosis. J. Can. Assoc. Radiol., *10*:24, 1959.
71. Wagner, G. P., et al.: Renal vein thrombosis; a roentgenologic diagnosis. J.A.M.A., *209*:1661, 1969.
72. Gyepes, M. T., et al.: Epinephrine-assisted renal venography in renal vein thrombosis. Radiology, *93*:793, 1969.
73. Robinson, T., and Rabinowitz, J. G.: The nephrotic syndrome. Radiol. Clin. North Am., *10*:495, 1972.

74. Emmett, J. L., and Witten, D. M.: *Clinical Urography,* 3rd ed. Philadelphia, W. B. Saunders Company, 1971, Vol. II.
75. Harrow, B. R., Sloane, J. A., and Salhanick, L.: Etiology of the hydronephrosis of pregnancy. Surg. Gynecol. Obstet., *119*:1042, 1964.
76. Dure-Smith, P.: Pregnancy dilatation of the urinary tract. Radiology, *96*:545, 1970.
77. Bücker, J., and Sildiroglu, A. I.: Ureteral obstruction due to ovarian vein following pregnancy. Fortschr. Roentgenstr., *116*:357, 1972.
78. Dejdar, R.: Roentgen findings in chronic pyelonephritis. Fortschr. Roentgenstr., *90*:196, 1959.
79. Kimmelstiel, P., Kim, O. J., Beres, J. A., and Willmann, K.: Chronic pyelonephritis. Am. J. Med., *30*:589, 1961.
80. Leadbetter, G. W., Jr., Duxbury, J. H., and Dreyfuss, J. R.: Absence of vesicoureteral reflux in normal adult males. J. Urol., *84*:69, 1960.
81. Gross, K. E., and Sanderson, S. S.: Cineurethrography and voiding cinecystography with special attention to vesicoureteral reflux. Radiology, *77*:573, 1961.
82. Garrett, R. A., Rhamy, R. K., and Carr, J. R.: Non-obstructive vesico-ureteral regurgitation. J. Urol., *87*:350, 1962.
83. Friedenberg, M. J., Eisen, S., and Kissane, J.: Renal angiography in pyelonephritis, glomerulonephritis and arteriolar nephrosclerosis. Am. J. Roentgenol. Radium Ther. Nucl. Med., *95*:349, 1965.
84. Hodson, C. J.: The radiological contribution toward the diagnosis of chronic pyelonephritis. Radiology, *88*:857, 1967.
85. Bliznak, J., and Ramsey, J.: Emphysematous pyelonephritis. Clin. Radiol., *23*:61, 1972.
86. Schmidt, J. D., Hawtrey, C. E., et al.: Vesicoureteral reflux. J.A.M.A., *220*:821, 1972.
87. Malek, R. S., Green, L. F., et al.: Xanthogranulomatous pyelonephritis. J. Urol., *44*:296, 1972.
88. Palubinskas, A. J.: Xanthogranulomatous pyelonephritis. Semin. Roentgenol., *6*:331, 1971.
89. Beachley, M. C., Ranninger, D., and Roth, F. J.: Xanthogranulomatous pyelonephritis. Am. J. Roentgenol. Radium Ther. Nucl. Med., *121*:500, 1974.
90. Rabinowitz, J. G., Kinkhabwala, M. N., et al.: Acute renal carbuncle. Am. J. Roentgenol. Radium Ther. Nucl. Med., *116*:740, 1972.
91. Evans, J. A., Meyers, M. A., and Bosniak, M. A.: Acute renal and perirenal infection. Semin. Roentgenol., *6*:274, 1971.
92. Caplan, L. H., Siegelman, S. S., and Bosniak, M. A.: Angiography in inflammatory space-occupying lesions of the kidney. Radiology, *88*:14, 1967.
93. Salmon, R. B., and Koehler, P. R.: Angiography in renal and perirenal inflammatory masses. Radiology, *88*:99, 1967.
94. Caro, G., Meissell, R., and Held, B.: Epinephrine-enhanced arteriography in renal and perirenal abscess. Radiology, *92*:1262, 1969.
95. Pancet, M. V.: Nephrocalcinosis: a clinicoradiologic study. Rev. Cubana Pediatr., *31*:255, 1959.
96. Kreel, L.: Radiological aspects of nephrocalcinosis. Clin. Radiol., *13*:218, 1962.
97. Engfeldt, B., and Lagergren, C.: Nephrocalcinosis: roentgenographic, biophysical and histologic study. Acta Clin. Scand., *115*:46, 1958.
98. Richardson, R. E.: Nephro-calcinosis with special reference to its occurrence in renal tubular acidosis. Clin. Radiol., *13*:224, 1962.
99. Pines, K. L., and Mudge, G. H.: Renal tubular acidosis with osteomalacia. Am. J. Med., *11*:302, 1951.
100. Courey, W. R., and Pfister, R. C.: Radiographic findings in renal tubular acidosis. Radiology, *105*:497, 1972.
101. Lindvall, N.: Renal papillary necrosis. A roentgenographic study of 155 cases. Acta Radiol. (supplement): 192, 1960.
102. Harrow, B. R.: Early forms of renal papillary necrosis. Am. J. Roentgenol. Radium Ther. Nucl. Med., *95*:335, 1965.
103. Harrow, B. R., et al.: Roentgenologic demonstration of renal papillary necrosis in sickle cell trait. N. Engl. J. Med., *268*:969, 1963.
104. Lalli, A. F.: Renal papillary necrosis. Am. J. Roentgenol., *114*:741, 1972.
105. McNulty, M.: Pyelo-ureteritis cystica. Br. J. Radiol., *30*:648, 1957.
106. Theros, E. G.: Pyeloureteritis cystica. Radiology, *94*:421, 1970.
107. Caffey, J.: Urinary obstruction. In *Pediatric X-ray Diagnosis,* 6th ed. Chicago, Year Book Medical Publishers, Inc., 1972.
108. Shanks, S. C., and Kerley, P.: Hydronephrosis and hydro-ureter. In *A Textbook of X-ray Diagnosis,* 4th ed. Philadelphia, W. B. Saunders Company, 1970.
109. Cukier, D. J., and Epstein, B. S.: Reversal of hydronephrosis due to extrinsic ureteral pressure from pelvic masses in women. Radiology, *78*:68, 1962.
110. Craven, J. D., Hudson, C. J., and Lecky, J. W.: A typical response of the kidney to period of ureteric obstruction. Radiology, *105*:39, 1972.
111. Melnick, G. S., and Bramwit, D. M.: Bilateral ovarian vein syndrome. Am. J. Roentgenol. Radium Ther. Nucl. Med., *113*:509, 1971.
112. Elkin, M.: Obstructive uropathy and uremia. Radiol. Clin. North Am., *10*:447, 1972.
113. Beck, J. J.: Acute radiation nephritis in childhood. Br. Med. J., *2*:489, 1958.
114. Jernigan, J. A.: Chronic radiation nephritis: a review of the literature with report of a case. Ann. Intern. Med., *51*:1084, 1959.

115. Aron, B. S., and Schlesinger, A.: Complications of radiation therapy: the genitourinary tract. Semin. Roentgenol., 9:65, 1974.
116. Harrow, B. R., Sloane, J. A., and Liebman, N. C.: Renal papillary necrosis and analysis: roentgen differentiation from sponge kidney and other diseases. J.A.M.A., 184:445, 1963.
117. Gardiner, J. H.: Radiologic observations associated with phenacetin overdosage. J. Can. Assoc. Radiol., 17:21, 1966.
118. Boyce, W. H.: Radiology in the diagnosis and surgery of renal calculi. Radiol. Clin. North Am., 3:89, 1965.
119. Vidal, B., and Englaro, G. R.: Radiological manifestations of polycystic kidney. Radiol. Med., 43:647, 1957.
120. Caffey, J.: Cystic disease of the kidney. In Pediatric X-ray Diagnosis, 5th ed. Chicago, Year Book Medical Publishers, Inc., 1967, p. 638.
121. Tucker, A. S., Newman, A. J., and Persky, L.: The kidney in childhood leukemia. Radiology, 78:407, 1962.
122. Hatfield, P. M., and Pfister, R. C.: Adult polycystic disease of the kidneys. J.A.M.A., 222:1527, 1972.
123. Post, H. W. A., and Southwood, W. F. W.: Technique and interpretation of nephrotomograms. Br. J. Radiol., 32:734, 1959.
124. Evans, J., and Chynn, K. Y.: Nephro-tomography in differentiation of renal cyst from neoplasm: a review of 500 cases. J. Urol., 83:21, 1960.
125. Gleason, D. C., et al.: Cystic disease of the kidneys in children. Am. J. Roentgenol. Radium Ther. Nucl. Med., 100:135, 1967.
126. Evans, J.: The accuracy of diagnostic radiology. J.A.M.A., 205:151, 1968.
127. Elkin, M., and Berstein, J.: Cystic diseases of the kidney — radiological and pathological considerations. Clin. Radiol., 20:65, 1969.
128. Grossman, H., Winchester, P. H., and Chisari, F. V.: Roentgenographic classification of renal cystic disease. Am. J. Roentgenol. Radium Ther. Nucl. Med., 104:319, 1968.
129. Rayfield, E. J., and McDonald, F. D.: Red and blonde hair in medullary cystic disease. Arch. Intern. Med., 130:72, 1972.
130. Mena, E., et al.: Angiographic findings in renal medullary cystic disease. Radiology, 110:277, 1974.
131. Newman, L., et al.: Unilateral total renal dysplasia in children. Am. J. Roentgenol. Radium Ther. Nucl. Med., 116:778, 1972.
132. Kyaw, M. M.: Roentgenologic triad of congenital multicystic kidney. Am. J. Roentgenol. Radium Ther. Nucl. Med., 119:710, 1973.
133. Palubnskas, A. J.: Medullary sponge kidney. Radiology, 76:911, 1961.
134. Lowen, W., and Smythe, A. D.: Cystic disease of the renal pyramids. Clin. Radiol., 15:271, 1964.
135. Grossman, H., and Seed, W.: Congenital hepatic fibrosis, bile duct dilatation, and renal lesion resembling medullary sponge kidney. Radiology, 87:46, 1966.
136. Morris, R. C., et al.: Medullary sponge kidney. Am. J. Med., 38:883, 1965.
137. Lalli, A. F.: Medullary sponge kidney disease. Radiology, 92:92, 1969.
138. Schmidt, M.: Medullary sponge kidney (German). Fortschr. Geb. Roentgenstr. Nuklearmed, 120:680, 1974.
139. Rabinowitz, J. G., Wolf, B. S., and Goldman, R. H.: Roentgen features of renal adenomas. Radiology, 84:263, 1965.
140. Khilnani, M. T., and Wolf, B. S.: Hamartolipoma of kidney: clinical and roentgen features. Am. J. Roentgenol. Radium Ther. Nucl. Med., 86:830, 1961.
141. Grabstald, H., Whitmore, W. F., and Melamed, M. R.: Renal pelvic tumors. J.A.M.A., 218:845, 1971.
142. Silbiger, M. L., and Peterson, C. C.: Renal angiomyolipoma. J. Urol., 106:363, 1971.
143. Reynolds, L. J., Fulton, H., and Snider, J. J.: Roentgenographic analyses of renal mass lesions. Am. J. Roentgenol. Radium Ther. Nucl. Med., 82:840, 1959.
144. Olsson, O.: Roentgen diagnosis of kidney tumors. Radiology, 1:163, 1961.
145. Hare, W. S.: Differential diagnosis of renal space occupying lesions J. Coll. Radiol. Aust., 5:68, 1961.
146. Bloom, V. R., and Middlemiss, J. H.: Diagnosis of malignancy of kidney, renal pelvis and ureter. Br. J. Urol., 33:56, 1961.
147. Boissen, E., and Folin, J.: Angiography in carcinoma of the renal pelvis. Acta Radiol., 56:81, 1961.
148. Phillips, T. L., Chin, F. G., and Palubnskas, A. J.: Calcification in renal masses: an eleven year survey. Radiology, 80:786, 1963.
149. Hope, J. W., Borns, P. F., and Koop, C. E.: Diagnosis and treatment of neuroblastoma and embryoma of the kidney, Radiol. Clin. North Am., 1:593, 1963.
150. Leitner, W. A., et al.: Limitation of angiography in renal mass evaluation. Arch. Intern. Med., 130:868, 1972.
151. Pick, R. A., Castellino, R. A., and Seltzer, R. A.: Arteriographic findings in renal lymphoma. Am. J. Roentgenol. Radium Ther. Nucl. Med., 111:530, 1971.
152. Cancelmo, J. J., et al.: Tumors of the ureter. Am. J. Roentgenol. Radium Ther. Nucl. Med., 117:132, 1973.
153. Heitzman, E. R., and Perchik, L.: Radiologic features of renal infarction. Radiology, 76:39, 1961.
154. Janower, M. L., and Weber, A. L.: Radiological evaluation of acute renal infarction. Am. J. Roentgenol. Radium Ther. Nucl. Med., 95:309, 1965.
155. Scatliff, J. H., Cuttino, J. T., et al.: Angiographic evaluation of renal infarction. Am. J. Roentgenol. Radium Ther. Nucl. Med., 108:674, 1970.

156. Marsh, A. P.: Primary diabetic pneumaturia diagnosed radiographically. N. Engl. J. Med., 262:666, 1960.
157. Seshanarayana, K. N., and Keats, T. E.: Spontaneous pneumopyelogram in a non-diabetic patient. Am. J. Roentgenol. Radium Ther. Nucl. Med., 107:760, 1969.
158. Caffey, J.: Congenital malformations. In Pediatric X-ray Diagnosis, 6th ed. Chicago, Year Book Medical Publishers, 1972.
159. Faegenburg, D., Bosniak, M., and Evans, J. A.: Renal sinus lipomatosis: demonstration by nephrotomography. Radiology, 83:987, 1964.
160. Poilly, J. N., Dickie, J. E. N., and James, W. B.: Renal sinus lipomatosis: A report of twenty-six cases. Br. J. Urol. 41:257, 1969.
161. Hodson, J.: Infections of the urinary tract. Semin. Radiol. 6:349, 1971.
162. Elliott, G. B., Path, E. R. C., et al.: Malacoplakia of the urinary tract. Am. J. Roentgenol. Radium Ther. Nucl. Med., 116:830, 1972.
163. Hynes, D. M., and Watkins, E. M.: Renal agenesis. Am. J. Roentgenol. Radium Ther. Nucl. Med., 110:772, 1970.
164. Mancha, E., et al.: Congenital renal hypoplasia. Am. J. Roentgenol. Radium Ther. Nucl. Med., 114:710, 1972.

SECTION

12

DISEASES OF THE DIGESTIVE SYSTEM

DISORDERS OF MOTILITY

Disorders of the Upper (Pharyngoesophageal) Segment

Dysphagia may occur as a result of weak and uncoordinated contractions of the pharyngeal musculature and the superior esophageal sphincter. These muscular disturbances may follow damage to the fifth, seventh, ninth, tenth, and twelfth cranial nerves, which are involved in the oropharyngeal phase of swallowing, or they may be caused by primary neuromuscular disease. Conditions that can cause upper segment dysphagia include pseudobulbar palsy, myasthenia gravis, dermatomyositis, and the muscular dystrophies.

Roentgenologic studies, especially cineradiography, help to demonstrate neurologic and myoneural causes of dysphagia, but they are of little help in determining the cause of the pharyngeal weakness or paralysis. The most frequent and reliable evidence is loss of movement or loss of proper sequence of movement in the oropharynx. Evaluation requires cineradiographic or videotape studies. There may also be retention of barium in the pyriform sinuses and valleculae, pharyngeal stasis, and aspiration of contrast material into the lungs. Prolonged retention in the pyriform recesses is abnormal and may be demonstrated by routine radiographic procedures.

In early or questionable cases, cineradiography is of decided value for demonstrating disorders of the pharyngoesophageal swallowing mechanism.[1, 2]

881

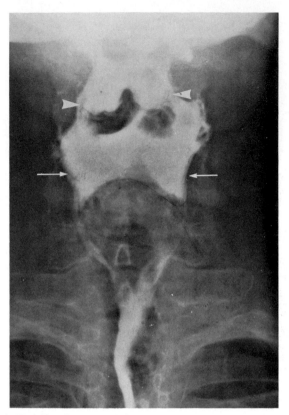

Figure 12–1 **Oropharyngeal Dysphagia: Pseudobulbar Palsy.** Several minutes after the ingestion of barium there is still retention of contrast material in the pyriform sinuses *(arrows)* and the valleculae *(arrowheads),* without evidence of mechanical obstruction. Such retention is abnormal. In this case the dysphagia developed after bilateral cerebral vascular accidents.

Cricopharyngeal Dysphagia

Prolonged and premature contraction of the cricopharyngeus muscle may lead to difficulty in swallowing. Inability of the muscles to relax produces localized narrowing and a smooth convex indentation of the posterior aspect of the barium-filled hypopharynx, generally at the level of C5–C6. This is best seen on lateral view. On anteroposterior view a lucent band is seen crossing the barium-filled esophagus, which is also somewhat narrowed in this view. The valleculae may appear distended, and aspiration into the trachea may occur. However, a small asymptomatic cricopharyngeal indentation is seen in almost half the population. Cinefluoroscopy is often necessary for demonstration of the smaller defects.

The cricopharyngeus dysfunction may contribute to development of a pulsion (Zenker) diverticulum.

The posterior location of the cricopharyngeal pressure defect distinguishes it from sideropenic web, which is usually anteriorly located.[3, 4]

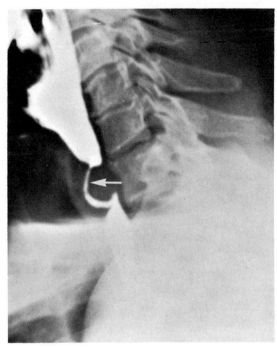

Figure 12–2 **Cricopharyngeal Dysphagia.** Roentgenogram of the neck after barium swallow reveals a localized narrowing and forward displacement of the posterior aspect of the barium-filled cervical esophagus *(arrow)* at the level of C6 due to prolonged contraction of the cricopharyngeus muscle.

Sideropenic Web

These bands arise in the anterior portion of the esophagus. They are most commonly found in the cervical esophagus and are frequently associated with iron deficiency anemia and dysphagia. The anterior location of the webs distinguishes them from cricopharyngeal narrowing. A high incidence of esophageal and pharyngeal carcinoma has been reported in patients with sideropenic webs.

With the greater use of cincradiography, an increasing incidence of webs is being reported. Many of these are found in persons with neither dysphagia nor anemia.[4-8]

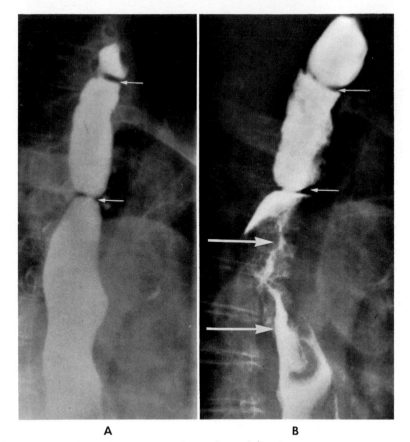

A   B

Figure 12–3 **Sideropenic Webs: Development of Esophageal Carcinoma.**

A, In a 50 year old woman who had severe microcytic anemia and dysphagia, there are two areas of esophageal narrowing due to webs. These appear as thin lucent bands *(arrows)* in the esophagus. They arise anteriorly and cause narrowing of the esophageal lumen.

B, One and one half years later, in addition to the webs *(small arrows),* there is an area of mucosal destruction and deformity *(large arrows)* caused by a carcinoma arising below the webs. The incidence of carcinoma in the pharynx and esophagus is significantly higher in patients with esophageal webs.

Disorders of the Lower (Esophagogastric) Segment

Diffuse Esophageal Spasm (Corkscrew Esophagus, "Curling")

In this neuromuscular disturbance there is a marked abnormality of peristalsis in the lower half or two thirds of the esophagus. Intermittent dysphagia and substernal pain are prominent clinical features. The peristaltic wave, which normally passes smoothly down to the esophagogastric junction, halts about the level of the aortic arch. Distal to this, the esophagus contracts diffusely and irregularly over its entire length and produces a series of alternating narrowed and wide areas, giving the so-called corkscrew appearance. The caudad passage of barium is delayed, or even reversed into the upper esophagus. These changes are best seen by fluoroscopy and are most clearly documented by cineradiography. Clinical, manometric, and radiographic improvement may occur after the administration of nitrites, especially nitroglycerin.

The distal esophageal wall is almost always thickened, sometimes massively, and may be identified by the increased soft tissue density between the intraluminal barium and the lung field.

A positive response to Mecholyl (increased pressure) is usual.

Diffuse esophageal spasm should be differentiated from tertiary peristalsis, which is not uncommon in asymptomatic older people. In tertiary peristalsis, the "curling" or corkscrew appearance is transient, esophageal emptying is usually not delayed, and there is no hypertrophy of the esophageal wall. (See *Presbyesophagus*, p. 886.)[9-12]

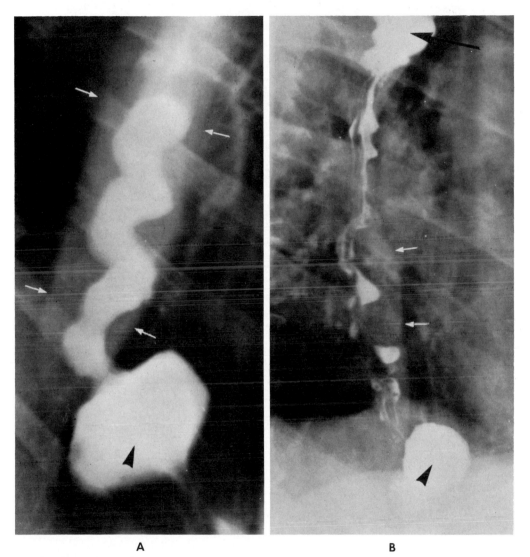

| A | B |

Figure 12-4 **Diffuse Esophageal Spasm.**

A, Esophageal study of a 56 year old man with dysphagia of several years' duration reveals a corkscrew appearance of the barium-filled lower esophagus. The soft tissue borders of the esophagus are easily identified *(arrows)* and define the marked thickening of the muscular walls. A persistent phrenic ampulla *(arrowhead)* is an unrelated finding.

B, The entire involved segment shows an irregularly contracted lumen with pouches of retained barium. This is due to the irregularity of the peristalsis, which may actually propel much of the contrast material in the reverse direction into the proximal esophagus *(black arrow).* The changes are caused by absence of a primary peristaltic wave below the level of the aortic arch. These physiologic alterations are best seen by cineradiography.

The abnormally thick esophageal wall is again apparent *(white arrows).* The phrenic ampulla *(arrowhead)* has partially emptied.

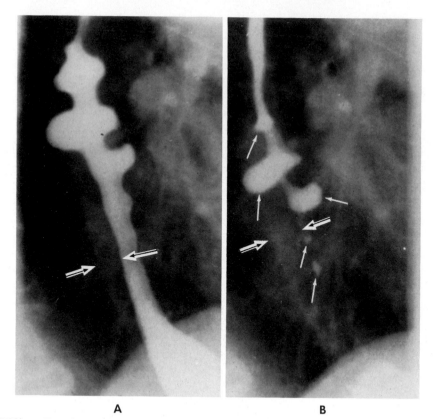

A   B

Figure 12–5   **Diffuse Esophageal Spasm with Dysphagia.**

A, The lower esophagus was narrow even when fully distended. Its wall is considerably thickened *(between arrows).* There are bizarre outpouchings of barium between the abnormal segmental contraction waves that have replaced normal peristalsis. The proximal esophagus was not dilated.

B, The pockets of barium have decreased in size but persist *(small arrows)* even after the lower segment has emptied. The esophageal wall *(between large arrows)* is even thicker than it was before emptying.

The thickened wall and the persistent pockets of barium distinguish diffuse lower esophageal spasm from ordinary asymptomatic tertiary waves.

Presbyesophagus

In many older individuals, there may be peristaltic abnormalities of the esophagus, most often with few or no symptoms.

Tertiary contractions of a long segment in the lower half of the esophagus are usually seen, but are transient. Infrequently, all peristalsis is diminished or absent and mild dilatation of the entire esophagus occurs, especially if associated with poor relaxation of the lower esophageal sphincter. Some dysphagia may be present, and the picture may mimic mild achalasia or a scleroderma esophagus.[2]

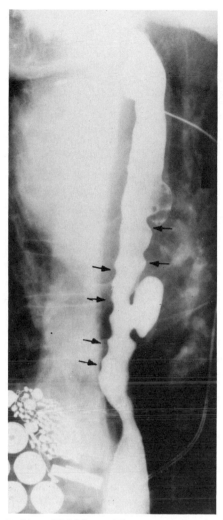

Figure 12–6 **Presbyesophagus in 75 Year Old Man.** There was no normal esophageal peristalsis, and ineffectual tertiary waves *(arrows)* are seen. The esophagus remained filled and mildly dilated. Dysphagia was present. In some cases, increased tone of the lower esophageal sphincter adds to the dysphagia.

Hypertensive Esophagogastric Sphincter

Spasm of the lower esophageal sphincter is usually a transient phenomenon and is considered to be of functional origin. Mild dysphagia or discomfort may accompany the spasm. It also occurs in nonfunctional conditions such as achalasia, Chagas' disease, and presbyesophagus, and after vagotomy.

During an episode, the extreme lower end of the esophagus remains contracted, holding up the barium column. As peristalsis becomes more vigorous, the spasm is overcome and emptying occurs. The peristaltic pattern is essentially normal in functional cases.[2]

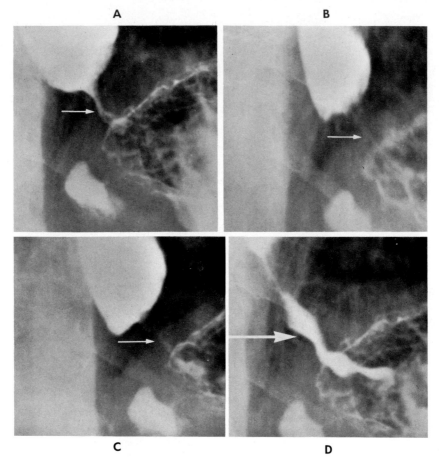

Figure 12–7 **Hypertensive Esophagogastric Sphincter: Esophageal Spasm with Dysphagia.**

   A, B, and *C,* There is an area of spasm in the distal esophagus *(arrows),* with proximal dilatation and a delay in barium emptying. No thickening of the esophageal wall is present.
   D, The distal esophagus is relaxed, and barium empties *(arrows).*

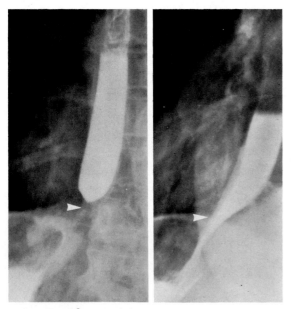

Figure 12–8 **Hypertensive Esophagogastric Sphincter: Esophageal Spasm with Transient Dysphagia.**

   A, Spasm of the distal esophagus *(arrowhead)* occurs during an episode of pain.
   B, Relaxation of the esophagus and emptying occur *(arrowhead)* after a short interval.

Achalasia of the Esophagus

Achalasia is a disorder of motility due to abnormalities of Auerbach's plexus that may lead to marked dilatation, elongation, and tortuosity of the esophagus. Characteristically, the failure of the cardioesophageal sphincter to relax causes a smooth, symmetric, tapered narrowing at the level of the diaphragm, with proximal esophageal dilatation. All degrees of dilatation are possible, depending on the duration and severity of the condition. Routine films frequently demonstrate diffuse widening of the mediastinum, often with a double contour almost invariably on the right; it is caused by the dilated fluid-filled esophagus. This widening generally extends to the diaphragm. An air-fluid level in the esophagus may be seen on erect views, and this helps distinguish achalasia from other causes of mediastinal widening. The gastric air bubble is small or absent.

Fluoroscopy reveals a decrease in or absence of the primary progressive peristaltic wave. Small amounts of barium may pass intermittently into the stomach as the terminal segment slowly opens and abruptly closes, but most of the barium remains in the uniformly dilated esophagus, even in the erect posture. In advanced cases, there is a massive dilatation and tortuosity of the esophagus, and the terminal narrowed segment may be at a right angle to the proximal segment. Repeated aspiration of esophageal contents may result in aspiration pneumonias and chronic pulmonary infiltrates.

Megaesophagus can also be a result of Chagas' disease, Riley-Day syndrome, scleroderma, or obstructing lesions in the vicinity of the cardioesophageal junction. Differentiation from carcinoma of the distal esophagus or gastric fundus is often difficult and may require esophagoscopy and manometric studies.

A lumen-obliterating contraction of the esophagus after subcutaneous Mecholyl (acetyl-β-methylcholine chloride) is fairly specific for achalasia, and can usually help distinguish achalasia from carcinoma or scleroderma.[13, 14]

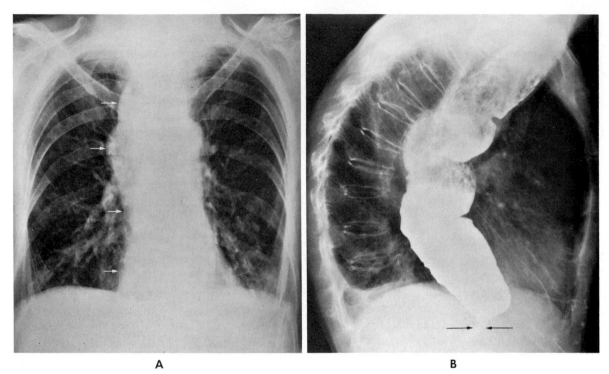

A   **B**

Figure 12–9 **Achalasia of Esophagus.**

A, This 77 year old woman had a long history of dysphagia and regurgitation. The density extending from the upper mediastinum to the diaphragm *(arrows)* is due to the dilated fluid-filled esophagus. No air-fluid level is seen.

B, Barium studies reveal a huge, dilated esophagus, containing nonopaque residue, tapering to the esophagogastric junction *(arrows).* The picture is characteristic of achalasia. The gastric air bubble is usually small or absent in advanced achalasia.

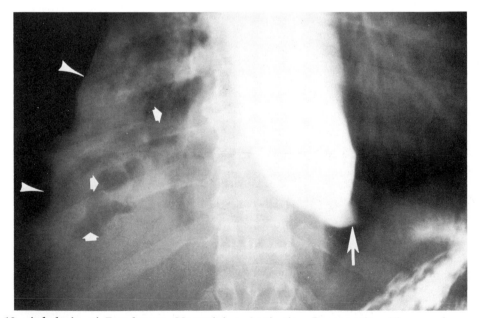

Figure 12–10 **Achalasia of Esophagus: Necrotizing Aspiration Pneumonia.** The esophagus is greatly dilated, tapering *(large arrow)* into a narrowed lower segment. The appearance is characteristic of achalasia.

The right lower lobe is atelectatic *(arrowheads)* and contains numerous irregular lucencies *(small arrows),* which were necrotic cavities.

This 41 year old man had severe achalasia for many years, and had numerous episodes of aspiration pneumonia, a common complication of this disorder.

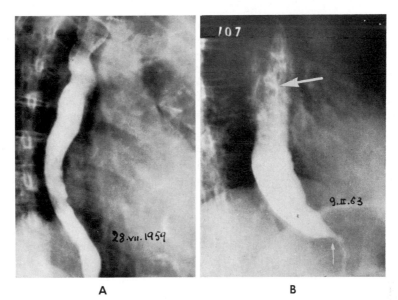

Figure 12–11 **Megaesophagus: Chagas' Disease.**

   A, The esophagus is not dilated, and normal peristaltic activity was observed. The esophagus was considered normal, although some clinical symptoms had already appeared.

   B, Five years later the esophagus is quite dilated and contains nonopaque residue *(large arrow),* and its lower end tapers *(small arrows).* Distinction from achalasia of the esophagus cannot be made roentgenologically.

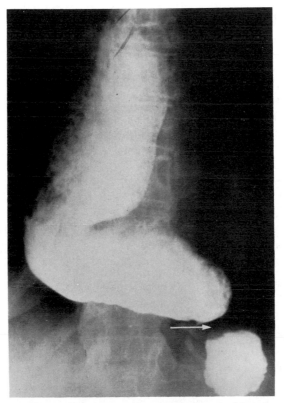

Figure 12–12 **Megaesophagus: Chagas' Disease.** The esophagus is dilated and tortuous, and the barium is mottled because of residual secretions and food. It tapers to a contracted lower esophageal segment *(arrow).* Although the appearance is characteristic of achalasia, it was due to Chagas' disease. (See also *Chagas' Disease,* p. 262).

Hiatal Hernia

There are three major types of hiatal hernia: sliding hernia, paraesophageal hernia, and hernia associated with a congenitally short esophagus.

The sliding hernia is the most frequent, representing approximately 75 per cent of cases. It is characterized by the intrathoracic location of the gastroesophageal junction. Radiographic diagnosis requires the demonstration of both gastric mucosa and the esophagogastric junction above the diaphragm. Gastric mucosal folds appear coarse, tortuous, and frequently scalloped, in contrast to the straight, fine, parallel esophageal folds. The esophageal hiatus is always widened. The distal esophagus frequently appears redundant. The hernia usually appears as a supradiaphragmatic pouch that does not show peristaltic stripping. The demonstration of an esophageal ring (Schatzki's ring or B ring), which marks the squamocolumnar junction, above the diaphragm associated with a widened hiatus indicates a hiatal hernia. Frequently, above the B ring, a second less pronounced ring (A ring) is seen which marks the tubulovestibular junction. Differentiation between sliding hernia and phrenic ampulla (see p. 897) may occasionally be difficult, but in the latter the hiatus is not widened.

Reflux of gastric contents into the esophagus occurs frequently in patients with sliding hernias, although it can occur in the absence of hiatal hernia. Reflux may lead to esophagitis, which is the cause of most clinical symptoms associated with the hernia (see p. 899). Esophagitis may lead to stricture and shortening of the esophagus.

In paraesophageal hiatal hernia, the cardioesophageal junction remains below the diaphragm, and a portion of the gastric fundus herniates into the chest alongside the distal esophagus. Plain films of the chest demonstrate this hernia as a round density posterior to the heart; occasionally it contains an air-fluid level. The normal gastric air bubble is often absent. Paraesophageal hernia generally is not reducible and may attain a huge size. Reflux rarely occurs. Occasionally, a lesser curvature ulcer develops in the herniated portion at the esophagogastric junction. It is often difficult to identify an ulcer in a hiatal hernia.

The congenitally short esophagus is the rarest type of hiatal hernia. It generally becomes symptomatic during the first five years of life. The hernia is fixed, and no alteration occurs with postural changes. There is almost always associated reflux and esophagitis. A short straight esophagus with a fixed hernia may represent a congenital lesion, but it may also represent the end result of a sliding hernia with shortening secondary to esophagitis. Some authorities doubt the existence of the congenitally short esophagus.

Occasionally one sees the combination of paraesophageal and sliding hiatal hernia. This usually occurs as a paraesophageal hiatal hernia in which the esophagogastric junction later ascends to lie above the diaphragm.[15-17]

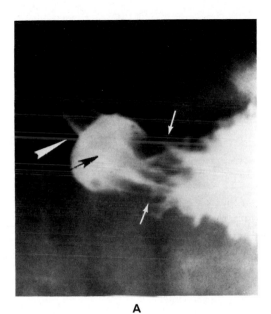

A

Figure 12–13 **Sliding Hiatal Hernia: Three Patients.**

A, The diaphragmatic hiatus *(white arrows)* is greatly widened, and the gastric mucosa extends into the hernial sac *(black arrow)*. The esophagogastric junction *(white arrowhead)* is above the diaphragm. The hernia was not apparent in the erect position.

Illustration continued on the following page

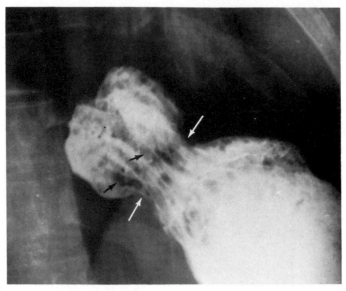

B

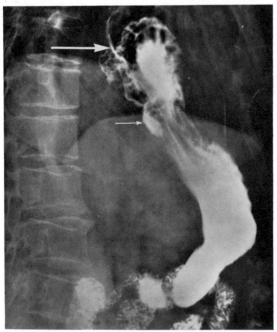

C

Figure 12–13   Continued

B, A large sliding hernia demonstrates the characteristic widened hiatus *(white arrows)* and the gastric mucosa *(black arrows)* in the hernial pouch. The hernia disappeared on erect films.

C, There is a gastric ulcer *(small arrow)* on the lesser curvature, just at the level of the widened hiatus. The heavy mucosal folds in the hernial sac are characteristic of gastric mucosa. The cardioesophageal junction *(large arrow)* is at the upper end of the hernial pouch.

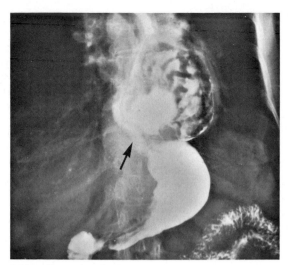

Figure 12–14 **Paraesophageal Hernia.**   The cardioesophageal junction is in normal position below the diaphragm *(arrow)*. The fundus has herniated through the esophageal hiatus and lies alongside the distal esophagus.

The features are characteristic of paraesophageal hernia.

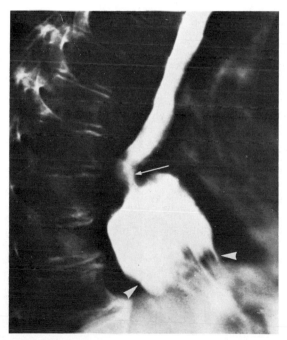

Figure 12–15 **Congenital Short Esophagus.**   The distal esophagus is narrowed *(arrow)* due to esophagitis, and the entire esophagus is shortened. A large hernia is seen above the diaphragm *(arrowheads)*. The hernia was not reducible in any position.

Although there is a superficial resemblance to sliding hernia, the extreme shortening of the esophagus and the persistence of the hernia in the erect position favor the diagnosis of a congenitally short esophagus. A history of symptoms early in childhood confirms this impression.

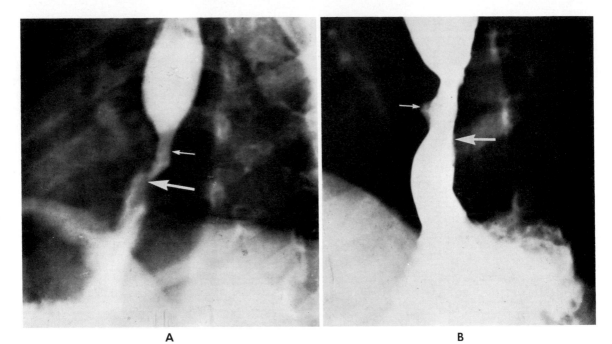

Figure 12–16 **Congenital Short Esophagus in a Symptomatic Child.**

A, There is stricture of the distal esophagus *(small arrow).* The proximal esophagus is dilated. The cardioesophageal junction *(large arrow)* remains fixed above the diaphragm.

B, Following an episode of bleeding 11 years later, an ulcer is seen *(small arrow)* in the narrowed area of the esophagus. Note dilatation of the proximal esophagus. The position of the cardioesophageal junction is unchanged *(large arrow).*

Recurrent esophagitis and ulceration are fairly frequent complications of a congenital short esophagus. (Courtesy Emile Gilbrin, Paris, France.)

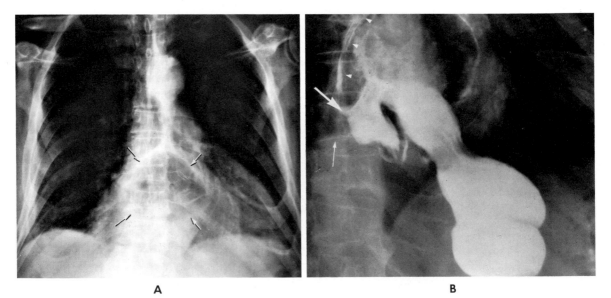

Figure 12–17 **Mixed Hernia.**

A, In posteroanterior view, a round lucency *(arrows)* posterior to the heart represents air within a large hiatal hernia. This appearance suggests a large paraesophageal hiatal hernia.

B, Gastrointestinal study shows that the fundus has herniated through the esophageal hiatus to lie alongside the distal esophagus *(arrowheads).* This is the usual appearance of a paraesophageal hernia; however, the cardioesophageal junction *(large arrow)* lies just above the diaphragm *(small arrow),* so that the hernia is of the mixed type.

Phrenic Ampulla

The phrenic ampulla is a physiologic ovoid dilatation between the distal tubular esophagus (A zone) and the diaphragm. The ampulla normally remains distended for a short time after contraction of the tubular esophagus, and then contracts and empties.

In normal individuals, the phrenic ampulla can remain filled during prolonged inspiration and may mimic a hiatal hernia. However, in the ampulla, only esophageal mucosa can be demonstrated, the dilatation is transient, and the esophagogastric junction can be demonstrated below the diaphragm. There is no widening of the esophageal hiatus.

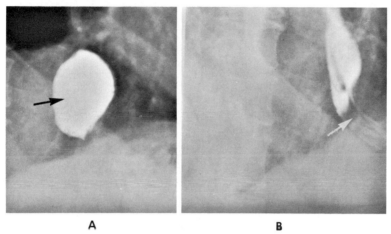

A   B

Figure 12-18 **Phrenic Ampulla.**

These films were taken with the patient holding his breath in inspiration.

A, The lower end of the esophagus (ampulla) is dilated *(arrow).* Note the contracted segment below the ampulla.

B, There is prompt emptying of the ampulla as the lower end of the esophagus relaxes *(arrow).*

A slowly emptying ampulla can be mistaken for a sliding hernia, but careful fluoroscopic observation will avoid this error.

Lower Esophageal (Schatzki's) Ring

The lower esophageal (B) ring is a localized area of restricted distensibility rather than a true contracture. It is a mucosal ring and not a muscular constriction. Most investigators believe that it marks the squamocolumnar junction. When this ring is found above the diaphragm, it usually indicates the presence of a hiatal hernia.

The Schatzki ring is found up to 5 cm. above the diaphragm and is best seen when the esophagus is fully distended with barium. It often cannot be demonstrated in the partially contracted esophagus. Radiographically it appears as a narrow annular constriction defect surrounding the entire esophagus. It may simulate a true annular constriction from a peptic esophagitis, but the latter is usually longer, more irregular, and does not produce a disc-like defect in the distended esophagus. Although usually asymptomatic, the ring can cause dysphagia, particularly if the lumen of the fully distended esophagus is narrowed to less than 13 mm. The presence of Schatzki's ring is a helpful landmark for radiographic identification of a small hiatal hernia.

Sometimes a transient and less well-defined second ring, called the A ring, is seen a short distance above Schatzki's ring. It marks the junction of the tubular and vestibular portion of the esophagus and is also called the inferior esophageal sphincter.[18-21]

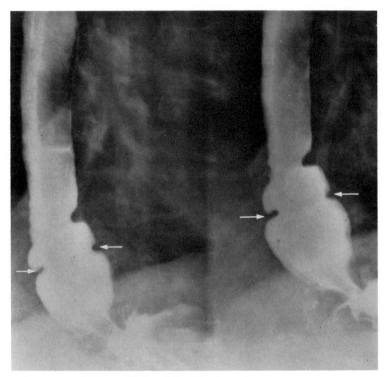

Figure 12–19 **Lower Esophageal Ring (Schatzki's Ring).** The ring appears as symmetric indentation defects *(arrows)* in the distended lower esophagus. It represents the esophagogastric junction, and the pouch below is a small hiatal hernia. The indentation proximal to the Schatzki ring is a transient second, or A, ring, which represents the sphincter between the tubular esophagus and the ampullary esophagus.

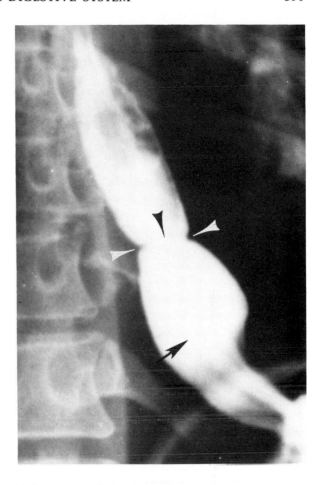

Figure 12–20 **Lower Esophageal Ring (Schatzki's Ring): Hiatal Hernia.** A characteristic thin ring is indenting *(white arrowheads)* and encircling *(black arrowhead)* the esophagus and marks the proximal end of a hiatal hernia *(arrow)*.

The Schatzki ring is seen only when the esophagus is distended. Only rarely will it compromise the esophageal lumen to any significant degree.

Esophagitis and Reflux Esophagitis

Inflammation of the lower esophageal segment is usually due to reflux of gastric acid contents. Reflux is most often associated with a hiatal hernia but can also be due to a dysfunction of the lower esophageal sphincter, persistent vomiting, and increased intra-abdominal pressure in obesity or pregnancy.

In reflux esophagitis, the esophagus may appear radiographically normal in a high percentage of symptomatic patients, since involvement is usually limited to the mucosa. A hiatal hernia or fluoroscopic evidence of reflux may be the sole finding. Deeper inflammatory changes in the lower esophagus may lead to focal spasm, abnormal peristalsis, local lack of distensibility, and delay in emptying. The motor changes are best demonstrated on cineradiographic or videotape studies.

Severe inflammatory involvement may cause coarsened, thickened folds and somewhat fuzzy serrated lower esophageal margins. With progression, the lumen may become narrowed by persistent spasm and have a granular mucosal appearance. Discrete ulcerations can develop. If fibrous contracture eventuates, the luminal narrowing is gradual, smooth, and tapering, with no mucosal detail. Proximal dilatation may be seen. At times, the appearance simulates carcinoma.

Esophagitis, ulceration, and eventual stricture can also occur some distance above the esophagogastric junction with ectopic gastric mucosa or in Barrett's heterotopic columnar epithelium. The latter may actually be due to metaplasia from chronic irritation and is often associated with a hiatal hernia. Other causes of diffuse or focal esophagitis include prolonged intubation, ingestion of chemical irritants, and candida infection.

In reflux esophagitis without decisive radiographic findings, the administration of 0.1N hydrochloric acid with the barium can sometimes produce significant motor disturbances of the lower esophagus and a reproduction of clinical symptoms, all of which may disappear after ingestion of antacids. (Ingestion of water while recumbent may help demonstrate reflux from the barium-filled fundus.) However, definitive diagnosis in most cases requires endoscopic detection of the mucosal inflammation. (See also Figs. 12–78 and 12–79).[16, 18-20, 22-24]

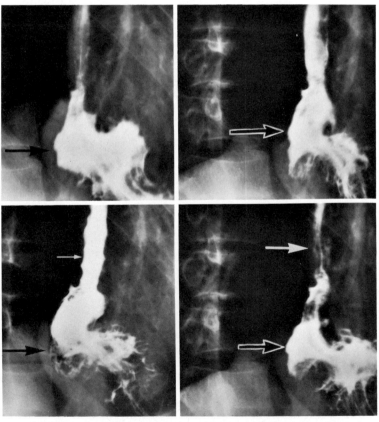

Figure 12–21 **Reflux Esophagitis and Hiatal Hernia.** The hernia is of moderate size *(black arrows)*. The esophagogastric junction is above the diaphragm, and the mucosal folds are coarse. Serial films demonstrate esophageal spasm and irritability. The esophagus has irregular serrated edges *(small white arrow)*, and the folds are broad, thick, and indurated *(large white arrow)*. Fluoroscopy demonstrated reflux of barium into the distal esophagus.

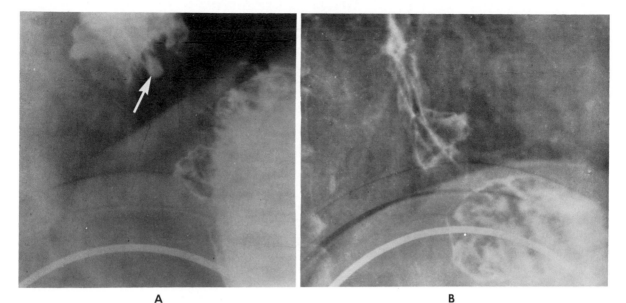

A   B

Figure 12–22   **Hiatal Hernia: Ulceration.**

A, There is an ulcer crater *(arrow)* above the diaphragm in the herniated portion of the stomach.

B, Following therapy, the ulcer has disappeared, and the mucosal pattern of the herniated portion of the stomach is normal.

Both ulceration and malignant neoplasms may arise within the herniated portion of the stomach. Mucosal distortion makes detection difficult, and multiple studies may be needed to establish the diagnosis.

Lower Esophageal Dysphagia Due to Systemic Disease

Systemic diseases that can cause faulty peristalsis or abnormal tone of the lower esophageal sphincter, which leads to dysphagia, include scleroderma, diabetic or alcoholic neuropathy, parkinsonism, multiple sclerosis, amyotrophic lateral sclerosis, pseudobulbar palsy, myotonia atrophica, dermatomyositis, and familial dysautonomia (see under specific headings).

Disorders of Gastroduodenal Motility

Acute Gastric Dilatation

Atony and dilatation of the stomach in the absence of mechanical obstruction is usually a postoperative complication, but it may also occur in diabetes, immobilization by cast, intra-abdominal inflammatory disease (usually pancreatitis), neurologic conditions such as tabes dorsalis and the post-vagotomy state, hypokalemia, and after severe trauma. It is also a frequent development in patients receiving oxygen nasally. Acute dilatation may cause a shock-like picture. Radiographic recognition and prompt decompression are often urgent.

There is a huge gastric shadow containing air, fluid, and retained food. When the patient is supine, the fluid-filled stomach may appear as a large upper abdominal mass displacing the intestines caudad. When large amounts of air are present, the entire stomach may be outlined. On erect or decubitus views, air-fluid levels may be seen. A barium study may be necessary to exclude mechanical obstruction and sometimes to unequivocally identify the dilated aperistaltic stomach.[25, 26]

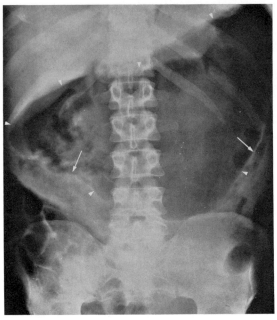

Figure 12–23 **Acute Gastric Dilatation.** In a film made 24 hours after abdominal surgery, a greatly distended stomach is outlined by air (*arrowheads*). The transverse colon is displaced caudad (*arrows*). Immediate decompression of the stomach via gastric tube is imperative.

Acute Gastric Volvulus

Gastric volvulus is usually secondary to hiatal herniation, eventration, or rupture of the diaphragm, although occasionally it is idiopathic. Invariably there is associated elongation of the various gastric ligaments.

Volvulus refers to obstruction due to twisting of the bowel; *torsion,* to twisting without obstruction.

Gastric volvulus may be classified according to the axis and direction of rotation. In organoaxial volvulus the rotation takes place around the long axis, an imaginary line from the cardia to the pylorus. In mesenteroaxial volvulus the rotation is at right angles to the long axis of the stomach. Combined volvulus is also possible.

In a mesenteroaxial volvulus the supine view discloses a distended fundus, generally in the left upper or mid abdomen, with smooth convex borders. In the erect views there are two or, rarely, three fluid levels. One level is in the cardia and another is in the antrum, which is now above the fundus; rarely, a third level may be found in the body of the stomach.

In organoaxial volvulus, complete obstruction of the lower esophagus is seen following barium ingestion, whereas in mesenteroaxial or combined volvulus the esophagus is patent and the actual point of twisting may be demonstrated.

Occasionally ischemic strangulation and necrosis can occur.[27-29]

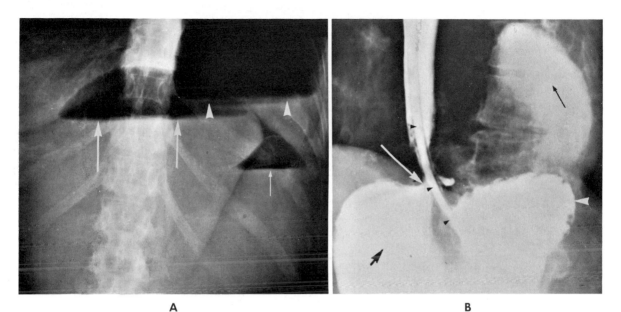

A   **B**

Figure 12-24 **Gastric Volvulus: Two Cases.**

A, In erect view there are three large fluid levels in the mid and left upper quadrant: one in the fundus *(large arrows),* another in the antrum of the stomach *(arrowheads),* and a third in the body of the stomach *(small arrow).* This is combined volvulus.

B, In the second case, barium studies with the patient lateral demonstrate the site of the twist *(white arrow).* The body of the stomach *(large black arrow)* lies anterior to the fundus *(white arrowhead).* Some barium has passed by the obstruction and is in the gastric antrum *(small black arrow),* above the diaphragm. There is a tube in the esophagus and gastric cardia *(black arrowheads).* (Courtesy Dr. A. Dick, Sunderland, England.)

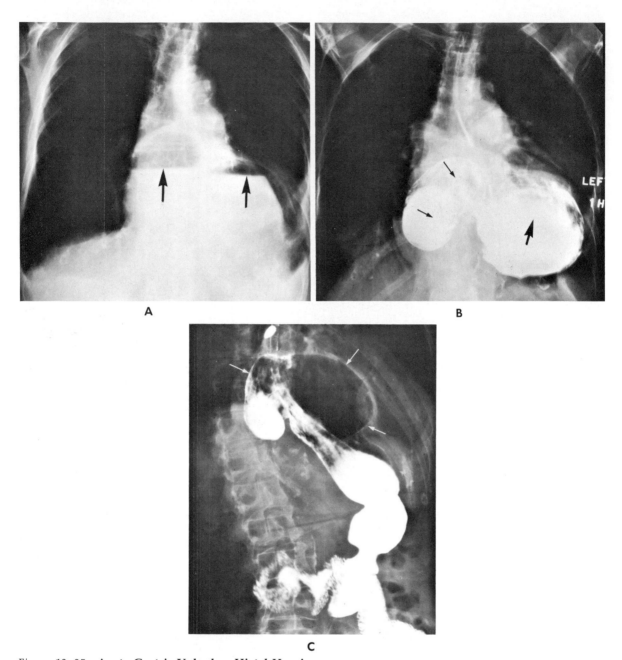

A

B

C

Figure 12–25 **Acute Gastric Volvulus: Hiatal Hernia.**

This 65 year old woman, known to have a large hiatal hernia, was admitted after two days of persistent vomiting.

A, Erect chest film reveals two distinct fluid levels *(arrows)* above the diaphragm.

B, Barium introduced through a gastric tube discloses complete obstruction of the distal stomach. Both the fundus *(large arrow)* and the distal half of the stomach *(small arrows)* are above the diaphragm.

C, After surgical correction of the volvulus, the pre-existing hiatal hernia *(arrows)* appears above the diaphragm, as it did before the volvulus. The rest of the stomach is now below the diaphragm, and emptying proceeds normally.

Most cases of acute gastric volvulus occur through the hiatus of a pre-existing hiatal hernia.

Pyloric Stenosis in the Adult

Pyloric stenosis in the adult is probably unrelated to infantile hypertrophic pyloric stenosis. It is due to hypertrophy of the pyloric muscle, which may either be idiopathic or result from previous pyloric channel ulcer disease or gastritis.

The pyloric canal is elongated and narrowed and may have an upward curve. A crevice may be present near the midportion of the greater curvature, representing the gap between the hypertrophied muscle bundles. A biconcave indentation due to impression by the hypertrophied muscle may be seen on the base of the duodenal bulb (umbrella defect). Flexibility of the walls is decreased, but intact mucosal folds can be demonstrated. There may be partial or complete obstruction of the stomach. In many cases it is difficult to differentiate narrowing due to pyloric hypertrophy, from the fibrotic scarring of inflammatory antral-pyloric disease or from an encircling malignancy. Cineradiography may be helpful. Laparotomy is frequently necessary for diagnosis.[30, 31]

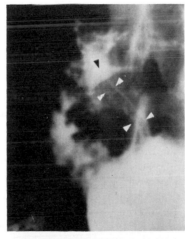
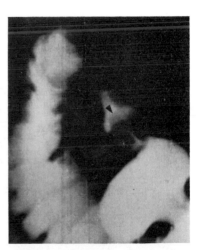
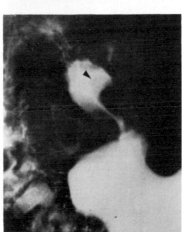
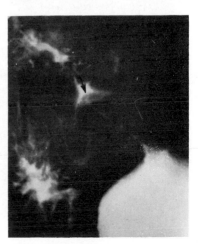

Figure 12–26 **Hypertrophic Pyloric Stenosis in Adult.** A 60 year old man without prior gastrointestinal symptoms developed progressive nausea and vomiting over a two-week period.

A composite made from four different films shows persistent narrowing and elongation of the pyloric and prepyloric area. A characteristic double barium track is seen (*white arrowheads*), and the umbrella defect (*black arrowheads*) from projection of the hypertrophied muscle into the base of the duodenal bulb is constant. Note the slight upward bowing of the elongated pyloric channel. The stomach was dilated and partially obstructed.

In spite of the brief acute history, the roentgen findings were considered characteristic of adult hypertrophic pyloric stenosis; this diagnosis was confirmed by surgery.

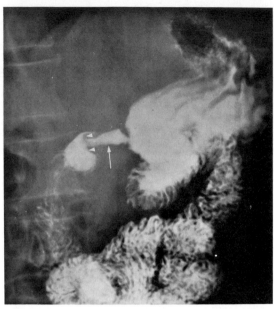

Figure 12-27 **Pyloric Stenosis in Adult.** There is elongation and narrowing of the pyloric canal *(arrow)* in a 47 year old man. An umbrella defect seen in the base of the duodenal bulb is due to indentation by the hypertrophied pyloric musculature *(arrowheads)*. There was minimal gastric obstruction.

Infantile Hypertrophic Pyloric Stenosis

This condition occurs early in the neonatal period and generally requires surgery for relief.

In about one fourth of cases, the plain abdominal film will show a gas-distended hyperperistaltic stomach in an otherwise relatively gasless abdomen. This finding is highly suggestive of the diagnosis.

On the upper gastrointestinal study there is persistent narrowing of the gastropyloric and prepyloric segments. The narrowing appears as a thin elongated string 1 to 2 cm. long. Gastric emptying is always delayed; from 6 to over 24 hours may be required for complete emptying if vomiting does not occur during the study.

The narrowed segment shows no significant peristalsis and appears rigid. It is usually slightly curved with an upward concavity. Frequently a double track of barium outlines the narrowed segment; this is virtually a pathognomonic finding.

The proximal stomach is usually not significantly dilated, and at its junction with the narrowed area there is an abrupt peak. A squared-off appearance and a shoulder indentation on the antrum results from the pressure of the proximal end of the hypertrophied muscle. A concave impression, also due to the hypertrophied muscle, may be seen on the base of the duodenal bulb.

Severe and prolonged pylorospasm can produce a similar appearance, but the double barium track in the narrowed area is not seen.

After pyloroplasty and clinical recovery there may be little change in the narrowing, but the double track will be absent, and gastric emptying will approach normal.[13, 32-34]

Figure 12–28 **Infantile Hypertrophic Pyloric Stenosis.**
Four hours after ingestion of barium, only a small amount has left the slightly dilated stomach. The pyloric-prepyloric area is persistently elongated and narrowed and contains two distinct tracts of barium *(small white arrowheads).* The junction of the antrum and the narrowed segment is peaked *(black arrowhead).* The shoulder impression *(arrow)* on the antrum has a sharp upper point *(large arrowhead),* characteristic of extrinsic pressure from the hypertrophied muscle. The duodenal bulb was not filled on this film.

The persistently elongated and narrowed pyloric-prepyloric segment with a double barium track, the shoulder impression, and the delayed gastric emptying are characteristic of hypertrophic pyloric stenosis in infancy. Other changes include indentation of the base of the duodenal bulb and triangular outpouching of barium in the pylorus, due to a cleft between the muscle bundles.

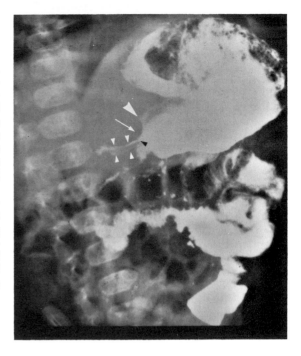

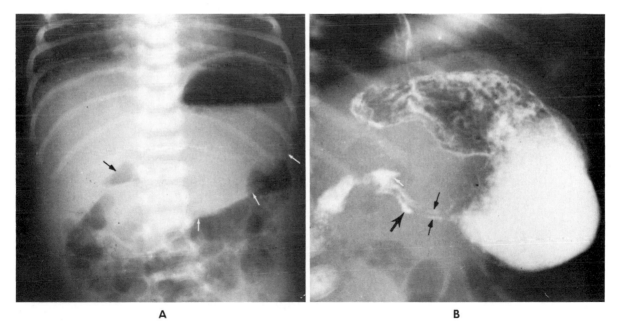

A   **B**

Figure 12–29 **Infantile Hypertrophic Pyloric Stenosis.**

A, The erect abdominal film, made several hours after feeding, reveals a dilated stomach *(white arrows)* filled with fluid. The fundal gas bubble is very large. The duodenal bulb is also gas filled *(black arrow).*

B, Barium study shows an elongated narrowed pylorus and antrum, with a double track sign *(small black arrows).* A characteristic barium spur *(large black arrow)* is seen in the prepyloric area of the greater curvature. A small umbrella defect at the base of bulb *(white arrow)* is due to the hypertrophied muscle.

Mallory-Weiss Syndrome

Originally this syndrome comprised massive gastrointestinal hemorrhage from a tear of the gastric mucosa near the esophagogastric junction. Severe emesis usually precedes the tear. However, the mucosal rent can also be entirely in the lower esophagus, or wholly intragastric. The hemorrhage can range from mild to massive. In a very small percentage of cases after the administration of oral contrast material (barium or water-soluble contrast) there will be a radiographically detectable linear collection of contrast material. Occasionally, if bleeding ceases, an irregular outpouching of the contrast material appears in the lower esophagus. In the vast majority of cases, however, gastrointestinal contrast studies are negative, and endoscopic examination will detect the linear tear.

During active bleeding, celiac angiography will disclose extravasation of contrast material into the lower esophagus or cardiac end of the stomach.[35-38]

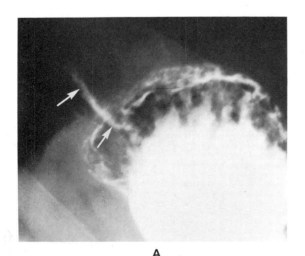
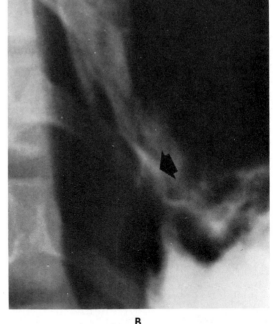

A   B

Figure 12–30   **Mallory-Weiss Syndrome: Two Cases.**

A, Upper gastrointestinal study of a 34 year old man following an episode of severe hematemesis reveals a persistent thick streak of barium (*arrows*) in the lower esophagus extending into the esophagogastric junction. This streak persisted after the rest of the esophagus emptied. This long tear of the esophagus was also seen during endoscopy and necessitated surgery.

B, Esophagogram of a 20 year old man with persistent emesis followed by hematemesis reveals an irregular streak of barium (*arrow*) along the distal esophagus. The tear was also seen endoscopically and was repaired surgically.

Since most of the cases of Mallory-Weiss syndrome are due to very superficial tears, roentgenologic demonstration of the tear itself is rare. (Courtesy Dr. M. Sparberg, Chicago, Illinois.)

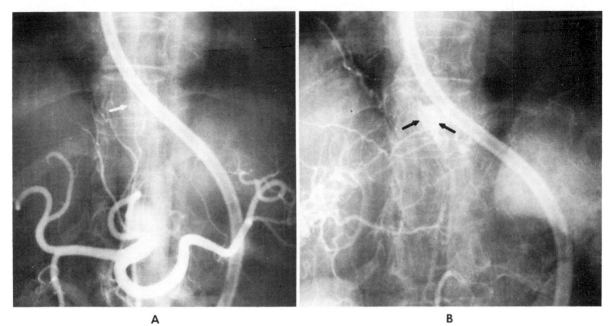

A   B

Figure 12–31 **Mallory-Weiss Syndrome: Celiac Arteriogram.**

A, During the early arterial phase, a faint opacification is seen *(arrow)* adjacent to the nasogastric tube.

B, In the later phase, contrast material has appeared in the lower esophagus *(arrows),* clearly indicating a bleeding site in the lower esophagus.

Megaduodenum

Idiopathic megaduodenum is probably secondary to aperistalsis resulting from abnormalities of the myenteric plexus. The idiopathic form must be distinguished from duodenal dilatation associated with other conditions. When megaduodenum is caused by pressure from the superior mesenteric artery, the dilatation diminishes considerably in the prone position. When it is associated with the Zollinger-Ellison syndrome, there is evidence of inflammation or ulceration. Megaduodenum is often encountered in scleroderma, but in these cases there are additional clinical and roentgenologic findings. Megaduodenum has also been observed in patients with granulomatous enteritis.[39]

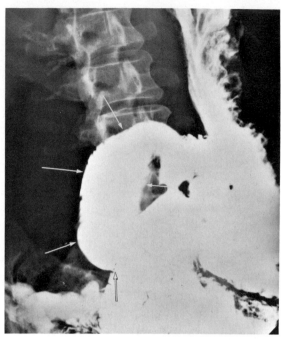

Figure 12–32 **Megaduodenum.** A 54 year old woman experienced periodic nausea and vomiting. The duodenum is large and atonic but not obstructed *(arrows)*. The dilated loop remains unchanged in all positions. This type of megaduodenum should be differentiated from that caused by mesenteric artery pressure on the third portion of the loop; in the latter, peristalsis is active and the obstruction is decreased in the prone position. Megaduodenum may occasionally occur in scleroderma.

Annular Pancreas

This rare anatomic anomaly can cause complete obstruction in the mid-descending duodenum during the first days or weeks of life indistinguishable radiographically from duodenal atresia or stenosis.

However, it may be asymptomatic until adult life, when epigastric pain, vomiting, and occasionally bleeding occur. Radiographically, there will be a narrow annular extrinsic defect in the upper or mid-descending duodenum with dilatation proximally. In about 30 per cent of patients, a complicating ulcer in the duodenal bulb is found. The band-like defect of annular pancreas usually can be distinguished from narrowing due to cicatricial postbulbar ulcer or primary duodenal neoplasm.[40, 41]

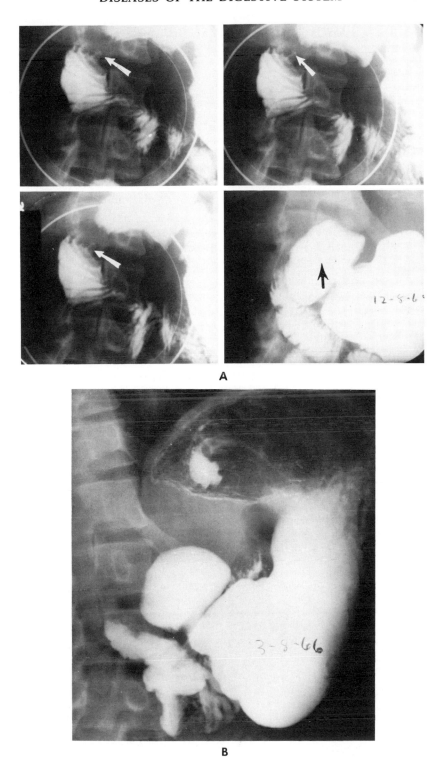

Figure 12–33 **Annular Pancreas in Adult.**

A, Gastrointestinal study of a 29 year old woman with a long history of recurrent nausea and vomiting reveals an area of narrowing *(white arrows)* in the duodenum just distal to the somewhat dilated bulb *(black arrow).*

B, Three months later, the findings are unchanged; the bulb and stomach are still moderately dilated.

At surgery, an encircling annular pancreas obstructing the duodenum was found.

Disorders of Intestinal Motility

Chronic Constipation

Chronic constipation may be caused by mechanical obstruction, such as carcinoma, stricture, or extrinsic pressure on the colon; these conditions are usually easily demonstrable on barium enema studies. When chronic constipation in adults is due to functional causes or improper bowel habits, the barium enema often reveals a dilated tortuous colon and rectum filled with feces. These findings may simulate those of congenital megacolon (Hirschsprung's disease); in congenital megacolon, however, the rectum is usually not distended with feces, except in the uncommon anorectal agangliosis.

Chronic constipation may be complicated by fecal impaction, which occurs when the feces in the rectum or sigmoid become dehydrated and sufficiently hardened to produce partial or complete obstruction. Barium enema will generally disclose the fecal nature of the intraluminal mass, especially in rectal impactions. Sigmoid impaction can produce complete obstruction that may radiographically simulate a tumor. In children, impactions in the sigmoid may displace and compress the lower ureters, causing stasis and dilatation of one or both upper urinary tracts.[42]

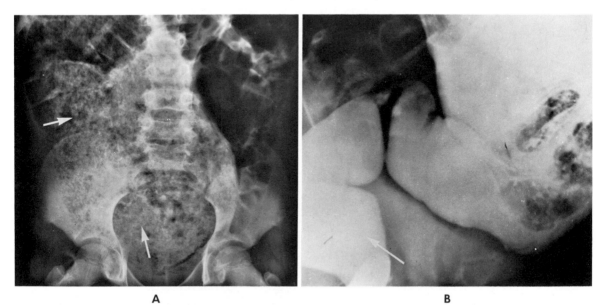

A   B

Figure 12–34 **Chronic Constipation: Atonic Colon.**

A, The greatly distended colon is filled with feces, which have a characteristic mottled appearance *(arrows).*

B, In enlarged view of rectum *(arrow)* and sigmoid there is no evidence of a narrowed aganglionic segment. The rectal ampulla balloons adequately.

In chronic constipation there is usually a tortuous, redundant, moderately dilated colon, which is filled with feces from the rectum to the cecum and empties poorly. The presence of a fecal-filled rectum helps differentiate chronic constipation from Hirschsprung's disease.

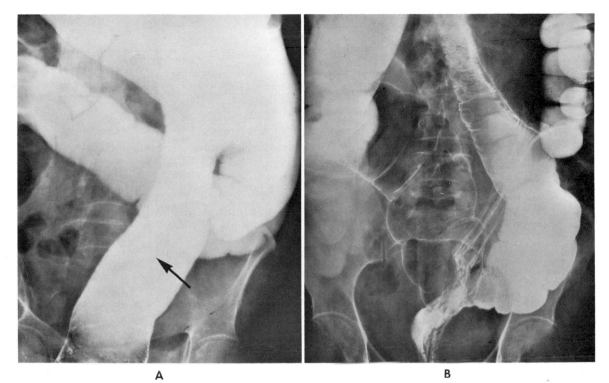

A   B

Figure 12–35 **Chronic Constipation: Acquired Megacolon.**

   A, This 69 year old woman had a history of constipation for 20 years. Barium enema study demonstrates a greatly dilated colon with a long sigmoid *(arrow),* loss of haustral markings, and redundant flexures. The cecum and ascending colon were incompletely filled even after instillation of 3½ quarts of the barium preparation.

   B, Film made following evacuation discloses considerable residual dilatation of the entire colon with air and barium. The cecum and ascending colon are now opacified.

   Megacolon resulting from chronic constipation may occasionally decrease or disappear if normal bowel habits can be reestablished.

Figure 12–36 **Chronic Constipation: Sigmoid Impaction: Barium Enema.** A 56 year old man with a history of chronic constipation experienced obstipation of one week's duration. The barium column is obstructed at the sigmoid because of a mass *(large arrows)* that fills the lumen. A small amount of barium has seeped beyond the obstruction and demonstrates a large mass of feces *(small arrows).*

   The absence of deformities of the bowel wall and the accumulation of feces proximally, coupled with this history, suggested the diagnosis of fecal impaction, which was confirmed. While a large polypoid villous adenoma might produce a similar picture, it does not usually obstruct.

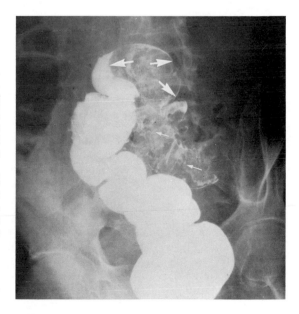

Cathartic Colon

The prolonged use of laxatives may lead to mucosal atrophy and neuromuscular changes in the colon.

Radiographically, the changes are most apparent in the right colon, especially the cecum and ileocecal valve, and consist of loss of haustral pattern, some shortening, and occasional dilatation. The cecum appears shortened and may become conical. With more extensive changes the colon distal to the cecum may appear tubular. Transient areas of narrowing are seen. Poor mucosal detail and some irregularity may appear on the postevacuation film. No ulcerations are present. The rectum and sigmoid are generally spared.

Radiographic resemblance to chronic or burned-out ulcerative or granulomatous colitis is generally clarified by the lack of shortening, the distribution, and the clinical history.[43, 44]

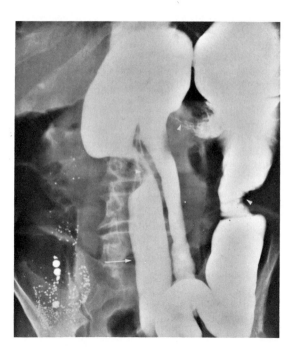

Figure 12–37 **Cathartic Colon.** Haustral markings are virtually absent *(arrows)*; however, the colon is elongated and the walls are distensible, distinguishing this condition from ulcerative colitis. Abnormal areas of contraction *(arrowheads)* are occasionally seen in the cathartic colon.

Irritable Colon

This condition cannot be diagnosed radiographically, but barium enema is important mainly to rule out other causes of the symptoms During barium enema there may be rapid filling, areas of irritability and spasm, and increased segmentation. These roentgen changes may be significant if the patient experiences distress corresponding to the clinical complaints. However, even in normal asymptomatic persons, colonic irritability and spasm during a barium enema study are often encountered, perhaps due to the use of preparatory laxatives and enemas. In some patients prediverticulosis (p. 931) may be an organic manifestation of the irritable colon syndrome.[45, 46]

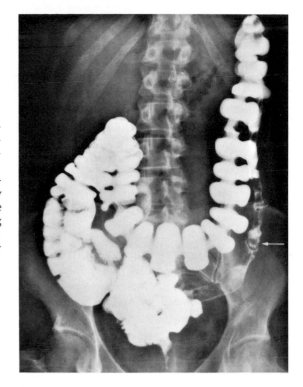

Figure 12–38 **Irritable Colon.** The strongly contracted descending colon *(arrow)* is periodically relaxed. The patient experienced pain during the contractions.

There is no organic or mucosal abnormality. Haustral markings in the remainder of the colon are very prominent. Although this picture is not diagnostic, the correlation of colonic spasm with symptoms arising during the examination may be confirmatory, especially if the patient indicates that he has had similar clinical symptoms.

Mechanical Obstruction of the Small Intestine

The roentgenogram generally reveals some evidence of obstruction within four to six hours after the onset. The earliest change seen is gaseous distention of a few small bowel loops proximal to the site of obstruction. Air-fluid levels may be seen in erect or decubitus views. Normally, fluid levels are not found in the small intestine distal to the duodenum. With progression of the obstruction, more loops become visible, and dilatation increases. The distended loops tend to curve upward, and air-fluid levels appear at various heights even in the same loop, giving rise to a stepladder appearance. Loops that are completely filled with fluid show neither gas nor fluid levels, so that recognition is extremely difficult.

The thin soft tissue stripe between adjacent gas-filled small bowel loops represents the thickness of the walls of these loops. In simple obstruction, this soft tissue stripe retains its normal appearance; with inflammation, exudation, and thickening of the bowel wall, the stripe is widened, so that the space between adjacent gas shadows becomes wider.

Absence of gas in the large intestine in cases of distended small bowel is characteristic of simple mechanical obstruction of the small bowel. Visualization of significant amounts of gas in the large intestine indicates that the obstruction is recent or that it is incomplete, or that there has been severe vascular damage to the small intestine leading to paralytic ileus and dilatation of the large intestine.

Small bowel loops may be differentiated from large bowel by their more central location and by the transverse stripes of the valvulae conniventes, which traverse the entire small bowel wall. These soft tissue stripes are closer together than the haustral markings of the colon. Serial examinations are frequently necessary to judge the course of an obstruction and to confirm the diagnosis.

In closed loop obstruction, which occurs in volvulus or incarcerated hernia, the bowel loop is obstructed at two points. Roentgenographically, closed loop obstruction may be indistinguishable from simple mechanical obstruction. Often, however, the distended loop is curved upon itself, and the soft tissue stripe of bowel wall between the gas-filled loops can be traced to the point of volvulus. The picture is often complicated by compromise of the blood supply to the affected loop, which can lead to thickening of the bowel wall and even to secondary paralytic ileus of the small and large bowels. If the affected loop becomes completely filled with fluid, it may appear as a soft tissue mass — a so-called pseudotumor.

Other findings resulting from ischemia or gangrene of a loop include loss of normal small bowel markings, a fixed distended loop that does not change in location or appearance over a number of days, and evidence of intraperitoneal fluid resulting from peritonitis.

The severity of the symptoms may help distinguish closed loop obstruction with compromise of the blood supply from simple mechanical obstruction. Water-soluble opaque materials can be given by mouth, but they rarely help to delineate the site and nature of the obstruction. If large bowel obstruction can be excluded, oral barium can be a definitive diagnostic agent.[47, 48]

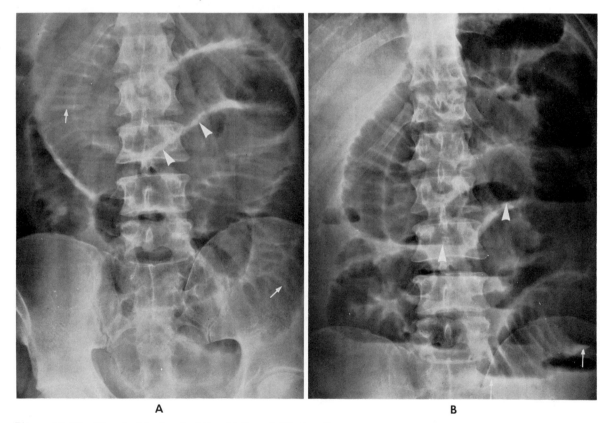

A   B

Figure 12–39 **Simple Mechanical Small Bowel Obstruction.**

A, There is marked, uniform distention of the small bowel. The linear densities *(arrows)* traversing the bowel gas are the valvulae conniventes; these identify the distended loops as small bowel. No gas is present in the large intestine. The soft tissue line *(arrowheads)* between adjacent loops is of normal thickness.

B, Erect view shows multiple air-fluid levels creating a stepladder effect *(arrowheads* and *arrow).*

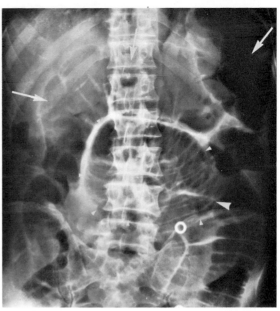

Figure 12–40 **Mechanical Small Bowel Obstruction: Volvulus.** In a 57 year old man, supine view reveals a distended loop of small intestine that has twisted and folded back upon itself *(small arrowheads)*. This represents the volvulus. The point of twisting is indicated by the large arrowhead. The other dilated small bowel loops and the dilatation of the large intestine *(large arrows)* are caused by secondary paralytic ileus.

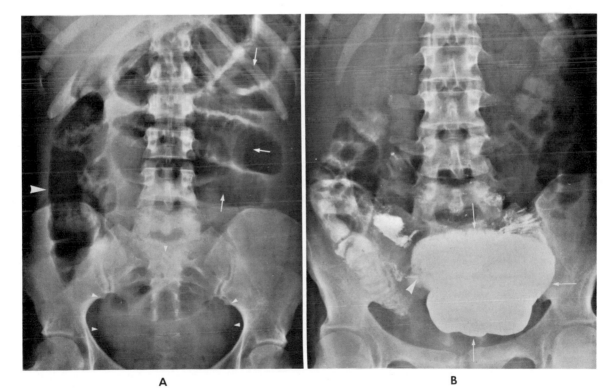

A   B

Figure 12–41 **Mechanical Small Bowel Obstruction: Volvulus: Pseudotumor.**

   A, A 27 year old female had distention and pain, and a lower abdominal mass was present. There are distended loops of small intestine *(arrows)*, and a vague soft tissue mass is seen in the lower abdomen *(small arrowheads)*. This is due to a fluid-filled volvulus (pseudotumor). Gas in the large intestine *(large arrowhead)* indicates that the obstruction is not complete.

   B, Barium meal examination demonstrates the volvulus *(arrows)* filled with barium. The point of twisting can be identified *(arrowhead)*. Some barium has entered the colon.

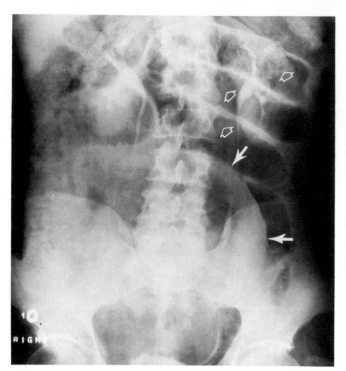

Figure 12–42 **Mechanical Small Bowel Obstruction: Volvulus and Gangrene: Pseudotumor.** Urographic film of a 56 year old man with acute onset of abdominal pain and vomiting reveals a normal urinary tract. However, there are several loops of distended small bowel *(open arrows)* and a soft tissue mass *(arrows)* in the lower abdomen. Some gas and fecal material are seen in the colon.

The soft tissue mass was fluid-filled small bowel loops that had become gangrenous several hours after volvulus.

Mechanical Obstruction of the Large Intestine

Mechanical obstruction of the large intestine is characterized by dilatation of the colon proximal to the site of obstruction. The distention usually ends near the site of obstruction, and the colon distal to the obstruction is usually collapsed and free of gas. Long fluid levels may be present. With a competent unyielding ileocecal valve, distention may become so extreme that perforation of the cecum may occur. If the ileocecal valve is incompetent, small bowel dilatation may be so great that the appearance simulates obstruction of the small intestine. This situation is most frequently found with a right-sided lesion.

Obstruction is most often due to neoplastic or inflammatory disease or to volvulus. Other less common causes include incarcerated hernia, fecal impaction, and extrinsic pelvic tumors. Toxic megacolon, Hirschsprung's disease, and segmental vascular occlusion of the colon can lead to large bowel distention simulating mechanical obstruction.

A barium enema study usually can be safely performed in a case of suspected large bowel obstruction, and the cause and site of the obstruction generally are readily demonstrated.[47]

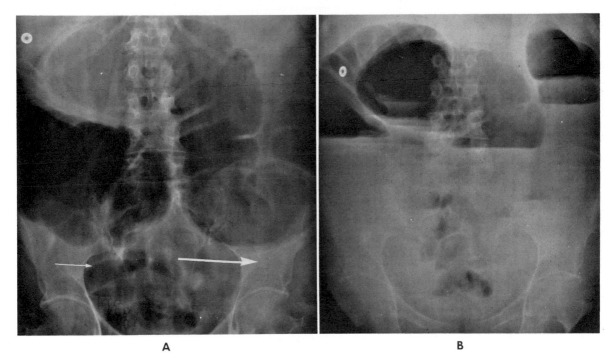

A   B

Figure 12–43 **Mechanical Large Bowel Obstruction.**

A, There is distention from the mid descending colon to the level of the cecum. There is no colonic gas below the mid descending colon *(large arrow),* and the rectal ampulla is empty. The gas in the pelvis is in the small bowel, owing to an incompetent ileocecal valve *(small arrow).*

B, In the erect view there are numerous fluid levels in the distended colon.

At surgery, an obstructing carcinoma of the mid descending colon was found.

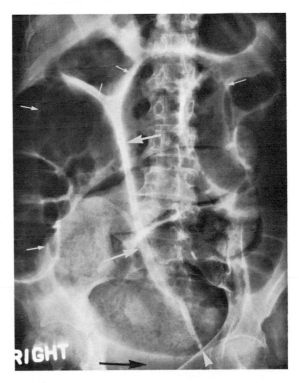

Figure 12–44 **Volvulus of Sigmoid.** A huge distended sigmoid loop has twisted and folded back upon itself *(small arrows).* The soft tissue stripe *(large white arrows)* represents the adjacent walls of the distended sigmoid; the lower portion of this stripe is at the point of twisting *(arrowhead).* The rectum is empty *(black arrow).* The portion of the colon proximal to the volvulus is also obstructed and distended with gas. In lateral decubitus views (not shown), many fluid levels were visualized.

Twisting of the sigmoid on its mesentery generally occurs when the mesentery is long and mobile. A closed loop obstruction results.

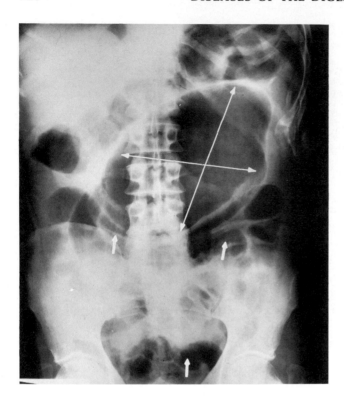

Figure 12–45 **Acute Volvulus of Cecum.** The huge gas shadow in the mid- and left upper abdomen *(double-arrow lines)* is a greatly distended cecum that has undergone volvulus. Some distended small bowel loops are seen *(arrows)*.

Characteristically, in cecal volvulus the distended cecum lies in the upper quadrant.

Pneumatosis Intestinalis

Air in the intestinal walls (pneumatosis) may appear as multiple subserosal cysts (pneumatosis cystoides) and/or as linear collections in the submucosa or subserosa. The condition may be idiopathic or secondary to bowel disease.

The idiopathic form is usually seen in asymptomatic individuals and is generally of the discrete cystic type. It usually occurs in an otherwise normal colon and generally disappears spontaneously. The secondary type is more often linear and is associated with small bowel disease, especially scleroderma or other collagen diseases. More acute bowel insults, such as infarctions, inflammatory necrosis, or obstruction, can also lead to linear pneumatosis, generally with serious prognosis.

Because of overlying bowel gas, the discrete lucent cysts may be difficult to identify without barium studies. If large, they may cause scalloping and multiple defects in the barium column, simulating polyposis or the thumbprinting of ischemic bowel disease. The extension of the discrete lucencies beyond the barium into the soft tissues will identify the lesions radiographically. The linear gas shadows are more easily recognized on plain films, appearing as a lucent line parallel to the bowel gas shadow.

Recurrent or persistent but asymptomatic pneumoperitoneum may result from rupture of the subserosal gas collections. An unexpected and asymptomatic pneumoperitoneum should initiate a search for underlying idiopathic pneumatosis intestinalis.

Pneumatosis of the esophagus and stomach can also occur but is quite rare.[49-56]

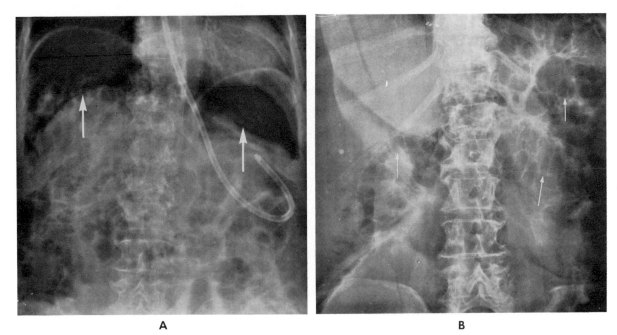

Figure 12–46 **Pneumatosis Intestinalis: Asymptomatic Pneumoperitoneum.**

A, Free air under both diaphragms *(arrows)* is secondary to a rupture of a cyst in the wall of the small intestine.

B, Recumbent view shows multiple gas-filled cysts *(arrows)*, which were in the wall of the small bowel.

Persistent or recurrent pneumoperitoneum in an asymptomatic patient suggests intestinal pneumatosis. The cysts are easier to identify when unobscured by intestinal gas, or on barium examination.

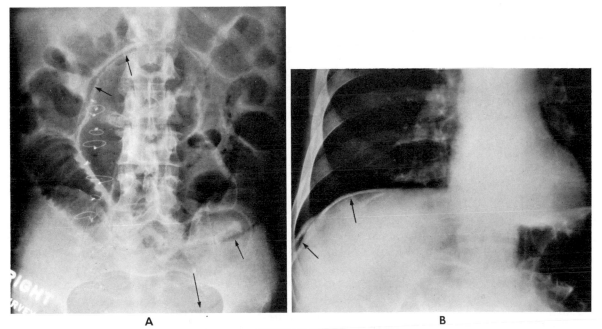

Figure 12–47 **Pneumatosis Intestinalis: Asymptomatic Pneumoperitoneum.**

A, Linear lucent streaks of varying lengths *(arrows)* are scattered throughout the small bowel walls. These are due to coalescence of individual cysts in the outer wall (subserosal). Individual cysts are present but difficult to identify because of overlying intestinal gas shadows.

B, Erect film reveals a small pneumoperitoneum, with free air *(arrows)* under the right diaphragm.

This patient had a long history of scleroderma with marked involvement of the small bowel and malabsorption (small bowel pattern shown in Fig. 3–3). The pneumatosis occurred late in the disease, and the pneumoperitoneum, which later became quite large, remained asymptomatic.

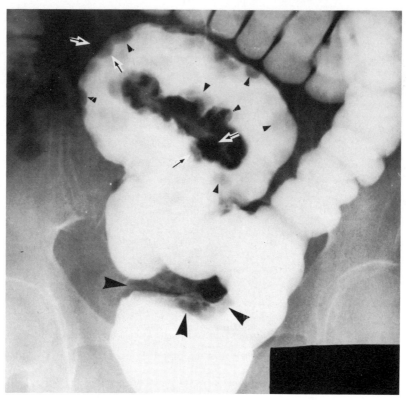

Figure 12–48 **Pneumatosis Intestinalis of Sigmoid.**   The patient was a middle-aged woman complaining of episodic diarrhea. Barium contrast study of the colon discloses multiple lucent defects of varying size *(small arrowheads)* limited to the sigmoid. These give the lumen a scalloped appearance. The lucent areas can be seen extending beyond the barium into the soft tissues *(black-white arrows),* a finding that identifies them as intramural gas cysts. A large gas cyst is deforming the rectosigmoid *(large arrowheads).* These gas cysts were also clearly seen on a plain film of the abdomen. At this time there was no evidence of pneumoperitoneum.

The radiologic appearance is characteristic of pneumatosis cystoides. However, failure to appreciate that the defects are lucent relative to the soft tissues might lead to an erroneous diagnosis of polyposis or vascular occlusion with thumbprinting. This form of pneumatosis is most frequently found in the sigmoid.

Paralytic Ileus

Paralytic ileus denotes the absence of significant intestinal propulsive peristalsis. It may be localized, due to regional inflammation, or generalized, as in peritonitis. Generalized ileus can also be due to trauma, neurogenic factors, certain drugs, and metabolic disturbances with electrolyte imbalance. Paralytic ileus may also be a complication of prolonged mechanical intestinal obstruction.

In generalized ileus there is usually uniform gaseous distention of both the large and small intestine. On postural films, air-fluid levels are commonly seen but they tend to be on the same level in each loop and are less numerous than in mechanical obstruction. If the ileus is due to peritonitis, the walls of the distended bowel become thickened and the properitoneal fat lines are obliterated. In early cases, especially during the early postoperative period, it may be difficult to distinguish radiographically between mechanical and paralytic ileus; serial films may be needed to make the distinction. Occasionally and atypically, there may be enormous distention of the large bowel with relatively little small bowel distention. In extreme cases, cecal perforation can occur. Often, barium enema studies must be made to rule out low large bowel obstruction, which can give a somewhat similar gas pattern.

Localized ileus of the small and, occasionally, the large bowel may occur in the vicinity of an acute inflammatory intra-abdominal condition such as appendicitis, cholecystitis, and pancreatitis. Radiographically there is a persistent local gaseous distention of a bowel loop—the so-called sentinel loop—often with fluid levels.[11, 47, 57]

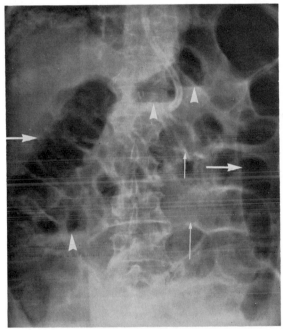

Figure 12-49 **Paralytic Ileus: Hypokalemia.**   Erect view demonstrates uniform distention of both the large (*large arrows*) and the small (*small arrows*) intestine. Some fluid levels are seen (*arrowheads*), but they are not prominent.

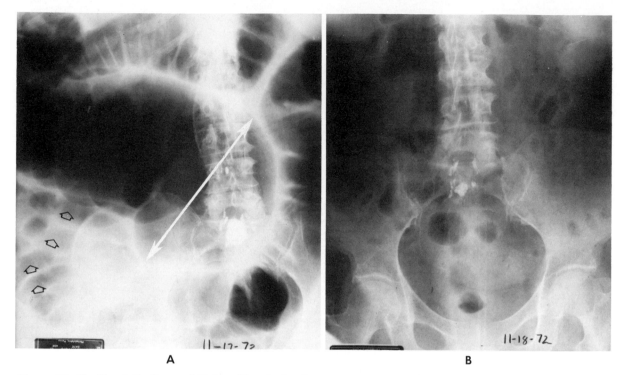

A   B

Figure 12–50 **Paralytic Ileus of Colon: Hypokalemia.**

A, The entire colon, including the rectum, is greatly distended. The cecum is enormously dilated (*double-headed arrow*). Some small bowel distention (*open arrows*) is also present. Barium enema study showed no obstruction.

The patient was markedly hypokalemic. Electrolyte infusion and rectal decompression were initiated.

B, Twenty-four hours later, the abdomen appears completely normal.

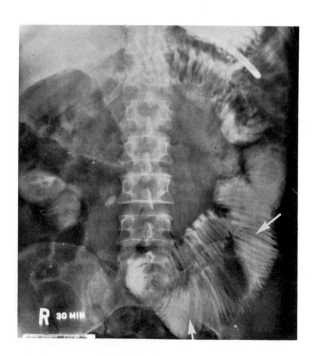

Figure 12–51 **Paralytic Ileus: Post Vagotomy.** A 30-minute film of a barium study of a patient who had recently undergone subtotal gastrectomy and vagotomy shows a dilated barium-filled jejunum (*arrows*). Peristalsis was absent, and the appearance was unchanged two hours later.

Gastric retention and paralytic small bowel ileus may temporarily occur following vagotomy.

Hirschsprung's Disease

In this disorder an aganglionic segment of colon prevents normal passage of peristalsis, and the colon becomes greatly dilated proximal to the aganglionic segment.

Most often the aganglionic segment is a short portion of sigmoid, but longer and more diffuse involvement can occur; the entire length of colon can be involved. The involved segment is usually of normal diameter and distensibility but appears to be relatively narrow by contrast with the dilated proximal colon. The demonstration of this disparity in size is essential in making the radiologic diagnosis, and a true lateral view of the pelvis is frequently needed to reveal the marked change in caliber. Demonstration of a definite transitional zone between the aganglionic segment and the dilated normal segment is the most important diagnostic point. There may be irregular and bizarre contractions in the aganglionic segment. Sometimes the aganglionic segment is almost impossible to demonstrate.

The above findings are the classic changes and are best seen in the older child. In infants and neonates, roentgen diagnosis is often difficult. The aganglionic segment may show nothing more than transient spasm. In an anorectal aganglionosis the narrowed rectum must be distinguished from congenital or inflammatory narrowing.

There is often retention of barium in the dilated colon for 24 to 48 hours after barium enema examination; this is especially frequent in infants. Occasionally there is evidence of an exudative enteropathy with a nodular edematous colon. The latter is secondary to obstruction, and the appearance of the involved segment superficially resembles ulcerative colitis.

Rarely, the entire colon of an infant is aganglionic, causing distention of the small bowel and vomiting. The colon on barium enema study may appear entirely normal, or may be small (microcolon); the radiographic picture is that of low small bowel obstruction without obvious colon disease.

The colon eventually becomes large, redundant, and almost constantly filled with feces; this may predispose to sigmoid volvulus. The rectal ampulla is usually empty, in contradistinction to the situation in chronic constipation, in which the rectal ampulla is dilated with feces.

Occasionally, a persistent megaloureter is encountered, due either to pressure from distended fecal-filled pelvic bowel or to an associated aganglionosis of the ureter.[58-60]

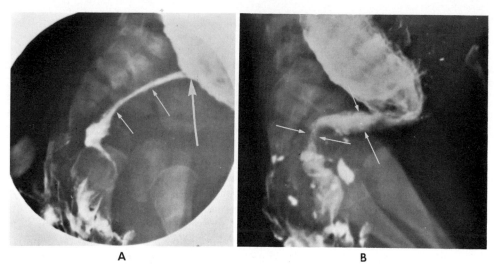

A   B

Figure 12–52   **Hirschsprung's Disease (Congenital Megacolon) in Two Patients.**

A, A 2 week old infant was constipated and vomited after feeding. Lateral view of the barium-filled colon shows a long narrowed aganglionic segment *(small arrows)* of the upper rectum and sigmoid. Note abrupt transition to the dilated proximal colon *(large arrow).*

B, In another patient, barium enema film demonstrates an aganglionic sigmoid segment *(arrows),* which, although of nearly normal caliber, appears narrow when compared to the dilated proximal colon.

In some cases of Hirschsprung's disease the aganglionic segment cannot be demonstrated radiographically; in such cases retention of barium for 24 to 48 hours after the enema examination, uniform dilatation of the colon, and an empty rectum suggest the diagnosis.

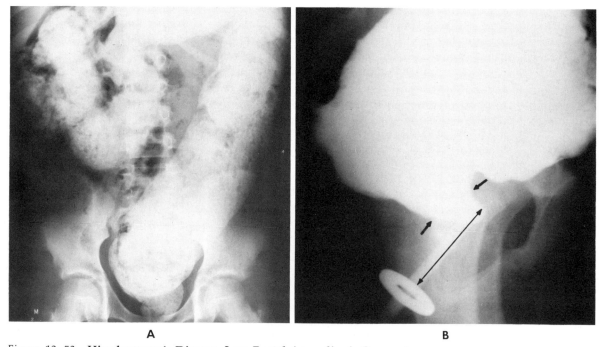

A   B

Figure 12–53   **Hirschsprung's Disease: Low Rectal Aganglionic Segment.**

A, Anteroposterior view during barium enema examination shows a feces-filled colon dilated down to the rectum.

B, Lateral film of the rectal area shows an increased distance between the anal marker and lower rectum *(double-headed arrow)* and narrowing of the lower rectal segment *(arrows).*

Hirschsprung's disease due to a low rectal aganglionic segment is not rare. An anal marker and lateral films are essential for adequate demonstration.

Figure 12-54 **Hirschsprung's Disease: Mega-loureter.** The greatly dilated left ureter seen on the excretory pyelogram had been present for a number of years in this 19 year old boy with anorectal Hirschsprung's disease. Pelvic and caliceal dilatation is minimal. Note that both lower ureters are laterally displaced by the dilated sigmoid and rectum.

Although some investigators believe that the megaloureter sometimes associated with Hirschsprung's disease is due to ureteral aganglionosis, most believe that it represents an incomplete obstruction by the persistently dilated feces-filled lower bowel. In constipated children with a dilated rectum or sigmoid, transient ureteral dilation often occurs.

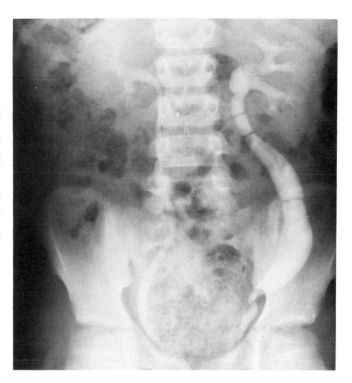

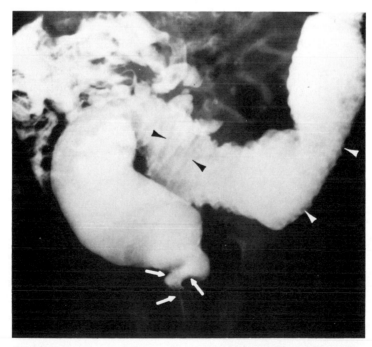

Figure 12-55 **Anorectal Hirschsprung's Disease: Exudative Enteropathy.** There is marked and persistent narrowing of the distal rectum and anus (*arrows*), which were the aganglionic segments.

In the dilated colon proximal to the narrowed rectum, the mucosal folds are greatly thickened (*black arrowheads*), somewhat resembling the valvulae conniventes of small bowel. The margins of the colon have become irregular (*white arrowheads*) owing to the edematous mucosal folds. The appearance suggests an inflammatory colitis (exudative enteropathy).

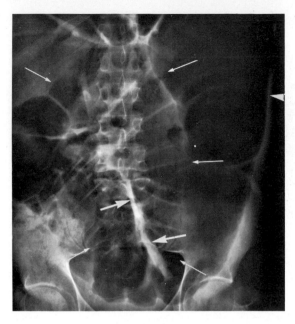

Figure 12–56 **Hirschsprung's Disease: Complicating Volvulus of Sigmoid.** A 30 year old man had Hirschsprung's disease and recent severe abdominal distention. The dilated and elongated double loop of sigmoid *(small arrows)* in the pelvis has twisted upon itself and has caused obstruction and dilatation of the proximal colon *(arrowhead)*. A white line *(large arrows)*, representing the double wall of the sigmoid, extends down to the point of obstruction. The rectum is empty below the point of obstruction.

The megasigmoid of Hirschsprung's disease is more prone to volvulus than is a normal sigmoid.

Diverticula of the Intestinal Tract

Zenker's Diverticulum (Pulsion Diverticulum)

A pulsion diverticulum occurs posteriorly in the lower cervical region at the junction of the cricopharyngeus and the inferior pharyngeal constrictor muscles. Dysphagia occurs when the diverticulum fills with food and secretions and impinges on the cervical esophagus. Recurrent aspiration pneumonia is a frequent complication.

Following a barium meal, the diverticulum appears as a rounded sac posterior to the esophageal lumen. It may reach 8 to 10 cm. in diameter. Larger diverticula may extend laterally into the neck or thoracic inlet and appear as mass densities in films of the chest. Occasionally a fluid level may be seen within the mass.[13]

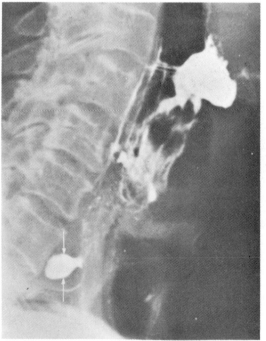

Figure 12–57 **Zenker's Diverticulum.** A smooth round outpouching arises posteriorly at the junction of the pharyngeal and cervical esophagus *(arrows)*. The diverticulum is small and is not significantly compromising the esophageal lumen.

Other Diverticula of the Esophagus

Traction diverticula of the middle third of the esophagus are the most frequent. These lesions appear as barium-filled sacs, with or without a neck, extending horizontally from the esophagus. Occasionally multiple lesions are seen. The traction diverticulum contains all esophageal muscular layers, empties readily, and is usually asymptomatic. The average size is 1 to 3 cm.

Epiphrenic diverticula are relatively rare. They develop in the lower esophagus, most often on the right. Sometimes they become quite large. They are pulsion diverticula, containing only mucosa and submucosa. Emptying is slow, and larger lesions are often associated with dysphagia, owing to esophageal compression. Neuromuscular dysfunction and hiatal hernia are often associated and are probably predisposing factors.[61]

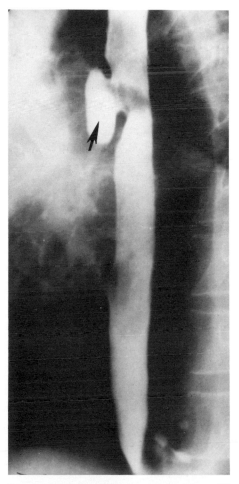

Figure 12–58 **Traction Diverticulum of Mid-Esophagus.** The barium-filled pouch *(arrow)* arising from the mid-esophagus has a neck and emptied readily. It contains all esophageal layers and is usually entirely asymptomatic.

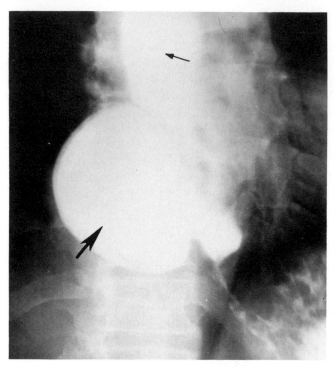

Figure 12–59 **Pulsion Epiphrenic Diverticulum of Lower Esophagus.**   This epiphrenic diverticulum *(large arrow)* is characteristically to the right of the lower esophagus. It is unusually large and is compressing the lumen, causing proximal esophageal dilatation *(small arrow).*

Epiphrenic diverticula are pulsion lesions which empty poorly and can cause dysphagia.

Gastric Diverticula

Diverticula occur in the stomach less frequently than in any other gastrointestinal organ. They are asymptomatic and are found in the juxtacardiac region, on the medial side. A small number occur in the prepyloric area.

Radiographically, the diverticulum appears as a characteristic outpouching, usually with a thin neck. Emptying readily occurs. Small diverticula in the prepyloric area may, at first glance, be mistaken for an ulceration, but identification is generally easy because of the absence of edema, spasm, and the other signs associated with ulcer disease. Occasionally, a small diverticulum may lie intramurally.[62]

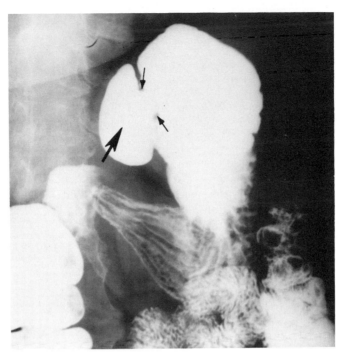

Figure 12–60 **Gastric Diverticulum.** The large smooth barium-filled pouch *(large arrow)* is connected to the cardiac portion of the stomach by a neck *(small arrows).* The location is characteristic of the majority of gastric diverticula, which are asymptomatic and of no particular clinical significance. Most gastric diverticula are smaller than the above.

Prediverticulosis and Diverticulosis of the Large Intestine

Prediverticulosis, or spastic colon diverticulosis, is an entity that has been confused roentgenographically with diverticulitis. The roentgen changes are confined to the sigmoid and, occasionally, the lower descending colon. The sigmoid appears narrowed and shortened with irregular borders. There are large wedge-shaped indentations, frequently asymmetric, giving rise to a sawtooth or palisade appearance. Diverticula are occasionally seen. The sawtooth appearance is due to thickening and shortening of the teniae, with subsequent shortening of the bowel and infolding of the mucosa. The heaped circular muscle projects into the lumen. These changes may precede formation of diverticula. Some investigators believe that prediverticulosis is a variant of the irritable colon syndrome.

Acquired diverticula of the large bowel are very common, especially among older persons, and the incidence and number of these diverticula increase with age. They are most frequent and numerous in the sigmoid and descending colon, but may occur in any portion of the colon. Like other acquired intestinal diverticula, they contain no muscular layer and empty poorly. The diverticula vary considerably in size, but unless inflamed, they produce no definite clinical symptoms. Occasionally bleeding may occur without inflammation.

Massive hemorrhage is sometimes due to a bleeding diverticulum, particularly in the right colon. Selective mesenteric arteriography is usually the only radiographic procedure that will disclose the exact bleeding point[63-66] and is of value in selecting the proper surgical approach.

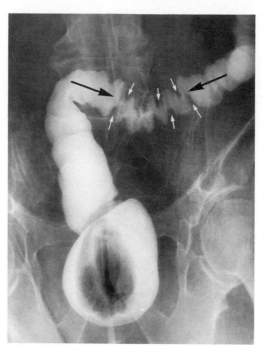

Figure 12–61 **Prediverticulosis of Sigmoid.**   The sigmoid is quite short, and one segment *(between black arrows)* shows the characteristic gross serrations of prediverticulosis. The wedge-shaped indentations *(white arrows)* between the "teeth" are due to thickening of the circular muscles and not to actual mucosal thickening. There are no diverticula.

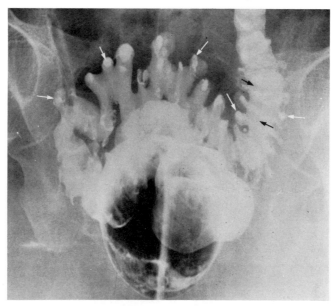

Figure 12–62 **Prediverticulosis and Diverticulosis of Sigmoid and Distal Descending Colon.**   In an angulated view of the sigmoid there is a relatively short sigmoid with the irregular serrations characteristic of prediverticulosis, similar to the appearance in Figure 12–61. Diverticula *(white arrows)* have developed in practically every projection between the thickened circular muscles. In the lower descending colon the appearance is more regular, due to more uniform circumferential muscular thickening *(black arrows).*

The areas of muscular thickening are sometimes erroneously interpreted as thickened mucosa from chronic inflammation.

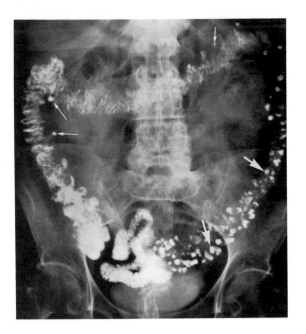

Figure 12-63 **Extensive Diverticulosis of Colon.** Postevacuation film following a barium enema shows numerous barium-filled diverticula diffusely spread throughout the sigmoid and descending colon *(large arrows)*. They are of fairly uniform size. A few diverticula are seen in the transverse and right colon *(small arrows)*.

Because of their inherent poor emptying, the diverticula remain filled after evacuation and are often seen most clearly on postevacuation films.

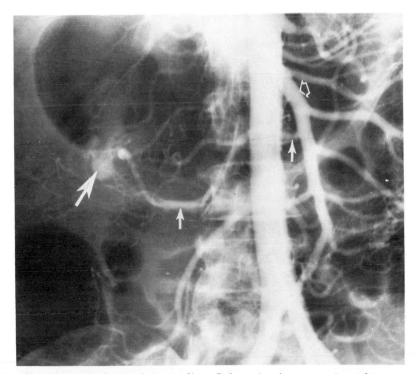

Figure 12-64 **Bleeding Diverticulum of Ascending Colon: Angiogram.** A midstream aortic angiogram made during severe unexplained rectal bleeding discloses extravasation of contrast material *(large arrow)* in the right upper quadrant. The involved vessel is the right colic branch *(small arrows)* of the superior mesenteric artery *(open arrow)*, indicating that the bleeding is in the right colon. Selective arteriography is usually necessary in order to demonstrate the bleeding site.

Surgery disclosed a bleeding diverticulum in the ascending colon.

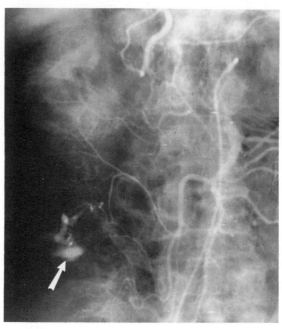

Figure 12–65 **Bleeding Diverticulum of Ascending Colon: Selective Superior Mesenteric Arteriogram.** Severe life-threatening gastrointestinal bleeding without localizing clinical symptoms was investigated by celiac and mesenteric arteriography. During the latter study, extravasation of dye into a pouch-like area *(arrow)* was observed. This proved to be a solitary bleeding diverticulum in the ascending colon.
  Diverticular bleeding is most likely to occur from a right-sided colonic diverticulum.

Meckel's Diverticulum

The congenital Meckel's diverticulum is usually found in the distal few feet of the ileum. Unlike acquired diverticula, Meckel's pouch always arises in the antimesenteric side of the ileum, and it contains all the muscular layers of the small bowel.

A nondiseased Meckel's diverticulum is rarely identified radiographically because its muscular coat permits rapid emptying of barium and because it can easily be mistaken for overlapping portions of a normal small bowel loop.

Recognition usually requires careful and repeated small bowel roentgen studies. The diverticulum may be found in any quadrant of the abdomen and frequently contains air mixed with barium. It usually appears as an oval or rounded pouch that may contain heterotopic gastric mucosa. Recognition of such mucosa may draw the radiologist's attention to an otherwise inconspicuous Meckel's pouch.

The most common complications are bleeding from ulceration, inflammation, obstruction, and perforation. The inflamed or ulcerated diverticulum can often be identified by a persistent air collection within the structure. Occasionally, enteroliths can be identified within the diverticulum. If causing obstruction or perforation, the diverticulum can generally not be recognized radiographically. If a bleeding diverticulum cannot be recognized on a small bowel study, mesenteric arteriography may identify a bleeding site in the ileum.[67-69]

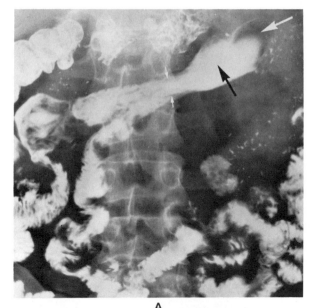

A

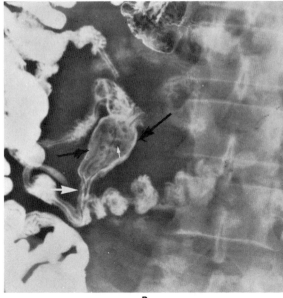

B

Figure 12–66 **Meckel's Diverticulum: Three Cases.**

The patients were young adults, and unexplained gastrointestinal bleeding was the chief clinical problem in each case.

A, A late small bowel film demonstrates a pear-shaped, barium-filled sac *(black arrow)* in the left midabdomen. Air is trapped in the diverticulum *(large white arrow)*. The neck is long and resembles normal small bowel *(small white arrows)*. The mucosal pattern is not well defined. (Courtesy Dr. A. Finkelstein, Philadelphia, Pennsylvania.)

B, The diverticulum *(black arrows)* is smaller and pear-shaped, and lies in the right midabdomen. The mucosal pattern *(small white arrow)* resembles gastric folds. The neck *(large white arrow)* of the diverticulum is narrow and contains normal small bowel mucosa.

C, The diverticulum *(arrows)* is low in the right pelvis, is round, contains folds like those of the stomach, and has a wide neck.

Note that in each of the three patients the diverticulum was in a different segment of the abdomen. (Courtesy A. S. Berne, Syracuse, New York.)

C

Diverticula of the Small Intestine

Diverticula are outpouchings of the mucosa through a small defect in the muscle coat. Almost all diverticula of the small bowel are acquired. They are found with increasing frequency in older individuals. The diverticula are usually found on the mesenteric side of the bowel and may vary considerably in size. Often they gradually increase in size over a period of years. Diverticula of the duodenum are very common, especially in the loop. Jejunal diverticula are considerably less common, and ileal lesions are very rare.

Diverticula empty poorly because of the absence of a muscular coat. Even when large, they are usually asymptomatic, but large collections of jejunal diverticula can cause stasis and bacterial overgrowth and sometimes can bring about the malabsorption syndrome and megaloblastic anemia.

The rare *intraluminal* duodenal diverticulum presents a characteristic radiographic appearance in which the diverticular wall appears as a lucent line within the barium-filled duodenum. It is a developmental anomaly and may be symptomatic.[70, 71]

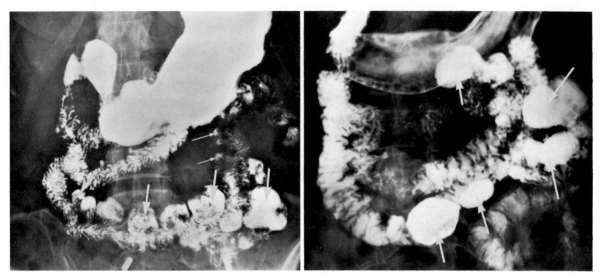

Figure 12–67 **Jejunal Diverticulosis: Two Cases.** Numerous jejunal diverticula *(arrows)* of varying size are seen, many of which contain filling defects due to retained food and secretions. These diverticula generally have a narrow neck.

Both patients had malabsorption.

Miscellaneous Disorders

Hypertrophy of the Ileocecal Valve

On barium enema films, the superior and inferior lips of the normal ileocecal valve may produce transverse or oval defects, usually on the medial side of the cecum, above and below the intramural portion of the terminal ileum.

Hypertrophy of the valve is not rare and is characterized by enlargement of one or both lips, sometimes accompanied by narrowing of the intramural portion of the terminal ileum. The hypertrophied valves are usually smooth in outline, although they may occasionally be lobulated. These changes are most often due to fatty infiltration. These defects may simulate a neoplasm, but generally their shape and location are quite characteristic.

The hypertrophied valve is usually asymptomatic although occasionally there may be recurrent right lower quadrant pain, suggesting appendicitis or regional enteritis. In some adults, enlargement of the valve is associated with intermittent ileocecal obstruction.[72-74]

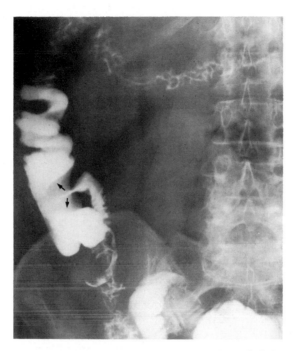

Figure 12-68 **Hypertrophied Ileocecal Valve.** The sharply marginated defects *(arrows)* above and below the intramural portion of the terminal ileum are the lips of a hypertrophied ileocecal valve. A normal valve is rarely more than half this size.

Gastritis

The roentgenogram is of limited value in the detection and evaluation of diffuse gastritis, since the radiologic appearance of the gastric folds correlates poorly with the gross, histologic, and gastroscopic mucosal findings.

In acute gastritis, no radiographic changes are usually seen; the superficial erosions are generally difficult to demonstrate. In severe acute phlegmonous gastritis, there may be persistent spastic deformities, disappearance of normal folds, and irregularities of the gastric margins — findings that can simulate extensive neoplasia.

In chronic hypertrophic gastritis the roentgenographic findings may vary from completely normal to greatly enlarged folds, especially in the fundus and proximal half of the stomach. No rigidity or contour deformities are seen. Secretions may or may not be increased. Giant hypertrophy of the folds is also found in Menetrier's disease (see p. 940). Lymphomatous or neoplastic submucosal involvement can sometimes closely simulate thickened folds; however, infiltrated folds cannot be obliterated by compression or by gastric distention, in contrast to noninfiltrated thickened folds.

In antral gastritis, roentgen changes are more frequent, since this area is narrower and more easily deformed. The folds may be thickened and distorted; antral folds over 5 mm. in width are suggestive of significant inflammatory involvement. Irregularities and narrowing of the antral contour may occur, sometimes closely simulating malignant disease. Normal antral distention is lacking. Often the distorted folds become attenuated and straightened during antral peristalsis, suggesting their nonmalignant nature.

In chronic atrophic gastritis the mucosal serrations along the greater curvature may be unusually small and regular. The fundus has a bald appearance, and a fine stippling may appear at the barium-air interface in the erect position (see p. 1137). The atrophic stomach of the elderly may also show limited distensibility, irregularity of the distal stomach simulating scirrhous carcinoma, and gastric retention. Achlorhydria is usually present.

Eosinophilic gastritis is discussed on page 124.

Cineradiography or videotape of the contrast-filled stomach can be extremely helpful in evaluating the changes in the folds during gastric motility, and in detecting subtle but significant alterations in peristalsis, especially in the lower half of the stomach.[63, 75-79]

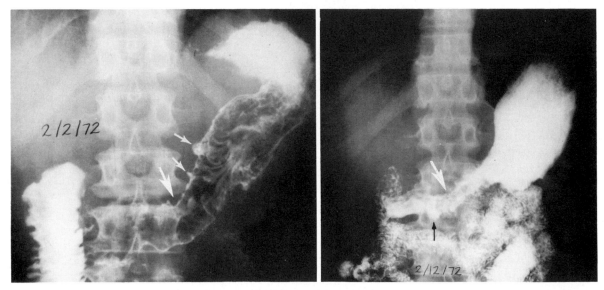

Figure 12–69 **Acute Phlegmonous Gastritis.**   The distal two thirds of the stomach is narrowed, spiculated, and irregular *(large arrows)*. The mucosal folds are virtually obliterated, and multiple ulcerations are apparent *(small arrows)*.

Severe edema and persistent spasm are responsible for this alarming appearance, which simulates an infiltrating neoplasm. Most often, acute gastritis produces only thickened folds with no significant changes.

The stomach became completely normal radiographically within a few weeks.

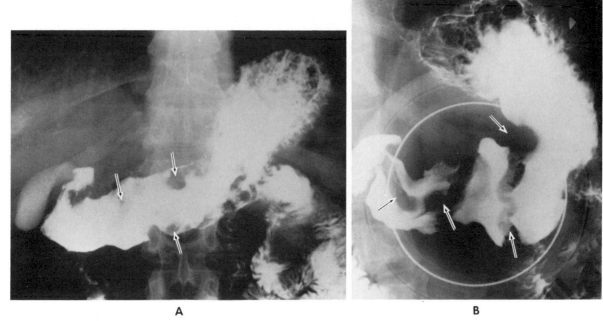

A   B

Figure 12–70 **Severe Hypertrophic Gastritis in a 60 Year Old Man.**

A, Posteroanterior film discloses distortion of the lower half of the stomach by multiple defects *(arrows).*

B, Oblique projection with compression shows huge folds *(arrows)* in the distal body and antrum. The mucosal pattern in the upper half of the stomach is entirely normal. The duodenum was normal.

The filling defects and contour deformity raised the possibility of a neoplastic process, but the pattern of the defects and their alteration during peristalsis were characteristic of greatly enlarged folds. Similar findings can occur in lymphomatous disease and in Menetrier's disease, although in the latter the fundus is usually involved. At surgery, a hypertrophic gastritis was found.

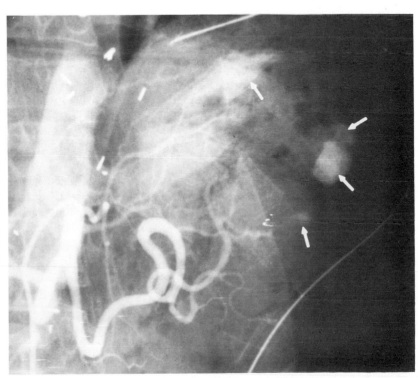

Figure 12–71 **Acute Hemorrhagic Gastritis: Angiogram.** Celiac angiography in an alcoholic with severe hematemesis reveals multiple collections of extravasated contrast material *(arrows)* in the gastric wall. The bleeding erosions were due to an acute alcoholic gastritis.

The superficial erosions of gastritis are almost impossible to demonstrate by barium studies.

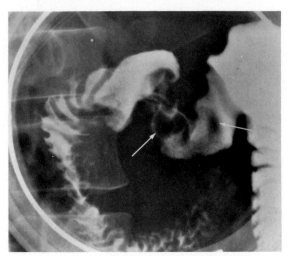

Figure 12–72 **Antral Gastritis.**   Mucosal folds are prominent in the antral portion of the stomach *(arrows)* and cause marked distortion and narrowing of the antrum. Serial films and fluoroscopy demonstrated alteration of the folds during peristalsis, which was considered to be evidence of benignity.

Frequently the lesions of antral gastritis cannot be radiographically distinguished from an infiltrating malignant neoplasm; cineradiography or interval radiographic studies may be required, and occasionally gastroscopy may be helpful. Surgical exploration is often performed when the diagnosis remains uncertain.

Giant Hypertrophy of the Gastric Mucosa (Menetrier's Disease)

This rare disease of unknown cause is characterized by enlargement of the gastric rugae and development of excess gastric mucus. It may be associated with the syndrome of multiple endocrine adenomatosis and may be a cause of hypoproteinemia. The patient may either be asymptomatic or have ulcer-like symptoms.

Radiologically, the marked enlargement of the gastric rugae is the most important finding. The enlarged tortuous folds may resemble the convolutional pattern of the brain. This characteristic appearance, however, is seen in less than half the cases. The giant rugae occur mainly in the greater curvature and proximal half of the stomach, the lesser curvature and the antral portion being less frequently and less extensively involved. The most frequent roentgenologic abnormality is the irregular and spiculated appearance of the greater curvature, which is indirect evidence of mucosal thickening. There is usually an abrupt transition between the abnormal and normal folds. An excess of gastric mucus is often present, lending a flocculated and reticular appearance to the barium. Occasionally thickening of the gastric wall may be demonstrated. Although no single sign is pathognomonic, combinations of these findings are highly suggestive.[80, 81]

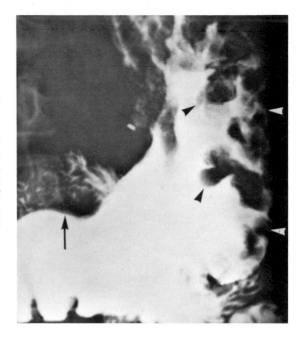

Figure 12–73 **Giant Hypertrophy of Gastric Mucosa (Menetrier's Disease).** The patient was a 42 year old man with a long history of epigastric pain, hypoalbuminemia, and edema. The gastric rugae *(black arrowheads)* are much enlarged, and the greater curvature is irregular *(white arrowheads).* The lesser curvature *(arrow)* is essentially normal in appearance. There is no evidence of flocculation of barium or thickening of the gastric wall. Giant folds are the outstanding feature of Menetrier's disease, yet without other corroborating findings they are not diagnostic. Similar giant folds may be found in lymphoma or gastritis.

Herniated Gastric Folds

Prolapse of antral gastric folds into the base of the duodenal bulb is a frequent finding, the significance of which is uncertain. Although usually asymptomatic, patients with this finding occasionally have ulcer-like symptoms.

On the roentgenogram, a lobulated filling defect, seen at the base of the duodenal bulb, gives rise to an umbrella defect. The herniated folds are generally most prominent during antral peristalsis and may disappear or decrease in size when the antrum is relaxed.

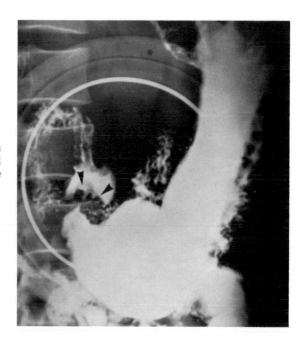

Figure 12–74 **Herniated Gastric Folds.** There is a symmetric indentation at the base of the duodenal bulb *(arrowheads),* due to herniated gastric folds. The patient was asymptomatic.

Hypertrophied Glands of Brunner

Brunner's glands occur in the submucosa of the duodenal bulb and in the prox- imal portion of the duodenal loop. When hypertrophied, they appear as multiple rounded radiolucencies, giving a cobblestone appearance to the barium-filled bulb and postbulbar area; they probably do not cause symptoms. The roentgen appear- ance is usually sufficiently characteristic for correct diagnosis. However, adenoma- tous hyperplasia of a single gland can produce a large duodenal filling defect that cannot be distinguished from a true tumor. It is postulated that the glands become enlarged in response to gastric hyperacidity.[82]

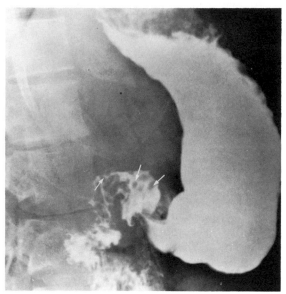

Figure 12–75 **Hypertrophied Glands of Brunner.** Multiple small discrete lucent defects in the duodenal bulb and the proximal loop *(arrows)* are due to hypertrophied Brunner's glands. The patient was asymp- tomatic.

Allergic or Angioneurotic Edema of the Gastrointestinal Tract

In some individuals with a history of angioneurotic edema, recurrent attacks of abdominal pain, nausea, and vomiting occur, lasting 1 to 5 days. These are as- sociated with focal areas of edema of the small bowel and occasionally of the colon.

The involved small bowel loops reveal thickened mucosal folds, spiculation, thumbprinting, and separation of loops by mural and mesenteric thickening, find- ings that simulate small bowel ischemia or intramural bleeding. Rapid disappear- ance of the symptoms and radiographic changes should suggest the diagnosis.

Focal areas of colonic involvement may show large submucosal defects or, if mucosal urticaria develops, may produce a striking and unique reticulated, blister- like pattern.

Occasionally, focal bowel edema may form a mass that can lead to intussus- ception.[83-85]

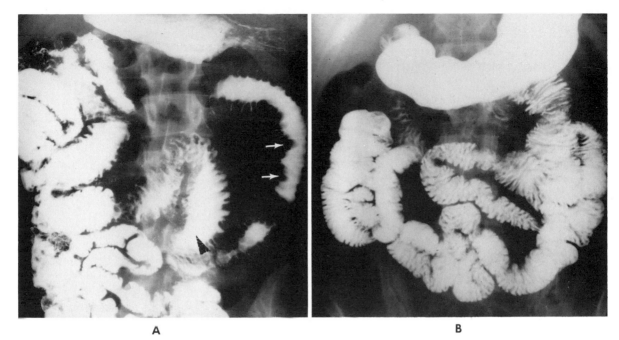

A   **B**

Figure 12–76 **Angioneurotic Edema of Jejunum.**

A, The proximal jejunal loop is edematous with thickened folds and thumbprinting *(arrows).* Distally, there is another widened edematous loop *(arrowhead)* with thickened folds. These loops were fixed.

The appearance of these loops is indistinguishable from an ischemic or hemorrhagic bowel.

B, Thirty-six hours later, the small bowel appears entirely normal. This 24 year old man has had repeated episodes of angioneurotic edema and recurrent attacks of abdominal pain and nausea that last from two to five days. (Courtesy Dr. K. D. Pearson, Santa Rosa, California.)

Figure 12–77 **Urticaria of Colon.** Barium enema made because of suspected cecal volvulus demonstrates the torsion point of the volvulus *(arrow).*

Of radiographic interest is the peculiar reticulated pigskin mucosal pattern *(arrowheads)* in the transverse colon and in the cecum just beyond the volvulus. This appearance has been reported to be characteristic of colonic mucosal urticaria, and in this case diagnosis was confirmed at surgery.

Although focal bowel urticaria can lead to intussusception, its relationship to the volvulus in this patient is not clear.

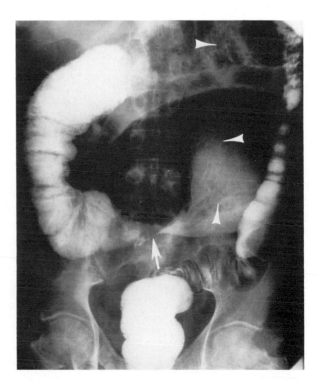

PEPTIC ULCER

Peptic Ulcer of the Esophagus

Benign ulcer of the lower third of the esophagus is most often a complication of reflux esophagitis, with or without hiatal hernia. The ulcer is frequently superficial and shallow and often may not be demonstrated radiographically. Signs of peptic esophagitis are usually present: an irritable distal esophagus with decreased distensibility, thickened folds, and a serrated indistinct border. The distal esophagus may show irregular peristaltic contractions and incomplete emptying. Stricture of the esophagus may eventually develop.

A constant crater must be demonstrated for definitive diagnosis. Mucosal folds radiating to the crater, and a spastic incisura on the opposite wall may be seen. Proximal dilatation is frequent. Rarely, perforation of the ulcer occurs.

A benign discrete ulcer of the lower esophagus located well above the esophagogastric junction is usually a Barrett ulcer, so called because it develops in heterotopic mucosa lined with columnar epithelium (Barrett's epithelium). Its higher location is its only distinctive radiographic feature. Diagnosis can often be confirmed by esophagoscopy. Barrett's epithelium may not be congenital but may develop as a consequence of reflux esophagitis.[16, 23, 63, 86]

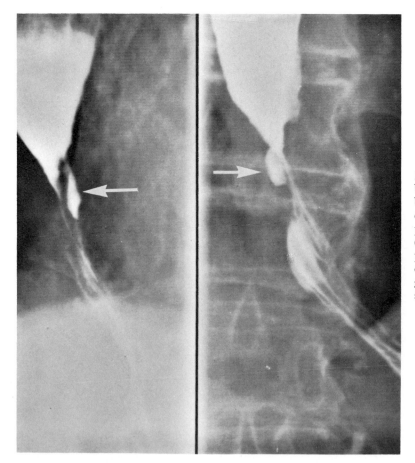

Figure 12–78 **Discrete Peptic Ulcer of Esophagus: Barrett's Ulcer.** A 56 year old man had dysphagia and lower substernal pain. There is a discrete ulcer (*arrow*) in the narrow lower esophageal segment, with moderate dilatation above it. Heterotopic gastric epithelium was demonstrated at biopsy.

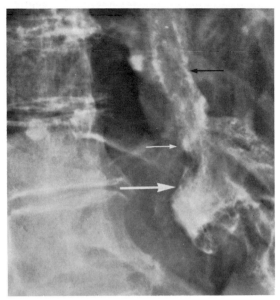

Figure 12–79 **Peptic Esophagitis.** The mucosa of the esophagus is irregular and swollen (*black arrow*), and the lower esophagus failed to become distended. These changes were due to reflux esophagitis. A hiatal hernia is present (*large arrow*), and reflux was demonstrated fluoroscopically. The outpouching (*small white arrow*) was an ulcer crater.

Benign Gastric Ulcer

Roentgenographic examination is the primary diagnostic tool for demonstrating gastric ulcers. It is also important in the recognition of complications, the evaluation of healing, and the differentiation of benign from malignant ulcers. Over 90 per cent of gastric ulcers can be shown radiographically; superficial gastric erosions and ulcers are usually not demonstrable. In 30 to 40 per cent of bleeding ulcers a crater may not be demonstrated, since it is filled with fibrin and clot. The vast majority of benign ulcers occur on the lesser curvature.

The benign ulcer arises in the mucosa and extends beyond the stomach lumen, whereas in carcinoma the primary process is a tumor growing within the wall and lumen of the stomach, with secondary ulceration within the tumor. Benign ulcer presents radiographically as a smooth, well-defined collection of barium projecting beyond the normal limits of the stomach. In profile, a thin radiolucent line measuring 1 to 2 mm. in thickness may be visible at the base of the ulcer. This lucent line (Hampton's line) is due to the thin overhanging marginal mucosa of the crater, and is probably the most reliable radiologic sign of a benign lesion. Another important sign of benignity is the presence of an ulcer collar. This is a lucent ring of thickened mucosa and submucosa between the ulcer niche and the stomach lumen, giving the ulcer a collar-button appearance. When visualized *en face,* the ulcer appears as a persistent rounded collection surrounded by a halo of edema. The presence of intact mucosal folds radiating to the ulcer crater and the absence of rigidity and infiltration are also important findings. An incisura is frequently found on the wall of the stomach opposite the ulcer crater. The incisura can occasionally be mistaken for a mass filling defect. Without multiple projections, a small gastric ulcer may be missed.

Pyloric channel ulcers are usually shallow but project beyond the lumen. The channel may be spastic, narrowed, and abnormally angulated, but often no narrowing is present. Radiating folds and a surrounding halo of edema are rarely seen. Healing and scarring can cause abnormal channel angulation and sometimes an obstructive stricture.

The size and location of the crater are of dubious value in differentiating benign from malignant ulcer, but statistically ulcers in the fundus or the cardia are more apt to be malignant. The most reliable evidence of benignity is the roentgenologic demonstration of complete healing. A decrease in the size of a crater may occur in a malignant ulcer, but there is almost never complete disappearance.

The most important finding in the diagnosis of malignant ulcer is the demonstration of a surrounding mass. There may also be distortion or destruction of the mucosal pattern, fixation, rigidity, and absence of peristalsis. The malignant ulcer tends to be within the confines of the stomach. Nodulation may occur at the base of the ulcer but is not a reliable indication of malignancy, since food or blood clot can simulate this appearance.

The overall accuracy of the radiologic differentiation of benign from malignant lesions approaches 90 per cent. Detection and correct interpretation of gastric lesions can be made in over 80 per cent of cases. Angiography is generally not reliable for differentiation between benign and malignant gastric ulcer. Fiberoptic endoscopy in expert hands will often be helpful in making the distinction. Endoscopy can also usually detect superficial or shallow ulcerations that are difficult to demonstrate radiographically.[76, 87-90]

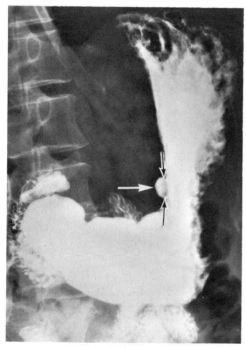

Figure 12–80 **Benign Gastric Ulcer.** A smooth circumscribed ulcer *(white arrow)* projects beyond the stomach. A thin radiolucent line (Hampton's line) *(black-white arrows)* is present at the base of the crater. This is the most reliable roentgenologic sign of benignity. There was no fixation or rigidity. Follow-up study after medical management indicated complete healing of the ulcer crater.

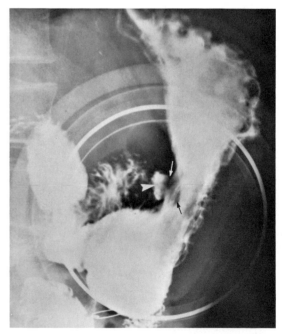

Figure 12–81 **Benign Gastric Ulcer with Ulcer Collar.** There is a large ulcer *(arrowhead)* with a lucent collar *(white arrow)* between the ulcer crater and the stomach wall. Thick edematous folds are present at the base of the ulcer *(black arrow).*

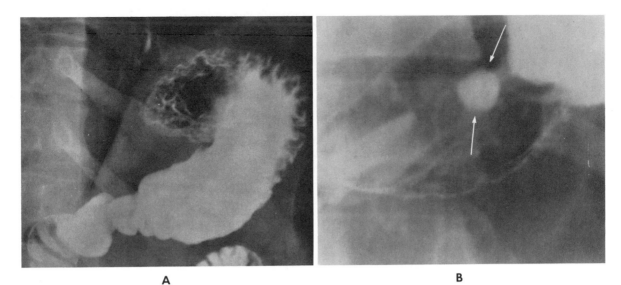

A   B

Figure 12–82   **Gastric Ulcer: Gastrointestinal Bleeding.**

A, Routine oblique view in upper gastrointestinal examination fails to demonstrate any abnormalities.

B, Supine, right posterior oblique projection (Schatzki's position) reveals accumulation of barium within an ulcer crater *(arrows).* No radiographic study of a patient with gastrointestinal bleeding is complete without a film done in the Schatzki position. In this position the lesser curvature of the stomach becomes dependent, and small ulcer craters in the lesser curvature, which are frequently not seen on other routine projections, are often visualized *en face.*

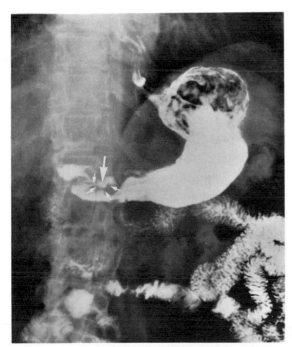

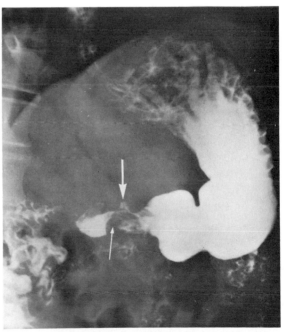

Figure 12–84 **Benign Antral Ulcer.** The ulcer crater *(large arrow)* projects onto the lesser curvature of the antrum. There is an incisura *(small arrow)* opposite the ulcer. The surrounding mucosa is thickened but intact, and the pyloric canal is somewhat eccentric due to spasm. There is no evidence of pyloric obstruction, and no rigidity was noted.

Figure 12–83 **Benign Prepyloric Ulcer.** There is a smoothly marginated prepyloric ulcer *(large arrow)* surrounded by thickened folds radiating to the crater *(small arrows).* The barium-filled spaces between the folds are thin and clearly outlined, indicating absence of infiltration.

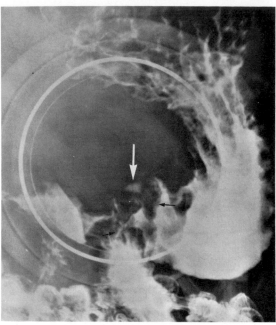

Figure 12–85 **Gastric Ulcer Associated with Gastritis.** There is an ulcer (*white arrow*) of the lesser curvature of the antrum. The mucosal folds are thickened and irregular (*black arrows*). The bizarre pattern of the antral mucosa, which is commonly seen in antral gastritis, makes differentiation from a carcinoma difficult. However, in antral gastritis the folds become thinner and more regular during peristaltic contraction of the antrum.

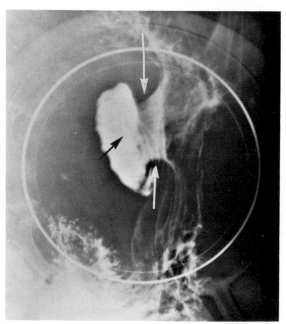

Figure 12–86 **Large Benign Ulcer of Lesser Curvature.** A huge ulcer (*black arrow*) projecting beyond the stomach gives a collar-button appearance (*white arrows*). It is difficult to evaluate the condition of the mucosa. Swelling and edema near the ulcer crater have caused apparent rigidity.

This type of ulcer is difficult to evaluate roentgenologically and must be followed closely. It was thought to be an ulcer crater of indeterminate type. At surgery it was found to be benign.

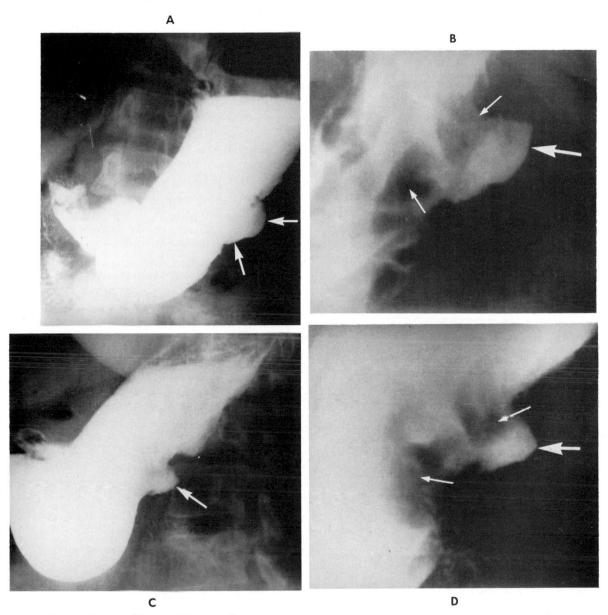

Figure 12–87   **Benign Ulcer of Greater Curvature.**

A and *B,* Films of the stomach of a 40 year old woman with upper quadrant pain disclose a large, smoothly marginated ulcer *(large arrows)* on the greater curvature. The ulcer projects beyond the confines of the rest of the lumen. The lucencies *(small arrows)* surrounding the ulcer represent edematous gastric folds.

C and *D,* After three weeks of antiulcer therapy, the ulcer *(large arrows)* has decreased to less than half its original size. The thickened folds *(small arrows),* however, persist. Note that the ulcer now no longer projects significantly beyond the other luminal margins. (This finding, if present originally, would be suggestive of malignancy.) Complete healing occurred within the next six weeks.

Formerly it was believed that ulcers on the greater curvature were more likely to be malignant than were ulcers on the lesser curvature. This assumption has not proved accurate. In current practice, surgical investigation is strongly recommended if any gastric ulcer does not heal completely in four to six weeks. Although malignant ulcers may decrease in size after medical treatment, complete healing rarely occurs.

Duodenal Ulcer

Over 90 per cent of duodenal ulcers arise in the first portion of the duodenum (the bulb). The only unequivocal diagnostic sign of active duodenal ulcer is the demonstration of an ulcer crater, which can be seen in about 80 to 90 per cent of the cases. The crater appears as a rounded or linear deposit of contrast material that is usually surrounded by lucent thickened folds often in a radiating pattern. When seen in profile, the ulcer appears to be a niche of barium projecting beyond the bulb. The ulcer may occur in any part of the duodenal bulb but is most frequently seen on the posterior wall. Multiple ulcerations can occur.

When the bulb is irritable and retains little barium, it may be difficult to demonstrate a crater. If the bulb is scarred, it may be difficult or impossible to differentiate the barium trapped between folds from an active ulcer crater.

A secondary sign of duodenal ulcer disease is deformity of the bulb due to edema and spasm of the muscularis. This causes straightening of the wall near the ulcer and formation of an incisura opposite the crater. If the ulcer is eccentric and near the base of the bulb, there may be apparent eccentricity of the pyloric canal. The mucosal folds of the bulb may be thickened and edematous, another secondary sign.

If an acute ulcer is superficial and confined to the mucosa, no deformity or other secondary signs are seen, and if the crater cannot be demonstrated, the study may appear completely negative. Secondary signs without a crater may suggest ulcer disease but are not diagnostic of active duodenal ulcer.

Tenderness and irritability of the bulb are unreliable signs to which little significance should be attached.

Occasionally a giant ulcer may involve the entire bulb area and simulate a deformed bulb. The unchanging appearance of the barium collection may provide the only clue.

Fibrosis and scarring occur with chronicity. This may result in relative narrowing, and the recesses at the base of the bulb may become enlarged and prominent, thus producing the so-called pseudodiverticulum. A bulb symmetrically narrowed in its midportion and associated with dilated fornices produces a cloverleaf deformity.

The complications of duodenal ulcer disease are discussed under *Complications of Peptic Ulcer*, page 958.[91, 92]

In the occasional case in which the presence of an active duodenal ulcer niche is radiographically equivocal, fiberoptic endoscopy may be more definitive.[91, 92]

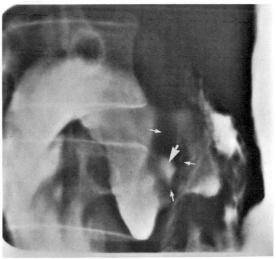

Figure 12–88 **Acute Duodenal Ulcer.** Enlarged view of the duodenal bulb and postbulbar area demonstrates an ulcer crater *(large arrow)* in the midportion of the bulb; it is surrounded by edematous folds *(small arrows)*. The absence of deformity suggests that this is a superficial and rather acute ulcer.

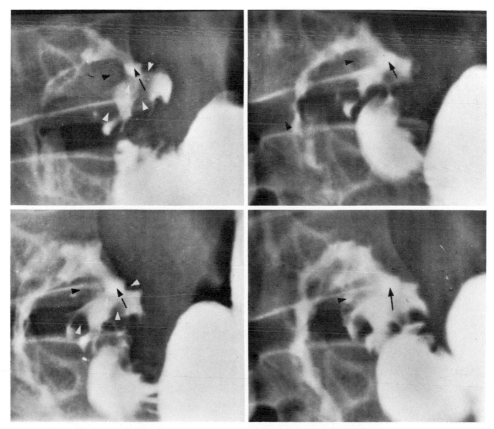

Figure 12–89 **Duodenal Ulcer.** A persistent ulcer crater is seen in the midportion of the bulb *(arrows)*. There is an incisura along the greater curvature of the bulb opposite the ulcer crater *(black arrowheads)*. The lucent areas *(white arrowheads)* surrounding and radiating toward the barium-filled crater are the thickened, edematous folds.

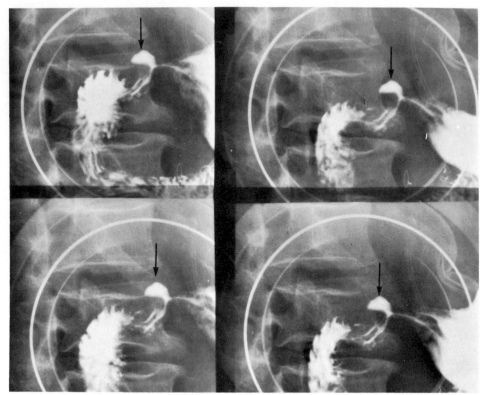

Figure 12–90 **Duodenal Ulcer: Deformed Bulb.** Serial compression films of the duodenal bulb demonstrate an accumulation of barium that represents an ulcer crater *(arrows)*. Deformity and scarring of the bulb are so severe that the rest of the duodenal bulb is not visualized.

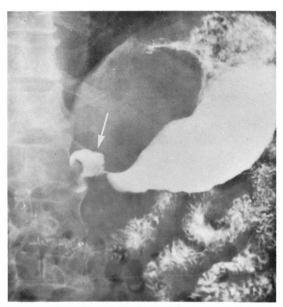

Figure 12–91 **Giant Duodenal Ulcer Simulating Deformed Bulb.** A huge ulcer crater has replaced the entire duodenal bulb *(arrow)* and grossly resembles a deformed bulb. However, ulcers like these do not change in form or empty during peristalsis, a fact which may help to distinguish them from deformed bulbs. Giant ulcers are quite rare, and are frequently mistaken for a deformed bulb.

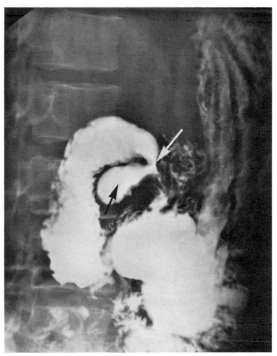

Figure 12–92 **Deformed Duodenal Bulb: Pseudodiverticulum.** There is an area of narrowing in the midportion of the bulb *(white arrow),* but an active crater cannot be demonstrated. The large barium-filled pouch *(black arrow)* at the greater curvature represents a pseudodiverticulum. In a severely scarred bulb without a definite crater, ulcer activity cannot be determined radiographically.

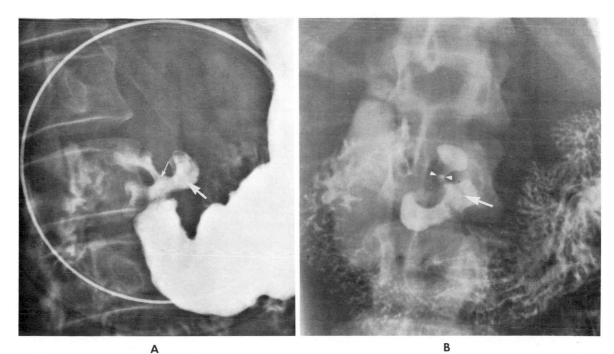

A   B

Figure 12–93 **Chronic Duodenal Ulcer Disease: Cloverleaf Deformity: Two Cases.**

A, The duodenal bulb *(large arrow)* is persistently deformed. The narrowed midportion *(small arrow)* compartmentalizes the rest of the bulb, producing the characteristic cloverlead bulb. No active crater was demonstrable, and the deformity was due to fibrosis and scarring.

B, In another patient who had recurrent symptoms of ulcer activity, the bulb *(arrow)* has a similar cloverleaf configuration. A small ulcer crater *(arrowheads)* can be seen in the narrowed midportion of the bulb.

The cloverleaf deformity is created by an ulcer in the central portion of the bulb; there is fibrotic contracture of the adjacent portions, leaving a narrowed midchannel. The cloverleaf bulb is only one of the numerous deformities produced by chronic ulcer disease.

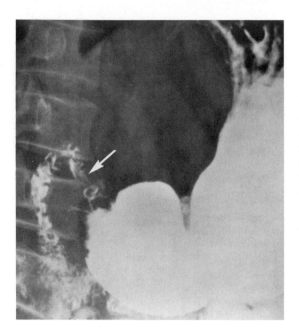

Figure 12–94 **Severely Scarred Duodenal Bulb with Unrelated Adenocarcinoma of Antrum.** The duodenal bulb *(arrow)* is severely scarred. No definite ulcer crater was seen. The patient presented with active gastrointestinal bleeding secondary to an active ulcer. At surgery a small adenocarcinoma was found in the pyloric area; roentgenographically it was not demonstrable. A duodenal ulcer was also present.

Recognition of an ulcer crater is often difficult or impossible in a severely deformed bulb. Comparison with prior films will usually prove helpful when searching for a recurrent ulcer.

Postbulbar Ulcer

These relatively rare ulcers are usually found on the inner aspect of the proximal portion of the descending duodenal loop, most often above the ampulla of Vater. These ulcers frequently cause recurrent bleeding. Definitive diagnosis can be made only by demonstration of the ulcer crater; localized narrowing due to spasm and irritability is often associated. In uncertain cases, hypotonic duodenography is usually very helpful. Healing is often followed by fibrotic stenosis of the proximal descending duodenum. The possibility of the Zollinger-Ellison syndrome (p. 955) should be considered when a postbulbar ulcer is discovered.[93-97]

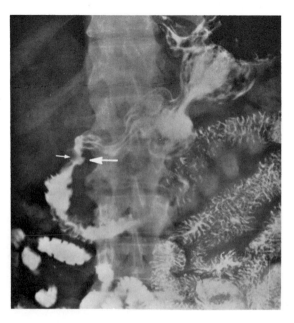

Figure 12–95 **Postbulbar Ulcer.** An ulcer crater is seen in profile *(large arrow)* in the proximal second portion of the duodenum. Incisura and mucosal edema *(small arrow)* of the opposite wall are demonstrated.

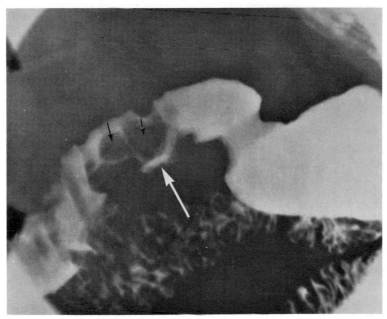

Figure 12–96 **Postbulbar Ulcer: Penetration.** Enlarged view of the duodenal area reveals a flat shallow ulcer *(white arrow)*. There is marked edema of the surrounding mucosa *(black arrows)*. At surgery the ulcer was found to have penetrated the head of the pancreas.

Zollinger-Ellison Syndrome

In this syndrome, due to non-beta cell islet tumors of the pancreas, there are a number of significant radiographic findings in the upper gastrointestinal tract. Elevated concentrations of gastrin are present in the tumor and serum.

There are one or more peptic ulcers, most frequently in the duodenal bulb but also in the stomach. About 75 per cent of ulcers are in these locations and are usually single. The others are in unusual locations from the postbulbar area to the upper jejunum. The ulcers show no distinctive roentgen features, but the more distal the ulcer is from the duodenal bulb, the more likely is the diagnosis of Zollinger-Ellison syndrome. The ulcers are extremely refractory to medical management. Occasionally giant ulcers are seen and should arouse suspicion. Early recurrence of large stomal ulcers is commonly encountered after surgery.

Usually there are excessive fasting gastric secretions and associated thickened folds. The highly acidic gastric contents often cause a chemical enteritis in the duodenum and even jejunum, evidenced by thickened valvulae with hazy margins (excessive secretions). The duodenal loop is often dilated and atonic (megaduodenum). In extreme cases, the appearance of the duodenum and jejunum may simulate granulomatous enteritis.

These findings in the duodenum and jejunum, when associated with one or more peptic ulcers, should suggest the possibility of Zollinger-Ellison syndrome. The Zollinger-Ellison syndrome may be a special form of the syndrome of multiple endocrine adenomatosis.

The pancreatic tumors—islet cell lesions—are generally small, and less than half are identified angiographically (pancreatic arteriography). The more vascular tumors produce a prolonged angiographic flush. Over half are malignant adenomas.[94, 95, 98-100]

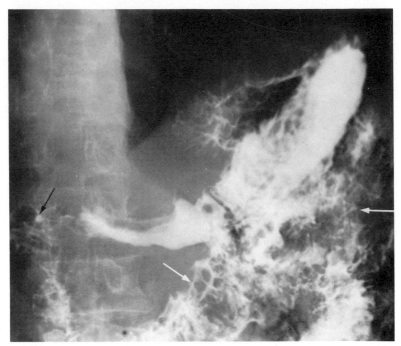

Figure 12–97 **Zollinger-Ellison Syndrome.** The jejunal folds are distorted, thickened, and rigid *(white arrows)*. An ulcer fleck is seen in the duodenum *(black arrow)*. The gastric folds are also thickened. The combination of jejunal changes and a peptic ulcer suggests the diagnosis. (Courtesy Dr. W. S. C. Hare, Melbourne, Australia.)

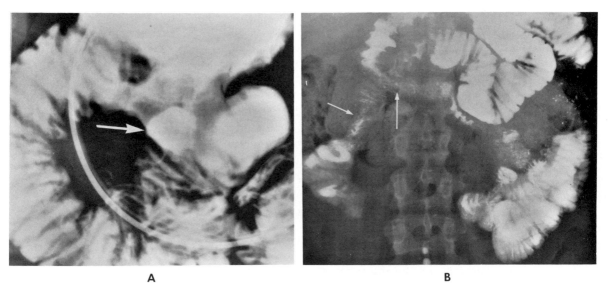

A   B

Figure 12–98 **Zollinger-Ellison Syndrome.**

A, In enlarged view of gastrectomy stoma there is a large marginal ulcer *(arrow)* that developed three months following gastrectomy.

B, The cobweb appearance of the jejunum *(arrows)* is due to inflammatory thickening of the valvulae. At surgery a pancreatic adenoma was found.

An ulcer recurring rapidly after surgery, and jejunal changes identified radiographically are characteristic of the Zollinger-Ellison syndrome.

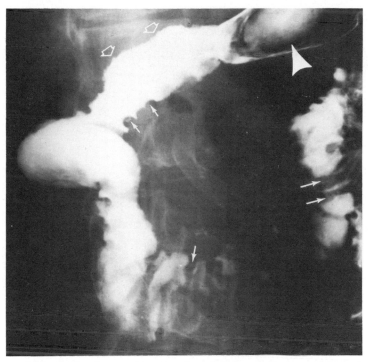

Figure 12–99 **Zollinger-Ellison Syndrome: Duodenal and Jejunal Changes.** The duodenal bulb (*arrow-head*) is not significantly deformed, but the duodenal loop and proximal jejunum show irritability, spasm, and coarsely thickened folds (*small solid arrows*). The multiple small irregularities in the postbulbar segment (*open arrows*) proved to be multiple small ulcerations.

In the Zollinger-Ellison syndrome, the highly acidic gastric contents cause a chemical inflammation in the duodenum and often in the jejunum.

Stress Ulcers

Ulcerations of the gastroduodenal area or rarely of other portions of the gastrointestinal tract can rapidly develop in patients under severe physiologic stress and are clinically manifested primarily by severe gastrointestinal hemorrhage. Stress ulcers are chiefly associated with sepsis, burns, pulmonary insufficiency, or severe trauma; they are also dreaded postoperative complications. Focal ischemia, often abetted by digitalis therapy, is thought to be a significant etiologic factor.

The ulcers are usually shallow, frequently multiple, and not surrounded by inflammatory induration. An erosive gastritis is often present. Upper gastrointestinal barium studies will disclose only 5 to 10 per cent of these stress ulcers, owing to their shallow nonindurated character. They may appear as shallow but persistent pools of barium, or as innocent looking barium smudges. Most often, however, no radiographic abnormalities are detected.

Gastroscopy may be extremely helpful, but blood and secretions in the stomach often obscure the finding. Sometimes the ulcerations may be in the mid-duodenum.

Localization of the bleeding area by celiac or selective arteriography is usually necessary in a severely bleeding patient with possible stress ulcer. Direct infusion of a vasopressor through the catheter may diminish or stop the bleeding. If surgical intervention is necessary, exact localization is extremely important.[101, 102]

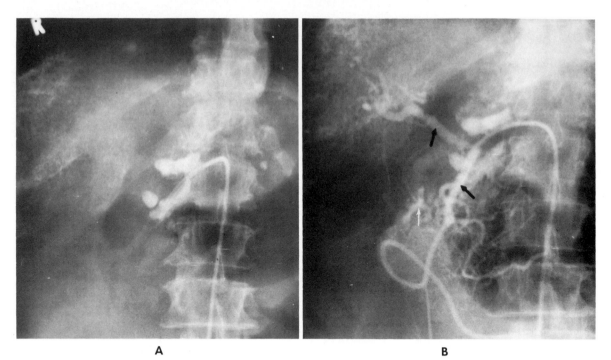

A   B

Figure 12–100   **Bleeding Stress Ulcer of Duodenum: Angiogram.**

   A, Preliminary film shows the catheter tip in the gastroduodenal artery. The densities near the catheter are due to a previous Thorotrast study with opacification of the lymph nodes.

   B, After injection of contrast material, the hepatic and gastroduodenal arteries are opacified *(black arrows).* An extravascular collection of contrast material *(white arrow)* is seen in the descending duodenum. This was the site of the bleeding stress ulcer.

   Bleeding stress ulcers are generally not visualized on barium contrast studies of the upper gastrointestinal tract. Angiography is usually performed as the primary procedure to identify the site of bleeding; prior barium studies may obscure significant angiographic findings.

Complications of Peptic Ulcer

Esophageal Stenosis Complicating Peptic Esophagitis and Peptic Ulcer of the Esophagus

   Stenosis of the lower esophagus following peptic ulcer of the esophagus is not infrequent; however, the most common cause of benign stricture is reflux esophagitis. The strictures are indistinguishable radiographically, but if a hiatal hernia is present below the stricture, reflux esophagitis is the probable cause.

   The stricture begins a short distance above the cardia and usually extends down to the esophagogastric junction. The esophagus is dilated above the stricture, and there is gradual tapering from the dilated to the narrowed segment. The stricture itself is usually fairly regular. Mucosal folds are few in number or totally absent. These features are characteristic of benignity, but occasionally an infiltrating malignant disease can mimic this appearance.

   Other causes of benign esophageal stricture include ingestion of caustic chemicals such as lye, prolonged intubation, and intensive radiation of the esophagus. These may occur in any portion of the esophagus. Esophagoscopy and cytologic washings are often necessary to rule out malignancy.[13, 86]

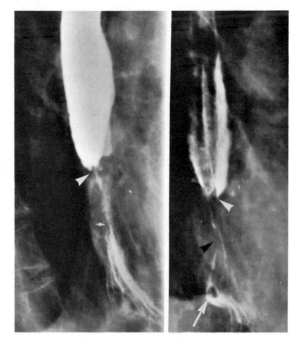

Figure 12–101 **Esophageal Stenosis from Peptic Esophagitis.**

A, The moderately dilated esophagus tapers to a stricture *(arrowhead).* The mucosal folds *(small arrow)* have been effaced.

B, Tapering is evident *(white arrowhead).* The stricture *(black arrowhead)* terminates in a hiatal hernia *(arrow).*

The hiatal hernia suggests that the stricture is due to reflux esophagitis, which often complicates sliding hiatal hernia.

Figure 12–102 **Esophageal Stenosis from Previous Peptic Esophagitis.** Proximal to the stricture there is pronounced dilatation of the normal esophagus, which then tapers to the strictured area *(arrow);* here it has been effaced, and the mucosal pattern is lacking *(arrowhead).* (Courtesy Dr. Arlyne Shockman, Veterans Administration Hospital, Philadelphia, Pennsylvania.)

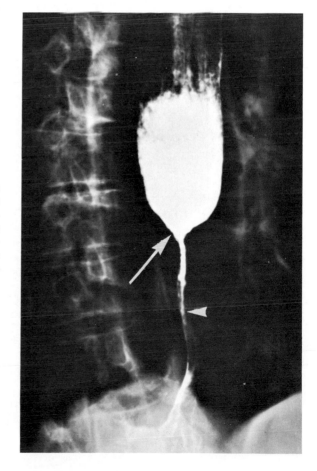

Gastroduodenal Stenosis

Stenosis is a fairly common complication of peptic ulcer disease; duodenal ulcer is the most frequent cause of gastric obstruction. The stenosis is due to scarring or inflammatory spasm or both. The bulb, if visualized, appears markedly distorted and narrowed.

Pyloric stenosis is generally secondary to scarring from previous pyloric ulcer disease. The stomach proximal to the narrowed area becomes dilated, and there is gradual tapering to the stenotic area. Lesser curvature gastric ulcers may result in shortening of the lesser curvature, with upward retraction of the antrum. Acute pyloric ulceration can cause sufficient edema and spasm to produce gastric obstruction. Differentiation from true stenosis can frequently be made only by observing the response to therapy. In an acute ulcer the obstruction is reversible.

The appearance of the stomach varies with the degree and duration of obstruction. Emptying time may be normal, but peristaltic activity may be increased. Frequently, the stomach can become dilated and atonic, with marked residual gastric secretions. A dilated stomach can attain huge proportions and may fill the entire upper abdomen. Complete emptying may take several days.

It is frequently impossible to determine by barium studies whether severe obstruction is due to a duodenal or a gastric lesion. After a period of gastric rest and therapy, reexamination will probably demonstrate the nature and location of the obstruction.[13]

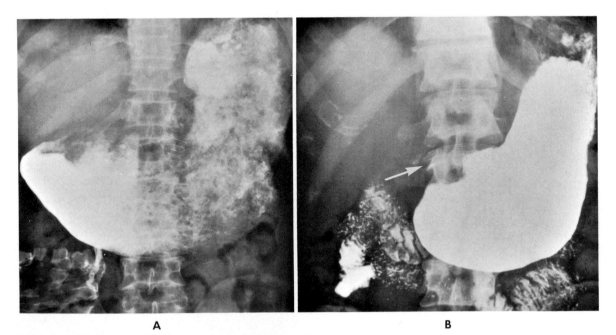

A   **B**

Figure 12–103   **Obstruction Secondary to Duodenal Ulcer Disease.**

A, Barium trickles from the dilated atonic stomach. There are marked residual secretions in the stomach, so that the barium has a mottled appearance. The site of obstruction is not apparent in this film. The patient was intubated to decompress and rest the stomach.

B, After four days of gastric rest, the study was repeated. It demonstrated a scarred deformed duodenal bulb *(arrow),* which was the site of the obstruction.

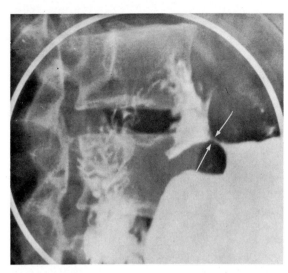

Figure 12–104 **Pyloric Stenosis.** Narrowed segment *(arrows)* at the pylorus merges smoothly with the dilated stomach. The lesser curvature of the stomach is shortened and elevated. Intensive medical therapy failed to bring about improvement. During surgery, fibrous scarring attributable to previous pyloric ulcer disease was found in the antrum.

Acute Perforation

A frequent complication of ulcer disease is perforation, which occurs most often in the pyloroduodenal area. Less commonly, a gastric ulcer may perforate.

Most intraperitoneal perforations occur on the anterior wall. Ulcers of the posterior wall tend to penetrate the pancreas, or they may perforate into the lesser omental sac or dissect along the retroperitoneal fascial planes.

Intraperitoneal perforation of the duodenum or stomach generally leads to pneumoperitoneum. With the patient in erect position, the free air is readily identified under the diaphragms as a crescentic area of lucency, without bowel markings, outlining the diaphragmatic leaf. Air may appear within one hour after perforation. As little as 2 cc. of air can be demonstrated. The patient should be seated or standing for at least five minutes before the films are made to allow the air to rise to the diaphragms. If the patient is too ill to stand or if the findings are questionable, a film should be obtained with the patient lying on his left side (left lateral decubitus film). Free air will collect in the region normally occupied by the liver, and possible confusion with gas-filled loops of bowel is avoided. If fluoroscopy is performed, limited diaphragmatic motion will be seen. A significant small bowel ileus usually does not occur in perforated peptic ulcer unless a complicating peritonitis develops. If free air is accompanied by an ileus soon after onset of clinical symptoms, the source of the perforation is more likely a colonic lesion.

No free air is demonstrated in about 25 per cent of the cases; in these patients, air instilled into the stomach via a tube will be detected in the peritoneal cavity.

When large amounts of intestinal contents have entered the peritoneum, air-fluid levels may be seen.[47, 103]

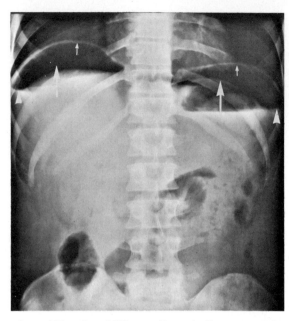

Figure 12–105 **Acute Perforation of Duodenal Ulcer.** Free air *(large arrows)* with fluid levels *(arrowheads)* has accumulated under each diaphragm. The free air is more easily identified on the right, where it is not confused with bowel or stomach air shadows. The diaphragms are outlined *(small arrows)* between the free air and the lung base.

Acute Hemorrhage

Gastroduodenal peptic ulcer disease is the most frequent cause of acute upper gastrointestinal bleeding. In about 80 per cent of cases gastrointestinal radiographic studies will disclose the suspected lesion. Radiography should be performed as soon as possible. Active bleeding requires selective angiography; barium studies are performed if the bleeding appears to be quiescent. The stomach should be lavaged to remove clots, which can simulate a gastric mass lesion or obscure an ulcer crater.

Other common sources of bleeding that can often be identified radiographically include esophageal varices, hiatal hernia, and gastric tumors. Erosive gastritis, superficial gastroduodenal erosions due to stress ulcerations, gastric varices, vascular malformations, small tumors of the small bowel, and a variety of rarer lesions can cause bleeding but are difficult or impossible to locate by conventional gastrointestinal studies.

The radiologic work-up of a patient with acute hemorrhage depends on the severity, duration, and activity of the hemorrhage. In massive continuing hemorrhage with active bleeding of over 1 ml. per minute, selective and subselective celiac and superior mesenteric arteriography will disclose the site of bleeding in a significant percentage of cases. Extravasation of the contrast material from the vascular tree into the stomach or small bowel localizes the site of bleeding. In addition, angiographic changes may indicate evidence of unsuspected varices, arteriovenous malformations or other abnormalities that may be the source of bleeding. The infusion of vasopressor drugs through the catheter may help stop or diminish the amount of bleeding.

If active bleeding has stopped or is not severe, barium studies of the gastrointestinal tract are indicated. Barium may obscure angiographic findings if given prior to angiography.[13, 104, 105]

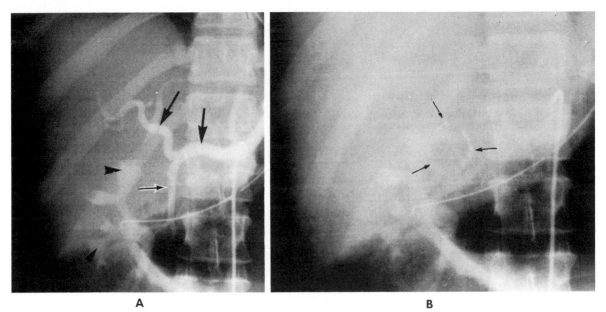

A   B

Figure 12–106 **Upper Gastrointestinal Hemorrhage: Localization by Celiac Arteriogram.**

A, Early film shows opacification of the hepatic artery *(black arrows)* and its gastroduodenal branch *(black-white arrow).* The pyelogram *(arrowheads)* is from a prior injection of contrast material.

B, Later film, made after disappearance of arterial opacification, shows a ring-like collection of contrast material *(arrows)* in the region of the duodenal bulb; this was the site of bleeding. The duodenal bulb is supplied by branches of the gastroduodenal artery.

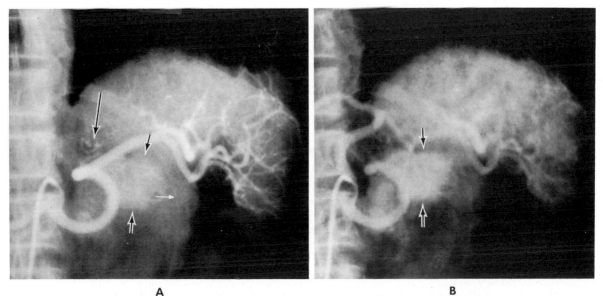

A   B

Figure 12–107 **Upper Gastrointestinal Hemorrhage: Localization by Celiac Arteriogram.**

A, Selective celiac arteriogram shows excellent opacification of the splenic artery and its branches. There is extravasation of contrast material *(short black-white arrows)* that arises from a tortuous gastric artery *(long black-white arrow).* The location of a faintly opaque gastric tube *(white arrow)* indicates that the bleeding is from the lesser curvature.

B, A few seconds later the extravasation has increased in amount and density *(arrows).* A large stress ulcer of the lesser curvature was found at surgery.

Lesser Sac Abscess

Posterior perforation of a peptic ulcer can produce air and fluid in the lesser omental sac. With the patient supine, a well-defined soft tissue density is seen occupying the position of the lesser sac, displacing the stomach forward, upward, and to the right. With the patient erect, air-fluid levels are seen extending across the midline in the region of the sac. The air in the distended lesser sac may extend up to the diaphragm. The fluid level is wider than that which occurs in the bowel, and there are no valvulae or haustral markings. On lateral decubitus films the air-fluid levels remain confined to the region of the lesser sac.[106, 107]

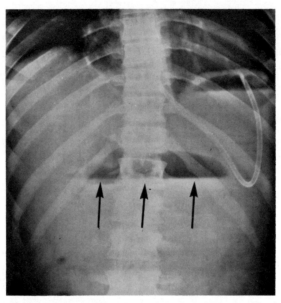

Figure 12–108 **Lesser Sac Abscess Due to Perforation of Gastric Ulcer.**   Gas has accumulated in the upper abdomen, and a fluid level extends across the midline *(arrows)* without evidence of bowel markings. The location of the gas and the long fluid level are characteristic of fluid in a lesser sac. The fluid was purulent.

Subphrenic (Subdiaphragmatic) Abscess

Localized subphrenic inflammation occurs most often as a complication of abdominal surgery or may be a sequela of a generalized peritonitis. It occurs more frequently on the right side. Fever and abdominal pain are the major symptoms.

The earliest radiographic finding is elevation and limited motion of the involved hemidiaphragm. A pleural reaction, with variable amounts of fluid, develops above the involved diaphragm. Sometimes, parenchymal basal densities due to compression atelectasis appear. By this time, the diaphragm is usually totally immobile and may even show paradoxical movement on respiration.

These findings may simulate pulmonary infarction, a postoperative pleuropneumonia, or reaction from surgical manipulation of the diaphragm. Sometimes, gas-forming organisms produce a diagnostic air-fluid level beneath the diaphragm. A left subphrenic abscess may be easier to recognize radiographically because it increases the distance between the diaphragm and the gastric fundus, and usually produces a pressure defect upon the upper portion of the stomach.

If the radiographic and clinical findings are inconclusive, a diagnostic pneumoperitoneum can be performed. Air will not accumulate under the involved diaphragm in the erect posture.

Postoperative elevation and fixation of a diaphragm associated with a pleural reaction is highly suggestive of subphrenic inflammation.[47, 108, 109]

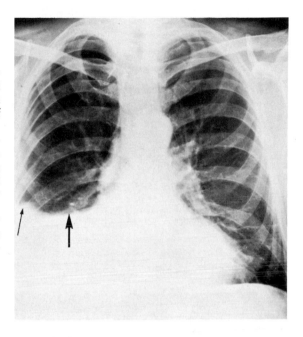

Figure 12-109 **Subphrenic Abscess: Postcholecystectomy.** One week after surgery there is pronounced elevation of the right diaphragm *(large arrow)*, which did not move with respiration. There is evidence of fluid in the right costophrenic angle *(small arrow)*.

When unexplained fever develops following abdominal surgery, elevation and fixation of a diaphragm (usually the right) is the earliest roentgenologic finding of subphrenic abscess. Pleural and parenchymal basal densities develop later and are strong confirmatory findings.

Basal densities and elevation of a diaphragm may be early findings in postoperative atelectasis, but some diaphragmatic excursion on respiration will distinguish this from a subphrenic abscess.

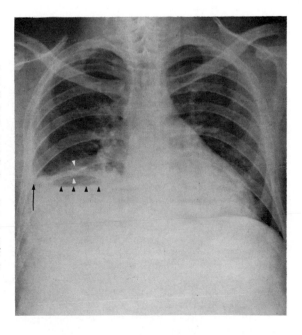

Figure 12-110 **Subdiaphragmatic Abscess Due to Ruptured Ulcer.** The right diaphragm is elevated, and there is a small amount of fluid at the costophrenic angle *(arrow)*. Several areas of parenchymal density are seen just above the diaphragm. There is an air-fluid level in the abscess *(black arrowheads)*. The diaphragm, outlined by the air in the abscess, is thickened and somewhat irregular *(white arrowheads)* as a result of the inflammatory process. There was no movement of the diaphragm on respiration.

Air-fluid levels in subdiaphragmatic abscess are seldom seen, and the diagnosis is usually made by observation of an elevated fixed diaphragm and the reactive pleural and parenchymal densities in the lung above the involved diaphragm. Complete fixation of the diaphragm helps distinguish subdiaphragmatic abscess from basal pleuropneumonia.

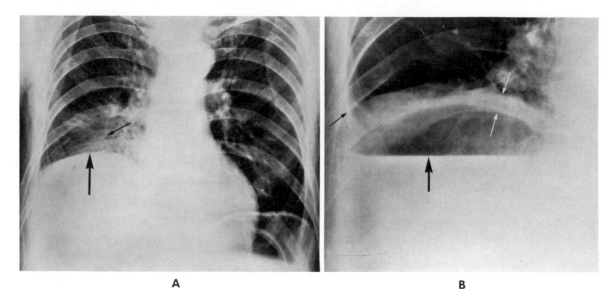

Figure 12–111   **Subphrenic Abscess: Postgastrectomy.**

A, Ten days after surgery there is marked elevation of the right diaphragm *(large arrow),* which remained fixed during fluoroscopy. Mottled linear densities at the right base *(small arrow)* simulate a pnuemonia. Only a small amount of fluid had developed, producing minimal blunting of the right costophrenic angle.

B, After surgical drainage, there is an air-fluid level in the abscess *(large black arrow),* which outlines the size of the abscess. The diaphragm is still elevated and fixed, and is greatly thickened *(white arrows).* Some pleural fluid persists *(small black arrow),* but the parenchymal reaction has subsided.

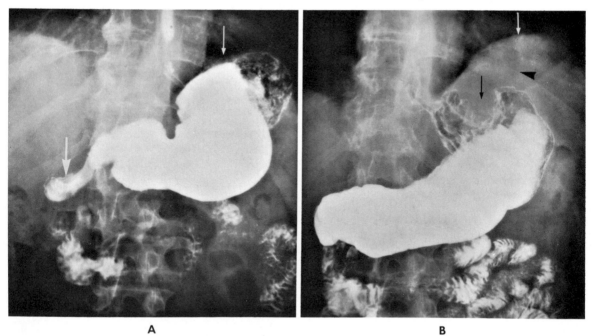

Figure 12–112   **Chronic Left Subphrenic Abscess Following Perforation of Gallbladder.**

A, The pyloroduodenal area is distorted *(large arrow),* due to a local abscess from the perforated gallbladder. The gastric fundus is in normal position *(small arrow)* directly beneath the left diaphragm. Surgery performed shortly after this study disclosed a local abscess around the gallbladder.

B, Four months later, after bouts of fever and recurrent episodes of pain in the left upper abdomen, there is elevation of the left diaphragm *(white arrow),* which was completely fixed on fluoroscopy. There is evidence of increased soft tissue between the diaphragm and the fundus *(arrowhead).* This was a chronic thick-walled subphrenic abscess.

The defect in the fundus *(black arrow)* was due to extrinsic pressure from a border of the abscess. Absence of significant reaction in the left lower lung field attests to the chronicity of the abscess.

Chronic Perforation

Peptic ulcers may penetrate the muscularis and serosa to form a pocket or abscess, or they may extend into adjacent viscera. On erect films an air-fluid level will often identify the pocket. Barium usually fills the pocket during gastrointestinal examination. These abscesses or pockets usually retain barium and remain unchanged long after gastric emptying.

If an abscess pocket is sealed off from the lumen, it may appear radiographically as a soft tissue mass producing pressure upon the stomach or duodenum.

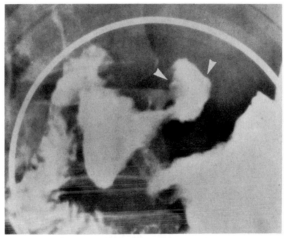

Figure 12–113 **Chronic Perforation of Duodenal Ulcer.**   The ulcer has penetrated the lesser recesses of the bulb (*arrowheads*). Although it resembles a pseudodiverticulum, this pocket remains filled with barium when the rest of the bulb contracts and empties.

Chronic Posterior Penetration into the Pancreas

Peptic ulcers of the duodenal bulb that penetrate into the head of the pancreas produce a localized pancreatitis and often cause a change in the patient's pain complex.

In addition to evidence of duodenal ulcer disease and bulb deformity, changes secondary to inflammation of the head of the pancreas may be noted. There is pressure on, and effacement of, the folds on the inner aspect of the postbulbar area and in the proximal descending duodenal loop. Rigidity of the loop is frequently noted.[110]

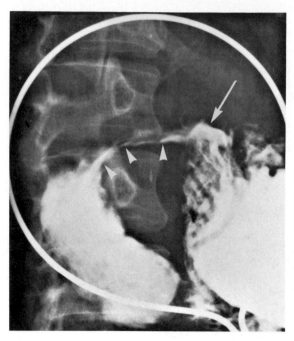

Figure 12-114 **Chronic Posterior Penetration into Head of Pancreas.** There is evidence of chronic ulcer disease with a deformed duodenal bulb *(arrow)*. The duodenal loop is stretched and the duodenal folds are effaced because of pressure *(arrowheads)*. Surgery revealed that the ulcer had penetrated into the head of the pancreas. Duodenal deformity associated with local loop changes strongly suggests posterior penetration of an ulcer.

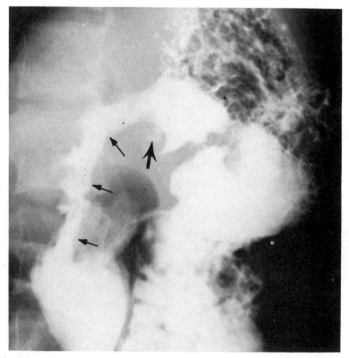

Figure 12-115 **Chronic Posterior Penetration into Head of Pancreas.** The posterior ulcer crater arising from the bulb is easily identified *(large arrow)*. The descending duodenum shows a smooth inner border with absence of normal medial folds *(small arrows)* and irregularities of the lumen. The latter findings were due to pancreatitis secondary to posterior penetration of the ulcer into the pancreatic head.

Marginal (Stomal) Ulcer

Ulcers that occur just distal to the stoma in patients who have undergone gastrectomy for peptic ulcer are termed *marginal* or *stomal* ulcers. A high incidence is found in patients with the Zollinger-Ellison syndrome. Only approximately 50 per cent of the ulcers can be demonstrated radiographically; therefore, negative findings do not conclusively eliminate the possibility of marginal ulceration in a patient who had undergone gastrectomy and who has a history of pain and/or hemorrhage. Endoscopy may clarify the diagnosis.

Positive radiologic diagnosis requires demonstration of the ulcer crater, which is most frequently on the dependent wall of the efferent loop of the jejunum adjacent to the stoma. The ulcer appears as a circumscribed dense collection of barium. Ulcers smaller than 5 mm. are rarely demonstrated. They can be as large as 50 mm. in diameter, and such large ulcers are frequently misdiagnosed as postoperative pouches. Rigidity of the jejunal wall may be the earliest and sometimes the sole finding of an anastomotic ulcer.

Secondary signs of marginal ulcer include obstruction of a previously patent efferent loop; spasm, edema, and narrowing of the jejunum; effacement of the mucosal folds in the region of the ulcer; and radiation of folds toward the region of the crater.

The diagnosis of postoperative jejunal ulcer and of other complications of ulcer is simplified if gastrointestinal films made within a month or two after surgery are available for comparison.[111, 112]

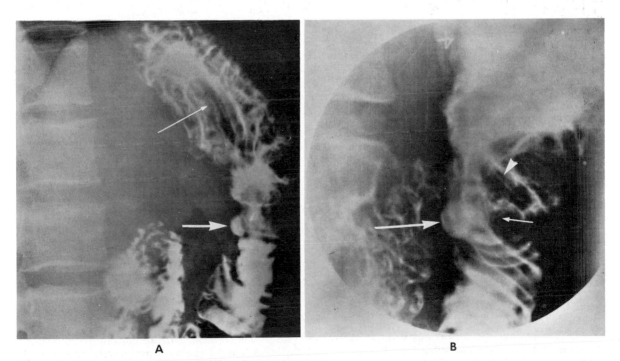

A   **B**

Figure 12–116 **Marginal (Jejunal) Ulcer Postgastrectomy.**

A, About two thirds of the stomach has been removed *(small arrow).* An ulcer crater *(large arrow)* can be seen in the dependent portion of the efferent loop near the stoma, a typical location of a marginal ulcer.

B, Enlarged view demonstrates the spasm *(small arrow)* and incisura on the wall opposite the ulcer crater *(large arrow).* There is edema and swelling of the mucosal folds *(arrowhead).*

Gastrojejunocolic and Gastrocolic Fistula

A gastrojejunocolic fistula can occur after gastrojejunostomy if a marginal jejunal ulcer develops and then penetrates into the adjacent transverse colon.

These fistulas are most readily uncovered by barium enema examination, during which the barium is seen passing from the transverse colon to the stomach or jejunum. Demonstration of the fistula by oral barium meal examination is often unsuccessful.

A gastrocolic fistula is due most often to a colonic carcinoma in or near the splenic flexure.[113]

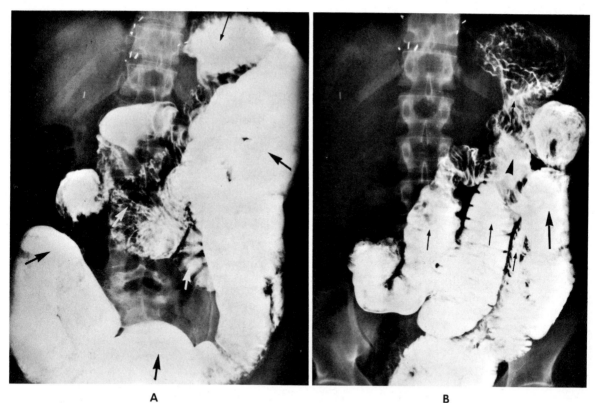

A   **B**

Figure 12–117 **Gastrojejunocolic Fistula: Barium Enema.**

A, This patient had a previous subtotal gastrectomy for duodenal ulcer. Barium has entered the stomach *(small black arrow)* and small bowel *(white arrow)* during a barium enema examination. The colon is outlined by large black arrows.

B, Postevacuation film clearly indicates filling of the small bowel and stomach *(small arrows).* Accumulation of barium at the gastrojejunal anastomosis *(black arrowhead)* represents a large marginal jejunal ulcer that has extended into the colon *(large arrow).*

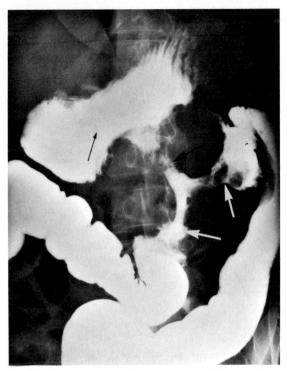

Figure 12–118 **Gastrocolic Fistula Secondary to Carcinoma of Colon.** Annular carcinoma of the transverse colon *(white arrows)* has invaded the stomach, producing a fistulous tract *(large black arrow)* from the colon to the stomach *(small black arrow).*

Hourglass Deformity

Hourglass deformity is a descriptive term applied to a bilocular stomach. It is usually due to chronic gastric ulcer disease with associated scar formation and shrinkage of the wall. When the scarring occurs in the midportion of the stomach, the greater curvature is generally drawn toward the lesser curvature, leading to asymmetric narrowing. Local muscular spasm may aggravate the deformity.

A similar deformity can result from an annular infiltrating carcinoma in the midportion of the stomach, but evidence of malignant infiltration usually aids in making the distinction radiographically.[13]

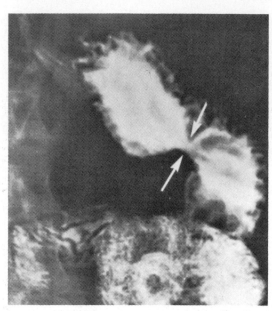

Figure 12–119 **Hourglass Deformity.** The stomach is bilocular as a consequence of scarring caused by a chronic benign ulcer on the lesser curvature. There is eccentric narrowing *(arrows)*. There is no evidence of infiltration, and the mucosa is intact.

Afferent Loop Syndrome

When the afferent loop of a gastrojejunostomy is dilated and empties poorly, it may be obstructed at the anastomosis or proximal to the anastomosis. The former is difficult to demonstrate radiologically, since the block prevents filling of the afferent loop, and occasionally a normal afferent loop may not fill because it is filled with secretions. When obstruction is proximal to the anastomosis, the barium fills a short segment of the loop up to the point of narrowing and obstruction. A third type of this syndrome, in which there is no organic obstruction, results from faulty anastomosis that causes the gastric contents to enter preferentially the afferent instead of the efferent loop. In this case the dilated afferent loop fills rapidly during barium meal examination and remains filled for an inordinate length of time. Obstruction of the efferent loop from a marginal ulcer or from edema will also lead to preferential filling of the afferent loop; this will radiologically simulate a true afferent loop syndrome.[114, 115]

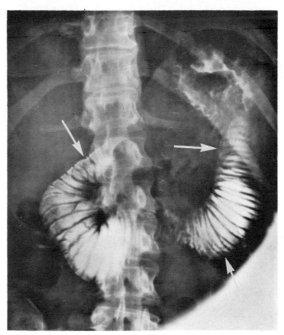

Figure 12–120 **Afferent Loop Syndrome: Faulty Anastomosis.** The barium-filled afferent loop is considerably dilated *(arrows)*. Very little barium has entered the efferent loop. The patient was relieved of clinical symptoms after surgical resetting of the gastrojejunostomy.

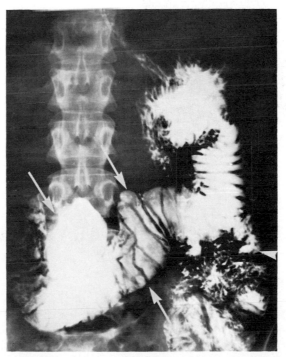

Figure 12–121 **Afferent Loop Syndrome.** The afferent loop is considerably dilated *(arrows)*; it fills rapidly and remains filled after gastric emptying. The efferent loop is patent *(arrowhead)* and of normal caliber. Surgical resetting of the anastomosis was necessary for relief of symptoms.

Jejunogastric Intussusception

This infrequent but serious complication of gastrojejunostomy may occur as early as one week or as late as 25 years after surgery.

The acute episode is marked by severe symptoms of gastric obstruction. Oral barium study discloses a coiled-spring filling defect in the stomach; this is the intussuscepted jejunum. Gastric emptying is delayed or absent. Early surgical correction is necessary.

In the chronic, recurring form, roentgenologic diagnosis can be made only during the episode of acute intussusception.[116]

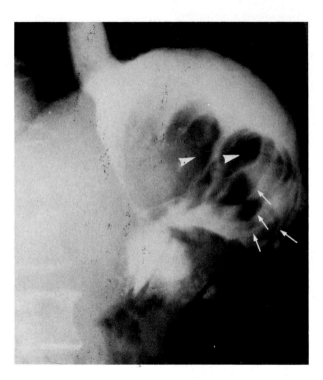

Figure 12–122 **Acute Jejunogastric Intussusception.** A 51 year old man developed increasing pain, vomiting, and hematemesis 10 years after a subtotal gastrectomy (Billroth II) for duodenal ulcer.

Barium study revealed a large mass of jejunum within the stomach. The jejunal folds are edematous *(arrowheads),* and the valvulae have the coiled-spring appearance *(arrows)* characteristic of intussuscepted small bowel. Obstruction was complete.

This acute intussusception of the jejunum through the stoma into the gastric pouch required immediate surgery. (Courtesy Drs. D. K. Dolan and R. E. Hockman, Iowa City, Iowa.)

DISEASES OF MALABSORPTION

Intestinal Malabsorption

Intestinal malabsorption is an extremely complex disorder associated with a great variety of symptoms, biochemical abnormalities, and causes. Radiologic abnormalities of the small bowel are very frequently associated, but malabsorption can exist without discernible small bowel changes. There is no good correlation between the appearance and severity of the small bowel alterations radiographically and the degree of clinical malabsorption.

For purposes of classification, the majority of the small bowel changes seen in patients with the malabsorption syndrome can be divided into several radiographic groups. However, it must be emphasized that the radiographic appearance may bear no relationship to the physiologic mechanism and to the degree of malabsorption. Hence, any radiographic classification is entirely arbitrary.

Virtually all the diseases and conditions in the following classification will be discussed and illustrated elsewhere under the specific condition or disease.

1. *Celiac-sprue pattern.* This is characterized by moderate dilatation of many of the small bowel loops, segmentation (discontinuous large segments), areas of effacement of the mucosal folds (moulage), and thickened folds in some of the segments. Alteration of motility, particularly hypomotility, and evidence of hypersecretion also occur. The most frequent and constant abnormality, however, is mild dilatation, which is best seen in the duodenum and mid and distal jejunum; it is often associated with areas of thickened folds. This deficiency pattern is nonspecific and can occur in a variety of conditions, including the "sprue" group (celiac disease, nontropical sprue, and tropical sprue), some severe parasitic infections, pancreatic insufficiency, hypoparathyroidism, and chronic small bowel ischemia.

2. *Infiltrative pattern.* This refers to conditions in which the small intestinal folds and often the bowel wall are diffusely thickened, usually by some infiltrative process. Prominent in this group are Whipple's disease, lymphosarcoma and reticulum cell sarcoma of the small bowel, amyloidosis, and intestinal lymphangiectasia.

3. *Other specific small bowel lesions.* This group includes many diverse conditions such as multiple jejunal diverticula, the blind loop, small bowel fistulas, scleroderma of the small bowel, extensive regional enteritis, other specific inflammatory enteritides, eosinophilic gastroenteritis, and mastocytosis.[117-121]

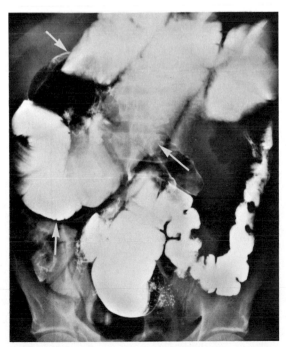

Figure 12–123 **Malabsorption: Blind Loop.** The greatly dilated loop of ileum *(arrows)* resulted from an end-to-side ileotransverse colostomy. The loop remained filled after evacuation, and alterations in bacterial flora due to stasis caused malabsorption.

Celiac Sprue Disease (Sprue, Celiac Disease, Nontropical Sprue, and Tropical Sprue)

Varying degrees of small intestinal dilatation, segmentation, hypersecretion, and barium flocculation are the characteristic radiographic changes in the small bowel.

Dilatation is the most constant and significant finding; it is most apparent in the jejunum. The dilated loops contract poorly, and transit time is often prolonged.

Other findings include segmentation (separate large clumps of barium-filled bowel), flocculation and fragmentation of the barium (snow-flake appearance), a coarse granular appearance of the barium, and an amorphous pattern of some loops. These changes are due to hypersecretion. When a colloidal barium preparation is employed, these changes are much less apparent.

The valvulae in some areas appear straight and thinned; in other segments they may appear thickened. This is probably due to a surrounding layer of secretions and not true thickening. Nonobstructive transient small intussusceptions with a coiled-spring appearance can occur, but usually without symptoms.

Clinical remission may or may not be associated with improvement of the radiographic small bowel findings. It must be emphasized that the radiographic changes usually do not correlate accurately with the clinical severity of the malabsorption.[117-123]

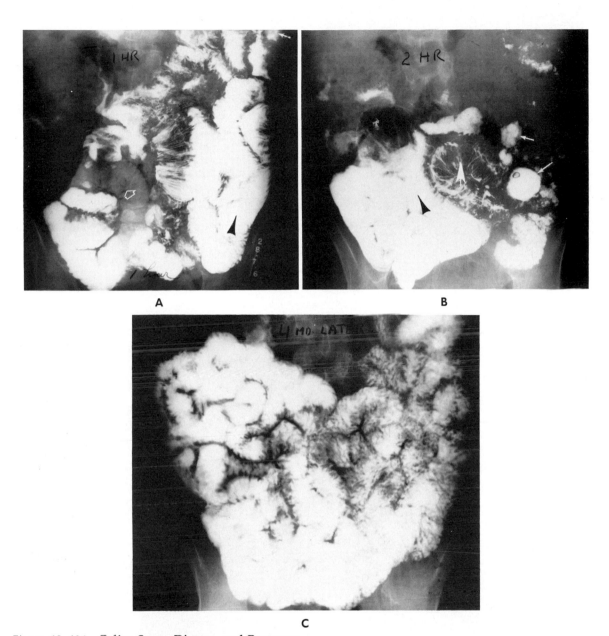

Figure 12–124 **Celiac-Sprue Disease, and Recovery.**

A and *B,* The one- and two-hour small bowel films reveal many mildly dilated loops *(black arrowheads),* discontinuous barium clumps *(small white arrows),* and hypersecretion as evidenced by fuzzy margins and barium dilution *(open white arrow).* The mucosal folds are not thickened, and transient small segments of mild intussusception are seen *(large white arrow).*

C, Four months later, after successful treatment, the small bowel pattern has returned to normal.

Mild dilatation, segmentation, evidence of hypersecretion, and transient areas of intussusception are classic characteristics of the sprue small bowel pattern.

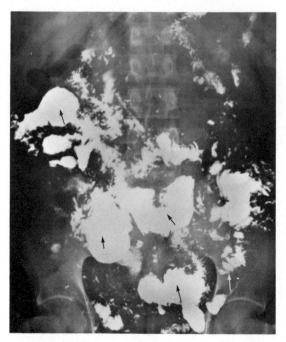

A

Figure 12–125 **Celiac-Sprue Disease.**

Various aspects of the deficiency small bowel pattern are illustrated in three cases.

A, There are numerous dilated loops *(black arrows);* in many of these the mucosal pattern has been effaced. Barium is distributed segmentally and discontinuously throughout the abdomen, and in some of these segments the mucosal folds are thickened *(white arrow).* Motility was decreased.

B, In addition to dilated segments and mucosal effacement *(large arrows),* there are large dilated loops of bowel that have thickened folds *(small arrows).* Segmentation is not prominent. There is flocculation of barium, and transit time was greatly delayed.

C, Dilatation is not a prominent feature *(black arrow),* but segmentation, flocculation, and discontinuity of loops are widespread. Much of the bowel mucosa is thickened *(white arrows).*

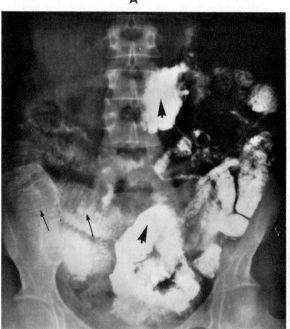

B

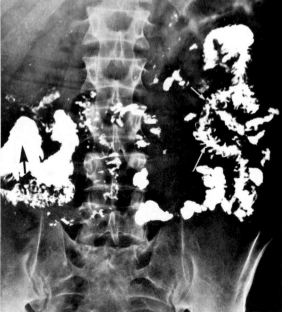

C

Whipple's Disease

This uncommon disease occurs most often in middle-aged males and is characterized clinically by malabsorption, abdominal symptoms, and polyarthralgia.

The significant radiologic findings are diffuse thickening of the mucosal folds and walls of the small bowel, most apparent in the jejunum. The thickened walls cause a characteristic separation of the loops in severe cases. There may be some evidence of hypersecretion. The lumen is normal or slightly dilated. In less advanced disease, thickening of the jejunal folds may be the sole finding. The absence of small bowel rigidity, spasm, or alterations of motility in Whipple's disease may help distinguish it from an inflammatory enteritis (giardiasis, eosinophilic gastroenteritis, and so on).

Similar small bowel infiltrative changes can be seen in intestinal lymphangiectasia, amyloidosis, lymphoma, and mastocytosis. Jejunal biopsy is usually necessary for positive diagnosis and will disclose the characteristic PAS-positive material. Dramatic decrease of the small bowel changes may occur after successful treatment.[124-126]

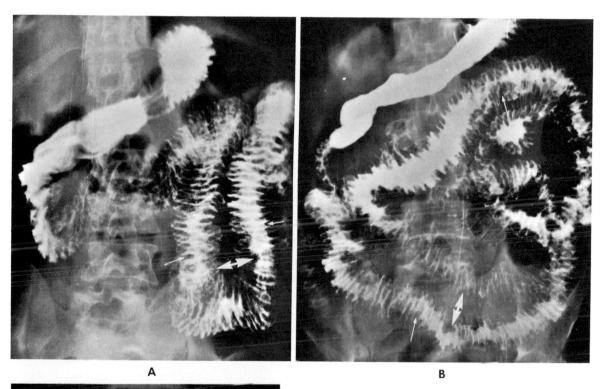

A   B

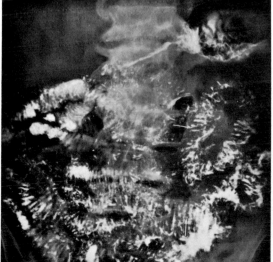

C

Figure 12–126 **Whipple's Disease in Two Patients.**

A and *B,* The infiltrated small bowel loops are dilated, and they have greatly thickened folds *(arrows)* which give them a spiculated appearance. The bowel walls are extensively infiltrated, so that the space between the lumina of adjacent loops *(double-headed arrows)* is much increased.

C, In another patient the small bowel changes are similar but less pronounced than in *A* and *B.* The thickened folds are indicated by the arrows.

In Whipple's disease the proximal loops of the small bowel are primarily affected. Similar changes occur in other conditions in which there is diffuse submucosal infiltration or thickening of the small bowel. (Courtesy Dr. G. Triano, Harrisburg, Pennsylvania.)

Intestinal Lymphangiectasia — Protein-Losing Enteropathy

Hypoalbuminemia in the absence of liver or renal disease may be due to loss of protein into the gastrointestinal tract. It can occur in adult sprue, diffuse ileojejunitis, Cronkhite-Canada syndrome, constrictive pericarditis, Menetrier's syndrome, and other diseases causing lymphatic obstruction of the intestinal tract. Malabsorption frequently is also present. In the absence of a well-defined gastrointestinal disorder, intestinal lymphangiectasia should be considered.

This idiopathic and probably congenital disorder — also known as exudative enteropathy of Gordon — is characterized by dilatation of the intestinal lymphatics. It usually occurs in individuals under age 25. Radiographically, the valvulae conniventes of the jejunum and, often, the ileum are greatly thickened. There may be little or no thickening of the bowel wall unless the serum albumin is below 2.5 gm. per 100 ml. The small bowel loops are otherwise normal, with no segmentation, dilatation, or deformity. Other hypoalbuminemic states, such as hepatic cirrhosis and nephrosis, can lead to small bowel edema and a similar radiographic appearance. Definitive diagnosis requires small bowel biopsy.

In many cases lymphangiography may disclose other lymphatic abnormalities in the extremities or abdomen, suggesting that the disorder is a systemic lymphatic dysplasia.[127-129]

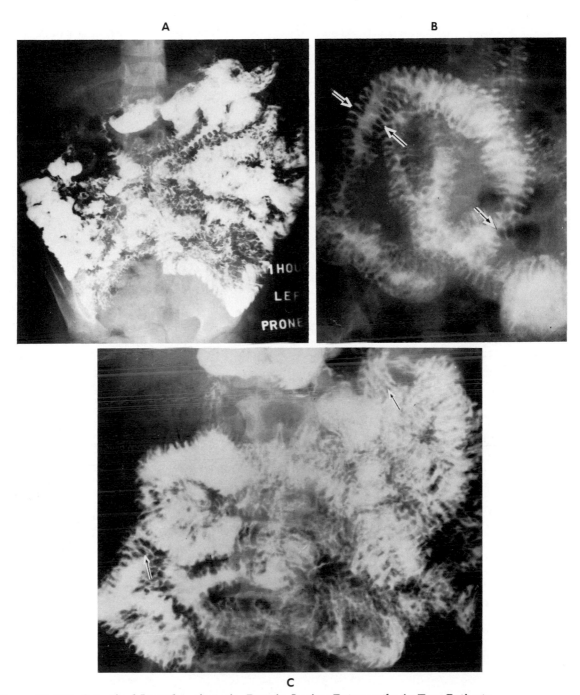

Figure 12-127 **Intestinal Lymphangiectasia: Protein-Losing Enteropathy in Two Patients.**

A and *B,* The mucosal folds (valvulae conniventes) of the jejunum and ileum are diffusely thickened *(arrows),* which is the characteristic feature of intestinal lymphangiectasia. The striking biconcave defects produced by the thickened folds is better seen in the localized view of the jejunum in *B*. (Courtesy Dr. O. Pock-Steen, Copenhagen, Denmark.)

C, In a 2 year old child with intestinal lymphangiectasia, there are identical small bowel changes. Arrows indicate thickened mucosal folds of the small bowel.

Disaccharide Malabsorption

Malabsorption of a disaccharide is due to a deficiency of its specific disaccharidase. The small bowel is normal both radiologically and histologically. However, if a large quantity of the specific, offending sugar (usually lactose or sucrose) is added to a barium-water mixture, the small bowel becomes dilated, the contrast material is diluted, and motility is increased. These changes result from entrance of fluid into the small bowel, whose content has remained hypertonic because of the nonhydrolyzed, unabsorbed sugar. This diagnostic test is fairly specific provided there is no other associated small bowel disease.[130-132]

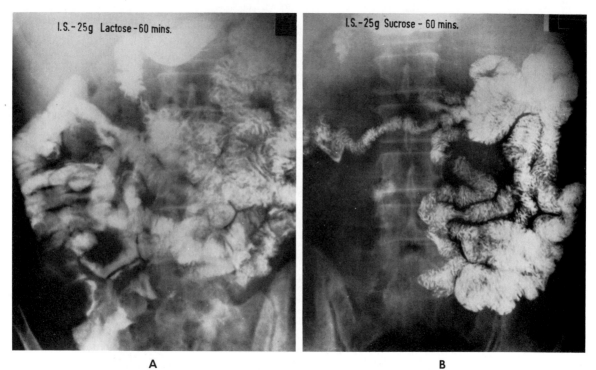

A   B

Figure 12–128 **Disaccharidase Deficiency: Lactose Malabsorption.**

A, A film made one hour after oral administration of a barium-water mixture containing lactose shows dilatation and hypermotility of the small bowel. There is also dilution of the contrast material, which produces poor mucosal definition.

B, Sucrose, absorbed normally by this patient, was used instead of lactose. At one hour the small bowel has completely normal appearance and motility. (Courtesy Dr. J. W. Laws, London, England.)

DISEASES OF THE PANCREAS

Radiology of the Pancreas

Investigation of suspected pancreatic disease may require abdominal films, upper gastrointestinal series, angiography, transhepatic cholangiography, pancreatography, and ultrasound studies.

Abdominal film can reveal pancreatic calculi, evidence of local ileus in acute pancreatitis, and a soft tissue mass if a large pseudocyst is present.

The upper gastrointestinal series can disclose indirect signs of a pancreatic disorder, such as impressions upon the duodenum in chronic pancreatitis or carcinoma of the pancreatic head, widening of the loop in pseudocyst or large carcinoma, and edematous duodenal folds in acute pancreatitis. Pressures on the stomach can occur from pseudocysts or a greatly edematous pancreas. If the duodenal findings are equivocal, hypotonic duodenography will often provide clarification.

Pancreatic angiography can often demonstrate an otherwise undetectable pancreatic tumor, and it often but not always can distinguish between carcinoma and the indurated mass of chronic pancreatitis. Pseudocysts are readily identified by angiography.

In the jaundiced patient, transhepatic cholangiography can often help distinguish between a common duct stone or biliary duct tumor and extensive obstruction of the common duct by a pancreatic mass.

The newer technique of endoscopic retrograde cholangiopancreatography, which involves catheterization of the ampulla via a duodenoscope, appears to be helpful in demonstrating inflammatory and neoplastic pancreatic lesions.

Ultrasonography can generally distinguish a pancreatic pseudocyst from a solid mass.[133]

Acute Pancreatitis

Depending on the severity of disease, roentgenologic changes are seen in the abdomen, the upper gastrointestinal tract, and, less frequently, the chest. Bone lesions can occur but are rare.

Abdominal films are usually normal, but they may show a nonspecific localized dilatation of an upper abdominal small bowel loop that frequently contains fluid—the sentinel loop. The duodenal loop is often distended by air, and this is a more definitive finding. Localized distention of the transverse colon, often to the splenic flexure (colon cutoff sign) is a suggestive but infrequent finding. A generalized ileus may be apparent in severe cases. Mottled areas of decreased and increased density due to edema and saponification of retroperitoneal fat are occasionally seen. Sometimes pancreatic calcifications, indicative of chronic relapsing pancreatitis, are present; this is a significant clue to the diagnosis.

Chest findings include elevation of the left diaphragm, which occurs in almost one third of cases, and linear inflammatory strands or pleural fluid, or both, at the left lung base. These findings are sometimes bilateral.

Oral barium studies will often demonstrate changes in the duodenal loop. Pressure effects of its medial border, edematous folds, a swollen ampulla, and even widening of the loop may be seen. These changes may be best demonstrated by hypotonic duodenography. Prominent rugal folds may be apparent on the posterior and greater curvature of the stomach; these disappear with recovery. A greatly edematous pancreas can produce a sizable pressure defect on the posterior stomach, simulating a retroperitoneal tumor or pseudocyst. The radiographic changes in the duodenum or stomach are seen in about one half of the patients, if they are examined within a week after onset of the acute illness.

Spread of pancreatic enzymes along the mesenteric planes can cause inflammatory changes in the jejunum and, less often, in the ileocecal area and transverse colon. These changes range from transient spasm and edematous folds to obstructive strictures and even abscesses.

Pseudocysts may be early complications of acute pancreatitis. They can arise from any portion of the pancreas. Depending on their location they produce characteristic pressure deformities on the stomach, duodenal loop, or remainder of the small bowel (see p. 993).

A rarer finding consists of small intramedullary osteolytic areas in one or more long bones. Their cause is uncertain, but local ischemia or intramedullary fat necrosis has been postulated. These bone lesions may disappear, or they may eventually calcify with an appearance identical to ordinary calcified bone infarcts.

Opacification of the gallbladder during oral cholecystography is poor or absent, a situation that persists for weeks or months. However, the gallbladder often opacifies after intravenous cholecystography.

During pyelography there may be impaired excretion from the left kidney due to spasm or even thrombosis of the left renal artery. The latter can be demonstrated by renal arteriography.

Barium studies, although the most revealing, are often omitted because of the patient's acute condition. However, a combination of the roentgen findings in the abdomen and chest may suggest the diagnosis.

The endoscopic pancreatogram will often show localized filling of secondary ductules and/or an acinar blush. If there has been previous chronic pancreatitis, there may also be evidence of calculi and pseudocysts. However, in severe acute pancreatitis, the patient is often too ill for the endoscopic study.[133-141]

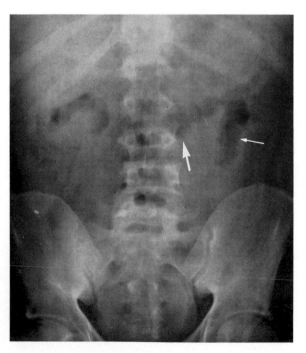

Figure 12–129 **Acute Pancreatitis: Localized Ileus (Sentinel Loop).** The short distended small bowel loop in the left upper abdomen *(small arrow)* persisted during several examinations. There is gas in the transverse colon *(large arrow),* but no distention. A sentinel loop, though frequently seen in acute pancreatitis, is nonspecific, being found in many other acute intra-abdominal inflammations such as cholecystitis and appendicitis.

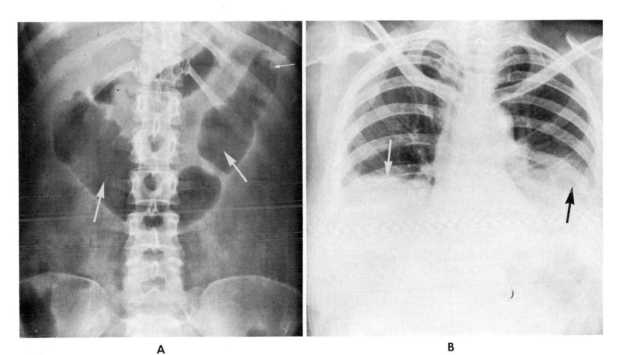

A   B

Figure 12–130 **Acute Pancreatitis: Colon Cutoff Sign, and Chest Findings.**

A, Almost the entire transverse colon is distended *(large arrows),* with a cutoff at the splenic flexure *(small arrow).*

B, There is a density at the left lung base, and the left costophrenic angle has been obliterated by fluid *(black arrow).* The right diaphragm is elevated, and plate-like atelectasis is seen at the right base *(white arrow).*

The colon cutoff sign associated with fluid in the chest, especially at the left base, strongly suggests acute pancreatitis.

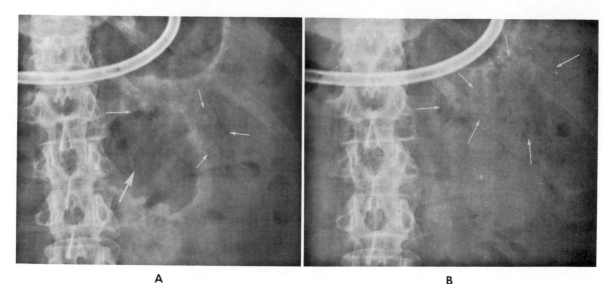

A   **B**

Figure 12–131   **Acute Pancreatitis: Secondary Retroperitoneal Abscess.**

A, A 56 year old man had acute abdominal symptoms and fever. There is a distended loop of small bowel *(large arrow)* in the left upper quadrant, and numerous small bubble-like lucencies *(small arrows)* lateral to the sentinel loop. A film of the chest demonstrated a small amount of fluid in the left pleural cavity. A tube is in the stomach.

B, Two days later the sentinel loop is not demonstrable, but the bubble-like gas shadows *(arrows)* are clearly shown. Barium enema study indicated that these gas shadows were outside the colon, and a diagnosis of retroperitoneal abscess was made.

At surgery, acute pancreatitis was found, in addition to a necrotic abscess with evidence of fat necrosis in the retroperitoneal space.

Small lucent shadows are characteristic of retroperitoneal air or gas and, as a rule, indicate a retroperitoneal abscess. Abscesses may develop rapidly following severe acute pancreatitis, and require surgical drainage. Radiographic diagnosis is based on recognition of extraluminal, small, bubble-like accumulations of gas.

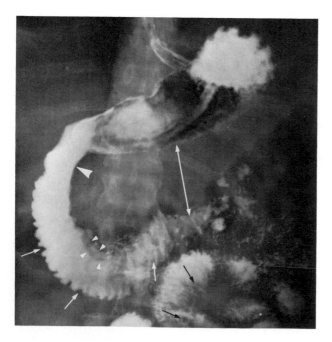

Figure 12–132   **Acute Pancreatitis: Oral Barium Study.** The duodenal loop is widened and dilated and contains thickened (edematous) folds *(small white arrows).* Pressure from the swollen pancreas has produced effacement of the folds along the inner aspect of the upper loop *(large arrowhead)* and a double border *(small arrowheads)* on the inner aspect of the third portion of the loop. The edematous pancreatic body causes an increased space *(double-headed arrow)* between the stomach and the distal loop. The jejunal mucosal folds are also somewhat edematous *(black arrows).*

The dilated loop, the edematous folds, and the evidence of pancreatic enlargement are highly characteristic of acute pancreatitis.

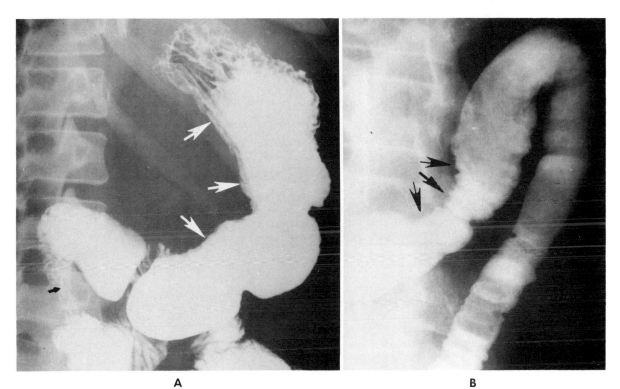

A   **B**

Figure 12–133   **Acute Pancreatitis of Body and Tail: Effect on Stomach and Colon.**

A, The lesser curvature of the stomach shows a persistent irregularity of its border *(white arrows)* owing to edema of its mucosa resulting from the adjacent inflamed body of the pancreas. Generally, these changes are best demonstrated on lateral film. The lesser curvature normally has a smooth sharp border.

Note the absence of changes in the duodenal loop *(black arrow),* since the pancreatic head was not involved.

B, A persistent pressure defect on a medial segment of the distal transverse colon is associated with a spiculated border *(arrows),* also due to an adjacent inflammatory mass arising from the pancreatic body. This effect, when more severe, can cause marked colonic spasm and produce the so-called colon cut-off sign on plain films.

Focal pancreatitis of the body without involvement of the head can occur but is uncommon.

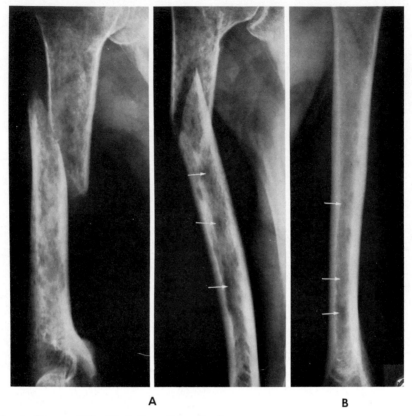

A   B

Figure 12–134   **Acute Pancreatitis: Medullary Bone Lesions.**

A, In the right humerus there are multiple, poorly defined intramedullary osteolytic areas *(arrows)* probably due to intramedullary fat necrosis. An old, ununited fracture is also present.

B, Similar but less striking lesions *(arrows)* are found in the distal femur.

The lesions in the right humerus are exaggerated by the associated osteoporosis of disuse from the old injury. (Courtesy Dr. J. L. Achord, Atlanta, Georgia.)

Chronic Pancreatitis

Chronic relapsing pancreatitis is characterized by recurrent acute attacks. Pancreatic calcifications develop in 20 to 40 per cent of cases and are virtually a pathognomonic finding. They may vary from a few discrete opacities in the pancreatic head, to extensive deposits that often spread to the body and tail. The calcium is mainly in the parenchyma but may also be within the ductile system (pancreatic lithiasis). On anteroposterior films, calcifications in the pancreatic head appear as small discrete irregular deposits in the vicinity of L1 or L2. During barium meal studies they are seen in the area surrounded by the duodenal loop.

The indurated pancreatic head may be enlarged and can produce pressure changes on the inner aspect of the loop, often with flattening of the medial folds. Distinction from pancreatic carcinoma may be difficult or impossible to make by means of the loop changes alone.

If severe pancreatic insufficiency has developed there may be a nonspecific celiac-sprue pattern associated with steatorrhea.

If obstructive jaundice occurs, a transhepatic cholangiogram will reveal a smoothly tapered and often undulant narrowing of the distal common duct, in contrast to abrupt cutoff and irregularity of the duct caused by pancreatic carcinoma; however, differentiation from carcinoma cannot always be made. Pancreatic angiography will sometimes help to make the distinction. Selective superior mesenteric and celiac arteriography frequently can confirm or suggest the diagnosis of pancreatitis. The most frequent findings in recurrent pancreatitis are a focal or generalized pancreatic blush and irregularity and beading of the small arteries. Occlusion of the splenic vein without encasement of the adjacent arteries is often found in pancreatitis of the tail or body. Sometimes, however, the angiographic findings may closely simulate those of pancreatic neoplasm.

In a small percentage of cases, irregular intramedullary calcific areas are found in the distal portion of one or more long bones; these are indistinguishable from calcified bone infarcts. They are thought to be healed calcified areas of intramedullary fat necrosis from prior acute pancreatitis.

The presence of pancreatic calcifications simplifies interpretation of abdominal and chest findings (see p. 983) during an acute flareup of chronic relapsing pancreatitis.

Endoscopic retrograde cholangiopancreatography is useful in diagnosis. Positive findings of duct abnormalities include diffuse narrowing, tortuosity, stenosis, dilatation, and abnormally filled branch ducts. Pseudocysts and ductile calculi can also be demonstrated in some cases.[142-146]

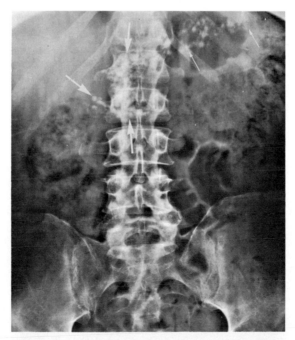

Figure 12–135 **Chronic Relapsing Pancreatitis: Extensive Pancreatic Lithiasis.** The pancreas is studded with calculi of varying sizes. All the calculi are within the ducts. The calcifications to the right of L2 and those overlying the spine *(large arrows)* are in the pancreatic head. From the area of the pancreatic head, calcifications extend upward and to the left, involving the body and tail of the pancreas *(small arrows)*. Most commonly the calcifications are found only in the pancreatic head and may be overlooked or mistaken for calcified mesenteric nodes.

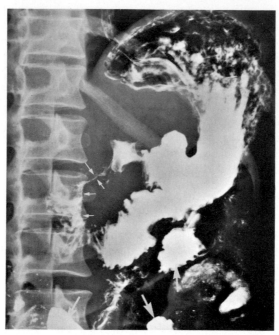

Figure 12–136 **Chronic Pancreatitis: Duodenal Loop Changes.** The mucosal pattern of the inner aspect of the duodenal loop is effaced, and extrinsic pressure is evident (*small arrows*). The lumen of the postbulbar area is considerably narrowed (*opposing small arrows*) by the indurated and enlarged pancreatic head. Pancreatic carcinoma can cause identical changes in the duodenal loop.

A small bowel deficiency pattern is demonstrated, with segmented and dilated loops (*large arrows*), some of which lack mucosal markings.

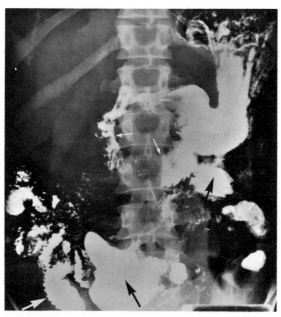

Figure 12–137 **Pancreatitis and Pancreatic Insufficiency: Malabsorption.** The deficiency pattern is evidenced by the dilated smooth segments (*black arrows*), thickened folds (*large white arrow*), and flocculation. The duodenal loop (*small white arrows*) is widened due to enlargement of the pancreatic head.

The deficiency pattern is not specific and is seen in many conditions associated with malabsorption; however, this pattern can occur without clinical malabsorption.

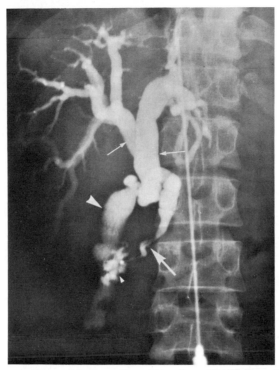

Figure 12–138 **Chronic Pancreatitis with Jaundice: Transhepatic Cholangiogram.** The biliary tree is clearly outlined. The dilated main hepatic bile ducts (*small arrows*) and the gallbladder (*large arrowhead*) are opacified. The lower end of the common duct (*large arrow*) is tapered, narrowed, and undulant. A small amount of opaque material has entered the duodenum (*small arrowhead*). There is no evidence of invasion or mass in the common duct; this finding helps differentiate chronic pancreatitis from pancreatic carcinoma.

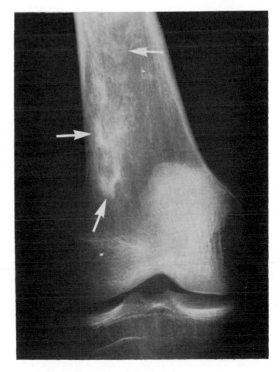

Figure 12–139 **Chronic Pancreatitis: Calcified Intramedullary Lesions.** Radiograph of the femur of a 35 year old man with chronic relapsing pancreatitis reveals irregular intramedullary calcifications (*arrows*). Biopsy showed large areas of necrotic fat cells surrounded by calcium deposits.

Radiographically, the appearance is indistinguishable from that of a calcified infarct. (Courtesy S. Bank, M.R.C.P., Capetown, South Africa.)

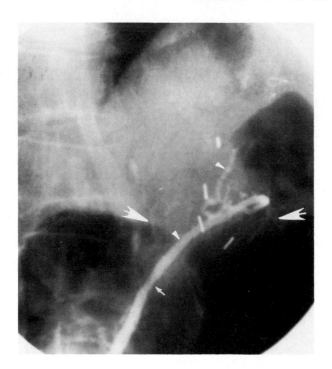

Figure 12–140 **Chronic Pancreatitis: Endoscopic Retrograde Pancreatography.** The pancreatic duct is mildly dilated and irregular, with areas of narrowing (*small arrow*) and beading (*arrowheads*). Many of the smaller ducts are filled (*large arrows*).

These ductal changes are characteristic of chronic pancreatitis. However, it is often impossible to distinguish chronic pancreatitis from pancreatic carcinoma by the appearance of the opacified pancreatic ducts alone.

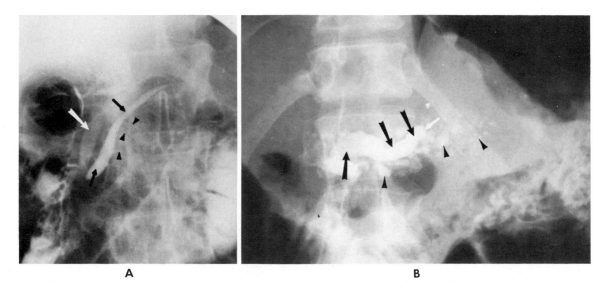

A   B

Figure 12–141 **Chronic Pancreatitis in Two Patients: Endoscopic Retrograde Pancreatography.**

In both these patients, the duodenoscope had been removed just prior to the radiographs.

A, The pancreatic duct is somewhat dilated proximally, and slightly irregular with some narrowing of its midportion (*black arrows*). There is filling of the branch ducts (*arrowheads*) all along the main duct. Incidentally, the common duct (*white arrow*) is also opacified.

B, In the second patient, there is extensive calcification of the pancreas (*arrowheads*). The pancreatic duct (*black arrows*), opacified via cannulation, is greatly dilated, somewhat irregular, and abruptly terminated (*white arrow*) by a duct calculus.

The various findings of chronic pancreatitis are illustrated in the above illustrations. These include pancreatic calculi, irregularities of the pancreatic duct, focal dilatations and narrowings, filling of the branch ducts, and calculous obstruction of the main duct. However, distinction from pancreatic carcinoma is often difficult or impossible.

Pancreatitis: Pseudocyst Formation

Pseudocysts usually result from recurring acute pancreatitis and, less often, after pancreatic trauma. They are loculated fluid collections arising from inflammatory processes, necrosis, or hemorrhage. They originate in any portion of the pancreas or adjacent tissue. Rapid enlargement is not unusual. They are usually not connected to the ductile system.

Although a soft tissue mass may be seen, most often recognition of the cysts depends on evidence of pressure and displacement of adjacent structures. A cyst in the head of the pancreas will usually cause pressure defects and may widen the duodenal loop; if arising from the body or tail the cyst may cause displacement and deformity of the stomach and the proximal jejunal loops. Colon displacement can also occur. Displacement of the left kidney or ureter is sometimes demonstrated on intravenous pyelogram, and compression of the portal vein may be seen on splenoportogram.

Pseudocysts are usually avascular, but they cause displacement of adjacent vessels on celiac or selective pancreatic angiograms. Most large cysts may be identified by this method. Sometimes the portal or splenic vein may be compressed or occluded. Splenomegaly and esophageal varices may then occur. Ultrasonography is useful in demonstrating the cystic nature of the mass lesion.[13, 142, 147, 148]

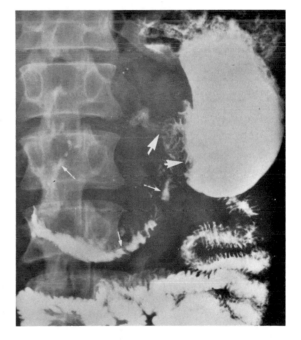

Figure 12–142 **Pseudocyst of Head of Pancreas.** The large mass has caused widening of the duodenal loop and presses on the inner wall of the loop *(small arrows)*. A pressure defect on the lower end of the stomach is also evident *(large arrows)*.

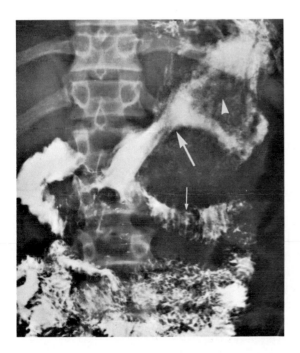

Figure 12–143 **Pseudocyst of Body of Pancreas.** A huge pseudocyst produces elevation of the body of the stomach *(large arrow)*, and depression of the duodeno-jejunal junction and the adjacent small bowel loops *(small arrow)*. The cyst has also created a large pressure defect on the body of the stomach *(arrowhead)*.

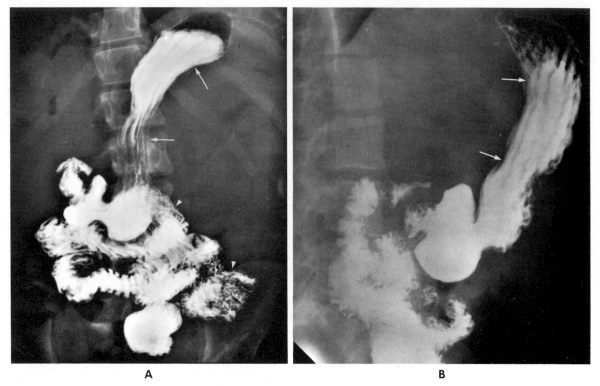

A   B

Figure 12–144   **Pseudocyst of Tail of Pancreas.**

A, The huge cyst causes displacement of the stomach medially *(arrows)* and the small bowel caudally *(arrowheads).*

B, In lateral view there is marked forward displacement of the upper half of the stomach *(arrows)* by the cyst, which is located in the retroperitoneal area behind the displaced stomach.

Figures 12–142 to 12–144 illustrate the characteristic displacement of the stomach and duodenum by large lesions of the head, body, and tail of the pancreas.

Cystic Fibrosis of the Pancreas (Mucoviscidosis)

In this hereditary disorder the basic physiologic abnormality is an increased viscidity of the mucus excreted by the exocrine glands. Characteristic changes in the sweat electrolytes are diagnostic. The viscid secretions result in a widespread bodily disorder most commonly and severely affecting the respiratory and gastrointestinal systems.

Pulmonary involvement is the most frequent and serious complication, appearing in infancy and childhood and usually causing death before the age of 30. Bronchiolar obstruction by viscid mucus can cause focal areas of atelectasis and recurrent pulmonary infections. Peribronchial involvement is most frequent in the perihilar and upper lobe areas. Radiographically the perihilar markings become stringy, thickened, and irregular, sometimes obscuring much of the cardiac borders (shaggy heart appearance). Hyperinflation always develops. Recurrent pneumonia and focal areas of atelectasis modify the picture. Eventually, permanent diffuse changes develop, owing to peribronchial fibrosis, emphysema, and bronchiectasis. These give rise to a characteristic roentgen picture of stringy, irregularly thickened markings, mainly perihilar and upper lobe, with severe hyper-inflation and cor pulmonale. Cardiac failure, often the terminal event, is evidenced mainly by cardiac enlargement. The congestive changes are masked on the radiograph by the underlying peribronchial densities.

In about 10 per cent of newborns with cystic fibrosis, thick mucus obstructs the small bowel—meconium ileus. Perforation and peritonitis may occur, and the extraluminal meconium may calcify, giving the characteristic picture of meconium peritonitis. A small bowel volvulus often is associated with the meconium ileus.

In older children or adults, large amounts of fecal material may accumulate in the terminal ileum and cecum and cause small bowel obstruction—the meconium ileus equivalent syndrome. A fecal bolus in the region of the terminal ileum is virtually pathognomonic of cystic fibrosis. Sometimes a persistent fecal collection in the cecum may cause a tumor-like defect in the cecum on the barium enema study. The viscid bolus may even cause intussusception.

Other abnormalities of the gastrointestinal tract occur in a high percentage of patients with cystic fibrosis. The commonest finding is an abnormal duodenal pattern, consisting of thickened mucosal folds, large nodular indentations, and, sometimes, a smudged, poorly defined mucosal pattern. Less often, thick coarsened folds are seen in the proximal jejunum, which may also be somewhat dilated. The classic small bowel malabsorption pattern with segmentation and flocculation is infrequently encountered in spite of the pancreatic enzyme deficiency. In older children, a nodular cobblestone pattern is often seen in the postevacuation colon film; this is due to redundant thickened colonic mucosa.

In a minority of cases, chronic plugging of the biliary canaliculi produces cirrhosis of the liver, with roentgen evidence of splenomegaly and esophageal varices. Mucoviscidosis has been postulated as an etiologic factor in the unexplained frequent association of adult emphysema and peptic ulcer, although this has not been corroborated.[149-156]

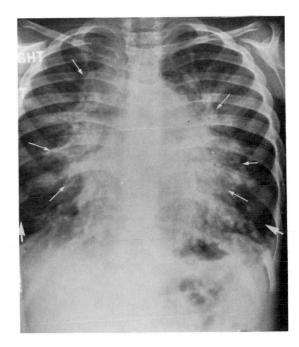

Figure 12–145 **Cystic Fibrosis: Pulmonary Changes in a Young Adult.** The heart shadow is obscured by stringy densities extending from the hila in all directions *(small arrows)*. These represent peribronchial infiltrates around the larger bronchi. There is hyperinflation at the bases *(large arrows)* with depressed diaphragms, an almost invariable finding in cystic fibrosis. Although these alterations are characteristic, pulmonary involvement is quite variable, and the pulmonary infiltrates change rapidly.

Extensive perihilar infiltrates that obscure the cardiac borders give rise to the shaggy heart appearance; this appearance is also seen in some cases of pertussis pneumonia. (See also Figure 9–11.)

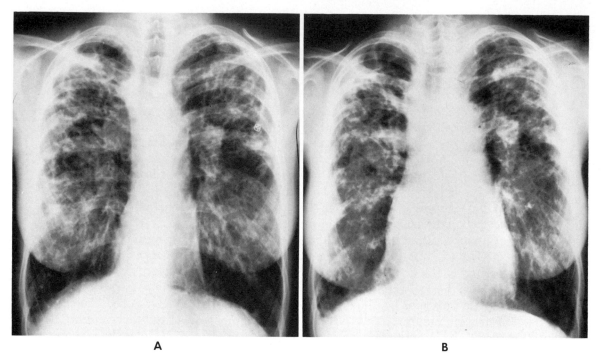

A   B

Figure 12–146   **Cystic Fibrosis: Right Heart Failure.**

A, In this 24 year old woman, the heart is small and the lung fields show the characteristic changes of advanced cystic fibrosis—hyperinflation and diffuse peribronchial thickening and infiltrates.

B, Clinical right heart failure developed six weeks later. The heart has become considerably enlarged, but the lung fields appear unchanged, with no apparent pulmonary or vascular signs of failure.

In cystic fibrosis patients, cardiac enlargement may be the only radiographic finding of right heart failure.

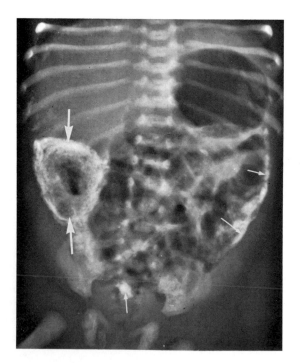

Figure 12–147   **Cystic Fibrosis: Meconium Peritonitis in an Infant.**   Uniform distention of both large and small bowel, which is characteristic of a toxic or paralytic ileus, is in this case due to chronic peritonitis.

The meconium, which has spilled into the peritoneum, has become calcified and can be seen along the lateral peritoneal wall (*small arrows*), as a large round accumulation beneath the liver (*large arrows*), and in the pelvis (*lower arrow*). These amorphous calcifications, when associated with ileus in a newborn infant, are diagnostic of meconium peritonitis.

The picture may also occur in a newborn with congenital strictures of the bowel which subsequently give rise to peritonitis, but in the majority of cases the cause is cystic fibrosis.

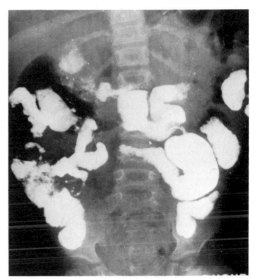

A

Figure 12–148 **Cystic Fibrosis: Malabsorption and Cor Pulmonale in a Child.**

A, A small bowel study of an unusually short-statured 6 year old with steatorrhea since infancy discloses a well-defined malabsorption pattern, with diffuse segmentation, numerous dilated loops, and effacement of mucosal folds (moulage).

B, A chest film is negative at this time. There had been relatively few respiratory episodes.

C, Eighteen months later, after repeated bouts of severe "bronchitis," there are diffuse interstitial densities throughout the lungs, and a marked enlargement of the main pulmonary artery *(arrow)*—a cor pulmonale. Hyperinflation was present although not readily apparent on the frontal film.

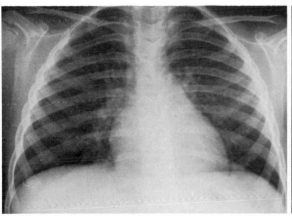

B

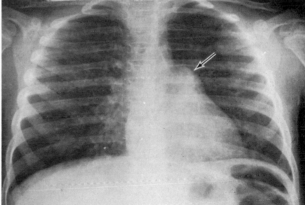

C

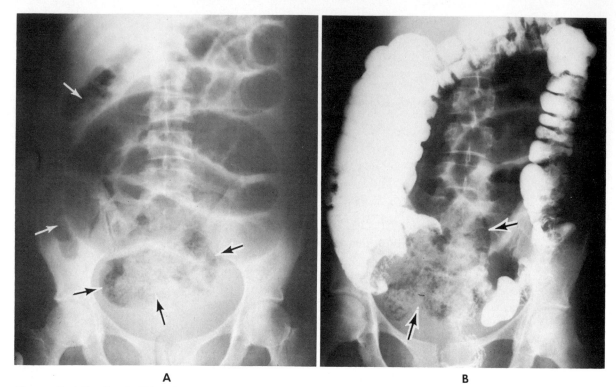

A   B

Figure 12–149 **Cystic Fibrosis: Meconium Ileus Equivalent Syndrome.**

A young woman with cystic fibrosis developed symptoms of intestinal obstruction.

A, Abdominal film reveals extensive small bowel distention, but there is a large collection of gas and feces in the lower abdomen *(black-white arrows),* suggestive of a sigmoid impaction. However, the large bowel *(white arrows)* is not dilated.

B, Barium enema shows that the "fecal" collection *(arrows)* is in the cecal and terminal ileum area, apparently obstructing the small bowel.

In older patients with cystic fibrosis, fecal inspissation and increased viscidity can occur in the cecum and extend into the terminal ileum to cause small bowel obstruction.

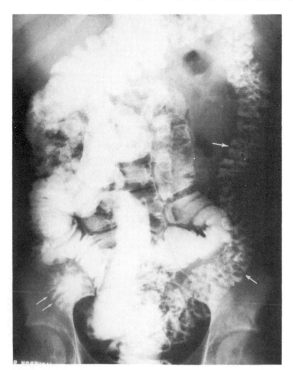

Figure 12–150 **Adult Cystic Fibrosis: Colon and Small Bowel Changes.** The mucosal folds in the descending colon are thickened and redundant, with a somewhat nodular appearance resembling polyps *(larger arrows).* The small bowel folds *(smaller arrows)* are similarly involved.

Changes in the colon and small bowel are found in about one third of older patients with cystic fibrosis and are due to increased numbers of goblet cells, distended mucosal glands, and adherent mucus.

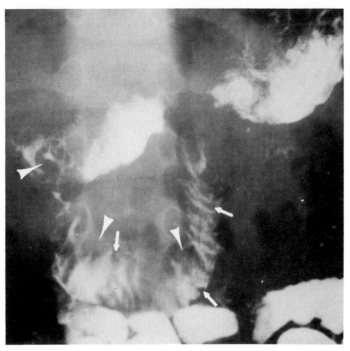

Figure 12-151 **Cystic Fibrosis: Duodenal Loop Changes.** The thickened mucosal folds *(arrows)*, the smudged appearance of the duodenum, and the nodular defects *(arrowheads)* are characteristic duodenal loop changes of cystic fibrosis.

Carcinoma of the Pancreas

In carcinoma of the head of the pancreas, suggestive findings on routine barium studies are seen in only about 50 per cent of cases. Early or small lesions rarely produce detectable roentgen abnormalities. Tumors of the body or tail become quite large before radiologic changes occur.

In carcinoma of the pancreatic head with jaundice, a frequent finding is a pressure defect on the distal duodenal bulb from dilatation of the common duct. Next in frequency is evidence of a mass pressing on the greater curvature of the gastric antrum. Often the changes in the duodenal loop are minimal and subtle: there are circumscribed indentations on the inner surface of the loop, effacement of the valvulae on the inner aspect, elongation and fixation of individual mucosal folds, and widening of the curve of the loop. With progression of the tumor, neoplastic invasion of the gastric antrum and duodenal loop may become apparent. The inverted figure 3 sign of Frostberg (i.e., indentations above and below the papilla of Vater) can be due to either neoplasm or inflammatory swelling of the pancreas; it is not as frequent as—nor is it the cardinal sign—it was initially considered to be.

When conventional barium studies in a suspected case are negative or equivocal, hypotonic duodenography should be performed. In this procedure, prolonged distention of the duodenal loop permits recognition of small and subtle loop changes from both extrinsic pancreatic pressure and intrinsic duodenal lesions.

Opacification of the common duct by oral or intravenous cholangiography in the absence of jaundice, or by transhepatic cholangiography in the presence of jaundice, often discloses the area of compression or invasion of the common duct.

In carcinoma of the body of the pancreas, a mass is frequently seen between the stomach and the duodenojejunal junction; the stomach is displaced upward and anteriorly and the duodenojejunal junction is displaced downward. Pressure and forward displacement of the upper half of the stomach can be seen with large lesions of the tail of the pancreas.

Angiographic studies for pancreatic carcinoma entail selective opacification of the hepatic, splenic, and superior mesenteric arteries and often subselective catheterization of the larger pancreatic arteries. Tumor vessels and staining are infrequent, since the tumor is often relatively avascular. Concentric narrowing and occlusion of the pancreatic arteries are helpful positive findings. Displacement and entrapment of other major arteries are significant. During the venous phase, there is often compression or occlusion of the portal or superior mesenteric vein from tumor of the head; in tumors of the body or tail, splenic vein involvement with numerous collaterals is frequent. Angiographic evaluation of the liver for metastatic disease should be made concurrently.

In spite of careful and extensive angiography, smaller pancreatic carcinomas are often difficult to detect.

Opacification of the pancreatic duct by direct catheterization through a duodenoscope may prove to be a helpful adjunctive procedure. Enlargement of the pancreas can frequently be demonstrated by ultrasonography.

In the presence of pancreatic mass or enlargement, pseudocyst or enlargement from chronic pancreatitis must be considered in the differential diagnosis. Ultrasound can usually distinguish a pseudocyst from a solid mass.[157-159]

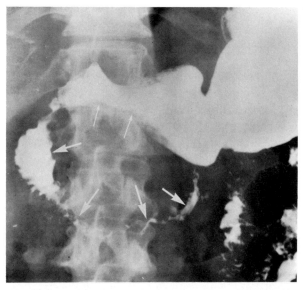

Figure 12–152 **Advanced Carcinoma of Head of Pancreas.** The greatly enlarged pancreatic head has produced a lobulated pressure defect on the greater curvature of the stomach *(small arrows);* this is often called the pad sign. Pressure changes are apparent also on the entire duodenal loop *(large arrows),* and there is marked enlargement and widening of the duodenal loop.

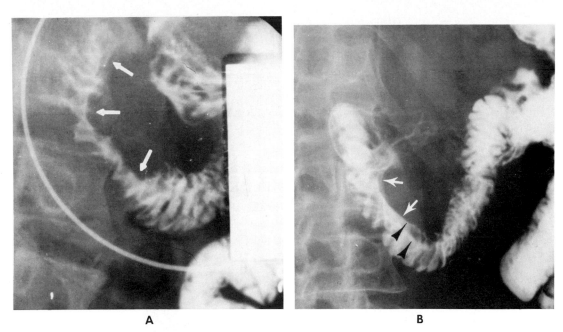

A   **B**

Figure 12–153   **Adenocarcinoma of Head of Pancreas.**

    A, Pressure defects on the medial aspect of the entire descending duodenal loop *(arrows)* are apparent. The lumen appears somewhat narrowed, and the normal mucosal pattern of the inner border is not seen.

    B, Hypotonic duodenography more strikingly demonstrates the large smooth pressure defect *(arrows)* and a double medial border *(arrowheads).*

    On a regular gastrointestinal study, the contractility of the duodenal loop may make identification of a pancreatic pressure defect difficult or impossible. Hypotonic duodenography, in which the loop is distended and noncontractile, permits positive identification of changes from extrinsic pancreatic pressure and from intrinsic duodenal lesions.

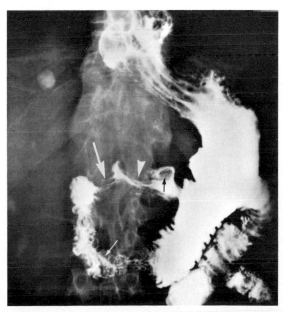

Figure 12–154   **Carcinoma of Head of Pancreas: Invasion of Gastric Antrum.**   The round defect in the antral portion of the stomach *(black arrow)* is due to invasion of the stomach by tumor, which has also produced a pressure defect more distally *(arrowhead).* A dilated common duct causes pressure just beyond the bulb *(large arrow).*

    The duodenal loop is somewhat widened, and there is evidence of pressure by a mass on the loop at the junction of the second and third portions *(small white arrow).* Sometimes this subtle alteration is the only finding, especially in early cases; it is often ignored, or is recognized only in retrospect.

    There is an unrelated large hiatal hernia, and an area of calcification in the base of the right lung.

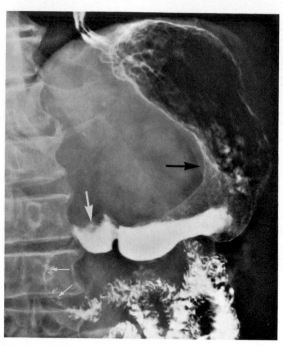

Figure 12–155 **Carcinoma of Head of Pancreas: Jaundice.** Pressure on the descending duodenal loop has caused effacement of the mucosal pattern on the medial aspect *(small arrows)*. The defect on the duodenal bulb *(large white arrow)* is from a dilated common duct. The liver is enlarged due to metastases, and presses upon the lesser curvature of the stomach *(black arrow)*.

Although the roentgenologic changes are not striking, the tumor was quite large.

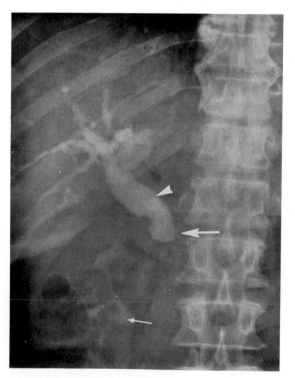

Figure 12–156 **Carcinoma of Head of Pancreas: Jaundice: Transhepatic Cholangiogram.** The common duct *(arrowhead)* is greatly dilated and is completely blocked *(large arrow)* at its lower segment. The obstructed area is irregular due to tumor invasion. The pyelogram *(small arrow)* results from the absorption of opaque material from the liver by the blood stream, and subsequent excretion by the kidneys.

A transhepatic cholangiogram in the presence of jaundice often allows differentiation of obstruction by calculus in the common duct, from obstruction by neoplasm of the common duct.

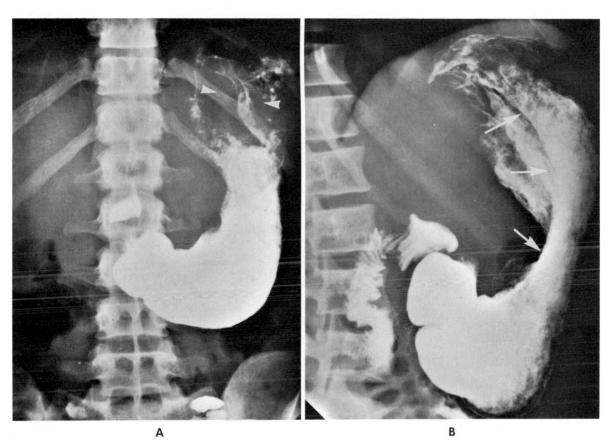

A   B

Figure 12-157 **Carcinoma of Tail of Pancreas.**

A, Large filling defects in the gastric fundus *(arrowheads)* simulate an intrinsic gastric lesion on anteroposterior view, but they are due to extrinsic pressure from a large carcinoma in the pancreatic tail.

B, Lateral film demonstrates extrinsic pressure deformity *(arrows),* due to the tumor, on the posterior wall of the stomach. The extent of the carcinoma can be surmised from these changes.

Tumors of the tail of the pancreas arise in the retroperitoneal space in the vicinity of the spleen and produce pressure effects on the gastric fundus; sometimes they displace the spleen.

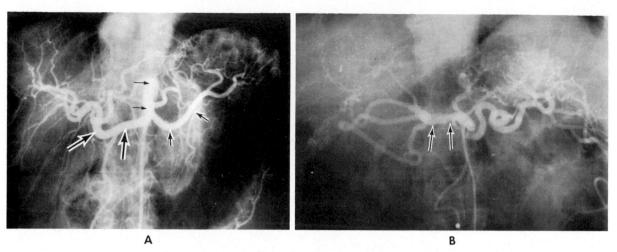

Figure 12–158 **Carcinoma of Body of Pancreas: Celiac Arteriogram.**

A, A normal celiac arteriogram shown for orientation and comparison illustrates a normal celiac artery *(black arrows)* containing the tip of the catheter. Its main branches, the hepatic artery *(large black-white arrows)* and the splenic artery *(small black-white arrows)* smoothly curve downward before coursing upward. All the vessels are smooth and regular.

B, Celiac arteriogram of a patient with backache and weight loss shows an elevated, irregular hepatic artery *(arrows),* which has been entrapped by a large carcinoma at the proximal portion of the pancreatic body. A prior barium gastrointestinal study was negative.

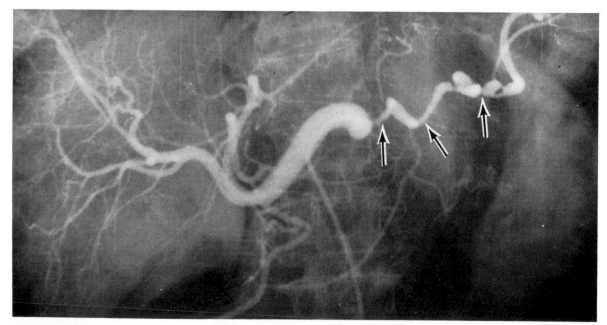

Figure 12–159 **Carcinoma of Body and Tail of Pancreas: Celiac Arteriogram.** The entire splenic artery is elevated, narrowed, and irregular. Its curves have become more angular *(arrows).* Almost the entire splenic artery was elevated and incarcerated by a large carcinoma of the body and tail of the pancreas.

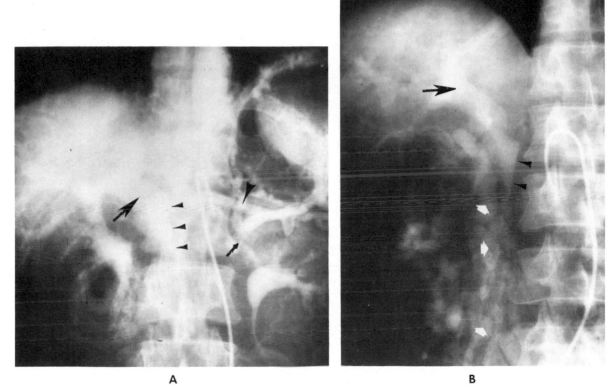

A   B

Figure 12-160 **Carcinoma of Pancreas: Obstruction of Splenic Vein and Superior Mesenteric Vein.**

A, Venous phase of celiac arteriogram shows an occluded splenic vein *(small arrow).* The portal vein *(large arrow)* is filled via a large collateral *(large arrowhead),* and there is evidence of mass pressure upon the portal vein *(small arrowheads).*

B, The venous phase of the superior mesenteric arteriogram shows filling of the portal vein *(black arrow)* by many collaterals *(white arrows),* but the superior mesenteric vein is occluded and not filled. The mass pressure on the portal vein *(arrowheads)* is again seen.

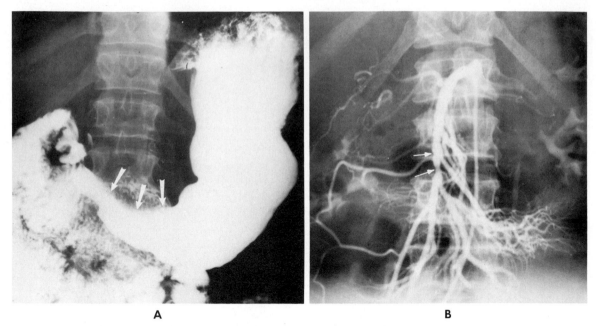

A   B

Figure 12–161   **Carcinoma of Body of Pancreas: Nonfunctioning Islet Cell Lesion.**

A, Gastrointestinal study in a 44 year old woman with epigastric pain shows evidence of a mass pressing upon the lesser curvature *(arrows)* of the distal third of the stomach.

B, Selective superior mesenteric arteriography discloses persistent irregularity, narrowing, and displacement to the right (entrapment) of the superior mesenteric artery *(arrows)*, indicative of a malignant pancreatic tumor.

INFLAMMATORY DISEASES OF THE INTESTINE

Regional Enteritis and Regional Colitis (Granulomatous Enterocolitis, Crohn's Disease)

Regional enteritis can occur at any age but is most common during the second and third decades. The most frequent site is the distal 12 inches of the terminal ileum, although any portion of the ileum or jejunum may be affected. Rarely, the stomach or duodenum is involved. In up to 40 per cent of cases the colon is also affected (regional enterocolitis). Involvement tends to be continuous in both the small and large bowel, but skip areas are frequent.

In regional enteritis the earliest radiographic findings are irritability and irregularly thickened folds in the affected segment. Later, the folds are effaced and the mucosa appears smooth and granular. Serrations due to small ulcerations are frequent. Progressive thickening of the bowel wall increases the space between adjacent loops and causes narrowing of the lumen. Superimposed prolonged spasm can produce an extremely narrow thread-like segment—the classic string sign. Fibrotic changes cause irreversibly fixed, narrowed, tube-like segments. Partial obstruction is common and may cause dilated proximal loops. Complete obstruction is unusual.

Inflammation and fibrosis often extend into the mesentery and mesenteric nodes, producing extraluminal masses that may displace or deform the cecum and adjacent ileal loops. Internal fistula formation between intestinal loops is fairly common but may be difficult to demonstrate. Fistulas to the skin, vagina, ureter, or bladder can also occur. Urinary tract involvement occurs in up to 10 per cent of cases, from either fistula formation or inflammation. In severe granulomatous enterocolitis, urography studies should be done.

Progress meal studies of the small bowel are necessary to disclose the full extent of small bowel involvement. Barium enema examination is also imperative because of the frequently associated colonic lesions.

Regional granulomatous colitis is the same pathologic process as regional enteritis. The colon may be involved alone, but ileal lesions are also present in a high proportion of cases. The right colon, especially the cecum and ascending colon, are the favorite sites, but any portion of the colon may be affected. Involvement of the entire colon and rectum occurs in up to 10 per cent of cases.

Radiographically, there is a distinct tendency toward eccentric involvement. The early findings are merely thickened folds and local irritability. Small nodular mucosal defects and small ulcerations produce fine serration of a wall. With progressive thickening of the wall and mucosa, nodular and often eccentric irregularities of contour appear. Pseudopolypoid mucosal thickening and deeper longitudinal and transverse ulcerations produce a cobblestone mucosa traversed by the barium-filled ulcer streaks. Eventually, the mucosa is totally effaced. Permanent areas of narrowing, deformity, or stricture can develop. Internal fistulas occur in almost half the cases. Pericolonic inflammatory masses sometimes develop. Occasionally an inflammatory pseudopolyp becomes quite large and simulates a true neoplasm. This usually occurs in the cecum.

A solitary segment of granulomatous colitis in the sigmoid may be indistinguishable from diverticulitis; biopsy is needed for correct diagnosis.

Gastric involvement is uncommon (less than 10 per cent) and is always associated with lesions of the ileum or colon. Involvement is almost always in the antrum, which appears narrowed and stiffened and may have a cobblestone mucosal pattern. Usually there is continuous involvement of the pylorus and proximal bulb, a highly suggestive appearance. Not uncommonly, the duodenal loop is also involved.

Although significant overlap exists between ulcerative colitis and granulomatous colitis both clinically and radiographically, certain radiographic features are more frequent in granulomatous disease. These include the predominant right-sided lesions with sparing of the distal colon, skip areas, eccentricity of wall involvement, long longitudinal ulcerations, strictures, fistulas, large irregular inflammatory polyps, ileal involvement, and the infrequency of toxic megacolon. Angiographic study of the colon is not generally helpful for distinguishing the two conditions.

It has been thought that bowel malignancy was not a complication of granulomatous colitis, but recent investigations suggest that rectocolonic carcinomas occur 20 times more often in patients with granulomatous disease than in a controlled population. Other rare complications are perforation, arthritis including sacroiliitis, liver disease especially pericholangitiis, and oxaluria with oxalate calculi.[160-169]

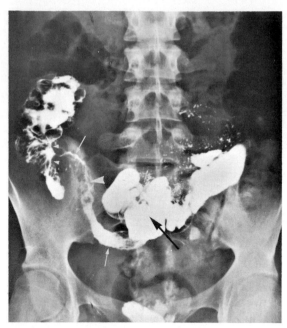

Figure 12–162 **Regional Enteritis: Terminal Ileum.** The distal 12 inches of terminal ileum *(small arrows)* are rigid, with thickened irregular folds distally *(large arrowhead)* and serrated margins proximally *(lower white arrow)*. The distal segment is narrow and stringy, and the ileocecal valve is thickened, producing indentations into the colon *(small arrowheads)*. There is dilatation from partial obstruction of the ileal loops *(black arrow)* proximal to the involved segment. The normal mucosal pattern is lacking throughout the affected segment.

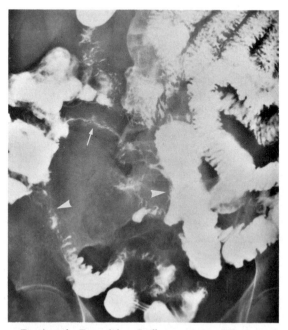

Figure 12–163 **Longstanding Regional Enteritis: Inflammatory Mass.** The diseased terminal ileum *(arrow)* is narrowed and irregular and has no mucosal pattern. It is elevated because of an inflammatory mass in the mesentery. The mass also displaces other loops of small bowel *(arrowheads)*. Such masses are not uncommon in protracted regional enteritis. Although the involved segment is persistently narrowed and fixed, there is only moderate dilatation of the proximal loops; complete obstruction is extremely rare.

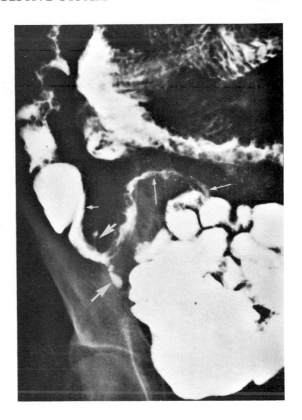

Figure 12–164 **Regional Enteritis: Fistulous Tracts.** A long segment of terminal ileum is diseased *(small arrows)*, with typical irregular narrowing, fixation, and loss of mucosal pattern. The involved loop is separated from the other loops by a thickened wall and mesentery. Barium projections *(large arrows)* from the ileum are fistulous tracts extending into the surrounding inflammatory mass. The uninvolved proximal ileum is dilated.

In this disease, fistulas may extend into inflammatory mesenteric masses, other small bowel loops, the sigmoid, the bladder, and even a ureter. External fistulas to the abdominal wall are not uncommon.

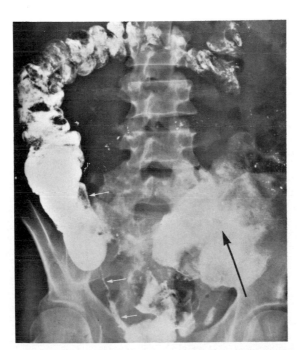

Figure 12–165 **Regional Enteritis: Matted Small Bowel Loops.** A long diseased segment of terminal ileum *(white arrows)* extends deep into the pelvis, where it is held by inflammatory adhesions. Inflammatory mesenteric involvement has produced matting. Many of the other ileal loops *(black arrow)* are matted because of a similar process, and were palpable in the left lower quadrant.

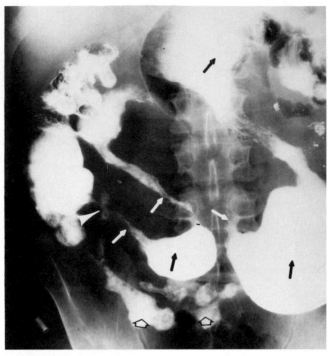

Figure 12–166 **Advanced Regional Enteritis.** The small bowel study discloses bizarre appearing structures, including many irregular inflammatory structures *(white arrows)*, greatly dilated segments *(black arrows)*, irregular, deformed loops *(open arrows)*, and a fistula between small bowel loops *(arrowhead)*. No mucosal pattern can be identified. The large spaces between loops are due to thickening of bowel walls and mesentery.

Virtually the entire small bowel was involved with granulomatous disease. Extensive involvement is often associated with malabsorption.

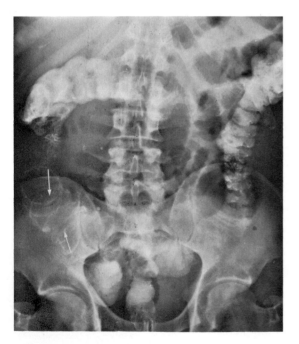

Figure 12–167 **Regional Enteritis: Intussusception of Inflammatory Mass.** A characteristic coiled-spring appearance in the right lower quadrant *(arrows)* on postevacuation barium enema film represents intussusception of the thickened terminal ileum through the ileocecal valve.

In adults, ileocecal intussusception is usually due to a mass that has been propelled into the colon by intense small bowel peristalsis. If the condition remains uncorrected, mechanical small bowel obstruction results. Surgical intervention becomes necessary if the intussusception does not correct spontaneously or by means of pressure exerted by a barium enema.

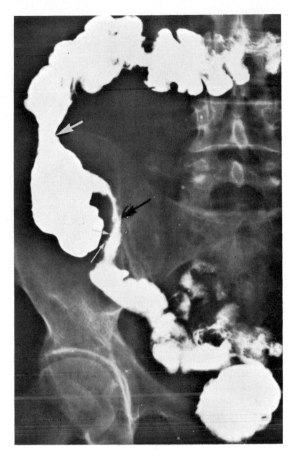

Figure 12–168 **Granulomatous Colitis and Enteritis.** The smooth narrow area in the midascending colon (*large white arrow*) represents chronic granulomatous colitis; this is the only area of colon involved. The terminal ileum (*black arrow*) is irregularly narrow, with small marginal ulcerations (*small white arrows*).

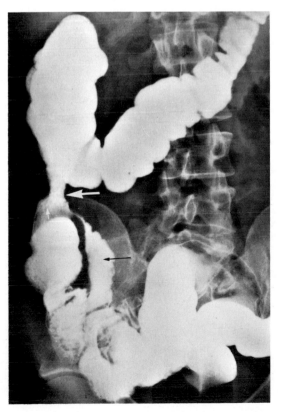

Figure 12–169 **Granulomatous Colitis in Ascending Colon.** The area just above the ileocecal region is smooth and narrow (*large arrow*). A cobblestone mucosa (*small white arrow*) can be seen throughout the involved segment. The terminal ileum (*black arrow*) is slightly dilated but otherwise normal. Differentiation between granulomatous colitis and ulcerative colitis often cannot be made by radiographic appearance, although involvement limited to the right colon strongly favors the diagnosis of granulomatous colitis.

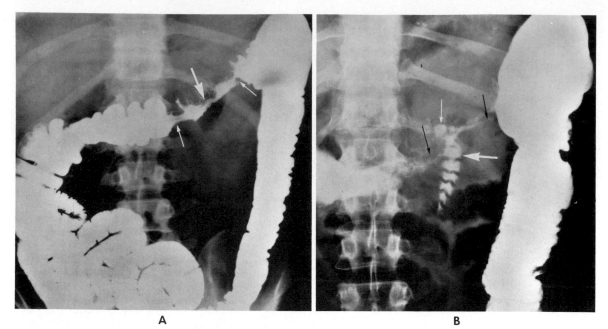

A   B

Figure 12–170   **Granulomatous Colitis of Transverse Colon, with Fistula Formation.**

A, There is segmental irregular narrowing of the transverse colon, with an abrupt transition to normal colon *(small arrows)*. Note the eccentric narrowing *(large arrow)* with multiple border irregularities, some of which were small ulcerations. The absence of shelving defects into the normal adjacent colon and the irritability of this segment fluoroscopically pointed to an inflammatory process.

The patient, a 31 year old man, experienced abdominal pain and lost much weight; the possibility of a malignant neoplasm was considered, but medical management was instituted.

B, Six months later, the segment has contracted further and is more distorted *(black arrows)*. A fistulous connection to the small bowel is demonstrated by direct barium flow from the lesion into a small bowel loop *(large white arrow)*. The round accumulation of barium *(small white arrow)* represents ulceration into the jejunum.

There had been no extension of the bowel involvement during the six month period, and this, together with the internal fistula, strongly suggested granulomatous colitis rather than segmental ulcerative colitis. The diagnosis was confirmed at surgery.

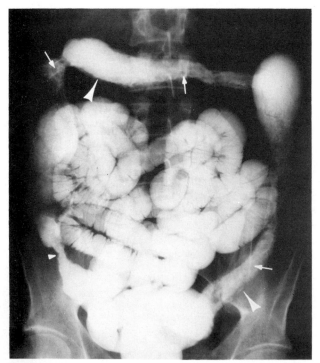

Figure 12–171 **Advanced Colitis: Granulomatous? Ulcerative?** The entire colon, except the rectum, is narrowed, shortened, and devoid of a normal mucosal pattern. Pseudopolyps *(arrows)* and ulcerations *(large arrowheads)* are present. A short segment of the terminal ileum *(small arrowhead)* is narrowed and has thickened walls.

Involvement of the entire colon by granulomatous disease (proved in this patient), although rare, can produce a radiographic appearance indistinguishable from that of advanced ulcerative colitis.

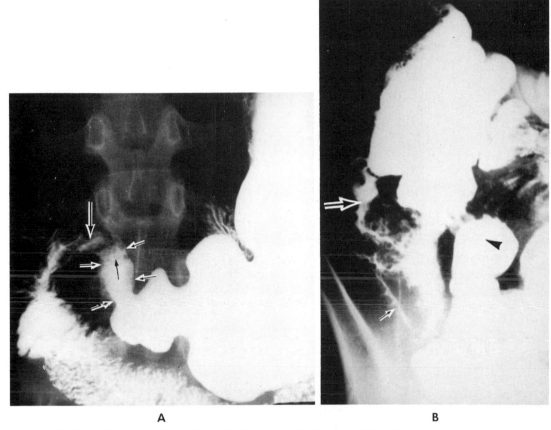

A   B

Figure 12–172 **Granulomatous Enteritis with Gastric and Duodenal Bulb Involvement.**

A, Upper gastrointestinal study in a 24 year old man with recurrent attacks of abdominal pain and moderate anemia reveals a stiffened narrowed antrum *(small black-white arrows)*. The involvement continues into the pylorus and duodenal bulb *(large black-white arrow)*. The narrowed deformed bulb can hardly be identified. The cobblestone mucosal pattern *(black arrow)* in the diseased antrum is strikingly similar to that seen in granulomatous colitis. A diagnosis of possible gastric and duodenal granulomatous disease was made, and a small bowel and colon study were suggested.

B, There is severe involvement of the cecum *(large arrow)* and terminal ileum *(small arrow),* and dilatation of the more proximal loops *(arrowhead).*

Gastric involvement in granulomatous colitis or enteritis, although rare, causes characteristic changes. The antrum, pylorus, and duodenal bulb are virtually always involved together, in a continuous fashion, and are narrowed and stiffened. Cobblestone gastric mucosal pattern can be seen in about half of these cases. In all reported cases with gastroduodenal involvement, ileal or colonic granulomatous disease was present.

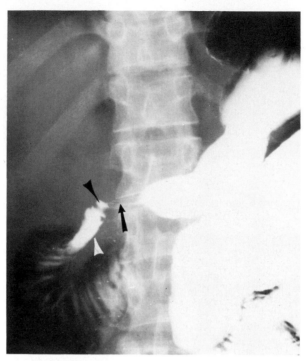

Figure 12–173 **Regional Enteritis: Gastric and Duodenal Involvement.** The gastric antrum is narrowed, with thickened folds *(arrow)*. The contracted fibrotic duodenal bulb *(black arrowhead)* is hardly recognizable, and the postbulbar duodenum *(white arrowhead)* is rigid and lacks a normal mucosal pattern.

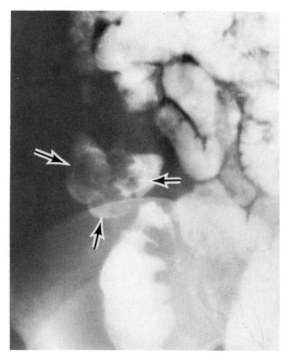

Figure 12–174 **Granulomatous Colitis: Giant Pseudopolyp in Cecum.** The large defect *(arrows)* in the cecum proved to be a giant pseudopolyp.

In regional granulomatous colitis, a persistent cecal mass could also be a giant fecal concretion proximal to a stricture, an unrelated adenomatous polyp, or a carcinoma.

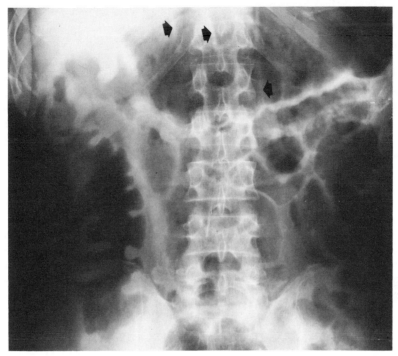

Figure 12–175 **Granulomatous Colitis: Megacolon.** Abdominal film of a young man with extensive granulomatous colitis shows a markedly distended transverse colon. Note the haustra (*arrows*) in the distended colon.

Toxic megacolon is extremely rare in granulomatous colitis in contrast to ulcerative colitis. Haustra are usually totally absent in the megacolon of ulcerative colitis, while defects due to pseudopolyps are common in the ulcerative but not granulomatous megacolon.

Ulcerative Colitis

In the early stages of this disease barium enema studies may appear negative, although irritability of the involved portions is common. The diagnosis of early ulcerative colitis is usually made by sigmoidoscopy. In somewhat more advanced disease, diagnosis can be readily made roentgenologically. Roentgen studies are most useful for determining the extent of involvement, the progress of the disease, and the complications.

The earliest roentgen changes are irritability, alterations of haustral markings, and tiny ulcerations. Instead of the normal smooth rounded sacculations, there may be flattening or squaring of the haustral outlines. Loss or alteration of the normal reticulated mucosal pattern may be seen on the postevacuation film. These changes are usually limited to the left colon. Of these early findings, only the ulcerations are characteristic, and even these may be simulated by barium-filled mucous glands in a normal colon. Often the soft tissue space between the anterior sacrum and the posterior rectum becomes widened due to a periproctitis. This may be a significant diagnostic clue.

As the disease progresses the roentgenologic appearance becomes more characteristic. The ulcers become larger. Some may burrow in the submucosa and develop a broad base and collar-button appearance. Edematous mucosal islands occur between ulcers, appearing as lucencies in the barium density. When numerous and fairly uniform, these produce the cobblestone appearance; with recurrent or continued disease they enlarge and become the characteristic pseudopolyps. The edematous nodules may disappear after a remission, but in the later stages of disease the pseudopolyps may persist because of fibrotic changes.

Often the bowel lumen narrows, the haustra disappear, and the bowel becomes shortened and rigid, presenting a tube-like appearance. The mucosal pattern is usually absent in this stage. Segmental strictures are uncommon, in contrast to granulomatous colitis.

The extent of the involvement is variable but is almost always continuous from the rectum proximally, and involvement of the entire colon is not unusual. Skip areas or single segment involvement above the sigmoid is quite rare, in contrast to granulomatous colitis. Not infrequently, back-lash involvement of the terminal ileum is seen, characterized by a thickened patulous ileocecal valve and a *dilated* stiff terminal ileum.

Among the complications detectable radiographically are colonic malignancy, acute toxic megacolon, and, rarely, fistula or pericolonic abscess.

There is a significantly increased incidence of colonic carcinoma in cases of longstanding ulcerative colitis. The carcinoma may be difficult to recognize radiologically, since it may resemble a strictured area or a large pseudopolyp. The average duration of the preceding colitis is over 10 years. The patients are usually young and the colitis frequently quiescent. The malignancy often is located in the right colon. Commonly, the lesions are long with irregular lumina and ragged edges. The ends may be cone-shaped, rather than abruptly narrowed with shoulder defects as in classic carcinoma. However, the defects may be similar to those seen in adenocarcinoma without ulcerative colitis. Any persistent narrowing should be viewed with suspicion.

Acute toxic megacolon is an uncommon but serious complication. There is pronounced distention, especially of the transverse colon. The pseudopolyps often appear as defects in the air column of the distended bowel, a highly suggestive finding. Toxic megacolon without pseudopolyps can also occur in other conditions, and on plain abdominal films distinction from a low mechanical large bowel obstruction may be difficult. Colonic perforation can occur, causing pneumoperitoneum and peritonitis.

Fistulas and pericolonic collections are much less common in ulcerative colitis than in granulomatous colitis.

Sclerosing cholangitis is a complication or associated disorder in about one per cent of patients. Other infrequent complications include pericholangitis, thromboembolic disease, arthritis including sacroiliitis, and nephrolithiasis.

The radiographic distinctions between ulcerative and granulomatous colitis are discussed under *granulomatous colitis* (see p. 1007).[67, 170–176]

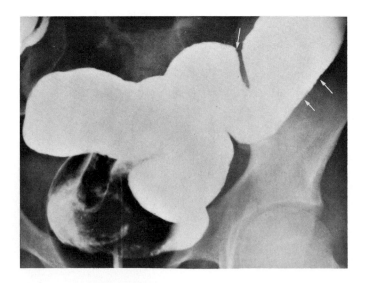

Figure 12–176 **Early Ulcerative Colitis: Sigmoid Ulcerations.** Barium enema examination was negative except for fine serrations in the sigmoid *(arrows),* which were due to small ulcerations. Evidence of ulcerative colitis was found on proctosigmoidoscopy.

Irritability and spasm of the sigmoid, and perhaps of the descending colon, are often seen in the early stage of the disease, but frequently the barium enema study is negative.

The fine serrations due to early ulcerations may be simulated by barium entering the mucous glands of a normal colon; hence, definitive diagnosis in many early cases must be made by proctoscopy and sigmoidoscopy.

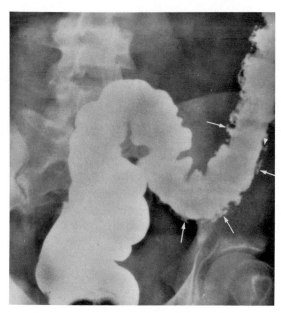

Figure 12–177 **Acute Ulcerative Colitis with Large Ulcerations.** The linear collections of barium *(arrows)* scattered diffusely along the margins of the sigmoid and descending colon were due to unusually large ulcerations that burrowed longitudinally beneath the mucosa *(arrowhead).*

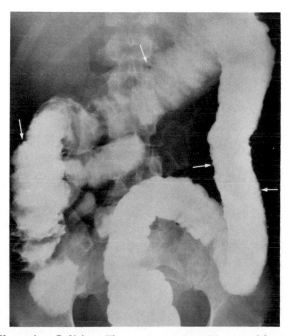

Figure 12–178 **Extensive Ulcerative Colitis.** The patient was a 26 year old man. Serrated margins, which involved practically every portion of the colon *(arrows),* were the result of extensive ulcerations. The thickened haustra and mucosal folds are most clearly seen in the transverse and right colon, presenting as lucent areas in the margins of the bowel.

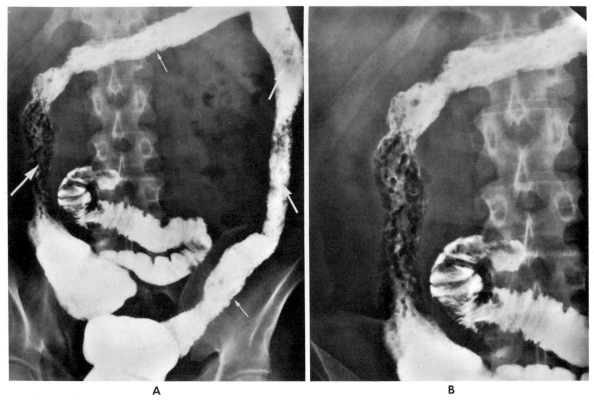

A   **B**

Figure 12–179 **Longstanding Ulcerative Colitis with Pseudopolyps.**

A, The entire colon is narrowed, rigid, and shortened. Haustra are absent.

The cobblestone appearance *(large arrows)* of multiple round defects is due to the innumerable pseudopolyps, which are hypertrophic areas of mucosa and submucosa. The pseudopolyps produce marginal defects *(small arrows)* along the colonic walls.

B, Enlargement of the right colon demonstrates the pattern of the pseudopolyps more distinctly.

The patient had a 15 year history of ulcerative colitis.

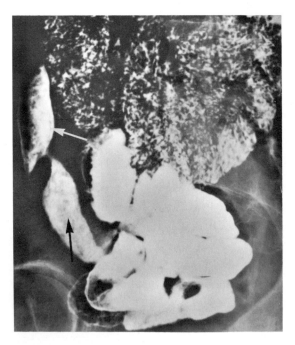

Figure 12–180 **Advanced Ulcerative Colitis: Terminal Ileum Involvement.** A small bowel study reveals a rigid and somewhat dilated terminal ileal segment *(black arrow)* with multiple small, round, lucent defects that represent thickened mucosa and submucosa. The distal inch of the ileum is narrowed. Barium has entered the cecum and ascending colon *(white arrow),* which also appear rigid. The cecal tip is contracted and tapered. Pseudopolyps in the cecum and ascending colon are well defined. Note the roentgenologic similarity between the diseased terminal ileum and the contracted right colon.

Terminal ileum involvement in advanced ulcerative colitis is termed back-lash ileitis. The segment is usually dilated and rigid, in contrast to the narrowed terminal ileum in regional enteritis.

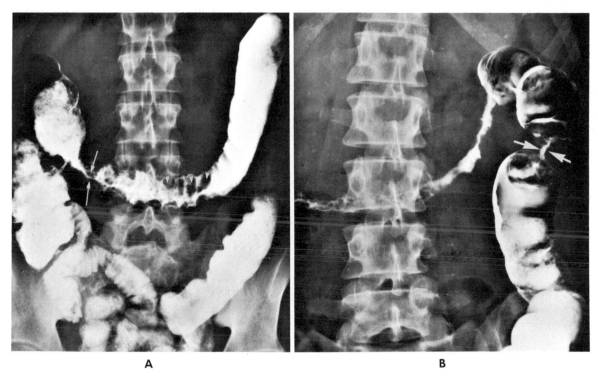

A   B

Figure 12–181   **Carcinoma of Colon Complicating Longstanding Ulcerative Colitis: Two Cases.**

A, Eccentrically narrowed area in the transverse colon *(arrows)* simulates a stricture, but proved to be a carcinoma. Note the unusually large pseudopolyps in the transverse colon *(arrowheads).*

B, An area of constriction more characteristic of neoplasm is seen in the descending colon *(arrows).* In this patient, changes of ulcerative colitis are seen most clearly in the transverse colon.

Both patients had had ulcerative colitis for over 10 years. In longstanding cases, any persistently deformed segment should be investigated for possible carcinoma.

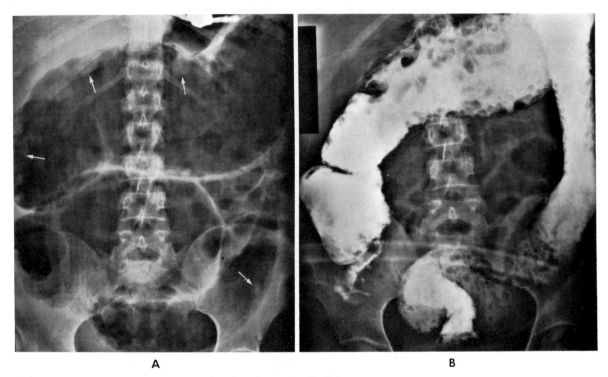

A   B

Figure 12–182 **Acute Toxic Megacolon in Ulcerative Colitis.**

A, Extreme gaseous distention of the entire colon is most marked in the transverse colon. The haustra are absent, and large pseudopolyps can be seen as defects extending from the wall into the air-filled lumen *(arrows).*

The patient had a long history of ulcerative colitis and was extremely toxic and febrile. The abdomen was greatly distended.

B, Barium enema made a few days later shows advanced ulcerative colitis involving the entire colon, with numerous large psuedopolyps, especially in the dilated transverse colon. Barium enema examination is rarely indicated in toxic megacolon.

Acute toxic megacolon is a rare but most serious complication; emergency management is necessary. Great distention of the colon, most pronounced in the transverse colon, and pseudopolyps visualized as defects in the air-filled colon are the roentgenologic findings that permit diagnosis even when no clear-cut history of ulcerative colitis is obtained. Less commonly, megacolon may be found in fulminating amebic colitis or granulomatous colitis.

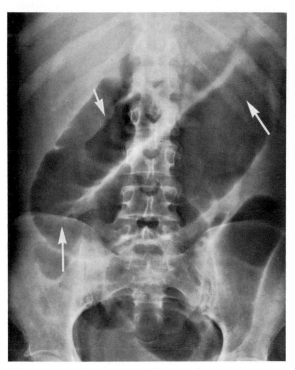

Figure 12–183 **Acute Toxic Megacolon Not Due to Ulcerative Colitis.** Marked distention of the colon, especially the transverse colon *(arrows)*, developed suddenly in a patient with an *E. coli* septicemia. The normal haustra and the absence of pseudopolyps may help distinguish megacolon due to other causes from the megacolon of ulcerative colitis.

Although acute toxic megacolon may develop in many diseases, it is most frequently seen in ulcerative colitis. The findings in toxic megacolon may be mistaken for those caused by low mechanical obstruction of the large bowel.

Appendicitis

Although the diagnosis of acute appendicitis is based primarily on clinical findings, roentgenograms may prove useful in corroborating the diagnosis and in demonstrating the presence of complications.

In a high percentage of cases, plain films reveal a distended loop of small bowel in the appendiceal area with or without fluid levels (sentinel loop). Less often, with the patient in upright position, there is a distended cecum containing fluid levels. A calcified fecalith in the appendix (appendolith) is associated with gangrenous appendicitis in a high percentage of cases. Radiographic recognition of an appendolith may therefore be of great significance. Barium enema examination should be avoided in acute cases because of the danger of perforation; if the examination is performed, visualization of the appendix virtually eliminates the diagnosis of acute appendicitis.

After perforation, generalized peritonitis with paralytic ileus (distended small and large intestines) may be seen; localized perforation leads to a periappendiceal abscess, which may present as a soft tissue mass or as an area of haziness in the right lower quadrant. The abscess may produce a pressure deformity on the cecum, which is seen either in the cecal air shadow on plain films or in the barium-filled cecum. Often there is small bowel distention due to mechanical small bowel obstruction. Free peritoneal air after rupture of the appendix is quite rare.[173, 177]

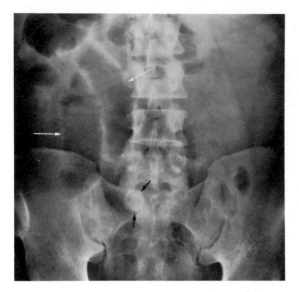

Figure 12–184 **Acute Appendicitis: Sentinel Loop and Fecalith.** In the right lower quadrant there is a distended loop of ileum (sentinel loop) *(white arrows),* which contained fluid levels in erect view.

The round density with the calcified rim *(black arrows)* is a fecalith in the appendix; when seen in conjunction with a sentinel loop, it suggests acute appendicitis.

A sentinel loop in itself is nonspecific, indicating the presence of a local intra-abdominal inflammatory condition such as appendicitis, cholecystitis, or pancreatitis.

Figure 12–185 **Acute Appendicitis: Distended Cecum with Fluid Levels.** There is a fluid level in the distended cecum *(large arrow),* as well as one in a descended loop of ileum *(small arrows)* (sentinel loop). Sentinel loop or distended cecum, or both, is seen only in severe and more rapidly progressive cases of acute appendicitis, and is suggestive of the diagnosis.

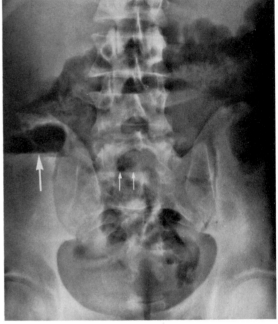

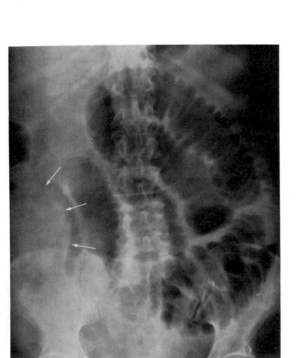

Figure 12–186 **Periappendiceal Abscess Producing Intestinal Obstruction.** A soft tissue mass in the right lower quadrant causes a curved pressure defect on the adjacent gas-filled small bowel loop *(arrows).* This mass was a periappendiceal abscess. Marked distention of the small bowel loops is due to an intestinal obstruction caused by pressure from the abscess.

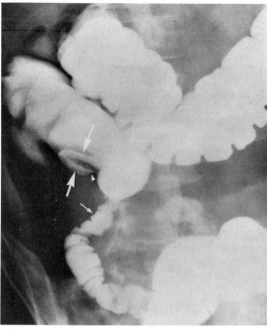

Figure 12–187 **Periappendiceal Abscess: Barium Enema.**   The cecum and terminal ileum *(small arrow)* are displaced medially by a right lower quadrant (periappendiceal) abscess. The appendix *(large arrows)* is partially filled with barium; its tip *(arrowhead)* is irregular and was imbedded in the periappendiceal abscess. Most often the appendix is not visualized.

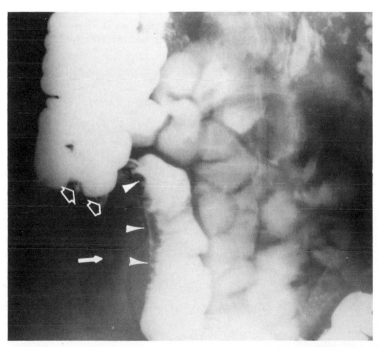

Figure 12–188 **Periappendiceal Abscess; Classic Findings.**   There is some deformity of the cecal tip *(open arrows)*, medial displacement and pressure on the lateral wall of the terminal ileum *(arrowheads)*, and a calcified appendolith *(solid arrow)*. These findings are virtually diagnostic of a periappendiceal abscess.

Diverticulitis

Diverticulitis can occur in any segment of the bowel, but the sigmoid and descending colon, respectively, are the most common sites. Sometimes a segment several inches long may be affected.

In uncomplicated inflammation of a diverticulum the early findings on barium enema examination are local irritability and spasm, usually with one or more associated diverticula. There may be prolonged spastic narrowing of the segment. These findings, however, may be transient and inconclusive. Later development of an intramural inflammatory mass will deform the wall, and the folds will be thickened.

Perforation or penetration of the infection can produce an extraluminal pericolonic inflammatory mass or abscess that can deform and compress one wall, often in an eccentric fashion. Narrowing occurs, and the folds are thickened but not destroyed. Sometimes small submucosal or subserosal fistulous tracts or a sinus tract can be demonstrated extending into the inflammatory mass. Fistulous connection to the bladder, vagina, or skin can occur. Typically, the lesion appears as a relatively long, narrowed, sometimes irritable segment in the sigmoid, with thickened mucosa, an extraluminal pressure deformity along a wall, and evidence of one or more diverticula within the segment. On plain film of the abdomen there may be a localized ileus (sentinel loop). In patients with suspected acute diverticulitis, barium enema study should be performed cautiously in order to avoid traumatic acute perforation.

Roentgenologic distinction from neoplasm may be difficult or impossible in some cases. Findings that favor the diagnosis of diverticulitis are preservation of the mucosal folds, gradual transition from diseased to normal colon, a rather long segment of involvement, and the presence of other diverticula.

A solitary area of segmental granulomatous colitis can also produce radiographic changes that cannot be readily distinguished from diverticulitis.

Acute diverticulitis of the right colon most often mimics acute appendicitis clinically. On barium enema study, there will be evidence of an eccentric mural defect or paracolic mass. The mucosal folds are intact but may be puckered or distorted. The offending diverticulum is usually obliterated and not seen. Radiographic differential diagnosis includes granulomatous or other infectious colitis, periappendiceal abscess, ischemic colitis, and neoplasm.[178-180]

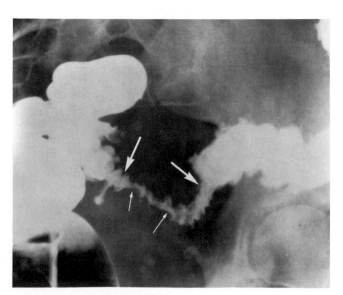

Figure 12–189 **Diverticulitis of Sigmoid.** The long narrowed segment of sigmoid *(between large arrows)* merges with normal colon at both ends. The mucosal folds are thickened but preserved. Numerous diverticula are seen proximal and distal to the narrowing. The curved impressions on the inferior border *(small arrows)* result from a peridiverticular inflammatory mass.

These findings are characteristic of diverticulitis and should not be misinterpreted as a malignant neoplasm.

Figure 12–190 **Diverticulitis of Sigmoid.** The long narrowed segment of diverticulitis contains mucosal folds that are thickened but intact. A number of small subserosal fistulous tracts are seen at the distal end of the lesion *(arrow).* There is gradual transition from diseased to normal sigmoid.

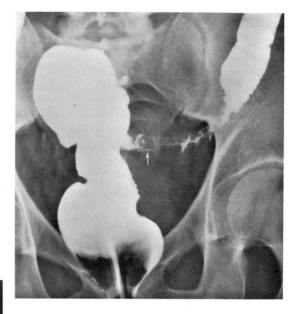

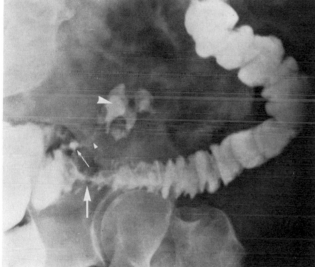

Figure 12–191 **Diverticulitis of Sigmoid: Sinus Tract and Abscess.** A narrowed segment of sigmoid *(large arrow)* contains a long diverticulum *(small arrow),* from which a sinus tract *(small arrowhead)* leads to an irregular barium-filled abscess cavity *(large arrowhead).*

Figure 12–192 **Diverticulitis of Descending Colon.** The short narrowed segment *(arrows)* in the descending colon was irritable, distensible at times, and tender. It never attained normal width during fluoroscopy. Although no diverticulum was demonstrable, a localized diverticulitis surrounded by a small peridiverticular abscess was found at surgery.

Local diverticulitis in which a diverticulum is not demonstrable may be indistinguishable from neoplasm or regional colitis.

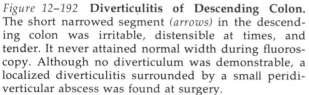
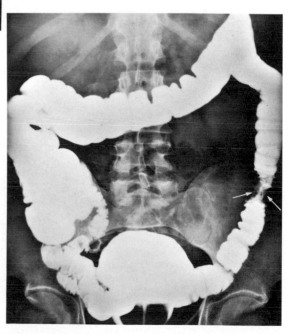

Infectious Colitis

Diffuse and segmental colitis due to specific infectious agents is discussed elsewhere. (See *Salmonella Infections,* p. 179; *Bacillary Dysentery,* p. 183; *Amebiasis,* p. 255; *Schistosomiasis,* p. 270, and *Intestinal Tuberculosis,* p. 201.) The radiographic changes can often simulate granulomatous and sometimes ulcerative colitis.

Necrotizing Enterocolitis of Infancy

This condition of uncertain origin can occur in utero or as late as 9 months of age; however, about 90 per cent of cases occur within 30 days of birth. Prematurity is a major predisposing factor.

Distention, vomiting, jaundice, and diarrhea are the usual symptoms. Bowel perforation is a common complication. Any or all of the small or large bowel can be involved; the ileum is the favorite site.

The roentgenographic abdominal findings are often pathognomonic. Distended loops of small bowel are usually seen. Pneumoperitoneum and pneumatosis intestinalis are found in about one third of the cases, and about half of these show air in the portal veins. A paralytic ileus picture, with intestinal pneumatosis, pneumoperitoneum, and gas in the portal vein, is a virtually diagnostic picture.

Only a small percentage of affected infants who develop pneumoperitoneum will survive. These newborn usually develop strictures and internal fistulas.

In milder cases without complicating pneumoperitoneum, recovery without surgery usually occurs.[181-183]

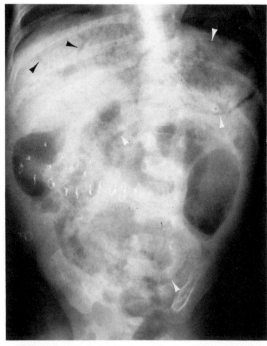

Figure 12–193 **Necrotizing Enterocolitis: Pneumatosis and Gas in Portal Vein.** In this 5 month old infant, there is diffuse dilatation of the bowel, with gas in the walls of the stomach and bowel *(white arrowheads).* Linear lucent streaks in the liver, extending to the periphery, are due to gas in the portal vein *(black arrowheads).*

The infant had congenital ileal atresia, and after neonatal surgery there were recurrent episodes of small bowel obstruction eventuating in fatal necrotizing enterocolitis.

Radiation Enterocolitis

See page 10.

Pseudomembranous Colitis

Pseudomembranous colitis is an uncommon acute inflammation of obscure origin. It can occur as a postoperative complication, or after antibiotic therapy, septicemia, or colonic obstruction. In almost half the cases, a staphylococcal organism is found.

The colon and distal ileum are most often involved, but the entire small bowel may be affected.

The abdomen film characteristically shows distention of the small and large bowel, and wall irregularities are usually apparent.

Barium enema studies reveal a shaggy irregular mucosa, often with nodular defects resembling pseudopolyps (probably due to pseudomembrane formation). Diffuse ulcerations are usually seen, often deeply penetrating. The appearance is usually indistinguishable from that of ulcerative or acute infectious colitis, and sometimes resembles ischemic colitis.

Ileal involvement consists of dilatation, thickened wall and folds—due to the pseudomembranes—and ulcerations.

Resolution may occur within a few weeks, but the condition may be fatal if untreated.[184-186]

The clinical history should aid diagnosis and distinction from other colitides.

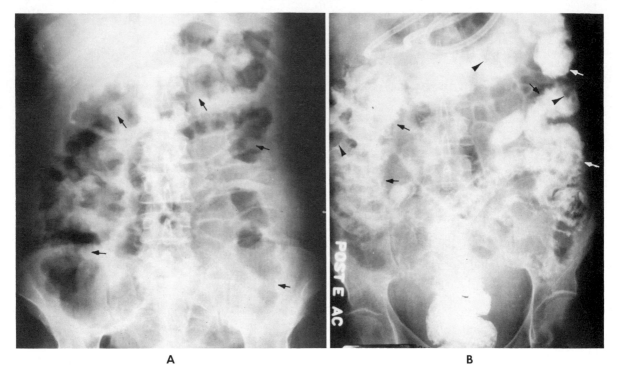

A   **B**

Figure 12–194 **Pseudomembranous Colitis.**

A, A 47 year old woman receiving clindomycin developed pain, diarrhea, abdominal distention, and rectal bleeding. An abdominal film reveals an ileus, with distention of both small and large bowel. Throughout the colon, irregularities and large defects are seen *(arrows).*

B, Barium enema discloses diffuse defects *(arrowheads)* and ulcer-like irregular projections *(arrows)* throughout the colon. The large defects were due to pseudomembranous plaques, producing a somewhat distinctive appearance. However, differentiation from acute ulcerative colitis with pseudopolyps or from acute bacterial colitis with extensive wall edema cannot be made solely from the radiographic appearance.

Evanescent Segmental Colitis

Evanescent segmental colitis occurs in young adults and is characterized by an acute onset of abdominal pain and diarrhea, often bloody. Radiographically, one or more segmental areas of spasm, thumbprinting, and often multiple ulcerations are seen, suggestive of focal granulomatous or ischemic colitis.

Clinical and radiologic recovery ensues within a few weeks without specific therapy.[187, 188]

A

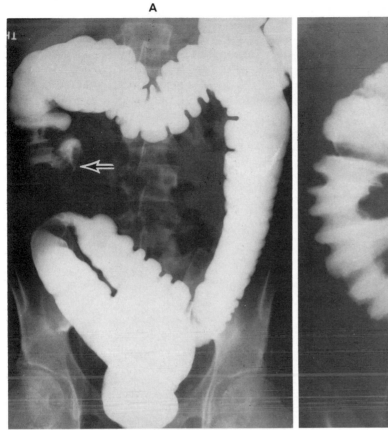

B

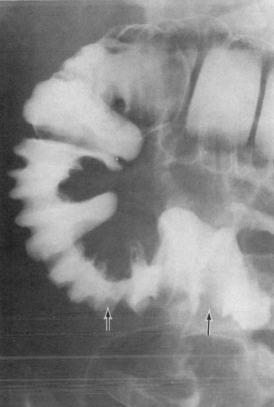

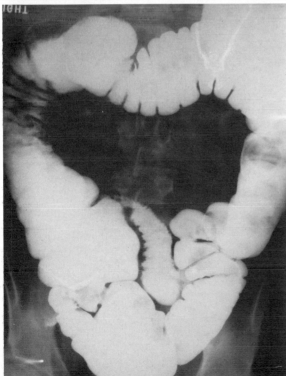

C

Figure 12–195 **Evanescent Segmental Colitis in 21 Year Old Man.**

A, There is spasm and irregularity in the ascending colon *(arrow).*

B, Marked irregularity, thickened folds, and thumbprinting are seen in the cecum and ascending colon *(arrows).*

C, The colon appears normal three weeks later.

The radiographic appearance and course of evanescent colitis are strikingly similar to those of ischemic colitis.

Colitis Cystica Profunda

This rare lesion of unsettled origin consists of submucosal mucoid-containing cysts up to 2 cm. in diameter. These nodular lesions may be diffusely scattered, but most often they are localized to the lower rectum or, less often, to the recto-sigmoid. Young adults are most commonly affected, presenting with a history of recurrent rectal bleeding, often associated with tenesmus, diarrhea, and mucus discharge.

Radiographically, the lesion appears as solitary or multiple polypoid nodules in the lower rectum. Although occasionally ulcerations may occur, the barium flecks are most often merely contrast material trapped between nodules.

The radiographic appearance can simulate villous adenoma, adenomatous polyps, lymphoma, carcinoma, or inflammatory granulomas. However, in a young adult with recurrent rectal bleeding and with diarrhea or tenesmus, a polypoid or multinodular rectal lesion is suggestive of colitis cystica profunda.[189, 190]

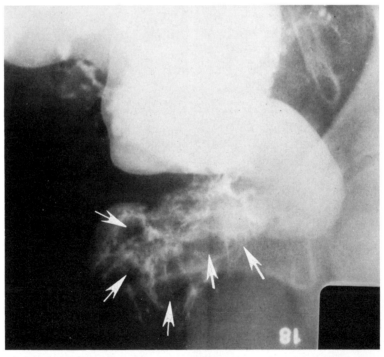

Figure 12–196 **Colitis Cystica Profunda.** Barium enema study of a 17 year old girl, with an eight year history of frequent rectal bleeding, shows an irregular, narrowed lower rectum. There are multiple nodular defects *(arrows)* within the lumen, with granular barium densities between the defects.

Primary Nonspecific Ulceration of the Small Intestine

Simple ulcers of the small intestine may be secondary to mesenteric thrombosis or embolism, polyarteritis nodosa, necrotizing arteriolitis, incarcerated hernia, or aortic surgery. A causal relationship has also been demonstrated between development of ulceration and prolonged ingestion of enteric-coated potassium chloride and thiazides.

Occlusion of a focal vascular segment of small bowel occurs most frequently in the distal jejunum or ileum. Subsequent mucosal edema and congestion lead to ulceration. The ulcer, being shallow, is usually difficult to demonstrate. A roentgen pattern indistinguishable from that of regional enteritis may develop, with thickened or effaced mucosa, narrowed loops, filling defects, and mesenteric thickening. These changes occur either alone or in various combinations, and they may be reversible.

A late sequela is the development of stenosis, which varies from a few centimeters to several feet in length. These stenotic segments usually have tapered margins, a tubular outline, and mucosal effacement. Proximal bowel dilatation can occur, and partial bowel obstruction may develop.[191-194]

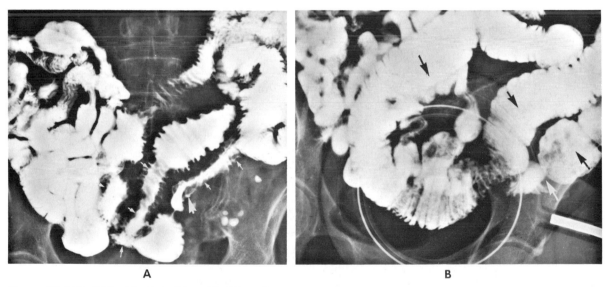

A   B

Figure 12–197 **Thiazide Enteritis with Ulceration.**

A, The patient was a 55 year old hypertensive receiving potassium chloride and thiazide. He developed abdominal pain and gastrointestinal bleeding. The small bowel studies demonstrate a long segment of diseased jejunum *(small arrows),* in which the mucosal folds are markedly thickened and edematous, and the lumen irregularly narrowed. The bowel wall is edematous, so that the space between the loops is increased. A shallow ulceration *(large arrow)* surrounded by thickened folds can be identified. Notice the similarity to regional enteritis. The remainder of the small bowel was normal.

B, A few weeks later a short segment of narrowing is seen *(white arrow)* with dilatation of the proximal loops *(black arrows).* The acute edema has subsided.

This appearance of stricture and partial obstruction is the usual finding in this condition; the earlier finding of acute edema of the bowel wall is present only during the acute ischemic phase. Similarly, the ulceration is usually not demonstrated radiographically once scarring and fibrosis ensue.

VASCULAR DISEASES OF THE INTESTINE

Acute Mesenteric Vascular Insufficiency

Acute ischemia of the small bowel can occur after occlusion of the superior mesenteric artery or its branches, after venous occlusion (10 per cent), or from severely reduced blood flow without actual occlusion. The findings on abdominal films may vary from an apparently normal gas pattern to a diffuse paralytic ileus with gas and fluid-filled small and large bowel loops. Frequently there is a marked discrepancy between the abdominal film findings and the desperately ill condition of the patient.

The gas-filled small bowel loops vary greatly in number, usually show air-fluid levels, and may be suggestive of mechanical obstruction in about one half of the cases. However, the affected segments tend to remain unchanged over multiple examinations, and often there is a scalloped appearance of the small intestinal walls due to mucosal edema and submucosal hemorrhage. Thickening and rigidity of the walls of the affected loops may occur. Sometimes, completely fluid-filled and airless loops may simulate a soft tissue mass (pseudotumor). Streaks of gas may appear in gangrenous walls of bowel and may extend into the portal venules, an ominous finding (see pp. 174–175). The colon cutoff sign — in which the small bowel and the right colon are distended up to Canon's point in the transverse colon — is suggestive evidence of mesenteric occlusion; unfortunately this sign is only infrequently encountered.

Abdominal aortography, preferably selective superior mesenteric arteriography, may demonstrate either total or segmental vascular occlusion or marked arterial narrowing with distinctly reduced blood flow. Focal acute arterial or venous occlusion may be difficult or impossible to demonstrate.

Barium studies are rarely done during the acute phase. The involved small bowel segments appear rigid, atonic, and somewhat dilated; the mucosal folds and bowel wall are thickened from edema; and characteristic thumbprint defects are usually seen. Barium will remain in the proximal affected loops for long periods because of absent peristaltic activity. The findings are quite suggestive, and barium studies should be performed when the diagnosis is in doubt.

The much less common occlusion of the inferior mesenteric artery (or vein) or its branches will lead to extensive or segmental infarction of the left colon and may produce characteristic changes on barium enema study (ischemic colitis). The infarcted area of the descending colon appears as a spastic, narrowed, and somewhat rigid segment with thickened folds and a scalloped contour. The proximal colon is usually dilated. The roentgenologic appearance is often similar to that of localized granulomatous or ulcerative colitis. If the involvement is severe, ulcerations and stenotic fibrosis can ensue. Less severe lesions may undergo complete recovery within weeks or a few months, with restoration of a normal colonic lumen and contour.

Angiographic studies are often unrevealing, especially in segmental ischemic colitis.

The clinical history, and the relatively rapid formation of a stricture or clearing of the lesion will differentiate the radiographic findings of ischemic colitis from granulomatous colitis.[195-202]

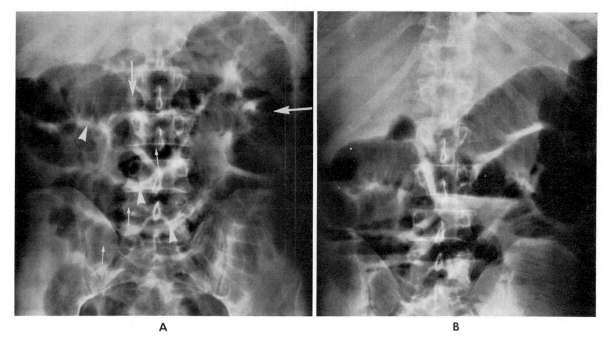

A B

Figure 12–198 **Acute Mesenteric Vascular Insufficiency.**

A, Both large bowel *(large arrows)* and small bowel *(small arrows)* are uniformly distended, with thickening between the bowel loops *(arrowheads)* due to edema of the bowel wall.

B, In erect view, long fluid levels are characteristic of severe paralytic ileus. The thickened bowel walls are again clearly demonstrated.

This picture of generalized ileus is frequently seen in mesenteric thrombosis, but the findings are variable; in some cases the gas pattern simulates that of mechanical obstruction, but without stepladder fluid levels.

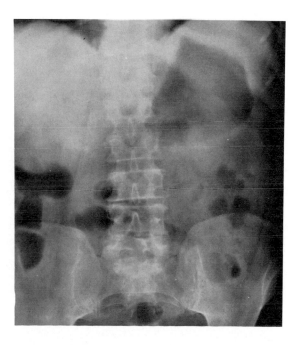

Figure 12–199 **Acute Mesenteric Vascular Insufficiency.** In recumbent view there are scattered gas-filled loops of large and small bowel without significant distention. Although the findings may be minimal, a history of acute abdominal crisis should suggest mesenteric vascular insufficiency.

Following mesenteric occlusion, the gas pattern in the abdomen is extremely variable. The finding of fixed, gas-filled small bowel loops on serial films is highly suggestive, but the clinical history is the most significant diagnostic aid. Diagnosis can often be confirmed by aortography.

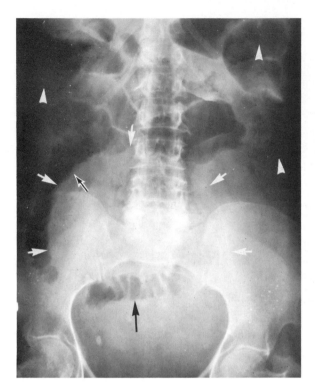

Figure 12–200 **Acute Mesenteric Occlusion: Pseudotumor.** This abdominal film of a 56 year old woman was made after 24 hours of severe abdominal pain, vomiting, and fever. The colon is distended with gas *(arrowheads),* and one small bowel loop with thickened valvulae conniventes *(black arrow)* is seen. These findings suggest an ileus. The soft tissue mass *(white arrows)* was thought to be a twisted or ruptured ovarian cyst but proved to be a pseudotumorous collection of edematous fluid-filled loops of infarcted small bowel. Note the streak of gas in the bowel wall *(black-white arrow).* (Courtesy Dr. J. D. Dunbar, Columbus, Ohio.)

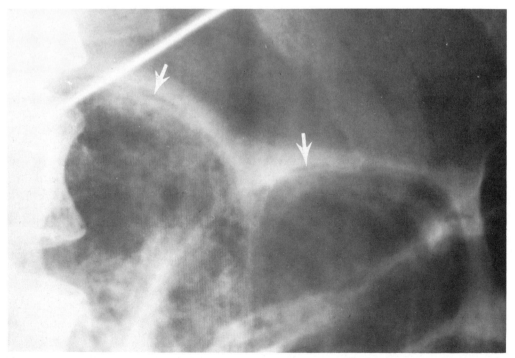

Figure 12–201 **Acute Mesenteric Occlusion: Bowel Gangrene and Pneumatosis.** Close-up view of distended small bowel loops reveals linear gas streaks (pneumatosis) in the walls *(arrows).*
    Gas-filled portal vein radicles in the liver were also seen radiographically in this patient.

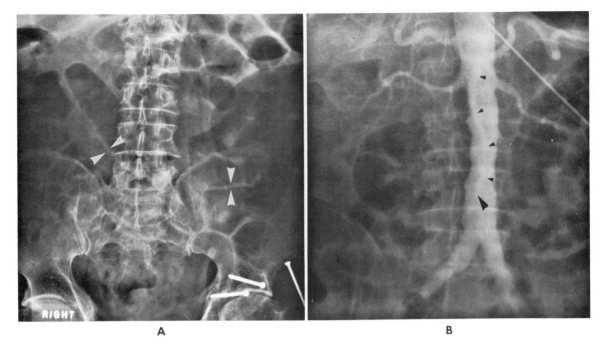

Figure 12-202 **Mesenteric Occlusion: Lumbar Aortogram.**

A, A 76 year old woman was acutely ill. Plain film demonstrates nonspecific ileus in which both large and small bowel are uniformly dilated. There is moderate thickening of the bowel wall *(arrowheads).*

B, The translumbar aortogram, the superior mesenteric artery *(small arrowheads),* which overlies the filled aorta, terminates abruptly *(large arrowhead).* Serial films failed to disclose filling of the distal branches of the superior mesenteric artery. Occlusion of the major branches of the superior mesenteric artery was found at surgery.

Figure 12-203 **Acute Mesenteric Occlusion: Early Small Bowel Findings on Barium Study.** Extensive edematous thickening of the mucosal folds *(arrowheads)* is demonstrated in many of the distended small bowel loops. Thumbprint defects due to submucosal hematomas *(white arrows)* can be identified. The other loops are dilated and atonic *(black arrows).*

Although contrast studies of the small bowel are rarely performed after acute mesenteric occlusion, the roentgen findings of extensive mucosal edema, intramural hematomas, and atonic, rigid, dilated loops are characteristic of acute arterial ischemia. (Courtesy Dr. J. D. Dunbar, Columbus, Ohio.)

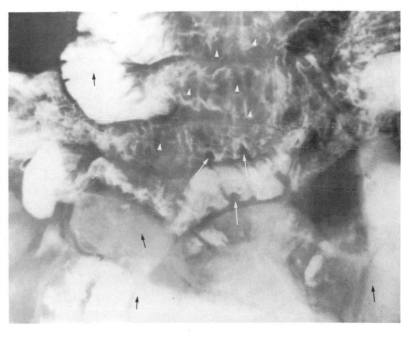

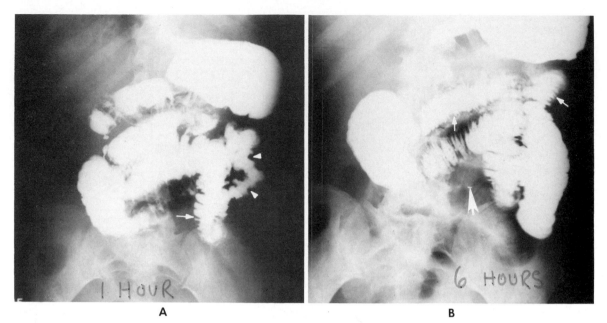

A   B

Figure 12–204 **Superior Mesenteric Artery Occlusion: Oral Barium Studies.** The one-hour film *(A)* and the six-hour film *(B)* are virtually identical. There has been no progress of the barium beyond the proximal jejunum, and the loops are atonic, dilated, and show thickened folds and spiculation *(small arrows).* A few areas of thumbprinting are seen *(arrowheads).* Some distal loops are dilated and filled with gas *(large arrow).*

Dilated atonic loops, marked delay in transit time, prominent thickened folds, spiculation, and thumbprinting are virtually diagnostic of acute small bowel ischemia. However, the barium may remain for long periods in the atonic bowel, preventing adequate angiographic visualization.

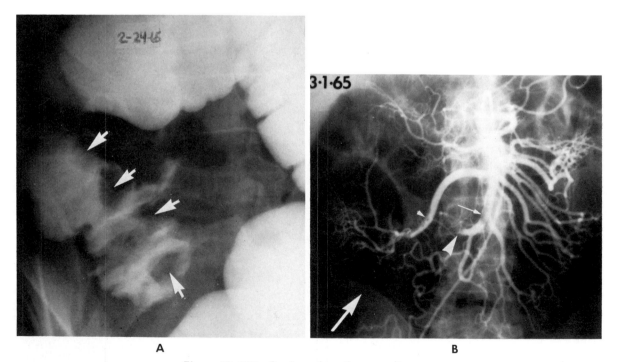

A   B

Figure 12–205   See legend on the opposite page.

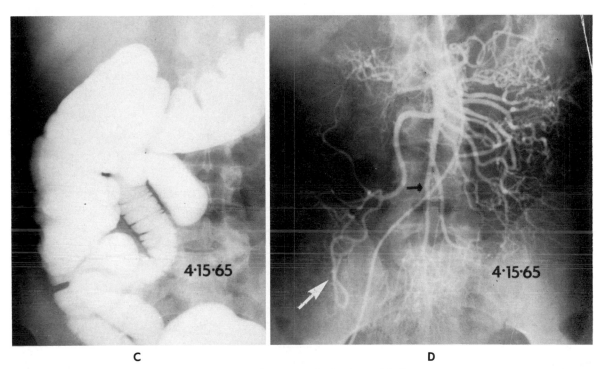

C

D

Figure 12–205 **Segmental Superior Mesenteric Artery Occlusion with Recovery.**

   A, A 45 year old man had leukocytosis and abdominal pain, which was later localized to the lower right quadrant. A barium enema exmination performed one day after onset of abdominal pain reveals irritability and deformity of the cecum and the proximal ascending colon. Multiple fingerprint defects *(arrows)* are due to submucosal hematomas.

   B, Selective superior mesenteric arteriogram discloses an irregular thrombus *(small arrow)* in the lower part of the arterial root. The ileocolic branch is completely occluded *(large arrowhead)* just distal to its origin, and there is very little vascularity in the ileocecal area *large arrow).* There are also a number of small thrombi *(small arrowhead)* in the right colic branch, but there is not complete occlusion of this branch.

   C, Six weeks later, after clinical recovery without surgery, barium enema study reveals a practically normal right colon and terminal ileum.

   D, A selective arteriogram now shows that the occluded ileocolic artery has thrombosed up to its origin *(black arrow),* but that adequate vascularity of the ileocecal area *(white arrow)* is now obtained by means of collaterals from the right colic artery. The clots in the right colic artery have disappeared. (Courtesy Dr. J. D. Dunbar, Columbus, Ohio.)

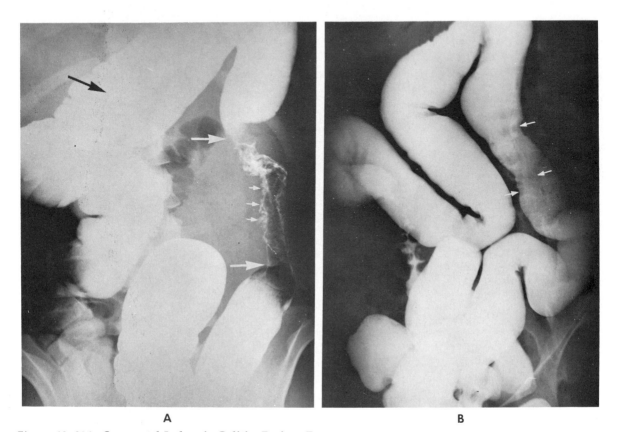

A   B

Figure 12–206 **Segmental Ischemic Colitis: Barium Enema.**

A, A young woman who had a collagen disease with widespread vascular disturbances developed sudden abdominal pain and bloody diarrhea. Barium enema study revealed irregular narrowing of a long segment of the descending colon *(between large white arrows)*. The mucosal folds were greatly distorted, and the contours *(small white arrows)* suggested ulcerations. This segment was rigid and did not retain barium. The proximal bowel is moderately dilated, particularly the transverse colon *(black arrow)*.

B, Two weeks later the clinical symptoms had cleared. The affected segment is distensible. There is still some mucosal swelling *(small arrows),* but the proximal colon is no longer dilated.

Within the following two weeks, the colon was normal on barium enema study. Although proof of occlusion was not obtained, the clinical and radiographic courses were typical.

Acute segmental ischemia of the colon is characterized by mucosal edema (thumbprinting, if extensive), irritability, and spasm. The involved segment may simulate granulomatous colitis radiographically. Recovery within six weeks is frequent but permanent fibrosis and stricture can sometimes occur.

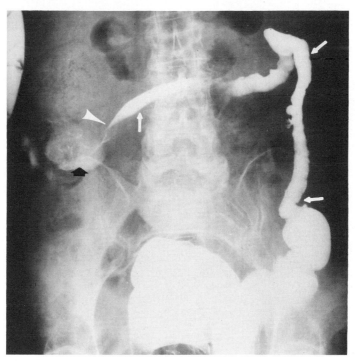

Figure 12–207 **Inferior Mesenteric Artery Occlusion: Stricture of Colon.** The transverse and descending colon are uniformly narrowed *(white arrows)* by fibrosis resulting from a prior acute ischemia. The proximal stricture *(arrowhead)* was severe enough to require a colostomy *(black arrow)*. The sigmoid and rectum appear normal.

Chronic Mesenteric Vascular Insufficiency

Abdominal pain due to vascular insufficiency is most frequently associated with narrowing of the lumina of the major intestinal arteries near their point of origin from the aorta. It is now believed that in gradual occlusive disease, at least two of the three major vessels (the celiac and the superior and inferior mesenteric arteries) must be significantly narrowed before symptoms appear. The mere demonstration of a stenotic or occluded major artery does not necessarily confirm an ischemic origin of the patient's symptoms, especially if large collateral vessels are opacified. However, compression of the celiac artery by a low lying medial arcuate ligament of the diaphragm can apparently cause ischemic symptoms, especially in patients under the age of 40.

Chronic mesenteric insufficiency may be progressive over a period of weeks or months and may lead to complete occlusion. In classic chronic mesenteric insufficiency, barium meal studies are essentially negative, although the deficiency small bowel pattern of malabsorption is occasionally seen. Arteriography is essential for diagnosis, and a lateral film is necessary, since the narrowing usually occurs near the point of origin of the vessels, which overlies the aorta on the anteroposterior view.

In patients with the medial arcuate ligament syndrome, lateral view discloses characteristic eccentric compression of the celiac artery along its superior border. This angiographic finding, however, is also encountered in asymptomatic individuals.[203-207]

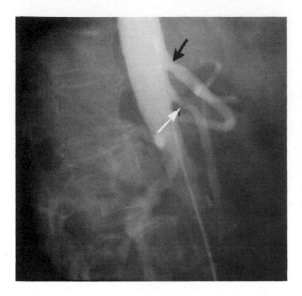

Figure 12–208 **Chronic Mesenteric Vascular Insufficiency: Aortogram.** Lateral view of an aortogram demonstrates narrowing of both the celiac axis *(black arrow)* and the superior mesenteric artery *(white arrow)* close to their aortic origins. Note slight poststenotic dilatation of the celiac artery. Without oblique or lateral views, these changes would probably not be appreciated. The patient had a history of chronic midabdominal pain, vomiting, and nausea occurring immediately after eating.

Gas in the Portal Vein

This is a rare and generally fatal complication of intestinal gangrene in which air or gas enters the portal circulation. It occurs in young infants with necrotizing enterocolitis and in older individuals with vascular ischemia and bowel infarction. Gas extends to the periphery of the liver and into the small venules. This condition should not be confused with air in the biliary tree, in which the arborizing air pattern is more central, is wider, and never reaches the periphery. Gas in the bowel walls can be demonstrated in a high percentage of cases with gas in the portal vein.[208-210]

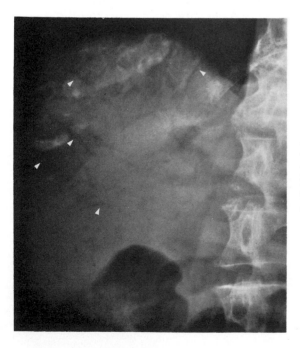

Figure 12–209 **Gas in Portal Vein.** A 77 year old woman developed mesenteric vein thrombosis and peritonitis. Film of right upper quadrant discloses gas in the branches of the portal vein system extending to the liver periphery *(arrowheads)*. This is a rare and usually fatal complication of intestinal gangrene.

Intramural Hematoma of the Duodenum

Bleeding into the duodenal wall can result from nonpenetrating abdominal trauma or spontaneously from a hematologic disorder or anticoagulation therapy. Persistent vomiting with or without abdominal pain is the usual symptom.

The findings on barium meal study are highly suggestive. The lesion involves the descending and transverse portions of the duodenum and is generally 10 to 20 cm. long. The proximal folds are thickened, and more distally the intramural mass widens the lumen and crowds the folds together into a coiled-spring appearance resembling intussusception. Obstruction to some degree is usually present. The hematoma is generally on the lateral aspect, in contrast to an ampullary or pancreatic tumor. If the hematoma is large, it may produce extensive pressure on the greater curvature of the stomach, may cause downward displacement of the transverse colon, or may even deviate the upper right ureter laterally.[211, 212]

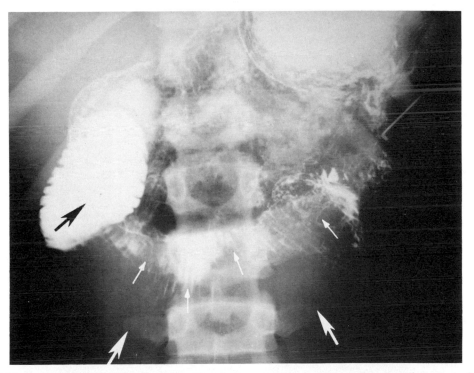

Figure 12–210 **Intramural Hematoma of the Duodenum.**   An upper gastrointestinal tract study of a boy with a two-week history of abdominal pain and vomiting following abdominal trauma reveals a dilated partially obstructed descending duodenum *(black arrow)*. Distally there is a soft tissue mass on the inferior surface of the duodenum *(large white arrows),* which is irregularly compressing, distorting, and elongating the mucosal folds *(small white arrows).*

The radiographic appearance is characteristic of an intramural mass; this was a huge hematoma.

DISEASES OF THE PERITONEUM AND MESENTERY

Ascites

Varying amounts of intraperitoneal fluid occur in many conditions, most commonly in hepatic cirrhosis, right-sided congestive failure, peritonitis, penetrating wounds of the abdomen, perforation of a peptic ulcer, and diffuse peritoneal metastases.

Massive ascites is usually easily recognized clinically. The radiographic findings of overall abdominal haziness, separation and floating of bowel loops, and increased pelvic density in the upright position are not very reliable, since obesity, technical radiographic factors, or some motion of the patient can cause similar findings. The more reliable findings in the supine radiograph are (1) increased distance between the properitoneal fat stripe and the ascending or descending colon (normally this space is no greater than 2 mm.), (2) a radiodensity above and around the bladder shadow, sometimes producing the "dog's ears" sign, and (3) obliteration of the lower lateral hepatic angle.

One or more of these signs may be present even with less than 800 ml. of intraperitoneal fluid or blood. The psoas lines remain intact in ascites; their obliteration occurs from retroperitoneal fluid or blood.[213]

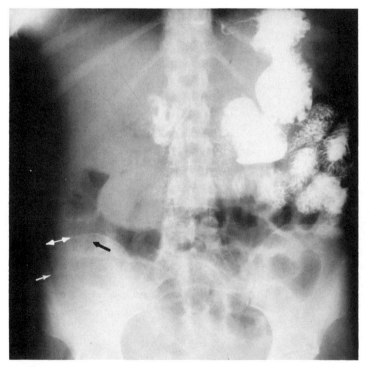

Figure 12–211 **Subclinical Ascites: Radiographic Signs.** There is an increased distance *(double-headed arrow)* between the properitoneal fat stripe *(white arrow)* and the gas-filled right colon *(black arrow)*, caused by fluid. Normally, the right colon and the fat stripe are contiguous (less than 2 mm. apart). The lower edge of the liver (hepatic angle) is obliterated by fluid.

The ascites, due to liver cirrhosis, was not clinically apparent.

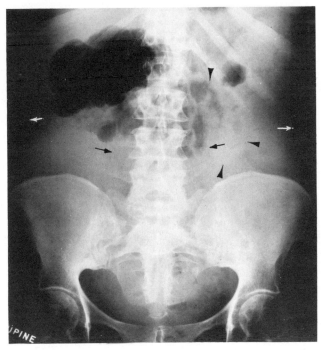

Figure 12–212 **Advanced Ascites in Cirrhosis.** The flanks are bulging *(white arrows)* but the flank fat stripe is not obliterated. The gas-filled bowel loops are bunched in the upper abdomen. The hepatic angle on the right is obliterated, but the retroperitoneal structures [psoas lines *(black arrows)* and the kidney shadow *(arrowheads)*] are visible.

Extensive ascites is readily recognized clinically, and the abdominal roentgen findings are merely corroborative.

Generalized Peritonitis

The radiographic picture is that of paralytic ileus: there is fairly uniform distention of both small and large bowel loops. Long fluid levels, which are not of the stepladder type, are seen in the erect view.

Eventually the walls of the small bowel become edematous, and the space between the loops increases. The properitoneal fat stripes are obliterated, a significant diagnostic sign. Radiographic evidence of ascites may be present.

If a ruptured viscus is the cause of the peritonitis, free air may be seen in the peritoneal cavity.

In children, a generalized peritonitis is sometimes accompanied by dilatation of the urinary tracts, probably due to inflammatory atony of the ureters.[47, 214]

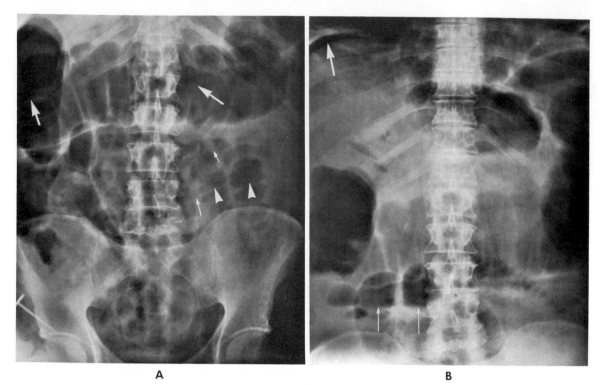

A   B

Figure 12–213   **Generalized Peritonitis Following Rupture of Appendix.**

A, There is uniform dilatation of the large bowel *(large arrows)* and small bowel *(arrowheads).* The increased space between the small bowel loops *(small arrows)* is due to edema of the bowel walls. The properitoneal fat line is obliterated.

B, Erect view shows free air under the right diaphragm *(large arrow).* The fluid levels in the loops in the lower abdomen *(small arrows)* are at the same level. This is characteristic of a paralyzed bowel, in contrast to a mechanical obstruction, in which the hyperperistalsis leads to fluid lines at various levels (stepladder effect).

Generalized Peritonitis: Abscess Formation

As generalized peritonitis subsides, localizing abscesses may occur in any portion of the abdomen. Thus, a pelvic abscess, subphrenic abscess, subhepatic or periappendiceal abscess may appear a few days or weeks after apparently successful treatment of peritonitis. The abscess is visualized roentgenologically as a mass, with displacement of adjacent bowel loops. Occasionally the abscess may occlude an adjacent small bowel loop and produce mechanical obstruction. Frequently there are multiple small lucencies within the abscess, permitting radiographic identification.

The radiographic findings in subphrenic abscess are discussed on page 964.

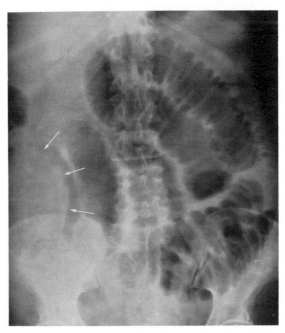

Figure 12–214 **Abscess in Right Lower Quadrant Following Peritonitis.** Following generalized peritonitis due to rupture of the appendix, a mass developed in the right lower quadrant and is seen pressing upon an adjacent small bowel loop *(arrows)*. Mechanical small bowel obstruction has developed, evidenced by the marked distention of the proximal small bowel loops.

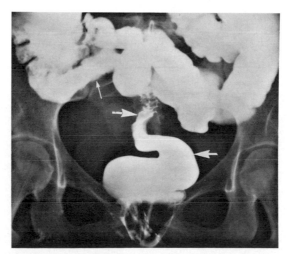

Figure 12–215 **Pelvic Abscess Following Pelvic Peritonitis.** A 26 year old woman had pelvic peritonitis following gonococcal tubo-ovarian disease. A barium enema study made two weeks later shows displacement of the sigmoid *(large arrows)* upward and to the left, and there was local irritability just beyond the rectosigmoid. The terminal ileum is also displaced upward *(small arrow)*. The changes were due to a localized pelvic abscess on the right side.

Tuberculous Peritonitis

See page 205.

Malignant Disease of the Peritoneum

Widespread seeding of the peritoneum with malignant cells and tissue most often occurs secondary to carcinoma of the stomach, colon, or ovary.

Roentgenologically there may be evidence of peritoneal fluid (ascites) and of multiple masses producing pressure defects on the small bowel. The small bowel loops may be separated by fluid or by direct infiltration of the small bowel wall by tumor. Infrequently, peritoneal metastases, usually from an ovarian malignancy, may calcify. Intraperitoneal introduction of water-soluble contrast medium can sometimes prove helpful in delineating and localizing large peritoneal metastatic masses.

Roentgenographic evidence of peritoneal involvement is occasionally the first evidence of a malignant condition, but more often the primary tumor is recognized before peritoneal implantation has become advanced.[13, 215, 216]

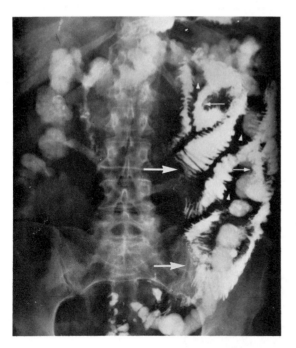

Figure 12–216 **Carcinomatosis of Peritoneum from Sigmoid Carcinoma.** Numerous masses in the mid-abdomen compress and displace the small bowel to the left (large arrows). The small bowel loops are separated by abnormally wide spaces (arrowheads), owing to the presence of fluid and tumor between them. There is localized pressure on some loops (small arrows) from smaller peritoneal and mesenteric tumor implants.

Roentgenologic evidence of multiple masses and fluid producing pressure defects and increased separation of the small bowel loops points to carcinomatosis of the abdomen.

Figure 12–217 **Massive Peritoneal Effusion from Pseudomucinous Cystadenocarcinoma of Ovary.** Haze over the abdomen and bulging of the flanks (arrows) are caused by intraperitoneal fluid and tumor masses; they displace the barium-filled stomach upward. There is unrelated rheumatoid spondylitis.

Similar peritoneal implants and fluid can result from rupture of a benign mucinous tumor of the ovary.

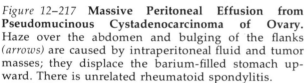

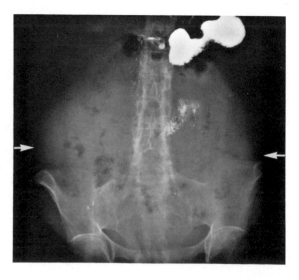

Figure 12–218 **Diffuse Calcified Peritoneal Metastases from Papillary Cystadenocarcinoma of Ovary.** There are diffuse sand-like calcifications *(large arrows)* scattered throughout the abdomen. These strongly resemble residual barium in the colon. However, careful scrutiny of the bowel gas shadows *(arrowheads)* suggests that the densities are not colonic; barium enema confirmed this.

There is also a more circumscribed calcification *(small arrow)* in the left lower quadrant; this was a discrete large tumorous mass.

Although calcified peritoneal carcinomatosis is rare and can be confused with colonic opacities, diffuse, psammoma body calcifications outside the colon are most often due to carcinomatosis from papillary cystadenocarcinoma of the ovary.

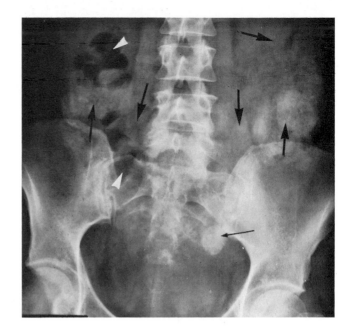

Mesenteric Cysts

Most mesenteric cysts are cystic lymphangiomas, probably related to a focal lymphatic abnormality. The latter may be developmental or acquired after surgical injury to lymphatics of the mesentery.

Although the cysts develop between layers of mesentery, they may be considered as benign peritoneal tumors. They may develop in any portion of the abdomen and are seen as round, sharply outlined anterior masses displacing the adjacent viscera, especially the small bowel. When small, the cysts are freely movable, but they may grow very large and become fixed. Calcification of the wall is not infrequent. The cysts rarely produce intestinal obstruction.[217, 218]

Figure 12–219 **Large Mesenteric Cyst with Calcification.** A huge soft tissue mass in the right midabdomen causes displacement of and pressure deformity on the barium-filled small bowel *(small arrows)*, and displaces the opacified gallbladder upward *(large arrow).* A portion of the cyst wall *(arrowheads)* is calcified. The ascending colon, which contains gas, is not displaced because it is retroperitoneal.

Even larger mesenteric cysts produce few clinical symptoms.

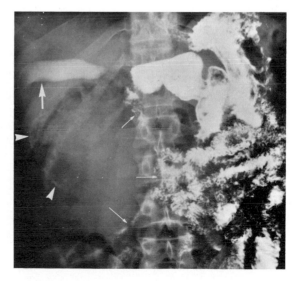

Retractile Mesenteritis (Mesenteric Panniculitis)

See page 118.

Subphrenic Abscess

See page 964.

NEOPLASTIC DISEASES OF THE ALIMENTARY TRACT

Carcinoma of the Esophagus

Carcinoma may develop in any portion of the esophagus: it is most frequent in the middle third, fairly common in the lower third, and least common in the upper third.

Like carcinoma elsewhere in the gastrointestinal tract, the lesion may be annular, polypoid, ulcerative, infiltrating, or a combination of these types. Usually, annular lesions are sharply demarcated and constrict the lumen, destroying the mucosal folds. The polypoid type produces intraluminal defects that often infiltrate the wall and destroy the mucosa. Occasionally, multiple small polypoid defects in a neoplastic lesion can simulate varices. The localized infiltrative lesion is hard to diagnose, since limited distensibility and decreased or absent local peristalsis may be the only changes. It may cause gradual narrowing of the lumen without a distinct transition zone, thereby making differentiation from peptic esophagitis difficult. In the ulcerating form of malignancy there is a crater surrounded by a mass that projects into the esophageal lumen. In all forms of esophageal carcinoma ulceration is not rare. Peristalsis through the involved area is diminished or absent.

Cineradiography or videotape is particularly useful in the diagnosis of esophageal carcinoma, as well as of most other problems of esophageal motility. These studies permit easy recognition of rigid areas in which there is no peristaltic activity, whereas on conventional films these areas are easily overlooked or misinterpreted.

When carcinoma of the lower esophagus extends into the cardia of the stomach, it may be impossible to determine whether the esophagus or the stomach is the primary site.

Obstruction of the lumen causes proximal dilatation of the esophagus, and aspiration pneumonitis may occur. Extension of the neoplasm to adjacent mediastinal structures can lead to fistula formation, especially into the tracheobronchial tree.[219-221]

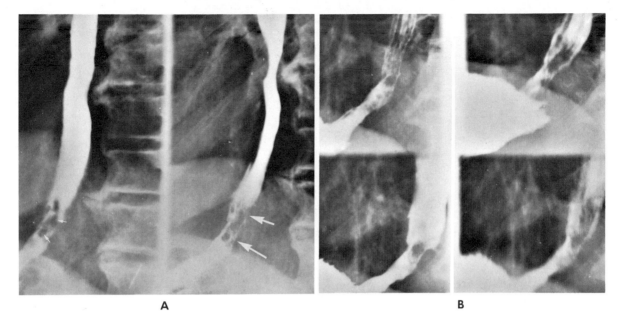

A   B

Figure 12–220 **Polypoid Adenocarcinoma of Lower Esophagus.**

A, Multiple small filling defects *(small arrows)* in the lower esophagus superficially resemble esophageal varices. There is no obstruction, but the posterior wall *(large arrows)* is somewhat irregular and appears rigid.

B, Serial study demonstrates that the segment is rigid and unchanged by peristalsis. This is strongly suggestive of neoplastic infiltration.

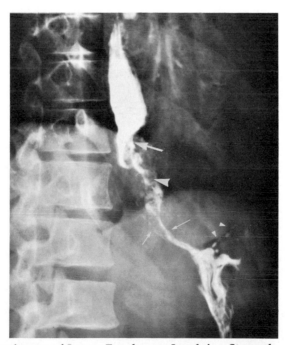

Figure 12–221 **Polypoid Carcinoma of Lower Esophagus, Involving Stomach.**   The lower esophagus is irregularly narrowed; neoplastic tissue has infiltrated and destroyed the mucosal folds *(large arrowhead)*. A large shelving defect (shoulder defect) projects into the esophagus above *(large arrow)*. The esophagogastric segment is narrowed *(small arrows)*, and a soft tissue mass of tumor *(small arrowheads)* has deformed the gastric fundus. There is a small amount of dilatation of the esophagus above the lesion.

It is often impossible to determine whether a carcinoma has originated in the stomach or in the lower esophagus.

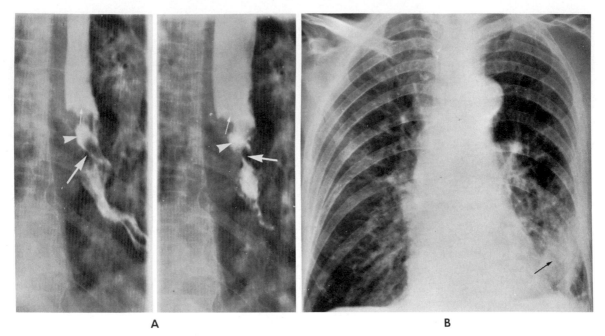

A   B

Figure 12–222 **Annular Ulcerating Carcinoma of Middle Third of Esophagus: Aspiration Pneumonitis.**

   A, The involved segment *(large arrows)* is irregular, narrowed, and deformed by filling defects, and the mucosa is distorted. A typical shelving defect *(small arrows)* is seen at the upper brim of the lesion. The barium accumulation *(arrowheads)* in the middle of the involved segment is due to an ulceration. The esophagus is distensible above the shelving defect.

   B, There is an area of aspiration pneumonitis *(black arrow)* at the left base. Aspiration pneumonitis from carcinoma of the esophagus occurs more frequently in upper esophageal lesions.

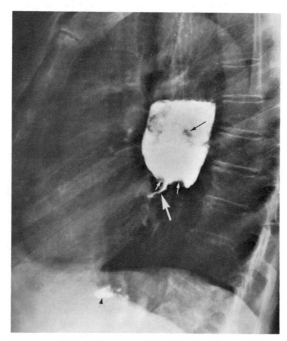

Figure 12–223 **Annular Carcinoma of Esophagus, with Obstruction.** Thread-like narrowing of the esophageal lumen *(large arrow)* is sharply demarcated from the dilated esophagus above by shelving defects *(small white arrows).* Only a trickle of barium *(black arrowhead)* has passed through the obstructed lumen in the cardia. Nonopaque food residue *(black arrow)* is present in the dilated esophagus.

   Generally, malignant neoplasms of the esophagus cause less obstruction and, consequently, less proximal dilatation than do inflammatory strictures or achalasia.

Leiomyoma and Leiomyosarcoma of the Esophagus

Leiomyoma is the most common benign tumor of the esophagus, although it is considerably less frequent than carcinoma. It causes an intramural extramucosal defect in the barium column, but there is preservation of mucosal folds. Over 90 per cent of leiomyomas occur in the middle or lower third of the esophagus.

There is usually a smooth crescent-shaped defect on one side of the lumen, and the linear mucosal folds are stretched. It may be difficult or impossible to distinguish between an extramucosal intramural lesion like leiomyoma and a defect due to extrinsic pressure. An intramural extramucosal defect generally produces an abrupt and sharply angled border with the barium column, in contrast to the gradual and smooth curve of an extrinsic lesion.

The roentgenologic changes caused by the rare leiomyosarcoma are similar to those of leiomyoma, since it remains a smooth extramucosal mass for a long time and mucosal destruction occurs late.

Dysphagia is the most common presenting symptom in both tumors.[222, 223]

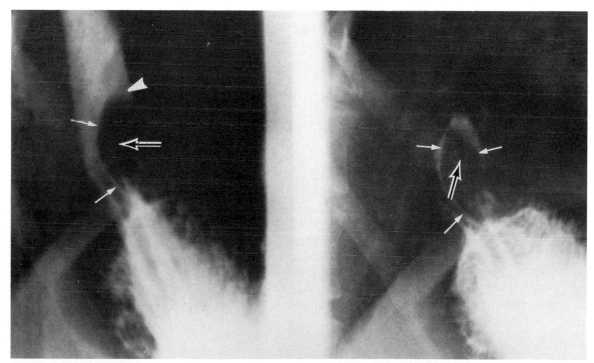

Figure 12–224 **Leiomyoma of Esophagus.** Esophagogram of a 34 year old man with a history of mild chronic dysphagia reveals a smooth eccentric defect *(black-white arrows)* in the lower esophagus; there is no obstruction. The mucosa is intact and curves around the lesion *(white arrows)*, findings indicative of a noninvasive extramucosal lesion. The sharp angle of barium at the edge of the mass *(arrowhead)* is characteristic of intramural origin. Leiomyoma is the most common benign intramural extramucosal lesion of the lower esophagus.

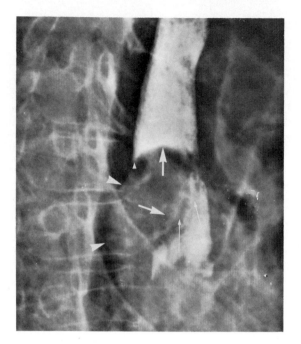

Figure 12–225 **Leiomyosarcoma of Midesophagus.** There is a smooth defect *(large arrows)* in the barium-filled esophagus; the posterior bulge of the smooth oval tumor can be seen as a soft tissue density *(large arrowheads)*. The mucosal folds are prominent and curved but appear a bit irregular *(small arrows)*, which suggests invasion. Note the acute angle of barium *(small arrowhead)* at the upper posterior border of the defect. This angulation is typical of an intramural extramucosal lesion; in extrinsic lesions the angle is obtuse.

The lesion was a leiomyosarcoma, but the roentgenologic findings were practically identical to those of leiomyoma although the soft tissue mass beyond the esophagus and suspicion of mucosal invasion suggested the possibility of a malignant lesion.

Carcinoma of the Stomach

The roentgenologic findings vary widely, depending on the size, location, and gross morphology of the tumor. The locations of gastric carcinoma, in decreasing order of frequency, are the antrum, the body, the cardia, and the fundus. Multiple lesions may occasionally be seen. The polypoid and fungating lesions appear as single or multiple filling defects, often with deformity of the gastric wall. Infiltrating lesions produce irregularities of the wall and destroy the mucosa. They occur most often on the lesser curvature.

Ulcerations frequently develop in gastric carcinoma, and radiographic distinction from benign ulcer is sometimes difficult or impossible. The malignant ulcer is generally flat, shallow, broad-based, and irregular; it does not extend beyond the gastric contour. A surrounding mass, adjacent infiltration, rigidity, and mucosal destruction are more positive signs of malignancy. However, the severe edema that may surround a benign gastric ulcer can produce a filling defect indistinguishable from a malignant mass. The size and the location of an ulcer are not accurate criteria for making the distinction. In uncertain cases, reasonably rapid healing of the ulcer and disappearance of surrounding defects under medical management favor benignity. A malignant ulcer may show improvement but does not heal completely.

The picture varies according to the location of the lesion. In the lower third of the stomach, polypoid or infiltrative luminal narrowing can lead to partial obstruction. In both the middle and lower thirds, rigidity is pronounced and peristalsis is absent. Malignant lesions of the fundus offer a diagnostic challenge inasmuch as they cannot be palpated and peristalsis is normally not present. Smaller fundal lesions may be overlooked radiographically. Air-contrast studies are of great aid in uncovering fundal lesions.

Widespread infiltrative carcinoma causes the stomach to be shrunken and rigid (linitis plastica). Often a rigid infiltrated antrum produces a widened patulous pyloric canal, with rapid emptying of the stomach.

Cineradiography or videotape is very helpful in detecting small infiltrating lesions, since it provides clear demonstration of peristaltic alterations and wall rigidity.[13, 87, 224-226]

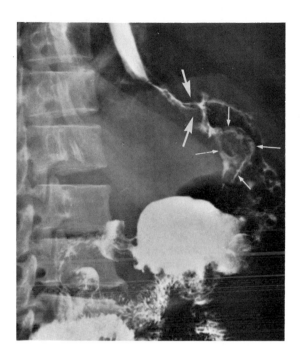

Figure 12–226 **Polypoid Carcinoma of Upper Third of Stomach.** A large irregular mass *(small arrows)* projects into the air-filled lumen of the upper portion of the stomach. Tumor extensions surround the cardia *(large arrows)* and have invaded the posterior soft tissues.

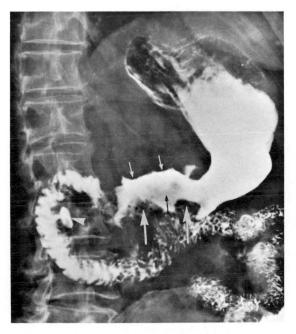

Figure 12–227 **Polypoid and Infiltrative Carcinoma of Gastric Antrum.** The gastric antrum is grossly deformed by large filling defects along the greater curvature *(large white arrows)*. The lesser curvature is rigid and irregular *(small white arrows)*, with intraluminal polypoid defects *(black arrow)*. An incidental duodenal diverticulum is noted *(arrowhead)*. The stomach is not dilated despite the extensive antral involvement; obstructive dilatation is much more common in benign prepyloric or duodenal ulcer.

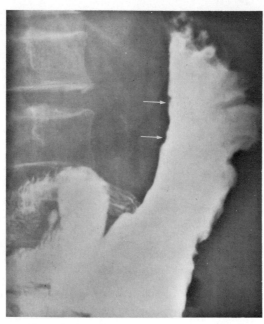

Figure 12–228 **Early Infiltrative Carcinoma of Lesser Curvature.** The lesser curvature area below the fundus was persistently irregular *(arrows)* throughout the examination. No mass or filling defect is apparent. The lesion was an infiltrative carcinoma. Such lesions are difficult to diagnose, especially if they arise above the area of peristalsis. Purely infiltrative lesions of the upper stomach may be overlooked, even when fairly extensive.

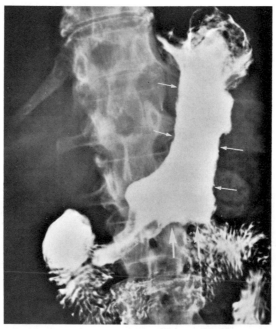

Figure 12–229 **Advanced Infiltrative Carcinoma of Stomach (Linitis Plastica).** The entire stomach except for the extreme fundus has been infiltrated. The walls are rigid and somewhat irregular, and the midportion of the stomach *(small arrows)* is fixed and narrowed. No mucosal folds are seen, nor is peristalsis evident, in this portion. There is a fixed deformity of the greater curvature in the preantral area *(large arrows)*, and the entire antrum is persistently narrowed and fixed, but patulous.

The absence of peristalsis (rigidity) is an important feature of infiltration even when irregularities of the wall are not obvious.

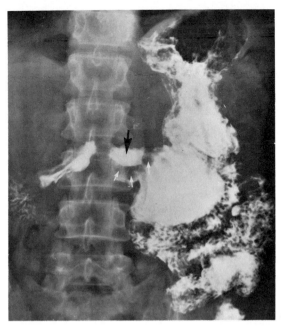

Figure 12–230 **Ulcerating Carcinoma of Gastric Antrum.** The antrum is narrowed, and the large ulcer *(black arrow)* on the lesser curvature is surrounded by irregular lucent areas *(white arrows)*, which represent tumor masses.

The ulcer does not project beyond the stomach as do most benign ulcers; such confinement to the stomach is a radiographic criterion for a malignant ulceration, but radiographic distinction is sometimes impossible.

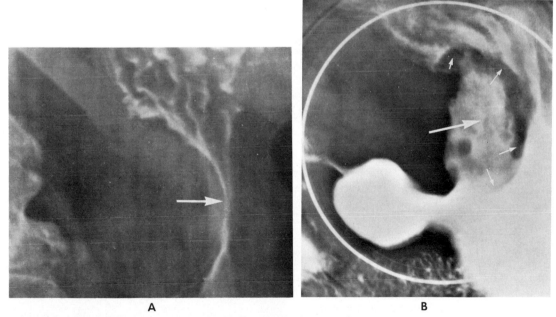

A   B

Figure 12–231 **Ulcerating Carcinoma of Middle Third of Stomach.**

A, In erect view pressure from a mass is evident on the lesser curvature *(arrow),* and the appearance suggests an extrinsic mass.

B, Recumbent view indicates that the pressure is caused by a huge ulcerating carcinoma of the lesser curvature. The large barium-filled area *(large arrow)* with irregular lucencies represents extensive ulceration; the irregular lucencies within the barium represent tumor masses; the remainder of the tumor mass is seen as a lucent band surrounding the ulcer *(small arrows)*. The gastric folds terminate abruptly at the site of the tumor. Peristalsis, which is absent along the lesser curvature adjacent to the lesion, is present in the uninvolved antrum.

Adenomatous Polyps of the Stomach

Polyps are found far less frequently in the stomach than in the colon, and they occur most commonly in patients with achlorhydria and pernicious anemia. Gastric polyps are also a prominent feature of the rare Cronkhite-Canada syndrome and rarely Peutz-Jeghers syndrome. Single polyps are most frequent, but multiple lesions are not rare. A stalk may be present. Polyps are most common in the antrum and are very rarely seen in the upper third of the stomach. A polyp, especially if it has a stalk, may prolapse into the duodenum and cause obstruction.

The polyps are seen as rounded lucencies in the barium-filled stomach, usually merging with the gastric folds; when thickened folds are viewed on end they can simulate a polyp. Pressure on the area may flatten heavy gastric folds, but a true polyp will maintain its roentgenologic appearance under pressure. If the polyp has a stalk and is movable, it may be mistaken for a foreign body. Polyps may bleed, but in most patients they produce no symptoms.[226-228]

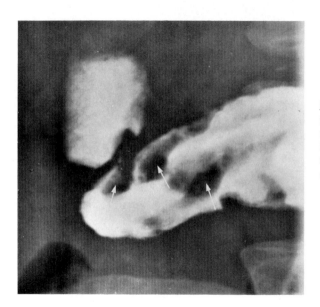

Figure 12–232 **Adenomatous Polyps of Gastric Antrum.** Film taken with compression demonstrates round defects *(arrows)* merging with the gastric folds. These were adenomatous polyps, but they might have been mistaken for heavy gastric folds on a film without compression.

Figure 12–233 **Polyposis of Antrum.** The numerous polyps present as round lucencies in the barium *(black arrows)* and as defects in the walls *(white arrows)*. Additional compression would permit clearer delineation of the lesions.

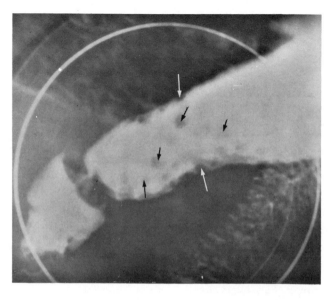

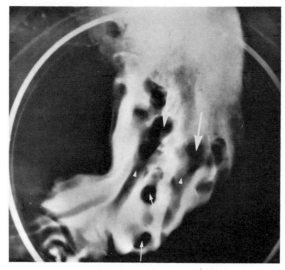

Figure 12–234 **Multiple Polyps of Body of Stomach.** The numerous round defects *(small arrows)* are characteristic of polyps. The polyps *(large arrows)* at the end of the thick folds *(arrowheads)* might readily be mistaken for folds seen *en face*. The patient had achlorhydria.

Leiomyoma, Aberrant Pancreas, and Other Extramucosal Gastric Lesions

Benign lesions that arise below the mucosa generally have a similar roentgenologic appearance and can rarely be distinguished from each other. Included in this group are leiomyoma, aberrant pancreas, lipoma, neurofibroma, leiomyoblastoma, and myoblastoma (granular cell tumor); leiomyoma and aberrant pancreas are the most common.

These extramucosal lesions appear as rounded, sharply defined wall defects without a pedicle. They stretch but do not destroy the mucosa. Except for the aberrant pancreas, which is almost never found in the proximal stomach, these benign tumors may occur in any portion of the stomach.

The leiomyoma and the very rare leiomyoblastoma may ulcerate centrally, producing a characteristic roentgenologic picture. Occasionally an antral leiomyoma may intussuscept into the duodenal bulb and cause gastric obstruction. A leiomyoma may sometimes extend entirely outside the gastric lumen and may produce little or no defect in the barium-filled stomach. The extragastric component may become quite huge, compressing the stomach and neighboring structures.

Aberrant pancreatic tissue produces a sharply rounded defect that is rarely greater than 2 cm. in diameter. The lesion is usually found in the antrum but may occur in the first or second portion of the duodenum. The umbilication or dimple around the small pancreatic duct, which arises from the nodule, may fill with barium and produce a characteristic roentgenologic appearance.[227, 229-231]

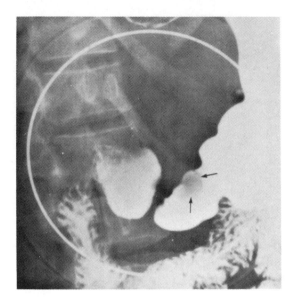

Figure 12-235 **Leiomyoma of Stomach.** The sharply demarcated lucency *(arrows)* along the lesser curvature of the antrum was a leiomyoma. It was entirely asymptomatic. There was no ulceration, and the mucosa was not destroyed. Radiographically, the tumor could not be distinguished from other intramural lesions.

A leiomyoma in the stomach may prolapse into the duodenal bulb. Since there is no stalk, the gastric wall also prolapses, thereby producing partial or complete obstruction, which, however, is usually temporary.

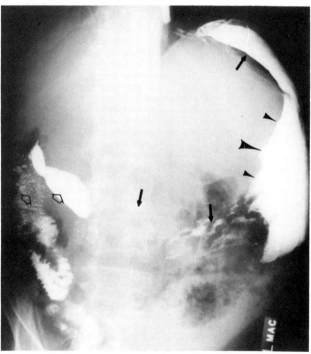

Figure 12-236 **Huge Leiomyoma of Stomach.** A large soft tissue mass is compressing and stretching the stomach *(black arrows).* The duodenal bulb and loop *(open arrows)* are displaced to the right. The irregularities of the lesser curvature *(small arrowheads)* mark the site of origin of the tumor. The ulceration *(large arrowhead)* was within the leiomyoma. Almost the entire tumor had extended extragastrically, a frequent characteristic of larger gastric leiomyomas.

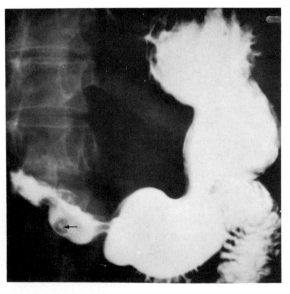

Figure 12-237 **Aberrant Pancreatic Nodule in Stomach.** A round sharply marginated defect in the gastric antrum contains a small central barium density *(arrow),* which is barium within the dimple containing the small pancreatic duct that arises from within the nodule.

Aberrant pancreatic nodules are also found in the duodenal bulb and proximal portion of the descending duodenal limb. In the stomach, the greater curvature of the antrum is the most common site. (Courtesy Dr. R. Rooney, Atlanta, Georgia.)

Leiomyosarcoma of the Stomach

The rare leiomyosarcoma arises as an intramural extramucosal lesion, indistinguishable from a leiomyoma. Later, ulceration and destruction of the mucosa may provide a clue to its malignant nature. The leiomyosarcoma may become lobular as it enlarges, and, like the gastric leiomyoma, it is also prone to ulceration and may have a large extragastric component. Over half the tumors are entirely exogastric, showing extrinsic pressure and stretching of the mucosal folds. A fistula into the tumor allows air or barium to enter the mass, a highly suggestive finding.[230-232]

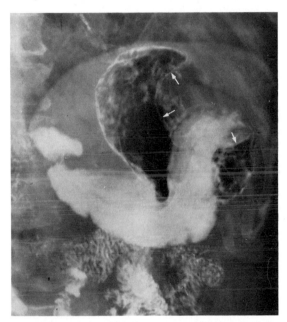

Figure 12–238 **Leiomyosarcoma of Stomach.** The large mass bulging into the stomach high on the greater curvature produces a smooth defect *(arrows)*. No ulceration is seen radiographically, although an ulcer was found at surgery. The mucosa is intact, and the appearance is characteristic of an intramural extramucosal mass.

Lymphosarcoma of the Stomach

This uncommon lesion usually has a roentgenologic appearance similar to that of an ulcerative or polypoid carcinoma, but it occurs in a younger age group. In a minority of cases there are greatly enlarged folds, occasionally with nodular lucencies, simulating the giant folds of gastritis. These are infiltrated areas, and, unlike ordinary thick folds, they do not disappear or straighten with external compression. Multiple ulcers are frequently seen and are strongly suggestive. The wall of the stomach may be thickened.

Direct invasion of the stomach can develop secondary to lymphosarcoma originating in the retroperitoneal space. The demonstration of additional tumors in other organs and tissues should suggest the possibility of lymphoma.[233, 234]

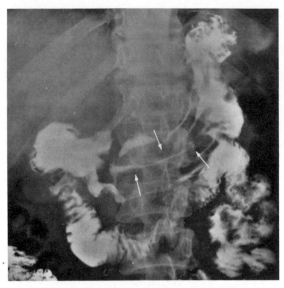

Figure 12–239 **Lymphosarcoma of Stomach.** Broad lucencies extending from the midstomach to the pylorus *(arrows)* were large folds infiltrated with lymphosarcoma. Their resemblance to ordinary enlarged gastric folds is striking. Although this appearance is characteristic of lymphosarcoma, it occurs in a minority of cases; most often the picture is indistinguishable from that of a carcinoma.

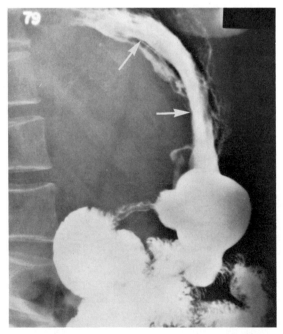

Figure 12–240 **Retroperitoneal Lymphosarcoma Displacing and Invading Stomach.** A large retroperitoneal mass, a lymphosarcoma, has displaced the body of the stomach anteriorly and produced a sharp indentation on its posterior wall *(arrows)*. The irregularities of the posterior wall *(between arrows)* were due to invasion and infiltration of the stomach by the lymphosarcoma.

Malignant Neoplasms of the Small Intestine

Primary malignancies of the small bowel make up less than one per cent of gastrointestinal neoplasms. Adenocarcinoma is the most common malignant tumor detected radiographically. Carcinoids are almost as frequent but are often too small to be seen on routine small bowel studies. The duodenum and jejunum are the most common sites of adenocarcinoma. Overall diagnostic accuracy is about 60 per cent, although 90 per cent of the tumors in the second portion of the duodenum may be demonstrated.

Radiographically, the carcinoma may be polypoid, annular, or infiltrative, or it may combine these features. The mucosa is distorted or destroyed, and the lumen is narrowed, often eccentrically, and irregularly. Obstruction, evident both clinically and radiographically, can occur intermittently. Malignant neoplasms of the small bowel are difficult to diagnose, especially if the lesion is not large and is not causing obstruction at the time of examination. Other primary malignant lesions, like leiomyosarcoma, are quite uncommon. Lymphosarcoma of the small intestine is discussed on page 1174.

Clinically, anemia, gastrointestinal bleeding, intermittent obstruction, and abdominal pain are the most frequent presenting symptoms.

Metastatic disease to the small bowel is rare. Occasionally a characteristic bull's eye appearance is seen. This occurs most often in metastatic melanoma and is due to central ulceration of a nodular metastasis in the mucosa. However, a metastatic lesion may have the radiographic characteristics of a primary malignancy.[235-239]

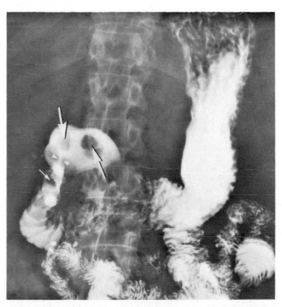

Figure 12–241 **Adenocarcinoma of Duodenum: Large Nodular and Infiltrative Lesion.** There are polypoid masses in the duodenal bulb *(large arrows)* and in the upper portion of the descending limb *(small arrow)*, and a constricting infiltration *(arrowheads)* at the postbulbar area. The lesion probably originated in the postbulbar area and spread proximally and distally. The second portion of the duodenum is one of the most common sites of small bowel neoplasm, but carcinoma originating in the duodenal bulb is very rare.

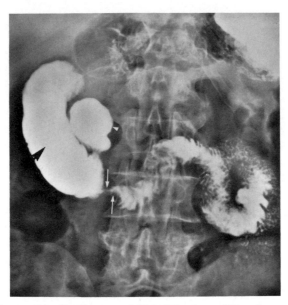

Figure 12–242 **Annular Obstructing Carcinoma of Third Portion of Duodenum.** The lesion has produced a "napkin ring" constriction of the duodenum *(white arrows)*, with polypoid masses encircling the lumen. There is a shoulder defect distally. The proximal descending duodenum *(black arrow)* is greatly dilated, and an incidental duodenal diverticulum *(arrowhead)* arising from the dilated loop is also distended.

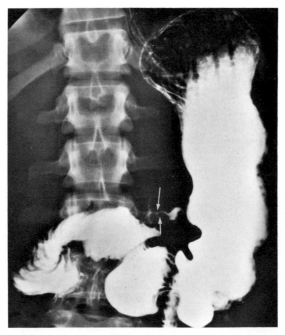

Figure 12–243 **Carcinoma of Fourth Portion of Duodenum.** The irregular stenosing lesion *(arrows)* is partly obscured by the barium-filled stomach and duodenal bulb. Proximally, the duodenum is moderately dilated.

    The fourth portion of the duodenum is frequently obscured by a barium-filled stomach or duodenal bulb. Persistent dilatation of the duodenum proximal to a lesion may often call attention to a lesion of the fourth part of the duodenum, hidden behind the barium-filled stomach.

Figure 12–244 **Adenocarcinoma of Proximal Jejunum.** Multiple nodular defects *(arrows)* in the jejunum just distal to the duodenojejunal junction (at ligament of Treitz) have destroyed and replaced the mucosal pattern. There is no obstruction or narrowing of the lumen. Such lesions produce few symptoms; occult bleeding may be the only clinical finding.

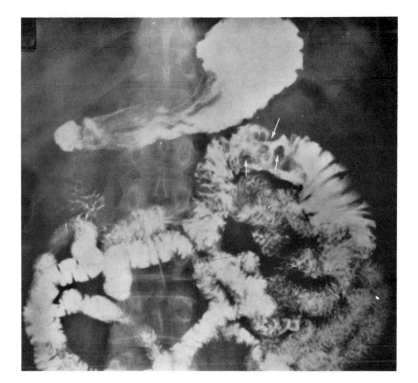

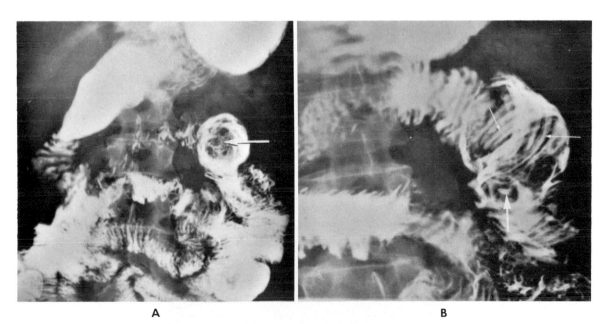

A   B

Figure 12–245 **Metastatic Malignant Melanoma of Small Bowel.**

A, A loop of ileum appears to be segmentally distended; it contains an irregular filling defect *(arrow)*.

B, A spot film of the area shows a dilated segment with a coiled-spring appearance *(small arrows)* due to intussusception of a tumor mass. The round defect with a central barium-filled umbilication *(large arrow)* is mucosal ulceration into a submucosal metastatic nodule—the bull's-eye appearance.

Although metastases to the small bowel are rare, the bull's-eye appearance suggests metastatic malignant melanoma. (Courtesy Dr. Arlyne Shockman, Veterans Administration Hospital, Philadelphia, Pennsylvania.)

Lymphosarcoma of the Small Bowel

See page 1174.

Benign Neoplasms of the Small Intestine

Benign tumors of the small intestine are relatively rare and usually solitary. Leiomyoma is the most common tumor, occurring most often in the jejunum. Adenomatous polyp is next in frequency and may be found in any portion of the small bowel. Lipoma and hemangioma are rare and usually not detected radiographically. All of these tumors are usually asymptomatic and do not undergo malignant degeneration, but occasionally they may bleed. Intussusception may occur, causing abdominal pain or intestinal obstruction.

During a progress barium meal examination, these lesions may cause filling defects in the barium column and appear as an intraluminal extramucosal mass or as a rounded or lobulated sessile or pedunculated intraluminal lesion. Occasionally there may be evidence of intussusception with a characteristic coiled-spring appearance. Sometimes a bleeding small bowel tumor may be localized by abdominal aortography.

Smaller lesions are generally not detected radiographically and are incidental findings at surgery or autopsy.

Multiple small bowel polyps may be seen in the Peutz-Jeghers syndrome (p. 1065) and in the Cronkhite-Canada syndrome (p. 1076).[235]

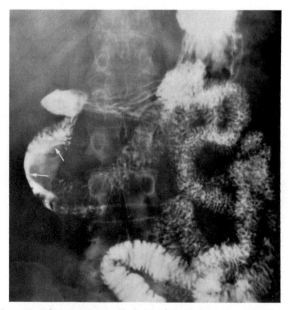

Figure 12–246 **Unusually Large Adenomatous Polyp of Duodenum.** A large lobulated mass in the descending duodenum has widened the lumen and produced a sharp lobulated filling defect *(arrows)*. Obstruction is absent despite the large mass. Intestinal polyps rarely attain this size.

Peutz-Jeghers Syndrome

Multiple polyps in the gastrointestinal tract associated with perioral pigmentation are the salient features of this familial condition.

Rectal bleeding and recurrent attacks of abdominal pain due to intussusception of the polyp are the principal symptoms.

The polyps occur most frequently in the ileum but may also occur in the jejunum, stomach, or colon. Radiographically there are multiple intraluminal defects in the small bowel and occasionally in the colon. These polyps vary from 0.1 to 3.0 cm. in diameter. They may be sessile or pedunculated. Histologically, the polyps are hamartomas, although some of the lesions, particularly those in the colon, are histologically indistinguishable from adenomatous polyps. The polyps rarely become malignant in contrast to some other forms of intestinal polyposis.[240-242]

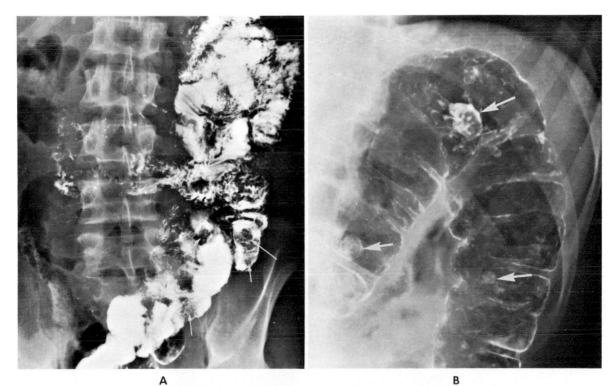

| A | B |

Figure 12–247 **Peutz-Jeghers Syndrome: Polyposis of Small Bowel and Colon.**

A, There are multiple filling defects *(arrows)* scattered throughout the small bowel. These polyps are often difficult to identify. There is no obstruction.

B, Air-contrast study of the colon demonstrates multiple defects in the air column due to polyps of varying sizes *(arrows).*

Carcinoma of the Colon

This is the most frequent malignant lesion of the intestinal tract. Although it may occur in any portion of the colon, the lesion is in the rectosigmoid region in about two thirds of cases, and in the cecum in about 10 per cent of cases. The barium enema, with an accuracy of over 90 per cent, provides a definitive examination for diagnosis of colonic tumors above the rectum.

The lesions may be annular, polypoid, or infiltrative, or may combine these characteristics. The annular lesion narrows the lumen abruptly. Generally, a portion of tumor projects into the normal area of colon, producing a shoulder defect. Annular lesions frequently cause obstruction. The polypoid lesion projects into the lumen as a nodular and often irregular mass; the cecum is a favored site. If the portion of the wall from which the tumor originates is visualized, infiltration may be evident. The mucosal pattern is generally destroyed in both the annular and polypoid type of lesion. A localized lesion infiltrating one wall will cause irregularity but is frequently unrecognized until narrowing occurs or intraluminal masses develop.

In general, roentgenologic diagnosis is not difficult provided oblique projections are employed to completely visualize redundant flexures.

Lesions of the rectosigmoid may easily be obscured by the anatomic angulation of this portion of the bowel. Lesions of the cecum are often difficult to demonstrate because the cecum is usually wide and capacious and often contains fecal material, which can obscure or simulate a lesion. Air-contrast studies are of considerable value for detecting these lesions. Repeated studies may be necessary before definitive diagnosis can be made. Complete obstruction of the large bowel by carcinoma is not uncommon. Ulceration and perforation are infrequent complications. An unusually high incidence of carcinoma is found in patients with long-term ulcerative colitis and in patients with familial polyposis.[13, 238, 243]

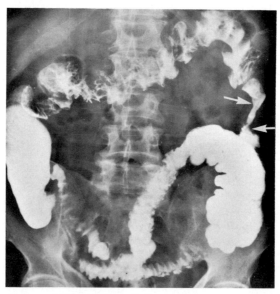

Figure 12-248 **Annular Carcinoma of Descending Colon.** The segment between the arrows is narrowed, irregular, and rigid, and shows loss of mucosal pattern. Note the abrupt transition to normal colon at the lower end, with a small shoulder defect *(lower arrow)*.

Annular lesions usually involve short segments of the colon.

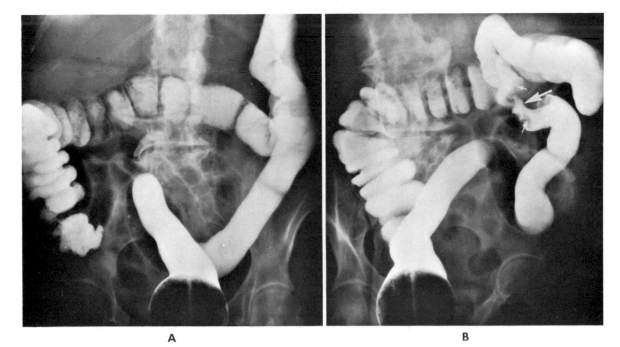

A   B

Figure 12-249 **Annular and Polypoid Carcinoma of Descending Colon.**

A, On filled posteroanterior film it is difficult to appreciate the lesion, which is obscured by the redundant splenic flexure.

B, Oblique view clearly demonstrates the irregular narrowed segment *(large arrow),* with polypoid masses *(small arrows)* projecting into the lumen above and below the constriction. This case exemplifies the necessity of obtaining oblique views during examination of the colon.

Figure 12-250 **Large Polypoid Carcinoma of Cecum.** The large lobulated defect in the cecum *(arrows)* was a polypoid carcinoma. It is difficult to distinguish from the numerous adjacent nodular defects, which are due to feces. Confirmation required reexamination after thorough cleansing of the bowel.

Polypoid cecal tumors are often masked by fecal contents.

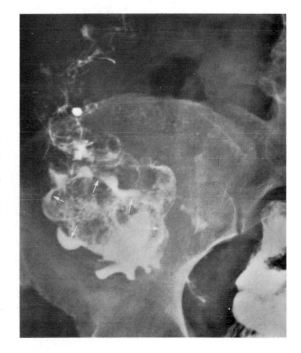

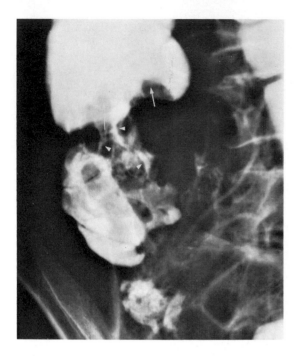

Figure 12-251 **Polypoid and Infiltrative Lesion of Cecum and Ascending Colon.** In the narrowed area the walls are irregularly infiltrated, with polypoid masses *(arrowheads)* replacing the mucosal folds. Extension of the masses produces large shoulder defects *(arrows)* in the proximal colon.

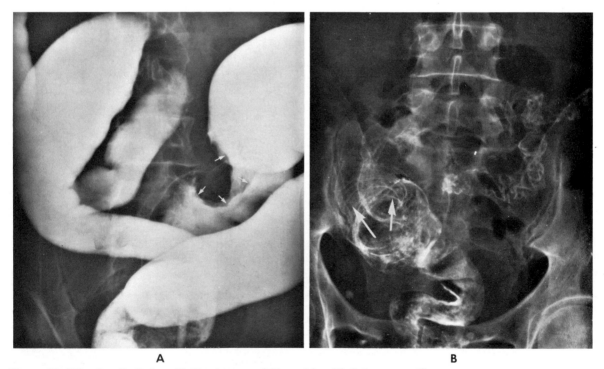

A   B

Figure 12-252   **Sessile Polypoid Carcinoma of Sigmoid, with Intussusception.**

A, There is a large polypoid eccentric mass defect *(arrows)* in the proximal portion of a redundant sigmoid. The borders of the defect are lobulated and irregular.

B, During evacuation, the tumor and its colonic segment have been propelled by peristalsis and have intussuscepted, as demonstrated by the coiled-spring appearance *(arrows)*. Often the intermittent intussusception of a small tumor is responsible for the initial clinical symptoms of episodic cramping pain.

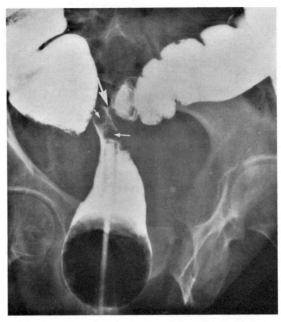

Figure 12–253 **Recurrent Carcinoma at Rectosigmoid Junction.** Barium enema examination four years following surgery discloses a smooth narrowed area at the rectosigmoid junction *(large arrow).* Polypoid defects with mucosal destruction are seen *(small arrows)* below the narrowed segment.

Postsurgical non-neoplastic narrowing and deformities often develop at the site of an anastomosis. A baseline barium enema examination after surgery will be helpful for later distinguishing between postsurgical narrowing and tumor recurrence at the anastomotic site.

Lymphosarcoma of the Colon

The uncommon lymphoma of the colon may be a primary tumor or a manifestation of diffuse systemic lymphoma. It can occur at any age.

Although the radiographic changes may be indistinguishable from those of a carcinoma, often there are some suggestive radiographic features. Frequently, lymphomatous involvement extends over a longer segment than carcinoma. There may be bulky irregular masses with one or more ulcerations. Submucosal involvement can give rise to diffuse nodules resembling polyposis, or may cause irregular thumbprinting with rigid thickened haustra suggestive of ischemic colitis. A solitary subserosal lymphomatous mass may simulate extrinsic pressure of a diverticular abscess; multiple subserosal masses resemble mesenteric metastasis.

Although by no means specific, any of these findings involving a long colonic segment should suggest the possibility of lymphoma.[244]

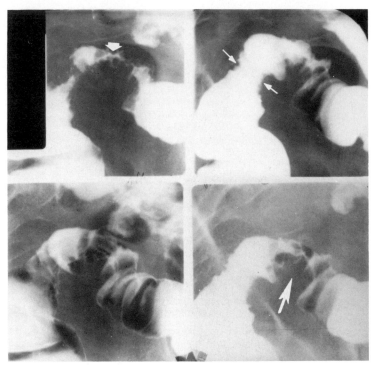

Figure 12–254 **Lymphosarcoma of Sigmoid in 57 Year Old Woman.** Serial films of the sigmoid reveal a larger nodular defect *(large arrow),* which has the appearance of a submucosal lesion. The overlying mucosa, however, is thickened and somewhat distorted *(small broad arrow).* Distal to the nodule, the sigmoid is spiculated *(small arrows),* slightly narrowed, and irritable. There was no obstruction.

At surgery, the entire area showed submucosal infiltration by a lymphosarcoma. The larger nodule had invaded the mucosa. An enlarged lymphomatous spleen was also found.

Usually a focal lymphosarcoma of the colon cannot be distinguished radiographically from a carcinoma. However, submucosal involvement, nodularity, and longer segment disease without obstruction are more often seen in lymphosarcoma.

Secondary (Metastatic) Neoplasms of the Colon

Metastatic disease to the colon can occur from direct extension, from intraperitoneal seeding, or from hematogenous neoplastic emboli.

The lesions to the colon due to direct extension or peritoneal seeding most often arise in the ovary, pancreas, stomach, uterus, or kidney and cause extrinsic crescentic defects upon the colon. Direct invasion characteristically causes fixation of the folds in transverse parallel arrangement. If invasive, a single metastatic lesion may be indistinguishable from a primary tumor. The embolic metastases occur most often from melanoma, breast, or lung malignancies. They usually grow from the submucosal layer into the lumen. Central ulceration is common, giving rise to a "bull's-eye" or "target" lesion, an appearance highly suggestive of metastatic disease. These lesions rarely obstruct but often cause bleeding.[245]

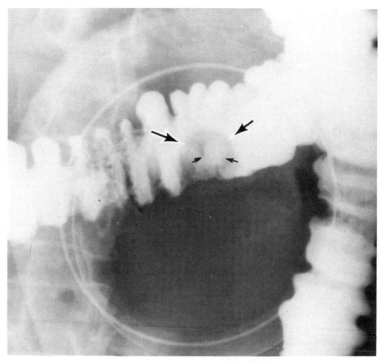

Figure 12–255 **Metastatic Melanoma to Colon.** The sharply circumscribed submucosal defect *(large arrows)* with central ulceration *(small arrows)* proved to be a metastatic lesion.

This bull's-eye appearance is characteristic (see also Fig. 12–245) of metastatic disease to the intestinal tract; larger infiltrating metastases, however, cannot be distinguished from primary neoplasm.

Endometriosis of the Colon

The fibrotic contractures resulting from pelvic endometriosis can involve the serosa of the adjacent rectum or sigmoid. This may cause fixation, kinking, and sometimes segmental bowel stenosis.

Actual growth of endometrial tissue in the wall of the rectum or sigmoid may produce an extrinsic mass defect. If the lesion bulges into the lumen, there is often palisading of the overlying mucosa, which usually remains intact. The radiographic findings may suggest an extrinsic mass, a wall tumor, a polypoid tumor, or carcinoma. Longer lesions with associated stenosis may even simulate an area of granulomatous colitis.

Accentuation and some enlargement of the lesion often occur if repeat barium enema is done during or just prior to menstruation—a suggestive finding.

A serosal, wall, or polypoid lesion in the sigmoid in a woman whose clinical symptoms are aggravated premenstrually is highly suggestive of endometriosis of the colon.[246–249]

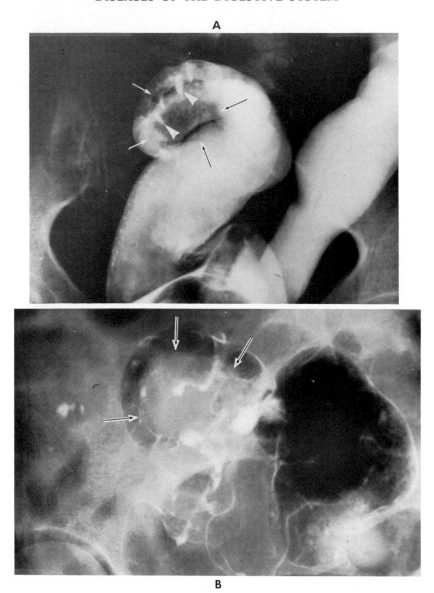

Figure 12–256   **Endometriosis of Sigmoid: Barium Enema.**

A 41 year old woman had been experiencing painful bowel movements and recurrent rectal bleeding three or four days prior to menstruation.

A, There is a large filling defect *(arrows)* in the distal sigmoid. The peculiar tooth-like barium projections *(arrowheads)* are probably part of the mucosa stretched over the mass.

B, The air-contrast film better delineates the size, shape, and smooth borders of the large submucosal endometrioma *(arrows).*

The extreme pain during the examination and the clinical history are helpful parameters for making a correct diagnosis.

Polyps of the Colon

Polyps are common in adults but rare in children. Single or multiple polyps can occur in any portion of the colon, but there is a predilection for the left colon, particularly the sigmoid. Polyps either can be completely asymptomatic or can cause recurrent painless rectal bleeding or mild obstructive symptoms.

A polyp may be sessile or pedunculated; the latter may have a stalk or pedicle up to a few inches in length. Small lesions are usually round or regular, but large polyps often become lobulated. Large numbers of polyps throughout the colon can occur in *Gardner's syndrome* (see p. 1415), *Peutz-Jeghers syndrome* (see p. 1065), *familial polyposis* (see p. 1074), and *Cronkhite-Canada syndrome* (see p. 1076).

Positive roentgenologic identification is often difficult, especially with small lesions. Small accumulations of fecal material can simulate the defect caused by a polyp, and large accumulations may completely obscure the lesion. In certain projections, diverticula, especially when coated with barium, simulate polyps. Moreover, clusters of diverticula can effectively conceal the polyp. Thus, repeated barium enema examinations with air-contrast studies and scrupulous cleansing of the bowel are necessary for accurate and positive diagnosis. The configuration of a polyp on a stalk in the barium or air column is quite characteristic, but it is prudent to demonstrate the lesion on two separate examinations before surgery is performed. A long stalk permits considerable change of location of the polyp in the various films.

Most polyps are benign adenomas, and their relationship to malignancy is controversial. However, the following roentgenologic criteria are generally accepted as definitive indication for surgery because of possible malignant change:

1. A polyp diameter greater than 10 mm.
2. Evidence of growth on serial studies.
3. Irregularities at the base or the periphery, or an unusually wide base.

Other benign tumors of the colon are considerably less frequent than polyps; of these, *lipoma* (Fig. 15-14) is the most common. *Carcinoid*, benign and malignant (Fig. 16-56), and *villous adenoma* (see p. 1077) are quite uncommon. The pseudopolyps of ulcerative colitis (Figs. 12-179 and 12-182) are readily distinguished from true adenomatous polyps by the associated changes of ulcerative colitis and by the absence of pedicles.[13, 63, 250, 251]

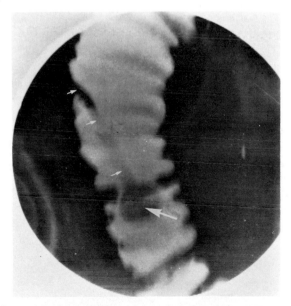

Figure 12-257 **Sigmoid Polyp with Long Stalk.** A compression film of the sigmoid made during barium enema demonstrates the smooth round defect of the polyp *(large arrow)* and the long pedicle *(small arrows)* leading to the point of origin in the bowel wall. The location of this polyp varied during the examination because of the long stalk.

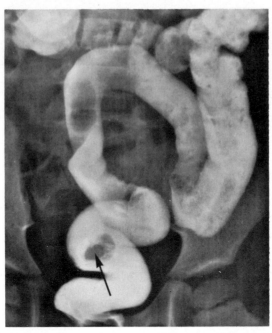

Figure 12–258 **Large Sessile Polyp.** The patient was a 4½ year old girl. The smoothly bordered defect *(arrow)* in the upper rectum was a large sessile polyp that caused rectal bleeding. Its appearance simulates the fecal collections often seen in the sigmoid; reexamination was needed for confirmation.

Rectal polyps are best diagnosed by proctoscopy, since smaller lesions of the rectum are usually not identified on barium enema study.

Familial Polyposis of the Colon

Innumerable polyps are scattered uniformly throughout the entire colon, and almost invariably malignant degeneration of one or more of these lesions occurs. Prophylactic colectomy is usually performed.

Rectal bleeding and diarrhea are the common symptoms.

The great number of small filling defects seen in the barium enema study makes diagnosis relatively easy, but occasionally all the lesions are tiny, resembling nodular mucosa rather than multiple polyps. In this case, especially if a history of familial polyposis cannot be elicited, a mucosal biopsy may be necessary for diagnosis. Nodular *lymphoid hyperplasia* of the colon may occasionally simulate polyposis.[252]

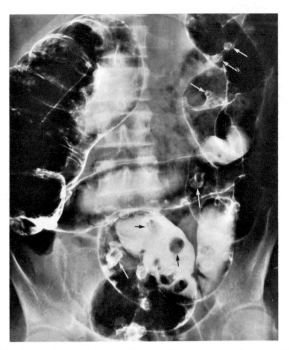

Figure 12–259 **Nonfamilial Polyposis of Colon.** The patient was a 44 year old man. A film made following air-contrast enema demonstrates numerous polyps of varying sizes, some of which are marked by arrows. The left side is more extensively involved.

In the air column the polyps are seen as a positive density *(white arrows),* but when surrounded by barium they present as a lucent defect *(black arrows).*

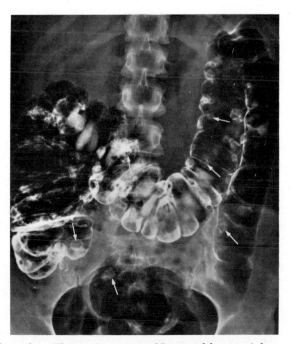

Figure 12–260 **Familial Polyposis.** The patient was a 35 year old man. A large number of polyps, some of which are indicated by arrows, are seen in air-contrast study. They are scattered uniformly throughout the colon. There was a family history of polyposis, but the patient refused colectomy. Malignant change in one or more polyps eventually occurs in a high percentage of patients with familial polyposis.

Cronkhite-Canada Syndrome

This rare syndrome of obscure origin is characterized by ectodermal changes (alopecia, nail atrophy, and hyperpigmentation), intestinal malabsorption, and protein loss. It usually appears in the sixth or seventh decade, with symptoms of abdominal pain and diarrhea.

Polyps are invariably present in the stomach and diffusely in the colon. Small intestinal polyps are less frequent, but coarsened mucosa and tiny radiolucencies are common.

The colon polyps are small and uniform, usually without pedicles. In the stomach, large or confluent polypoid masses may obscure the smaller lesions.

Many of the polyps appear to be cystic glandular dilatation rather than true adenomatous polyps. However, malignant degeneration can occur.[153, 253, 254]

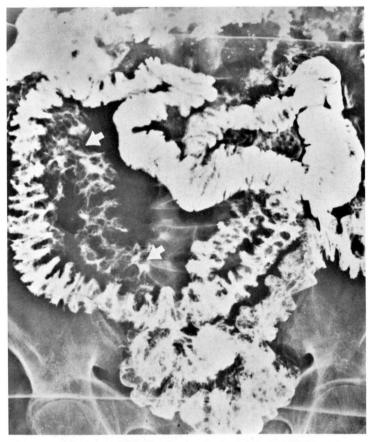

Figure 12–261 **Cronkhite-Canada Syndrome.** The folds of the small bowel are diffusely thickened *(arrows),* and multiple small radiolucent areas of mucosal hypertrophy can be seen. Diffuse gastric polyposis and scattered small colonic polyps were also present in this patient. (Courtesy Drs. R. Marshak and A. E. Lindner: *Radiology of the Small Intestine.* 2nd ed. Philadelphia, W. B. Saunders Company, 1976.)

Villous Adenoma

This tumor varies from 2 to 20 cm. in diameter, but is usually fairly large and soft. Approximately 80 per cent of lesions occur in the rectum and rectosigmoid, but they may appear in any portion of the gastrointestinal tract. A higher than expected incidence of villous adenoma occurs in the syndrome of multiple endocrine adenomatosis. A severe mucous diarrhea that can cause electrolyte depletion is the predominant symptom. About one half of the lesions are malignant.

Radiographically the smaller lesions resemble an ordinary sessile polyp. The larger lesions produce a characteristic irregular, shaggy filling defect. On profile view there is a shaggy appearance, with barium filling the spaces between the villi. *En face,* a bubbly appearance with multiple filling defects is typical; superficially it may resemble a fecal collection. The soft tumor may change shape during compression or on evacuation films. The bowel wall remains soft and contractile. Obstruction does not occur even with large lesions. The larger lesions have a higher probability of malignancy, but there are usually no clearcut radiographic distinctions between the benign and malignant villous tumor.[255, 256]

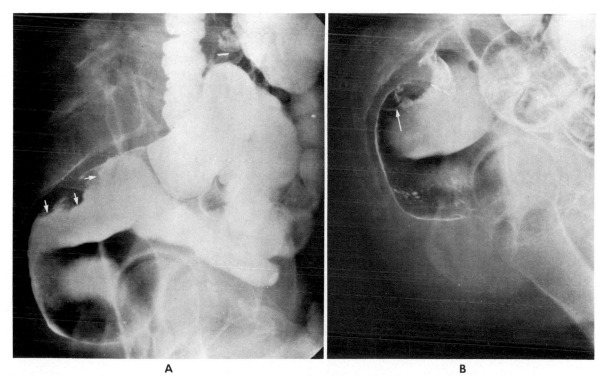

| A | B |

Figure 12–262   **Villous Adenoma of Rectum: Barium Enema.**

The patient was a 55 year old man.

A, Lateral view of barium enema study shows an irregular filling defect *(arrows)* on the posterior wall of the upper rectum. The barium seen projecting into the defect represents barium between the villi.

B, In lateral air view, alteration in shape of the adenoma can be seen *(arrows),* and small barium projections into the defect are again apparent.

The location of the lesion, the small barium projections into the defect, and the frequent alterations in shape are characteristic of villous adenoma.

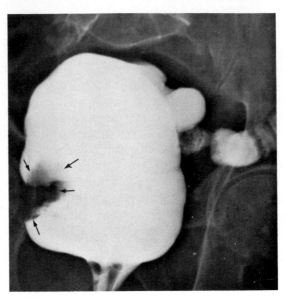

Figure 12–263 **Villous Adenoma of Rectum: Barium Enema.** The adenoma appears as a lobulated defect (*arrows*). The small barium projections into the defect are seen at the lower border of the lesion.

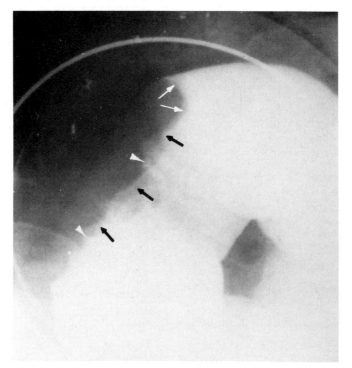

Figure 12–264 **Villous Adenoma of Sigmoid: Barium Enema: Close-up Compression View.** The filling defect has a fairly regular upper border (*white arrows*). However, the bulk of the defect has a very irregular margin (*black arrows*), with many small projections of barium (*arrowheads*) extending into the defect. The latter findings are highly suggestive of villous adenoma.

DISEASES OF THE GALLBLADDER AND BILE DUCTS

Chronic Cholecystitis: Cholelithiasis

The principal roentgenologic features are demonstration of calculi, or persistent nonvisualization of the gallbladder after oral cholecystography, or both.

If the gallbladder is not visualized after oral cholecystography, provided that malabsorption or liver impairment is not present, the patient probably has chronic cholecystitis and, usually, calculi. The density of the gallbladder is not a reliable criterion of function, and relatively faint opacification in the absence of calculi is not a dependable indicator of gallbladder disease.

Calculi are found in most cases of chronic cholecystitis. Only about 15 per cent of calculi are radiopaque and apparent on plain abdominal films. Occasionally, a stone that is not opaque but that contains gas-filled fissures is recognized on plain films. Most stones can be identified after cholecystography, which demonstrates their presence in over 95 per cent of cases. Erect or decubitus views during cholecystography are essential in order to see the layering of tiny nonopaque calculi; these might be missed on recumbent views. When oral cholecystography fails to opacify the gallbladder even after a repeat dose of the contrast agent, intravenous cholecystography is often effective provided that the cystic duct is not obstructed.

An infrequent finding on plain films is opacification of the gallbladder due to opaque milk of calcium bile. Chronic cystic duct obstruction is usually responsible for the high concentration of calcium carbonate in the bile, and sometimes an associated calculus is seen in the vicinity of the cystic duct. Another rare but striking finding in chronic cholecystitis is calcification of the gallbladder wall.[257, 258]

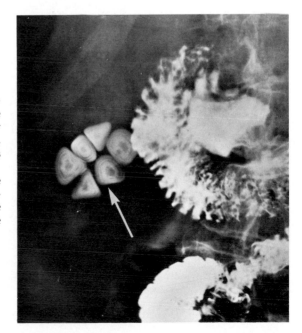

Figure 12–265 **Faceted, Laminated, Opaque Gallstones.** The six gallstones *(arrow)* collectively create the shape of a gallbladder. Each stone is concentrically laminated and has flat faceted borders. Obviously, such calculi have developed over a long period. This film was part of a gastrointestinal series.

Gallstone calcification has several patterns: there may be a partially calcified rim, a complete ring shadow, a calcified center in a stone that is otherwise nonopaque, or homogeneous calcification of the entire calculus.

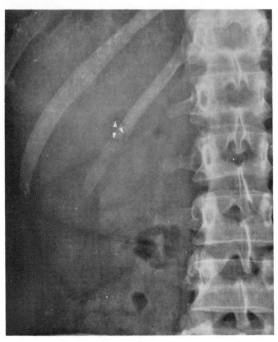

Figure 12–266 **Gas-Containing Gallstone.**   There are a number of small curvilinear lucencies *(arrowheads)* in the right upper quadrant; these are small gas pockets in a fissured gallstone. Although they are infrequently seen, such lucencies, which are often stellate, are characteristic and may be the only roentgenologic clue to the presence of gallstones on plain films.

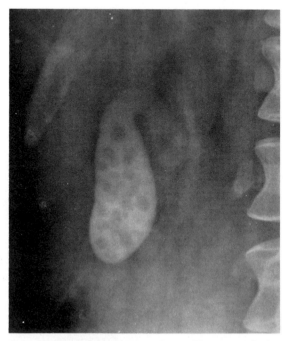

Figure 12–267 **Nonopaque Calculi: Oral Cholecystogram.**   The opacified gallbladder contains a large number of round filling defects scattered throughout the viscus. This is a recumbent view.

Such nonopaque calculi can be demonstrated only if the gallbladder is opacified. In many cases of chronic calculus cholecystitis, the gallbladder fails to be opacified after oral cholecystography and an intravenous study may be necessary to prove the presence of calculi.

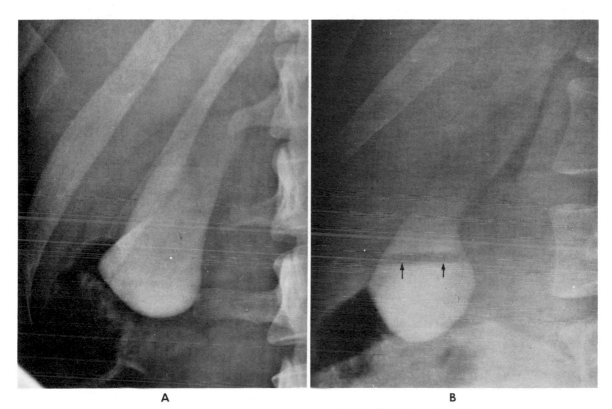

A   B

Figure 12–268 **Chronic Calculus Cholecystitis: Layering of Calculi in Erect Position.**

A, The recumbent cholecystogram demonstrates an opacified gallbladder in which are found ill-defined lucencies that resemble gallstones.

B, In erect view there is a translucent band across the gallbladder *(arrows)*. This represents a layer of small nonopaque calculi. These stones "float" at the same level, since they have identical specific gravities. Frequently no defects are detected in recumbent views, but a thin translucent layer of stones will become apparent on erect or decubitus views. Occasionally the tiny stones fall to the fundus of the gallbladder and produce a crescentic lucent band in the floor of the gallbladder in erect views. Unless an erect or decubitus film has been made, the cholecystogram is incomplete and does not exclude calculi.

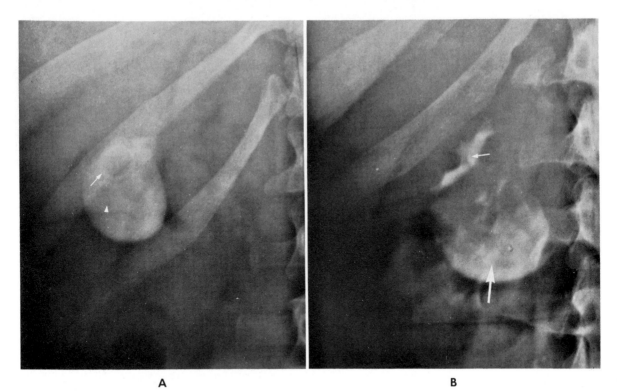

A   B

Figure 12–269 **Chronic Cholecystitis: Milk of Calcium Bile: Plain Film.**

    A, The gallbladder is diffusely opacified in plain film, simulating a cholecystogram. A calculus with cal-
cified rim *(arrow)* and a nonopaque calculus *(arrowhead)* can be identified in the milk of calcium bile.

    B, In erect view made during a urogram, the milk of calcium bile drops to the dependent portion of the
gallbladder *(large arrow).* The right renal pelvis is opacified *(small arrow),* since the film was part of a
pyleogram.

    Milk of calcium bile is generally the result of a partially obstructed gallbladder, which causes a high
concentration of calcium carbonate in the bile; the bile then becomes diffusely radiopaque.

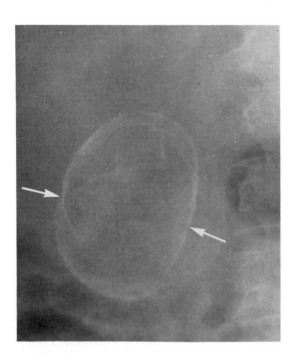

Figure 12–270 **Chronic Cholecystitis: Calcification of
Gallbladder Wall: Plain Film.** In the gallbladder wall
there is a well-defined shell of calcification *(arrows)*
that outlines the entire structure. This relatively rare
finding is indicative of a diseased gallbladder wall.

Acute Cholecystitis

About 80 per cent of cases are due to calculous obstruction of the cystic duct.

Plain abdominal films are usually unrevealing. Demonstration of opaque gallstones or a change of position of a previously observed gallstone may be significant, but only a minority of biliary calculi are radiopaque. The most frequent significant findings are distention of the second portion of the duodenum and localized small bowel distention (sentinel loop). These changes are due to local peritoneal irritation by a suppurative gallbladder.

If the obstructed gallbladder becomes distended, a soft tissue mass, often indenting the adjacent colon, may be apparent. Infrequently, the gallbladder may be outlined by intraluminal or intramural gas resulting from gas-producing bacilli.

Oral cholecystogram during the acute stage invariably fails to opacify the gallbladder. Intravenous cholecystography opacifies the common duct but not the gallbladder. If the gallbladder does opacify, the diagnosis of acute cholecystitis is questionable.

A localized pericholecystic abscess can occur, and this may sometimes be identified by the presence of small gas bubbles in the gallbladder area. Perforation can also produce roentgen findings characteristic of generalized peritonitis or subphrenic abscess.[259-261]

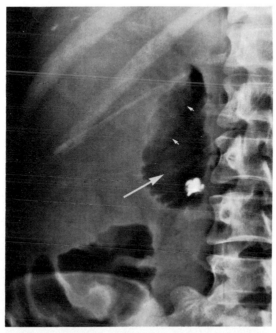

Figure 12–271 **Acute Cholecystitis: Local Ileus and Distended Gallbladder.** There is distention of a gas-filled loop (the descending duodenum) *(large arrow)*; one border of the distended gallbladder projects into the lumen *(small arrows)* of this loop. The opacity near the spine is residual barium from a previous study.

Cystic duct obstruction due to an impacted calculus almost always accompanies, and probably often precipitates, acute cholecystitis.

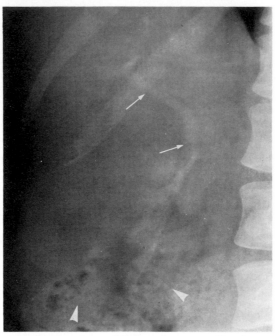

Figure 12–272 **Acute Cholecystitis: Intravenous Cholecystogram.**   One hour after an intravenous injection of opaque medium, the common duct is opacified *(arrows)* and appears normal. The gallbladder is not opacified either in this film or in films made as late as four hours after the injection. The contrast-filled bile, failing to enter the gallbladder, has passed directly into the small intestine, opacifying its contents *(arrowheads)*.

At surgery an acute suppurative cholecystitis and an obstructing calculus in the cystic duct were found.

Intravenous cholecystography is a valuable diagnostic aid in cases of suspected acute cholecystitis. If the common duct is opacified but the gallbladder is not, cystic duct obstruction is almost certainly present.

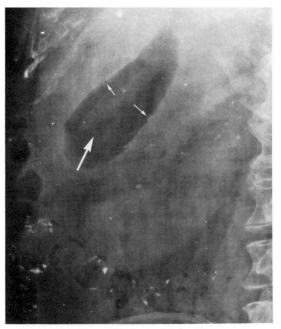

Figure 12–273 **Acute Emphysematous Cholecystitis in a Diabetic.**   The enlarged gallbladder is filled with gas *(large arrow)*. Irregularity of the wall *(small arrows)* is due to edema of the mucosa. The condition is encountered most frequently in diabetics. The gas-forming organism is usually *E. coli* or *C. welchii*. Often there is sufficient exudate in the gallbladder to produce a fluid level in erect view.

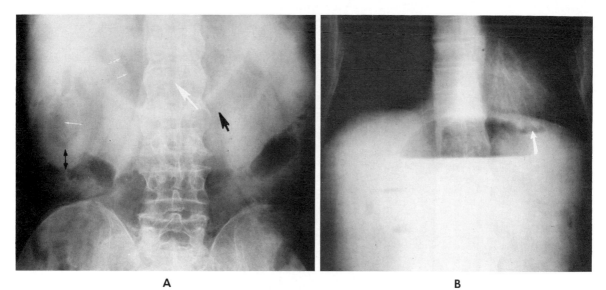

A   B

Figure 12–274   **Emphysematous Cholecystitis: Rupture Into Lesser Sac.**

A, Recumbent film shows a gas-filled gallbladder and common duct *(small white arrows).* The gallbladder lumen is somewhat irregular, and its wall is greatly thickened *(double-headed arrow).* A large midline collection of gas *(large white arrow)* is depressing the gastric air bubble *(black arrow).*

B, Erect film shows the large air-fluid collection in the lesser sac, extending across the midline. The gastric air bubble *(arrow)* is lateral to the lesser sac collection.

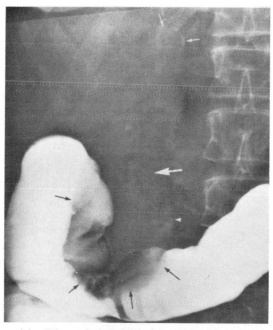

Figure 12–275   **Acute Cholecystitis: Distended Gallbladder: Stone in Cystic Duct.**   The greatly distended gallbladder has produced a pressure deformity on the barium-filled colon *(black arrows).* A sentinel loop of duodenum *(large white arrow)* signifies the acute inflammatory nature of the process. A portion of the gallbladder wall is seen through the air-filled loop *(arrowhead).* The obstructing opaque calculus in the cystic duct or neck of the gallbladder can be identified *(small white arrows)* by its partially calcified rim.

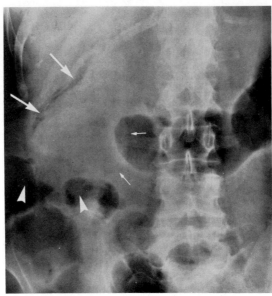

Figure 12–276 **Acute Suppurative Cholecystitis: Perforation into Gallbladder Bed.**   The distended gallbladder is seen as a soft tissue mass *(small arrows)* that depresses the gas-filled right colon *(arrowheads)*.
There are gas bubbles *(large arrows)* in the soft tissues along the lateral aspect of the gallbladder, indicative
of a gas-forming abscess adjacent to the gallbladder.

Gallstone Ileus (Biliary Fistula)

An inflamed gallbladder may adhere to an adjacent viscus and a gallstone
may ulcerate into the gastrointestinal lumen, producing a fistulous tract. The most
common site is the duodenal bulb, although the proximal duodenal loop, the hepatic flexure of the colon, and the antral portion of the stomach may occasionally be
the site. Intestinal gas passes through the fistula into the biliary tree, so that the
biliary ducts or the gallbladder, or both, are readily identified by the location and
shape of gas shadows.

A large gallstone that has entered the gastrointestinal tract may obstruct the
small bowel and produce characteristic roentgenologic findings. The calcified gallstone may sometimes be identified in the small bowel. When this is seen, the
diagnostic radiographic triad of gallstone ileus is complete: (1) air in the biliary
tree, (2) evidence of small bowel obstruction, and (3) opaque calculus in the small
intestine. Any two of these findings are sufficient for the diagnosis.[262, 263]

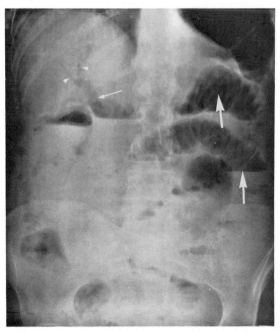

Figure 12–277 **Gallstone Ileus: Erect View of Abdomen.** The dilated small bowel loops *(large arrows)* with fluid level are characteristic of mechanical small bowel obstruction. The common duct *(small arrow)* and the hepatic ducts *(arrowheads)* are outlined by gas that has entered from the duodenum through the fistula. The obstructing calculus cannot be seen.

Although air in the biliary tree almost always indicates the presence of a biliary-intestinal fistula, air may also briefly be seen following biliary tract surgery. Biliary air and small bowel obstruction strongly suggest gallstone ileus, and identification of the gallstone within the intestinal tract makes the diagnosis virtually certain. Gallstone ileus is the cause of about 2 per cent of all cases of intestinal obstruction.

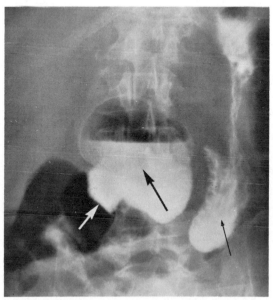

Figure 12–278 **Duodenal Obstruction Due to Ulcerated Gallstone.** The lower duodenal loop is obstructed *(white arrow)* by a large nonopaque gallstone that has ulcerated into the duodenal bulb. As the barium leaves the stomach *(small black arrow)*, it passes through the fistula into a greatly distended gallbladder, which contains an air-fluid level *(large black arrow)*. Surgical removal of the gallstone was followed by complete recovery.

Choledocholithiasis

Opacification of the common duct is required for visualization of nonopaque stones and for accurate localization of opaque calculi. If the oral cholecystogram opacifies the gallbladder, the common duct often becomes visible on the film made after ingestion of a fatty meal. When the gallbladder is not visualized or has been surgically removed, an intravenous cholangiogram will usually opacify the duct and demonstrate calculi unless there is jaundice. Tomography of the opacified common duct is of great value in delineating anatomic and pathologic changes. In the presence of obstructive jaundice, transhepatic cholangiography will opacify the biliary tree down to the point of obstruction. A calculus is distinguished from tumor by the upward convex contour of the calculous defect.

Endoscopic retrograde cholangiography will often clearly demonstrate a calculus in the opacified common duct.

On a barium study, an enlarged edematous duodenal papilla may be seen if a stone is impacted in the lower end of the common duct.

Direct injection of contrast material into the common and cystic duct during surgery (operative cholangiography) affords evidence of common duct stones. Postoperatively, the entire biliary tree may be opacified by means of a T-tube inserted into the common duct during surgery (T-tube cholangiography).

The common duct normally has a diameter of 12 mm. or less; the duct is considered to be dilated if the diameter is greater than 15 mm.[257, 264]

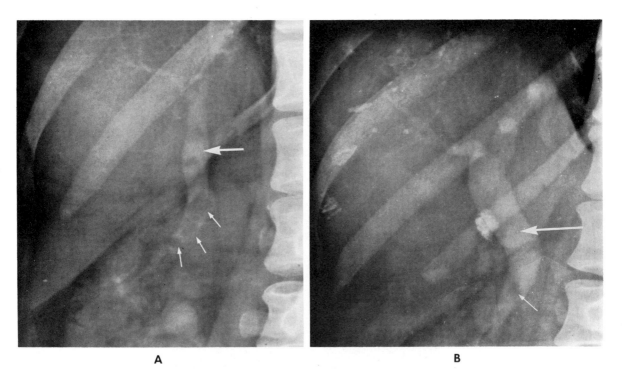

A   B

Figure 12–279 **Choledocholithiasis: Intravenous Cholangiogram.**

Each of these patients had had a cholecystectomy.

A, The common duct is well opacified *(large arrow)*. The multiple irregular persistent lucencies *(small arrows)* were calculi in the common duct.

B, The common duct is very clearly opacified *(large arrow)* and is dilated, measuring over 15 mm. in diameter. A single nonopaque stone *(small arrow)* is easily identified.

Frequently, visualization of the common duct following intravenous cholangiography is rather faint, and confusing gas shadows are present. In such cases, tomography of the duct often provides unobscured visualization.

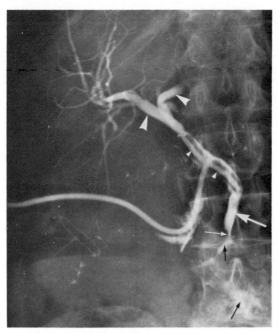

Figure 12–280 **T-Tube Cholangiogram: Normal Biliary Tree.** The T-tube *(small arrowheads)* in the common duct is surrounded by lucent bands that represent the thickness of the T-tube wall. The common duct is not dilated *(large white arrow),* and opaque material flows readily into the duodenum *(black arrows).* The normal narrowing of the distal end of the duct *(small white arrow)* is evident.

There is filling of the left and right hepatic ducts *(large arrowheads)* and of the intrahepatic branches from the right duct.

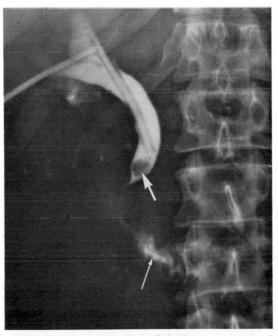

Figure 12–281 **T-Tube Cholangiogram: Common Duct Calculus.** An irregular round calculus produces a defect *(large arrow)* in the lower end of the dilated common duct. Some dye flows around the calculus into the duodenum *(small arrow).* This calculus would have been found during surgery by means of an operative cholangiogram.

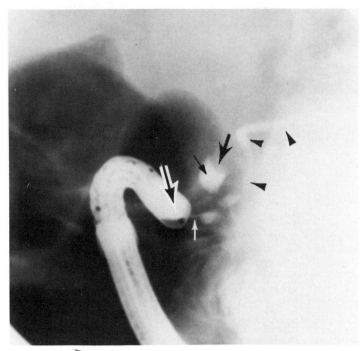

Figure 12–282 **Common Duct Stone Demonstrated by Transduodenal Cannulation of Ampulla.** The tip of the duodenoscope *(black-white arrow)* is in the descending duodenum, and its cannula *(small white arrow)* is in the ampulla of Vater. The lower end of the common duct *(small black arrow)* is filled, but the remainder is occluded by a calculus, which produces a characteristic curved defect *(large black arrow)*. The pancreatic duct *(arrowheads)* is opacified and appears normal.

Prior to this study, the patient, a 75 year old man with progressive painless jaundice, was thought to have a carcinoma of the pancreas.

Congenital Atresia of the Common Duct

This rare anomaly is always associated with unremitting jaundice from birth and hepatosplenomegaly. Theoretically, a transhepatic cholangiogram should opacify the biliary tree down to the point of atresia, but there are no reports of this procedure being performed in infants.

Direct injection of contrast material during laparotomy demonstrates the dilated and completely obstructed biliary tree. The lower end of the duct is the most common site of atresia.

Rachitic bone changes frequently develop (hepatic rickets), and in an infant with hepatosplenomegaly, persistent jaundice, and skeletal changes of rickets, obstructive malformation of the biliary tree should be suspected.[265, 266]

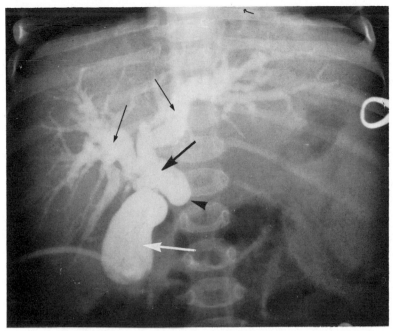

Figure 12–283 **Congenital Atresia of Common Duct.** The biliary tree, filled through a tube in the gall-bladder *(white arrow)*, is greatly dilated throughout. The common duct *(large black arrow)* is dilated and is completely obstructed because of atresia of the lower end *(arrowhead)*. There is uniform dilatation of the intrahepatic biliary tree *(small black arrows)*.

The liver extends across the midline, nearly to the left lateral wall. Left-sided liver enlargement is common in hepatomegaly.

Congenital Cystic Dilatation of the Common Duct (Choledochal Cyst)

This rare disorder of children and young adults is most frequent in the Oriental race. In Caucasians the disease has a distinct predilection for females (ratio of four to one).

Jaundice, abdominal pain, and a right upper quadrant mass constitute the diagnostic triad. In infants, before a mass is apparent the condition is often mistaken for biliary atresia.

A rounded right upper quadrant mass can usually be demonstrated radiographically; calcification does not occur. The cyst usually becomes quite large, and on barium meal studies there will be pressure on the duodenal loop with anterior and left-sided displacement of the distal stomach, the duodenal bulb, and the descending loop. The third portion of the duodenum is displaced downward.

Oral cholecystography is generally unsuccessful. Rarely, intravenous cholecystography with delayed films may opacify the cyst. Roentgen demonstration is generally made by operative cholangiogram or by percutaneous or operative injection of contrast material directly into the cystic mass. Transhepatic cholangiography and sometimes endoscopic retrograde cholangiography will opacify the cystic mass.[267–269]

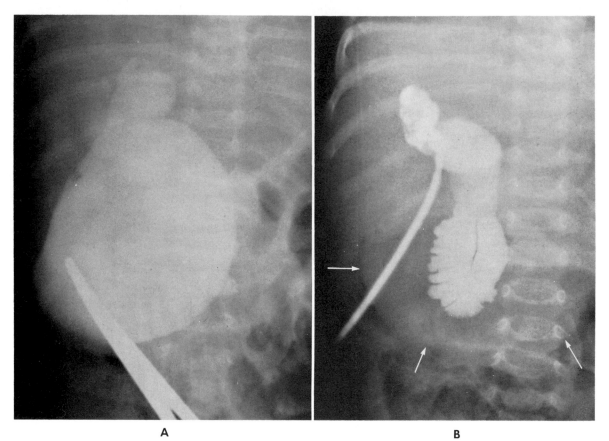

A   B

Figure 12–284   **Congenital Cystic Dilatation of Common Duct in a Female Infant with Jaundice.**

    A, Direct injection of contrast material during surgery demonstrates the huge cyst-like dilated common duct in the right upper quadrant.

    B, Following a bypass procedure the opaque material passes from the proximal common duct through the surgical anastomosis into the duodenum. The unresected cyst can be seen as a large soft tissue density *(arrows),* displacing the adjacent intestinal gas shadows.

Carcinoma of the Gallbladder

As a rule, roentgenology is not revealing until the lesion has become quite large and has extended to adjacent structures. Cholecystography, whether oral or intravenous, often fails to opacify the gallbladder even in relatively early cases and is therefore of little aid. Later, if the tumor obstructs the common duct, jaundice occurs, rendering such studies totally useless.

On barium studies, evidence of pressure and invasion of the distal duodenal bulb and postbulbar area is sometimes present, which rarely extends beyond the proximal descending duodenum. These findings occur in about a third of the cases and strongly suggest the diagnosis.

Often definitive diagnosis can be made by celiac and mesenteric arteriography. There may be enlargement and encasement of the cystic artery, with amputation of one or more branches. Neovasculature is usually seen, often with a blush in the gallbladder area. The gallbladder wall, often opacified during the venous phase, will be unevenly thick walled.

Endoscopic retrograde cholangiography may reveal deformities, compression, or even invasion of the common duct by an extrinsic mass.[270-272]

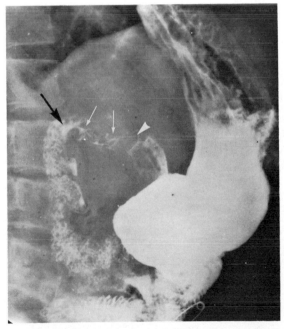

Figure 12-285 **Carcinoma of Gallbladder: Invasion of Duodenum.** The arrowhead marks the pylorus. There is evidence of a mass pressing upon the superior portion of the distal duodenal bulb and the immediate postbulbar area, with invasion and distortion of the mucosa *(white arrows)*; the segment is fixed and rigid. Characteristically, the involvement does not extend beyond the bend *(black arrow)* of the duodenal loop.

Although a distended gallbladder or common duct can produce pressure defects on the same segment of the distal duodenal bulb area, the absence of infiltration and invasive mucosal destruction helps distinguish a distended gallbladder from invasive gallbladder carcinoma.

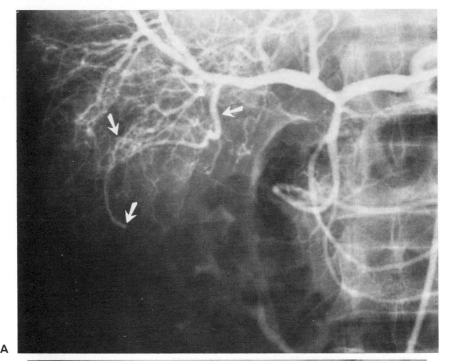

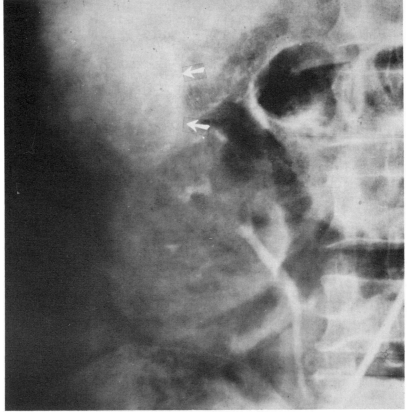

Figure 12–286 **Carcinoma of Gallbladder: Angiographic Findings.**

A, On celiac arteriogram, the cystic artery *(upper right arrow)* is dilated and draped around the gall-bladder. The posterior branch is abruptly occluded *(lower arrow)*. Neovasculature *(upper left arrow)* in the liver is due to extension of the carcinoma.

B, In the venous phase, an irregular and thickened gallbladder wall is opacified *(arrows)*. (Courtesy Dr. R. M. Abrams, New York, New York.)

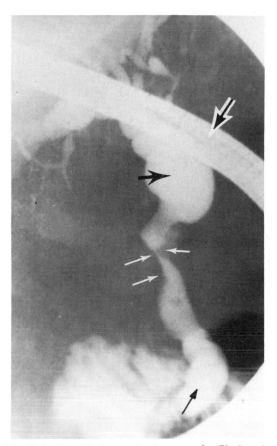

Figure 12–287 **Carcinoma of Gallbladder: Endoscopic Retrograde Cholangiopancreatography.** The common duct was opacified via duodenoscopic *(black-white arrow)* cannulation of the ampulla of Vater. The distal duct *(small black arrow)* appears fairly normal, but the midportion of the common duct is irregular, narrowed, and compressed by an extrinsic lateral mass *(white arrows)*. These changes were due to invasion of the common duct by a carcinoma of the gallbladder. The duct proximal to the involved segment is dilated *(large black arrow)*. The patient was jaundiced.

Benign Tumors of the Gallbladder

Polyps of the gallbladder are usually small and may be single or multiple. The most frequent lesions are cholesterol polyps and mucosal adenomas. Malignant change is extremely rare.

The polypoid lesions appear as fixed lucent defects in the opacified gallbladder. Profile views demonstrate their intimate relationship to the wall.

Adenomas are most often single and sessile and are most frequent in the middle third of the gallbladder. They are usually asymptomatic. Cholesterol polyps are frequently multiple, somewhat irregular in outline, and often associated with chronic cholecystitis. However, conclusive radiographic distinction between adenoma and cholesterol polyp is often impossible.

The fixed position of polyps and adenomas on recumbent, erect, and decubitus films will help distinguish them from calculi.[273, 274]

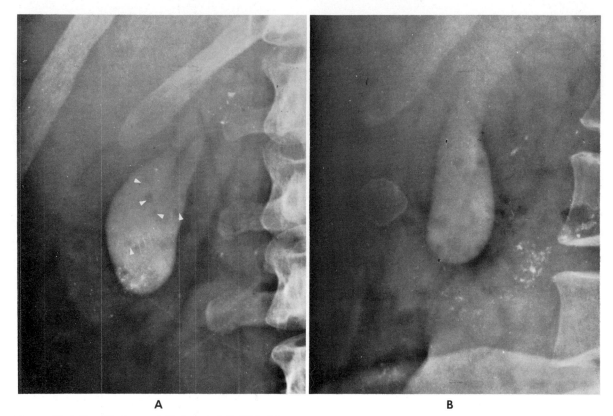

Figure 12–288   **Cholesterol Polyps of Gallbladder.**

A, Recumbent cholecystogram shows multiple small round defects *(arrowheads)* scattered throughout the gallbladder.

B, These defects maintain a fixed relationship to each other and to the gallbladder when the patient is in the erect position, whereas gallstones drop or become layered in the erect position.

Rarely, a single calculus impacted in the gallbladder wall retains its position and simulates an adenomatous polyp.

Adenomyosis (Intramural Diverticulosis) of the Gallbladder

This condition, generally considered to be degenerative rather than inflammatory, is due to hyperplasia of the gallbladder wall. There is focal proliferation of the epithelium and thickening of the muscular wall, which is associated with hernia-like outpouching of the mucosa. Localized outpouchings usually occur in the fundus but may develop along the entire wall; in the latter case they are also known as Rokitansky-Aschoff sinuses.

On cholecystography the diverticula are usually seen as small dye-filled densities outside the lumen, usually associated with a small intraluminal defect due to hyperplasia of the epithelium. The incidence of adenomyosis is higher in gallbladders with congenital and acquired narrowings and mucosal duplications. These lesions are far more common than is indicated by their infrequent appearance on the radiogram. They are best seen on a film of the contracted gallbladder, and sometimes can be visualized only on this film made following ingestion of a fatty meal. Dense opacification due to hyperconcentration and hypercontractility after the fatty meal is common and characteristic in adenomyosis.[275-277]

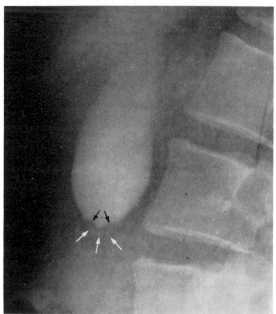

Figure 12–289 **Adenomyosis of Gallbladder Fundus.** There are a number of tiny dye-filled areas *(white arrows)* below the tip of the gallbladder, which are characteristic of intramural diverticula. The two defects *(black arrows)* bulging into the lumen of the dye-filled gallbladder are erroneously called the *adenomyomas,* an inaccurate term for localized hyperplastic epithelium. The condition is generally considered a form of chronic cholecystosis, and may or may not be clinically symptomatic.

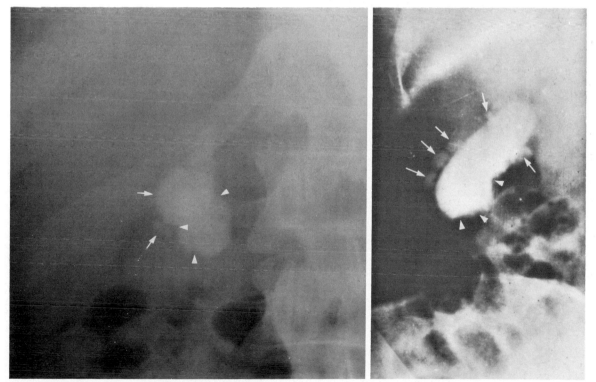

Figure 12–290 **Extensive Adenomyosis of Gallbladder: Two Patients.** Both gallbladders show numerous intramural diverticula of varying size *(arrows)*. Both have lost their normally smooth, regular contour. The walls are irregular and contain small indentations *(arrowheads)*, which are collections of hyperplastic epithelium, or "adenomyomas."

In adenomyosis, the gallbladder can usually be opacified by oral cholecystography. The roentgen appearance is characteristic and diagnostic.

Carcinoma of the Biliary Ducts and Ampulla of Vater

This lesion is quite rare and generally involves the main hepatic ducts or the common duct. Obstructive jaundice is almost always the presenting symptom; consequently, duct opacification, which is necessary for determining the nature and site of the lesion, cannot be obtained by oral or intravenous contrast studies. Transhepatic cholangiography usually discloses the lesion. Successful transduodenal cannulation may disclose a neoplastic involvement of the common or main hepatic duct.

Although carcinomas of the ampulla of Vater are duodenal tumors, they can be considered with bile duct lesions. Obstructive jaundice also is an early finding in ampullary carcinoma, even when the lesions are quite small.

If ampullary lesions are suspected, a careful examination of the barium-filled duodenal loop should be made by both routine barium examination and hypotonic duodenography. Small lesions usually produce no specific findings, or they may merely give rise to an innocent-appearing prominent ampullary lucency. Larger lesions produce a more pronounced defect in the region of the ampulla. They may also invade the bowel wall, causing irregular defects and infiltration typical of a malignant lesion in the small bowel.[278,279]

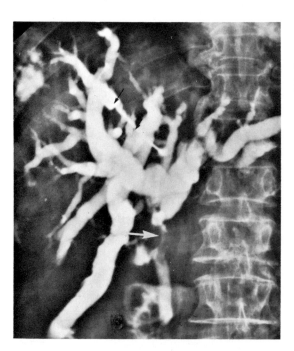

Figure 12–291 **Carcinoma of Common Duct in Patient with Jaundice: Transhepatic Cholangiogram.** The needle in the liver can be seen *(black arrows)* within a bile duct. The entire intrahepatic biliary tree is greatly dilated down to the area of constriction in the proximal common duct *(white arrow).* The involved segment is narrowed and irregular, and is the site of an infiltrating carcinoma.

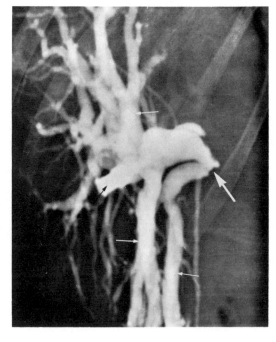

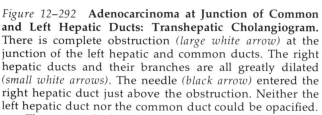
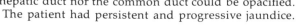

Figure 12–292 **Adenocarcinoma at Junction of Common and Left Hepatic Ducts: Transhepatic Cholangiogram.** There is complete obstruction *(large white arrow)* at the junction of the left hepatic and common ducts. The right hepatic ducts and their branches are all greatly dilated *(small white arrows).* The needle *(black arrow)* entered the right hepatic duct just above the obstruction. Neither the left hepatic duct nor the common duct could be opacified.

The patient had persistent and progressive jaundice.

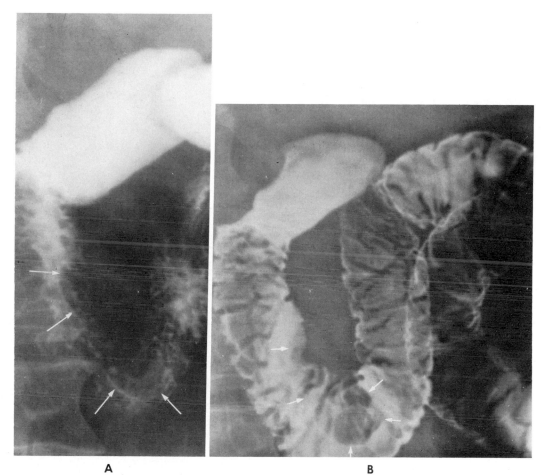

A   B

Figure 12–293 **Polypoid Carcinoma of Ampulla: Hypotonic Duodenogram.**

A, A routine gastrointestinal series shows a large pressure defect *(arrows)* on the inner aspect of the second and third portions of the duodenum, strongly suggestive of extrinsic pressure from a pancreatic carcinoma.

B, Reexamination of the duodenal loop by hypotonic duodenography (barium and air directly introduced via tube into a duodenum dilated by prior parenteral injection of propantheline bromide [Probanthine]) clearly indicates that the defect is an intraluminal lesion *(arrows)*. This was an unusually low carcinoma of the ampulla.

Hypotonic duodenography is of great value for clearly delineating intrinsic and extrinsic lesions of the duodenal loop.

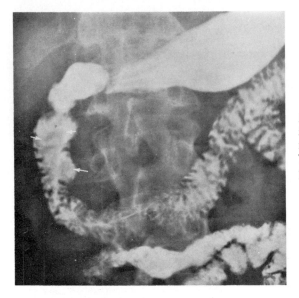

Figure 12-294 **Carcinoma of Ampulla of Vater.** The faint lucency *(arrows)* in the descending duodenum represents a lobulated tumor arising from the ampulla. The mass causes distention of the lumen. The mucosal pattern appears to be intact. Jaundice was present.

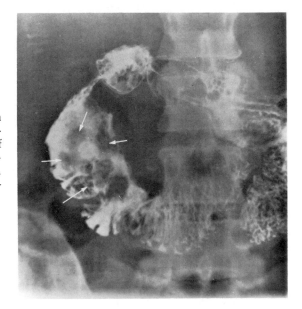

Figure 12-295 **Extensive Carcinoma Arising from Ampulla of Vater.** The descending duodenum is distended by a large polypoid mass *(arrows)*. The walls of the duodenal loop are rigid and irregular, showing extensive infiltration. The mucosal pattern is destroyed. Jaundice did not develop until the lesion was far advanced.

Primary Sclerosing Cholangitis

Primary sclerosing cholangitis, a rare condition of unknown origin, is characterized by progressive or intermittent obstructive jaundice due to an inflammatory fibrosis and stenosis of the bile ducts. In longstanding cases, pericholangitis and secondary biliary cirrhosis may develop. In about 25 per cent of cases there is an associated ulcerative colitis.

Operative or T-tube cholangiogram reveals irregular luminal narrowing, beading, and decreased arborization of the intrahepatic radicles. Rarely, the intrahepatic tree appears normal. In all cases, however, there is some stenotic involvement of the extrahepatic ducts (common hepatic and common bile ducts). Characteristically, there is little or no ductile dilatation, even proximal to a stenotic segment.[176, 280, 281]

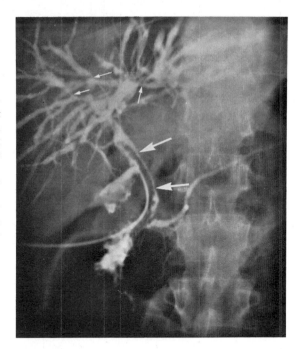

Figure 12–296 **Primary Sclerosing Cholangitis.** A T-tube cholangiogram in a chronically jaundiced patient reveals a somewhat narrowed and irregular common duct *(large arrows),* with more apparent narrowing proximally, in the common hepatic duct. Very little contrast material enters the duodenum.

The intrahepatic ducts are irregular and there are multiple areas of focal narrowing *(small arrows),* but proximal dilatation is minimal. The absence of greatly dilated intrahepatic ducts greatly decreases the chances for a successful transhepatic cholangiogram. (Courtesy Dr. W. Obata, San Francisco, California.)

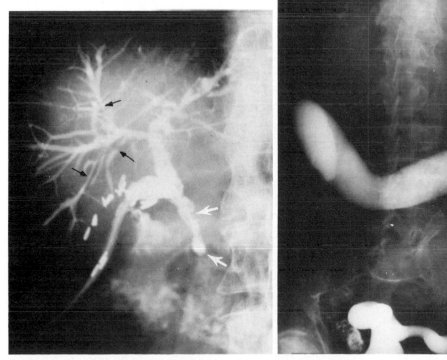

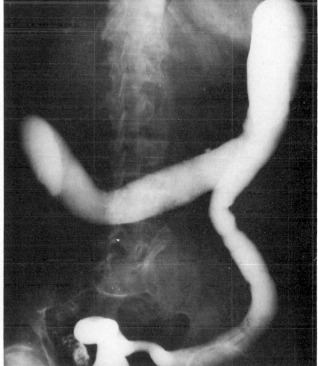

A   B

Figure 12–297 **Sclerosing Cholangitis in Chronic Ulcerative Colitis.**

A, T-tube cholangiogram discloses an irregular common duct with areas of narrowing *(white arrows).* Many areas of narrowing are also seen in the intrahepatic radicles *(black arrows).* Note absence of dilatation proximal to narrowing. This patient had recurrent episodes of jaundice.

B, Barium enema shows the characteristic shortening, narrowing, and anhaustral pattern of chronic ulcerative colitis.

Twenty-five per cent of cases of sclerosing cholangitis are associated with ulcerative colitis.

Primary Biliary Cirrhosis (Cholangiolitic Hepatitis)

The persistent jaundice of primary biliary cirrhosis (cholangiolitic hepatitis) results from a progressive chronic fibrosis of unknown origin, originating in and around the interlobular ducts and leading to regenerative nodules of liver tissue. The extrahepatic ducts are *not* involved, in contradistinction to sclerosing cholangitis.

Cholangiography (T-tube or operative) usually discloses diffuse or focal narrowing of the intrahepatic ducts, but without significant proximal dilatation. In some cases, the intrahepatic ducts appear normal. In all cases, however, the extrahepatic ducts remain uninvolved.

In both conditions, transhepatic cholangiography preoperatively is generally unsuccessful because of the absence of dilated intrahepatic ducts.[282]

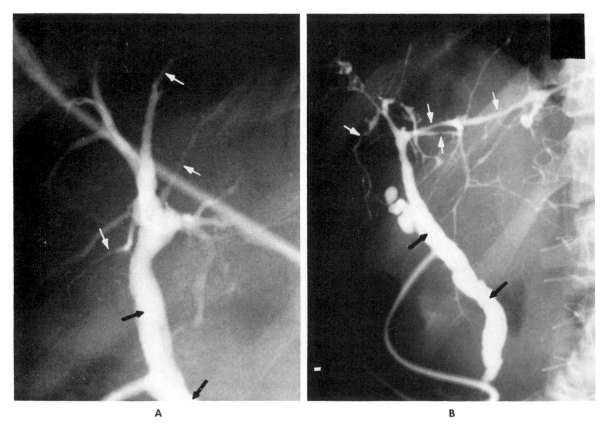

A   **B**

Figure 12–298   **Primary Biliary Cirrhosis (Cholangiolitic Hepatitis): Two Patients.**   The intrahepatic ducts show decreased branching and areas of diffuse and focal narrowing *(white arrows)*. The extrahepatic ducts *(black arrows)* are normal in both patients.

Patient *A* was a 25 year old woman; patient *B* was a 64 year old woman. (Courtesy Dr. Harley C. Carlson, Rochester, Minnesota.)

Cavernous Ectasis of the Intrahepatic Ducts (Caroli's Disease)

In this rare familial disease, there is segmental saccular dilatation of the intrahepatic bile ducts predisposing to cholangitis, gallstones, and liver abscess formation. Cirrhosis and portal hypertension do not occur.

Preoperative diagnosis is unlikely. A hepatic arteriogram will show displacement of vessels around large masses, indistinguishable from polycystic liver disease. Similar but smaller masses can occur in congenital hepatic fibrosis, and it is still uncertain whether Caroli's disease, polycystic liver, and congenital hepatic fibrosis are actually separate entities or stages of the same disease.

T-tube cholangiography will demonstrate the saccular dilatation of the bile ducts.[283]

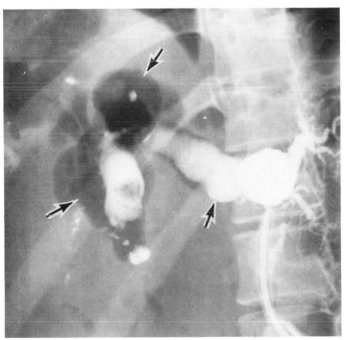

Figure 12-299 **Cavernous Ectasia of Intrahepatic Ducts (Caroli's Disease): Tube Cholangiogram.** The right intrahepatic ducts are dilated, and the communicating saccules are visualized *(arrows)*, some by contrast material and others by previously injected air. (Courtesy Dr. John A. Evans, Jersey City, New Jersey.)

DISEASES OF THE LIVER

Pyogenic Abscess of the Liver

Generally there is elevation and limited motion of the right diaphragm. If the abscess is in the upper portion of the liver, there may be some pleural reaction and areas of parenchymal density in the right lower lung field. These findings are similar to those of subphrenic abscess, but are considerably less marked. Occasionally, when gas-forming bacteria are responsible, an air-fluid level in the erect position will clarify the diagnosis. The liver is usually enlarged.

Hepatic angiography may help differentiate an intrahepatic abscess from a subdiaphragmatic abscess. Intrahepatic abscesses usually displace the hepatic arteries. During the hepatogram the abscess appears as an avascular area with a surrounding rim of hyperemic staining.[257, 284–286]

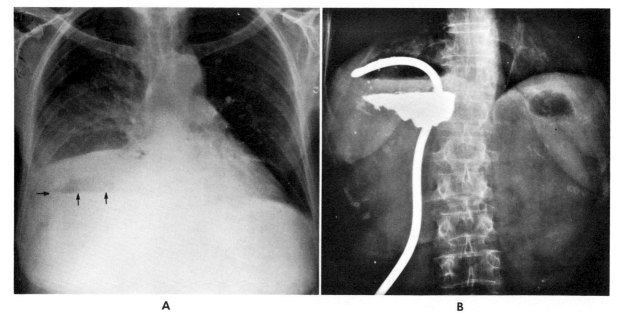

A   B

Figure 12–300 **Pyogenic Liver Abscess Due to E. coli.**

A, In erect view, the right diaphragm is elevated and there is blunting of the costophrenic angle. Respiratory movements of the right diaphragm were minimal. The large air-fluid level *(arrows)* in the upper portion of the liver density is diagnostic of an abscess. These findings are virtually indistinguishable from those of a subphrenic abscess.

B, Erect view made after instillation of iodized oil into the abscess through a drainage tube indicates full extent of the abscess. The oval air shadow and the bottom of the oil density mark the upper and lower boundaries of the abscess cavity.

Hepatic Venous Occlusion (Budd-Chiari Syndrome)

Occlusion of the major hepatic veins leads to congestive hepatomegaly, ascites, and abdominal pain—the Budd-Chiari syndrome. The cause of primary thrombotic occlusion of the hepatic veins is unknown. Secondary occlusion may result from polycythemia, intrahepatic diseases, or obstruction of the veins by tumor.

Roentgen diagnosis necessitates special and often multiple angiographic procedures.

Direct hepatic venography via catheter through the right atrium is the most informative procedure. Complete obstruction of a major vein is recognized by a spider-web venous vascular pattern radiating from the catheter tip, without opacification of the normal vein and its branches. With incomplete obstruction there may be opacification of a coarse network of smaller intrahepatic veins that tend to converge at the site of the junction of the hepatic vein and vena cava. If the catheter manages to traverse the narrowed segment, the proximal obstructed vein can be opacified, delineating the exact site of obstruction.

Indirect evidence of venous occlusion may be obtained by celiac or selective hepatic arteriography. The main and branch hepatic arteries are narrow, and there may be stretching of some smaller vessels. Some reverse flow into the vena cava may occur; this is a significant finding. The venous phase of celiac arteriography will often disclose evidence of portal hypertension, with reverse flow filling portions of the mesenteric, gastric, and esophageal veins.

Percutaneous injection of contrast material into the liver parenchyma (sinusoids) will opacify the hepatic veins and may demonstrate the site of venous obstruction (Ramsay and Britton). Reverse flow into hepatic lymphatics and portal vein, or through collaterals to an unobstructed hepatic vein, may occur.

In about 20 per cent of cases there is associated thrombotic occlusion or narrowing of the upper inferior vena cava; this is readily demonstrated by inferior cavography.[287-292]

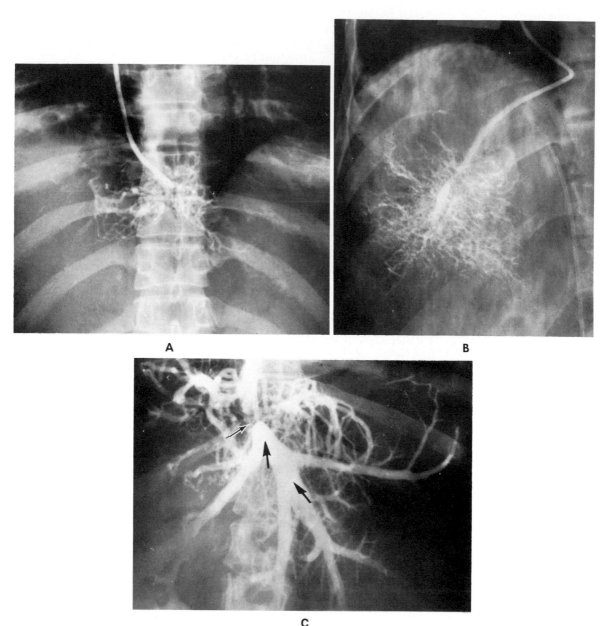

Figure 12–301 **Hepatic Vein Obstruction: Three Patients.**

In each of these three individuals with clinical manifestations of Budd-Chiari syndrome, a hepatic venogram was performed by passing a catheter through the right atrium into a main hepatic vein.

A, Occlusion of the left hepatic vein is disclosed by a spider-web vascular pattern replacing opacification of the left hepatic vein.

B, A similar vascular pattern replaces opacification of the right hepatic vein in another patient.

C, The catheter has passed through the obstructive narrowing of the left hepatic vein, and the proximal portion of the vein is greatly dilated *(black arrows)* proximal to the obstructive point *(black-white arrow).* Extensive collateral veins are bypassing the obstruction. (Courtesy Dr. L. Kreel, London, England.)

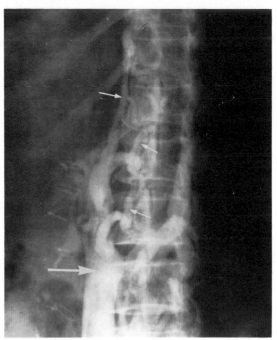

Figure 12–302 **Malignant Occlusion of Vena Cava: Cavagram.** The patient had developed ascites, jaundice, an enlarged liver, and abdominal pain.

The inferior vena cava *(large arrow)* was opacified to the level of L3; the contrast medium then entered the collaterals of the azygos venous system *(small arrows)*. No filling of the vena cava above L2–L3 was observed. The vena cava and hepatic vein were occluded by a retroperitoneal sarcoma.

In hepatic vein occlusion without caval occlusion, inferior cavography is not diagnostically helpful, since normally the hepatic vein does not fill with contrast material during this study. (Courtesy Dr. M. Levander, Stockholm, Sweden.)

Portal Venous Occlusion

Occlusions of the portal vein can be intrahepatic or extrahepatic, and can occur in a variety of conditions, both inflammatory and neoplastic. Thrombosis secondary to pre-existing portal hypertension is the most common cause.

Percutaneous splenoportography or, preferably, selective splenic or superior mesenteric arteriography (venous phase will opacify the portal system) will demonstrate nonfilling or an obstructive site of the portal vein. Abnormal collateral venous channels that are attempting to decompress the portal venous system by way of the systemic veins may be opacified. Occasionally a portal thrombus may calcify, producing a characteristic density on plain films of the abdomen.[289, 293, 294]

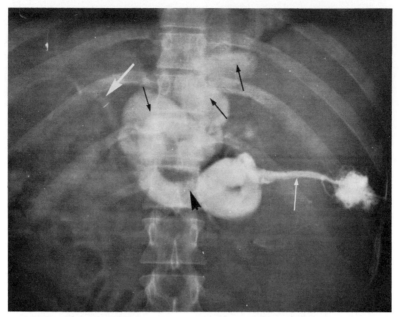

Figure 12–303 **Partial Occlusion of Portal Vein: Splenoportogram.** The splenic vein *(small white arrow)* enters the greatly dilated portal vein *(arrowhead)*. The contrast medium then passes into the dilated, tortuous, varicose collaterals *(small black arrows)*. An intrahepatic branch of the portal vein is filled *(large white arrow)*, but the remaining portal branches are not opacified.

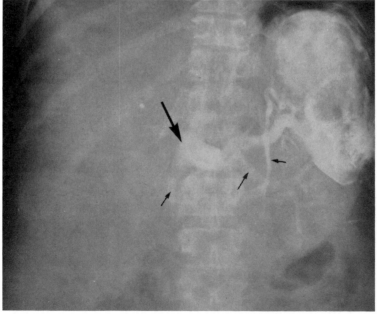

Figure 12–304 **Complete Occlusion of Portal Vein by Malignant Melanoma: Splenoportogram.** There is abrupt occlusion of the portal vein *(large arrow)*, which has been invaded by tumor. There is extensive collateral venous filling *(small arrows)* from both the splenic and portal veins.

Normally, no collaterals are filled during splenoportography.

Cirrhosis of the Liver

The findings in Laennec's cirrhosis are mainly the result of the portal hypertension; there are no findings in early cases.

Esophageal varices and, less often, gastric varices may be seen once the cirrhosis is established; indeed, bleeding from the gastrointestinal tract may be the first clinical manifestation. Varices usually occur in the lower third of the esophagus and appear as rounded defects in the barium column. Changes in size readily occur, and the varices usually disappear during peristalsis or deep inspiration, so that careful examination, including the Valsalva maneuver, mucosal relief studies, and multiple films, should be made. Nevertheless, roentgenologic demonstration of varices can be made in only about half the cases; negative findings therefore do not rule out varices. The gastric varices are frequently indistinguishable from prominent mucosal folds in the fundus and are difficult to diagnose in the absence of esophageal varices. In severe cases of portal hypertension, varices may extend into the upper esophagus.

Splenomegaly may be recognized on abdominal films in a high percentage of cases. Extensive ascites can produce a diffuse haze overlying the abdomen. Decubitus or erect films may show increased density in the dependent portion of the abdomen, confirming the presence of fluid. In massive ascites the diaphragms are elevated.

When the serum albumin level is 2 grams or less, there is usually edema of the small intestine characterized by slightly dilated loops, an increased space between the loops due to wall thickening, and uniform thickening of the mucosal folds. In severe cases a stacked-coin appearance is found. Associated ascites may or may not be present in these circumstances. An identical small bowel appearance due to intestinal edema can occur in other conditions with severe hypoproteinemia, such as nephrosis or intestinal lymphangiectasia.

In advanced cirrhosis the liver is shrunken and the right kidney and duodenal bulb may occupy an abnormally high position. On abdominal films these findings in conjunction with an enlarged spleen sometimes suggest the diagnosis of cirrhosis.

Occasionally, portal hypertension causes increased flow through the azygos system, in which case there is evidence of a dilated azygos vein on the frontal chest film.

Vascular changes within the liver and portal system reflect the extent and severity of the cirrhosis and can be evaluated by selective hepatic, splenic, or celiac arteriography.

Hepatic arteriography performed in the stage of fatty infiltration (precirrhotic) or of early hypertrophic cirrhosis discloses stretching and narrowing of all the vessels. In the fibrotic stage there is a nonspecific corkscrew arterial pattern reflecting the loss of liver volume. The extrahepatic arteries are often enlarged. The hepatic veins appear tortuous, narrow, and irregular.

During the venous phase of celiac or splenic angiography, there will be opacification of dilated splenic and portal veins, and retrograde filling of some portions of the mesenteric, gastric, and esophageal veins, with demonstration of esophageal or gastric varices. In the absence of portal hypertension, only the splenic and portal veins are opacified.

Splenoportography will also demonstrate these venous changes of portal hypertension, but this procedure has been largely replaced by the safer celiac arteriography.[295-300]

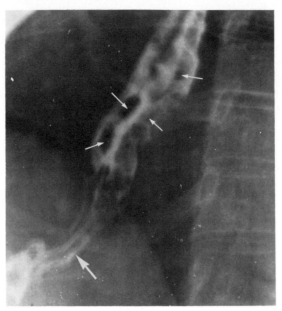

Figure 12–305 **Laennec's Cirrhosis: Esophageal Varices.** A mucosal study of the lower esophagus shows multiple oval tortuous filling defects *(small arrows)*, which are large varices. Such defects are absent in the contracted segment below *(large arrow)*; the varices are obliterated by peristaltic contraction.

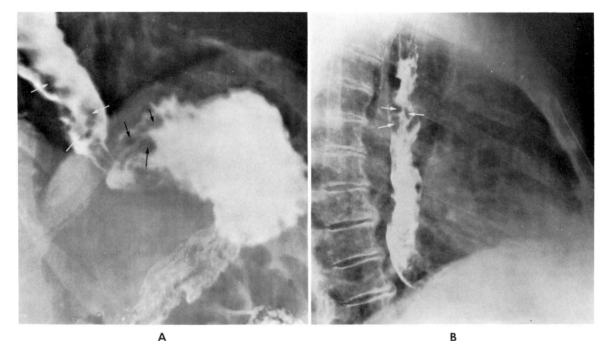

A   B

Figure 12–306 **Laennec's Cirrhosis: Extensive Esophageal and Gastric Varices.**

A, The circinate defects caused by varices are clearly evident *(white arrows)*; the lucencies in the gastric fundus *(black arrows)* were also due to varices, but resemble enlarged fundal mucosal folds.

B, Varices are present in the middle and upper esophagus *(arrows)*. High esophageal varices may occur in advanced cirrhosis with longstanding severe portal hypertension.

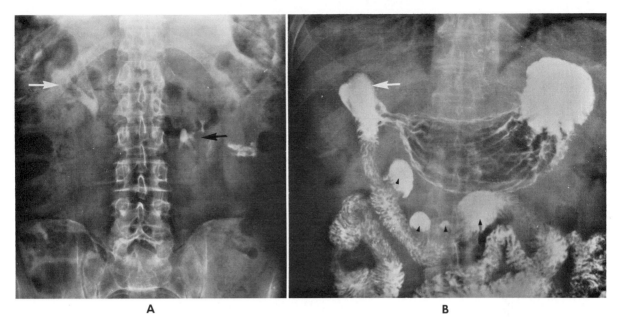

A   **B**

Figure 12–307   **Advanced Laennec's Cirrhosis: Shrunken Fibrotic Liver.**

A, The urogram demonstrates marked elevation of the right kidney *(white arrow),* compared to the normal position of the left kidney *(black arrow).* Normally, the right kidney is lower than the left.

B, The entire distal stomach and duodenal bulb *(white arrow)* are elevated and shifted to the right. Duodenal diverticula *(arrowheads)* were an incidental finding.

Elevation of the right kidney and the duodenal bulb is a consequence of the decreased volume of the liver.

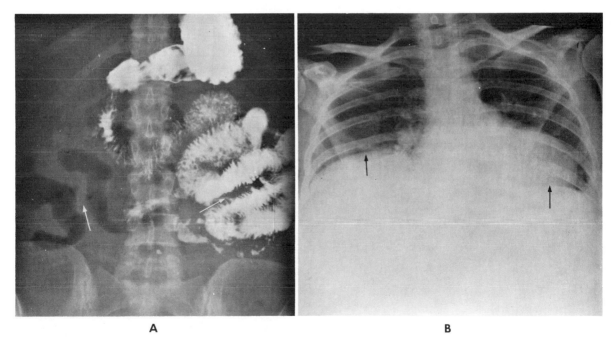

A   **B**

Figure 12–308   **Portal Cirrhosis: Ascites.**

A, The abdomen is hazy; the space between the air-filled and barium-filled small bowel loops *(arrows)* is increased because ascitic fluid is present between the loops.

B, The diaphragms are elevated *(arrows)* by the intra-abdominal fluid, so that the chest is shortened and the heart is horizontal.

Elevation of the diaphragms may result from intra-abdominal fluid, abdominal masses, or marked bowel distention. An infrapulmonic effusion may simulate an elevated diaphragm.

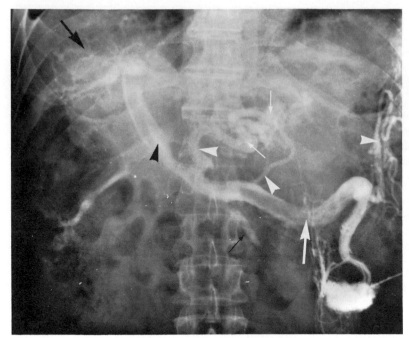

Figure 12–309 **Cirrhosis and Portal Hypertension: Splenoportogram.** In a normal splenoportogram, usually only the splenic and portal veins are opacified. In portal hypertension, the splenic *(large white arrow),* portal *(black arrowhead),* and intrahepatic veins *(large black arrow)* are dilated; they showed prolonged opacification. Numerous portal branches from the stomach *(white arrowheads)* and the distal inferior mesenteric vein *(small black arrow)* are opacified by reflux filling. Tortuous varicosities are identified in the dilated gastric veins *(small white arrows).* The distribution of the intrahepatic veins *(large black arrow)* indicates a small shrunken liver.

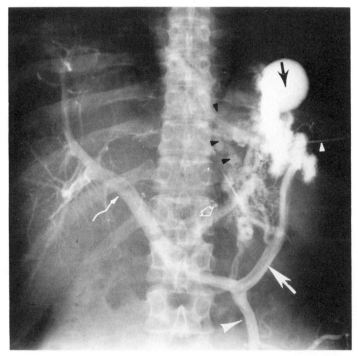

Figure 12–310 **Cirrhosis and Portal Hypertension: Splenoportogram.** Direct injection of water-soluble contrast material into the spleen *(black arrow)* via a needle catheter *(small white arrowhead)* has opacified the splenic *(large white arrow)* and portal *(undulating arrow)* veins. In a normotensive portal system, these are the only two veins opacified. However, increased portal pressure has led to retrograde filling of the superior mesenteric vein *(large white arrowhead),* a large gastric vein *(open arrow),* and other smaller veins. Varicosities *(black arrowheads)* are opacified in the stomach and lower esophagus.

The venous phase of a selective celiac or splenic arteriogram will duplicate the venous filling seen on splenoportogram.

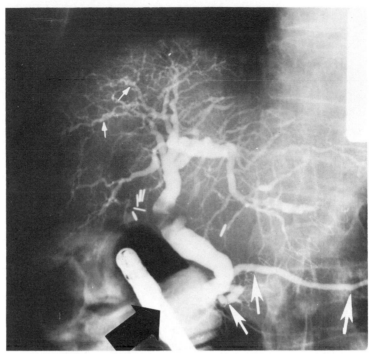

Figure 12-311 **Cirrhosis of Liver: Endoscopic Retrograde Cholangiopancreatography.** The duodeno-scope *(large black arrow)* is in the duodenum, and its catheter has been directed into the ampulla of Vater, permitting opacification of the entire biliary tree and pancreatic duct *(large white arrows)*.

The intrahepatic biliary branches show marked corkscrewing *(small arrows)*, suggestive of parenchymal liver atrophy and fibrosis.

The pancreatic duct has a smooth regular outline, and the pancreas was normal.

Dubin-Johnson Syndrome

In this condition of persistent nonhemolytic hyperbilirubinemia, oral cholecys-tography results in nonvisualization of the gallbladder in about 90 per cent of cases. Opacification of the gallbladder after rapid intravenous injection of cholangiographic contrast material often does not occur within the normal two-hour period but may be delayed up to six hours, probably because of the decreased excretory rate of the contrast material. This delayed intravenous opacification may be a pathognomonic feature of the syndrome.[301]

Focal Nodular Hyperplasia of the Liver

In young women who are taking oral contraceptives, solitary or multiple nod-ules may develop in the liver. These "tumors" histologically resemble focal nodular hyperplasia and are *not* adenomas.

Occasionally a focal nodule may become quite large. If in the left lobe of the liver, there may be radiographic evidence of an extrinsic mass effect on the stomach. However, smaller lesions can be detected by radioisotope scan or, preferably, hepa-tic arteriography. The latter study can define the site and size of these vascular nodules.

Although these nodules are often totally asymptomatic, acute massive in-traperitoneal hemorrhage from a ruptured nodule can occur.[302]

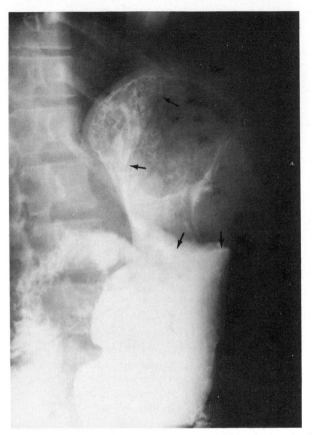

Figure 12–312 **Focal Nodular Hyperplasia of Liver.**   A 28 year old woman who had been using contraceptive pills for several years developed acute epigastric pain. The pain gradually disappeared.

Gastrointestinal radiographs reveal a large pressure defect on the anterior portion of the upper half of the stomach. Note the sharp borders *(arrows)* of the defect, and the absence of mucosal destruction, findings characteristic of noninvasive pressure from an extrinsic mass.

The mass proved to be a huge nodule of hyperplastic tissue, apparently the result of prolonged use of contraceptive pills.

Primary Hepatic Carcinoma (Hepatoma)

Nonspecific hepatomegaly is the most common finding on routine films. The area of liver density is increased, the right diaphragm is elevated, and usually there is evidence of pressure or displacement of the hepatic flexure of the colon and the lesser curvature of the stomach. Reactive densities may appear in the right lower lung field.

Irregular clusters of calcification within the tumor are infrequent in adults but relatively common in children (30 per cent of cases). In nearly half the affected children there is a severe generalized osteoporosis apparently due to a systemic protein deficit of hepatic origin.

Since cirrhosis of the liver is frequently associated with hepatoma, splenomegaly and esophageal varices are often present. Demonstration of esophageal varices in a patient with hepatomegaly is more suggestive of primary liver carcinoma than of ordinary cirrhosis, since in the latter the cirrhotic liver is usually small and fibrotic when varices develop.

Selective celiac or hepatic arteriography provides the most accurate diagnosis. Characteristically there are stretched, displaced, and enlarged intrahepatic arteries, abnormal neovasculature, small arteriovenous shunts, tumor stains, and blushes. Multinodular highly vascular foci are found in about half of the hepatomas. Defects will be apparent in the hepatogram phase.

A dense hepatogram showing tumor defect can also be obtained by injection of contrast material into the umbilical vein, but this study gives no information about the vascularity of any of the lesions.

Radioisotope scan is a safe and simple method for demonstrating a sizable mass within the liver.[278, 303–307]

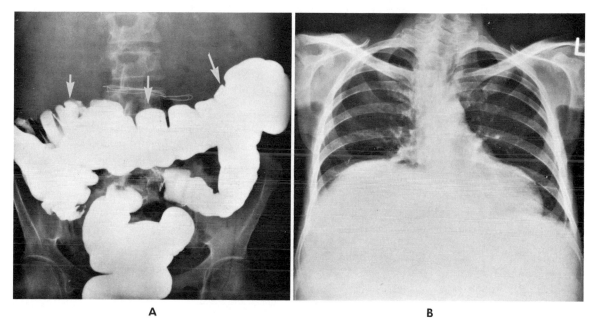

A   B

Figure 12–313 **Primary Carcinoma of Liver: Massive Hepatomegaly.**

A, Massive enlargement of the right and left lobes of the liver produces a homogeneous density of the upper abdomen, and the entire transverse colon is displaced downward *(arrows).*

B, The right diaphragm is considerably elevated by the massive liver.

These findings are indicative of pronounced nonspecific hepatomegaly, which may be due to many causes other than a primary hepatoma.

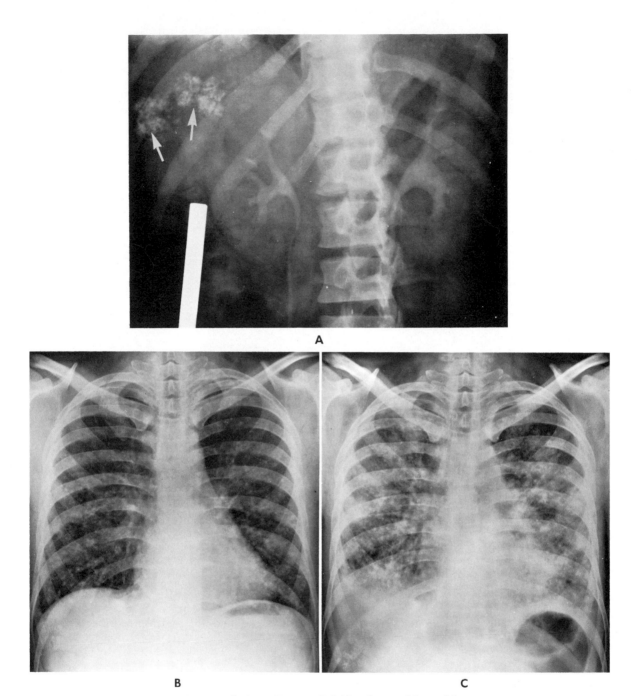

Figure 12–314 **Primary Carcinoma of Liver: Tumor Calcification and Lung Metastases.**

The patient was a 31 year old woman.

A, A portion of urogram shows that the liver is not enlarged, but there are clusters of amorphous calcification *(arrows)* in the liver area; these were within a highly anaplastic primary hepatoma.

Calcification occurs very rarely in primary liver carcinoma, but is somewhat more frequent in younger adults and children.

B, There are extensive small nodular infiltrates due to diffuse pulmonary metastases.

C, One month later, shortly before death, there is a great increase in the number of metastatic nodules and infiltrates.

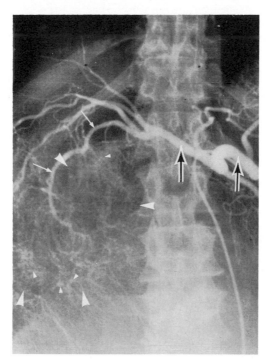

Figure 12–315 **Primary Solitary Carcinoma of Liver: Celiac Arteriogram.** The hepatic artery (*large arrows*) and the intrahepatic main branches are displaced upward by the tumor. The entire tumor area (*large arrowheads*) is extremely vascular, and the tumor vessels are irregular and bizarre. Irregular areas of pooling of dye or staining are apparent (*small arrowheads*). The hepatic artery (*large arrows*) and the tumor-feeding artery (*small arrows*) are both somewhat dilated. The corkscrew, tortuous appearance of some of the intrahepatic arteries is due to the associated cirrhosis. There was early opacification of the veins (not shown), indicative of intratumoral arteriovenous shunts. (Courtesy Dr. James J. Pollard, Boston, Massachusetts.)

Metastatic Disease of the Liver

Routine radiographic studies are of limited value for detecting metastatic lesions of the liver. There may be nonspecific hepatomegaly. Very rarely a metastatic lesion will calcify, and these lesions are almost invariably from a colonic carcinoma. Calcified breast carcinomatous metastases have also been reported. The calcifications are usually punctate, granular, and in clumps.

Liver scan is currently the favorite procedure for disclosing hepatic metastases.

Definitive roentgen diagnosis can often be made by celiac or hepatic arteriography. Multiple tumor vessels and tumor stains and scattered areas of stretching and distortion of the intrahepatic vessels are characteristic and diagnostic. If the metastasis is avascular, it appears as a lucent filling defect during the hepatographic phase and may not be distinguishable from a cyst or nonmalignant tumor.

Occasionally, widespread hepatic metastases can lead to esophageal varices.[215, 278, 289, 308]

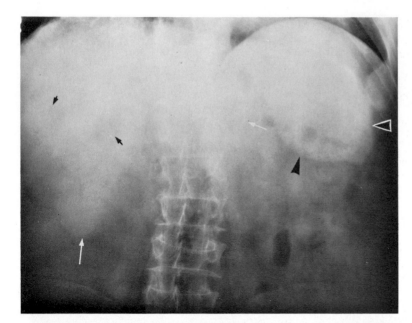

Figure 12–316 **Metastatic Malignant Neoplasm of Liver: Hepatosplenogram.** The liver *(white arrows)* and spleen *(black arrowheads)* are opacified following thorium dioxide (Thorotrast) hepatosplenography. There are a number of vague irregular defects in the liver opacity *(black arrows)*. These represent metastatic malignant masses.

This study was performed many years ago, before the dangerous late effects of Thurotrast were appreciated.

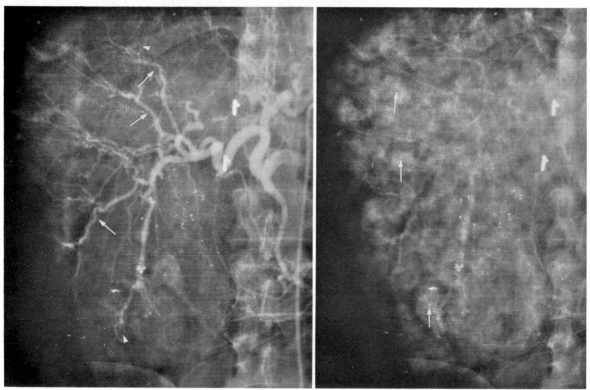

A   B

Figure 12–317 **Widespread Metastatic Disease of Liver: Angiogram.**

A, Film made during opacification of the intrahepatic arterial tree (celiac arteriography) demonstrates stretching and tortuosity *(arrows)* of many hepatic vessels, and numerous areas of abnormal smaller vessels *(arrowheads),* which suggest multiple tumors.

B, During the late capillary phase, numerous dense tumor stains *(arrows)* of varying size are seen; this finding is characteristic of widespread metastatic disease. At surgery a primary malignant carcinoid of the ileum was found.

Abnormal vessels and staining during hepatic angiography are specific for malignant neoplasms of the liver. There may also be displacement and stretching of the vessels around a liver mass. (Courtesy Dr. R. A. Nebesar, Boston, Masschusetts.)

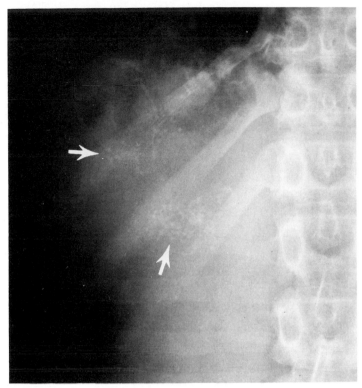

Figure 12–318 **Calcified Carcinomatous Metastasis to Liver.** Scattered punctate granular calcifications are seen in the mid- and upper liver area *(arrows)*. These were within metastases from a colon carcinoma (adenocarcinoma).

Although calcified metastases are quite rare, their punctate appearance is rather characteristic, and the vast majority are from a mucinous carcinoma of the colon.

REFERENCES

1. Donner, M. W., and Siegel, C. I.: The evaluation of pharyngeal neuromuscular disorders by cinefluorography. Am. J. Roentgenol. Radium Ther. Nucl. Med., *92*:299, 1965.
2. Zboralske, F. F., and Dodds, W. J.: Roentgenographic diagnosis of primary disorders of esophageal motility. Radiol. Clin. North Am., 7:147, 1969.
3. Hampton, J.: Cricopharyngeal dysphagia. Am. J. Roentgenol. Radium Ther. Nucl. Med., *84*:1028, 1960.
4. Clements, F. L., Cox, G. W., et al.: Cervical esophageal webs – a roentgen-anatomic correlation. Am. J. Roentgenol. Radium Ther. Nucl. Med., *121*:221, 1974.
5. Brunton, F. S., and Eban, R. E.: Sideropenic webs in men. Br. J. Radiol., *33*:723, 1960.
6. Bothwell, T. H., and Thomas, R. G.: Sideropenic dysphagia. S. Afr. Med. J. *32*:614, 1958.
7. Seaman, W. B.: The significance of webs in the hypopharynx and upper esophagus. Radiology, *89*:32, 1967.
8. Waye, J. D., Pitman, E. R., and Kruger, K. F.: Esophageal web and colitis. Am. J. Gastroenterol., *57*:248, 1972.
9. Johnstone, A. S.: Diffuse spasm and diffuse muscle hypertrophy. Br. J. Radiol., *33*:723, 1960.
10. Westgaard, T., and Keats, T. E.: Diffuse spasm and muscular hypertrophy of the lower esophagus. Radiology, *90*:1001, 1968.
11. Gonzalez, G.: Diffuse esophageal spasm. Am. J. Roentgenol. Radium Ther. Nucl. Med., *117*:251, 1973.
12. Orlando, R. C., and Bozymski, E. M.: Clinical and manometric effects of nitroglycerine in diffuse esophageal spasm. N. Engl. J. Med., *289*:23, 1973.
13. Bockus, H. L.: *Gastroenterology,* 3rd ed. Philadelphia, W. B. Saunders Company, 1975.
14. Ennis, J. B., and Lewicki, A. M.: Mecholyl esophagography. Am. J. Roentgenol. Radium Ther. Nucl. Med., *119*:241, 1973.

15. Hagarty, G.: Classification of esophageal hiatus hernia with special reference to sliding hernia. Am. J. Roentgenol. Radium Ther. Nucl. Med., *84*:1056, 1960.
16. Wolf, B. S., Marshak, R. H., and Som, M. L.: Hiatus hernia; role in peptic esophagitis and peptic ulceration of the esophagus. Am. J. Roentgenol. Radium Ther. Nucl. Med., *79*:741, 1958.
17. Stilson, W. L., Sanders, I., et al.: Hiatal hernia and gastroesophageal reflux. Radiology, *93*:1323, 1969.
18. MacMahon, E., Schatzki, R., and Garey, J.: Pathology of a lower esophageal ring: report of a case with autopsy, observed for nine years. N. Engl. J. Med., *259*:1, 1958.
19. Schatzki, R.: The lower esophageal ring. Am. J. Roentgenol. Radium Ther. Nucl. Med., *90*:805, 1963.
20. Heitmann, P., et al.: Simultaneous cineradiographic-manometric study of the distal esophagus: small hiatal hernias and rings. Gastroenterology, *50*:737, 1966.
21. Goyal, R. J., Glancy, J. J., and Spiro, H. M.: Lower esophageal ring. N. Engl. J. Med., *282*:1355, 1970.
22. Jordon, P. H., Jr., and Longhi, E. H.: Diagnosis and treatment of an esophageal stenosis in a patient with Barrett's epithelium. Ann. Surg., *169*:355, 1969.
23. Crummy, A. F.: The water test in evaluation of gastric-esophageal reflux. Radiology, *87*:501, 1966.
24. Palmer, E. B.: The hiatus hernia–esophagitis-esophageal stricture complex. Am. J. Med., *44*:566, 1968.
25. Leigh, T. F.: Acute gastric dilatation. J.A.M.A., *173*:1376, 1960.
26. Doppman, J. L., and Johnson, R. H.: The mechanism of shock in acute gastric dilatation. Br. J. Radiol., *42*:613, 1969.
27. Dick, A.: Volvulus of the stomach with diaphragmatic hernia. Clin. Radiol., *14*:149, 1963.
28. Rennell, C. R.: Foramen of Morgagni hernia with volvulus of the stomach. Am. J. Roentgenol. Radium Ther. Nucl. Med., *117*:248, 1973.
29. Wastell, C., and Ellis, H.: Volvulus of the stomach: A review. Br. J. Surg., *58*:557, 1971.
30. Desmond, A. M., and Swynnerton, B. F.: Adult hypertrophy of the pylorus. Br. Med. J., *1*:968, 1957.
31. Bateson, E. M., et al.: Radiological and pathological observations in a series of seventeen cases of hypertrophic pyloric stenosis in adults. Br. J. Radiol., *42*:1, 1969.
32. Haran, P. J., Darling, D. B., and Sciammas, F.: The value of the double-track sign as a differentiating factor between pylorospasm and hypertrophic pyloric stenosis in infants. Radiology, *86*:723, 1966.
33. Riggs, W., and Long, L.: The value of the plain film roentgenogram in pyloric stenosis. Am. J. Roentgenol. Radium Ther. Nucl. Med., *112*:77, 1971.
34. Cremin, B. J., and Klein, A.: Infantile pyloric stenosis: a 10 year survey. S. Afr. Med. J., *42*:1056, 1968.
35. Sparberg, M.: Roentgenographic documentation of the Mallory-Weiss syndrome. J.A.M.A. *203*:151, 1968.
36. Baum, S., et al.: Mallory-Weiss syndrome. Surgery, *58*:797, 1965.
37. Carr, J. C.: The Mallory-Weiss syndrome. Clin. Radiol., *24*:107, 1973.
38. Watts, H. D., and Admirand, W. H.: Mallory-Weiss syndrome: A reappraisal. J.A.M.A., *230*:1674, 1974.
39. Faigenberg, D., and Bosniak, M.: Duodenal anomalies in the adult. Am. J. Roentgenol. Radium Ther. Nucl. Med., *88*:642, 1962.
40. Lloyd-Jones, W., Mountain, J. C., and Warren, K.: Annular pancreas in the adult. Ann. Surg. *176*:163, 1972.
41. Moresi, H. J., and Ochsner, S. F.: Megabulbus of the duodenum in the adult. Report of a case associated with annular pancreas and ulceration. Am. J. Dig. Dis., *9*:170, 1964.
42. Shopner, C. E.: Urinary tract pathology associated with constipation. Radiology, *90*:865, 1968.
43. Marshak, R. H., and Gerson, A.: Cathartic colon. Am. J. Dig. Dis., *5*:724, 1960.
44. Lemaitre, G., et al.: Radiologic aspects of chronic colitis due to laxative abuse. J. Belg. Radiol., *53*:339, 1970.
45. Lunsden, H.: The irritable colon syndrome. Clin. Radiol., *14*:54, 1963.
46. Gramiak, R., Ross, P., and Olmstead, W. W.: Normal motor activity of human colon. Am. J. Roentgenol. Radium Ther. Nucl. Med., *113*:301, 1971.
47. Frimann-Dahl, J., Jr.: *Roentgen Examination in Acute Abdominal Diseases,* 2nd ed. Springfield, Charles C Thomas, Publisher, 1960.
48. Shauffer, I. A., and Ferris, E. J.: The mass sign in primary volvulus of the small intestine in adults. Am. J. Roentgenol. Radium Ther. Nucl. Med., *94*:374, 1965.
49. Druckmann, A., et al.: Pneumatosis of the intestines. Am. J. Roentgenol. Radium Ther. Nucl. Med., *86*:911, 1961.
50. Meihoff, W. E., Hirschfield, J. S., and Kern, F.: Small intestinal scleroderma with malabsorption and pneumatosis cystoides intestinalis. J.A.M.A., *204*:854, 1968.
51. Seaman, M. W., Fleming, R. S., and Beker, D. H.: Pneumointestinalis of the small bowel. Semin. Roentgenol., *1*:234, 1966.
52. Mueller, C. F., Morehead, R., et al.: Pneumatosis intestinalis in collagen disorders. Am. J. Roentgenol. Radium Ther. Nucl. Med., *115*:300, 1972.
53. Bryk, D.: Unusual causes of small bowel pneumatosis: Perforated duodenal ulcer and perforated jejunal diverticula. Radiology, *106*:299, 1973.

54. Jaffe, N., Carlson, D. H., and Vawter, G. F.: Pneumatosis cystoides intestinalis in acute leukemia. Cancer, *30*:239, 1972.
55. Bell, R. S., Graham, B., and Stevenson, J. K.: Roentgenologic and clinical manifestations of neonatal necrotizing enterocolitis. Am. J. Roentgenol. Radium Ther. Nucl. Med., *112*:123, 1971.
56. Vanasin, B., Wright, J. R., and Schuster, M. M.: Pneumatosis cystoides esophagi. J.A.M.A., *217*:76, 1971.
57. Goldstein, H. M., and Sankaran, B. S.: Colonic ileus: an atypical form of adynamic ileus. J.A.M.A., *230*:1008, 1974.
58. Evans, W. A., and Willis, R.: Hirschsprung's disease: roentgen diagnosis in children. Am. J. Roentgenol. Radium Ther. Nucl. Med., *78*:1024, 1957.
59. Schey, W. L., and White, H.: Hirschsprung disease. Am. J. Roentgenol. Radium Ther. Nucl. Med., *112*:105, 1971.
60. Sane, S. M., and Girdany, B. R.: Total aganglionosis coli. Radiology, *107*:397, 1973.
61. Bruggeman, L. L., and Seaman, W. B.: Epiphrenic diverticula: an analysis of 80 cases. Am. J. Roentgenol. Radium Ther. Nucl. Med., *119*:266, 1973.
62. Eells, R. W., and Simril, W. A.: Gastric diverticula. Am. J. Roentgenol. Radium Ther. Nucl. Med., *68*:8, 1952.
63. Margulis, A. R., and Burhenne, H. J.: *Alimentary Tract Roentgenology*. St. Louis, The C. V. Mosby Co., 1967.
64. Smith, C. C., and Christensen, W. R.: Colonic diverticulosis. Am. J. Roentgenol. Radium Ther. Nucl. Med., *82*:996, 1959.
65. Baum, S., Rosch, J., et al.: Selective mesenteric arterial infusions in management of massive diverticular hemorrhage. N. Engl. J. Med., *288*:1269, 1973.
66. Casarella, W. J., Kanter, I. E., and Seaman, W. B.: Right sided colonic diverticula as cause of acute rectal hemorrhage. N. Engl. J. Med., *286*:450, 1972.
67. Berne, A. S.: Meckel's diverticulum: x-ray diagnosis. N. Engl. J. Med., *260*:690, 1959.
68. Dalinka, M. K., and Wunder, J. F.: Meckel's diverticulum and its complications, with emphasis on roentgenologic demonstration. Radiology, *106*:295, 1973.
69. Muroff, L. R., Casarella, W. J., and Johnson, P. M.: Preoperative diagnosis of Meckel's diverticulum. J.A.M.A., *229*:1900, 1974.
70. Polachek, A. A., et al.: Diverticulosis of jejunum with macrocytic anemia and steatorrhea. Ann. Intern. Med., *54*:636, 1961.
71. Heilbrun, N., and Boyden, E. A.: Intraluminal duodenal diverticula. Radiology, *82*:887, 1964.
72. Grayson, C. E.: Enlargement of the ileocecal valve. Am. J. Roentgenol. Radium Ther. Nucl. Med., *79*:823, 1958.
73. Klotz, E., and Gumrich, H.: Differential diagnosis of benign space-occupying processes of the cecum. Fortschr. Roentgenstr., *113*:20, 1970.
74. Berk, R. N., and Lasser, E. C.: *Radiology of the Ileocecal Area*. Philadelphia, W. B. Saunders Co., 1975, p. 21.
75. Bertine, L.: Gastritis: a medical dilemma. Radiology, *78*:627, 1962.
76. Hines, W. B., Kerr, R. M., et al.: Roentgenologic and gastrocamera correlation in lesions of the stomach. Am. J. Roentgenol. Radium Ther. Nucl. Med., *113*:129, 1971.
77. Daweke, H., Hinssen, M., and Stolze, T.: Chronic gastritis: its diagnosis and clinical significance. Radiologe, *12*:155, 1972.
78. Turner, C. J., Lipitz, L. R., and Pastore, R. A.: Antral gastritis. Radiology, *113*:305, 1974.
79. Bryk, D., and Elguezabal, A.: Atrophic stomach of the elderly. Am. J. Roentgenol. Radium Ther. Nucl. Med., *123*:236, 1975.
80. Reese, D. F., Hodgson, J. R., and Dockerty, M. D.: Giant hypertrophy of the gastric mucosa. Am. J. Roentgenol. Radium Ther. Nucl. Med., *88*:619, 1962.
81. Burns, B., and Gay, B. B.: Menetrier's disease of the stomach in children. Am. J. Roentgenol. Radium Ther. Nucl. Med., *103*:300, 1968.
82. Berman, V., and Goldberg, M. J.: Hyperplasia of Brunner's glands. Br. J. Radiol., *32*:241, 1959.
83. Pearson, K. D., Buchignane, J. S., et al.: Hereditary angioneurotic edema of the gastrointestinal tract. Am. J. Roentgenol. Radium Ther. Nucl. Med., *116*:256, 1972.
84. Berk, R. N., and Millman, S. J.: Urticaria of the colon. Radiology, *99*:539, 1971.
85. Johnson, T. H., and Caldwell, K. W.: Angioneurotic edema of the colon. Radiology, *99*:61, 1971.
86. Hebestreit, H. P., and Lütgemeier, A. F.: Benign stenosis of the esophagus in ectopic gastric mucosa. Fortschr. Roentgenstr., *115*:419, 1971.
87. Dodd, G. D., and Nelson, R. S.: The combined radiologic and gastroscopic evaluation of gastric ulceration. Radiology, *77*:177, 1961.
88. Wolf, B. S., and Bryk, D.: Simple benign prepyloric ulcer. Am. J. Roentgenol. Radium Ther. Nucl. Med., *86*:50, 1961.
89. Boijjsen, E., and Reuter, S. R.: Angiography in diagnosis of chronic unexplained melena. Radiology, *88*:686, 1967.
90. Boijjsen, E., Wallace, S., and Kanter, E.: Angiography in tumors of the stomach. Acta Radiol. (Diagn.), *4*:306, 1966.
91. Teplick, J. G., and Haskin, M. E.: Duodenal ulcer disease. Med. Sci., *1*:82, 1962.
92. Belber, J. P.: Endoscopic examination of the duodenal bulb: a comparison with x-ray. Gastroenterology, *61*:55, 1971.

93. Cooke, L., and Hutton, C. F.: Post-bulbar duodenal ulcer. Lancet, *1*:754, 1958.
94. Hare, W. S. C.: Zollinger-Ellison syndrome. J. Coll. Radiol. Austral., *4*:84, 1960.
95. Missakian, M. M., Carlson, H. C., and Huizenga, K.: Roentgen findings in Zollinger-Ellison syndrome. Am. J. Roentgenol. Radium Ther. Nucl. Med., *94*:429, 1965.
96. Rodriguez, H. P., Aston, J. K., and Richardson, C. T.: Ulcers in the descending duodenum. Am. J. Roentgenol. Radium Ther. Nucl. Med., *119*:316, 1973.
97. Tréheux, A., Fays, J., and Velut, A.: The use of hypotonic duodenography in the diagnosis of post-bulbar ulcers. Ann. Radiol., *12*:451, 1969.
98. Nelson, S. W., and Christoforidis, A. S.: Roentgenologic features of the Zollinger-Ellison syndrome. Semin. Roentgenol., *3*:254, 1968.
99. Gray, R. K., Rösch, J., and Grollman, J. H.: Angiography in the diagnosis of islet-cell tumors. Radiology, *97*:39, 1970.
100. Zboralske, F. F., and Amberg, J. R.: Detection of the Zollinger-Ellison syndrome: The radiologist's responsibility. Am. J. Roentgenol, Radium Ther. Nucl. Med., *104*:529, 1968.
101. Baum, S., Ward, S., and Nusbaum, M.: Stress bleeding from mid-duodenum. Radiology, *95*:595, 1970.
102. Lucas, C. E., et al.: Natural history and surgical dilemma of stress gastric bleeding. Arch. Surg., *102*:266, 1971.
103. Keeffe, E. J., and Gagliardi, R. A.: Significance of ileus in perforated viscus. Am. J. Roentgenol. Radium Ther. Nucl. Med., *117*:275, 1973.
104. Nusbaum, M., et al.: Demonstration of intra-abdominal bleeding by selective arteriography. J.A.M.A., *191*:389, 1965.
105. Koehler, P. R.: Demonstration of massive acute hemorrhages of the gastrointestinal tract with arteriography. Fortschr. Geb. Roentgenstr. Nuklearmed., *110*:1, 1969.
106. Mellins, H. Z.: The radiologic signs of disease in the lesser peritoneal sac. Radiol. Clin. North Am., *2*:107, 1964.
107. Faegenburg, D., et al.: Colon bacillus pneumonia: a complication of lesser sac abscess. Am. J. Roentgenol. Radium Ther. Nucl. Med., *107*:300, 1969.
108. Dineen, P., and McSherry, C. K.: Subdiaphragmatic abscess. Ann. Surg., *155*:506, 1962.
109. Sanders, R. C.: Post-operative pleural effusion and subphrenic abscess. Clin. Radiol., *21*:308, 1970.
110. Teplick, J. G.: Duodenal loop changes in posterior penetration of duodenal ulcer. Ann. Intern. Med., *44*:968, 1956.
111. Ellis, K.: Gastro-jejunal ulcer. Radiology, *71*:187, 1958.
112. Schatzki, R.: The significance of rigidity of the jejunum in the diagnosis of postoperative jejunal ulcers. Am. J. Roentgenol. Radium Ther. Nucl. Med., *103*:330, 1968.
113. Thaeng, R. H., Hodgson, J. R., and Scudamore, H. H.: Gastro-colic and gastro-jejunocolic fistulas. Am. J. Roentgenol. Radium Ther. Nucl. Med., *83*:876, 1960.
114. Kinsella, V. J., and Hennessy, W. B.: Gastrectomy and the blind loop syndrome. Lancet, *2*:1205, 1960.
115. Burhenne, H. J.: Iatrogenic afferent loop syndrome. Radiology, *91*:942, 1968.
116. Dolan, K. D., and Hockman, R. E.: Jejunogastric intussusception ten years after surgery. J.A.M.A., *205*:178, 1968.
117. Booth, C. C.: Classification of malabsorption syndrome. Br. J. Radiol., *33*:201, 1960.
118. Laws, J. W., and Pittman, R. G.: Radiologic investigation of malabsorption syndrome. Br. J. Radiol., *33*:211, 1960.
119. Triano, G. J.: Small bowel in Whipple's disease. Am. J. Roentgenol. Radium Ther. Nucl. Med., *87*:717. 1962.
120. Martel, W., and Hodges, F. J.: Small bowel in Whipple's disease. Am. J. Roentgenol. Radium Ther. Nucl. Med., *81*:623, 1959.
121. Nicolette, C. C. and Tully, T. E.: Duodenum in celiac disease. Am. J. Roentgenol. Radium Ther. Nucl. Med., *113*:248, 1971.
122. Ruoff, M., Lindner, A. E., and Marshak, R. H.: Intussusception in sprue. Am. J. Roentgenol. Radium Ther. Nucl. Med., *104*:525, 1968.
123. Isbell, R. G., Carlson, H. C., and Hoffman, H. N.: Roentgenologic-pathologic correlation in malabsorption syndrome. Am. J. Roentgenol. Radium Ther. Nucl. Med., *107*:158, 1967.
124. Clemett, A. R., and Marshak, R. H.: Whipple's disease. Radiol. Clin. North Am., *7*:105, 1969.
125. Marshak, R. H., and Lindner, A. E.: *Radiology of the Small Intestine.* Philadelphia, W. B. Saunders Co., 1975.
126. Phillips, R. L., and Carlson, H. C.: The roentgenographic and clinical findings in Whipple's disease. Am. J. Roentgenol. Radium Ther. Nucl. Med., *123*:268, 1975.
127. Marshak, R. H., et al.: Protein disorders of the gastrointestinal tract; roentgen features. Radiology, *77*:893, 1961.
128. Pock-Steen, O. C.: Roentgenologic changes in protein-losing enteropathy. Acta Radiol. (Diagn.), *4*:681, 1966.
129. Shimkin, P. M., Waldmann, T. A., and Krugman, R. L.: Intestinal lymphangiectasia. Am. J. Roentgenol. Radium Ther. Nucl. Med., *110*:827, 1970.
130. Laws, J. W., and Neale, G.: Radiological diagnosis of disaccharidase deficiency. Lancet, *2*:139, 1966.
131. Thompson, J. R., and Sanders, I.: Lactose-barium small bowel studies. Am. J. Roentgenol. Radium Ther. Nucl. Med., *113*:255, 1971.

132. Rosenguist, C. J., et al.: Intestinal lactose deficiency. Radiology, *102*:275, 1972.
133. Rohrmann, C. A., Silvis, S. E., and Vennes, J. A.: Evaluation of the endoscopic pancreatogram. Radiology, *113*:297, 1974.
134. Bockus, H. L.: Acute inflammation of the pancreas. Gastroenterology, *34*:467, 1958.
135. Shallenberger, P. L., and Kaff, D. F.: Acute pancreatitis. Ann. Intern. Med., *48*:1185, 1958.
136. Cantwell, D. F., and Pollock, A. V.: Radiology of acute pancreatitis. Clin. Radiol., *10*:95, 1959.
137. Poppel, M. H.: The roentgen manifestations of pancreatitis. Semin. Roentgenol., *3*:227, 1968.
138. Achord, J. L., and Gerle, R. D.: Bone lesions in pancreatitis. Am. J. Dig. Dis., *11*:453, 1966.
139. Myers, N. N., and Evans, J. A.: Defects of pancreatitis on the small bowel and colon. Am. J. Roentgenol. Radium Ther. Nucl. Med., *119*:151, 1973.
140. Balthazar, E., and Henderson, N.: Prominent folds of the posterior wall and lesser curvature of the stomach: a sign of acute pancreatitis. Radiology, *110*:319, 1974.
141. Myers, M. A., and Evans, J. A.: Effects of pancreatitis on the small bowel and colon. Am. J. Roentgenol. Radium Ther. Nucl. Med., *119*:151, 1973.
142. Leger, L., and Crismer, R.: Roentgen diagnosis of chronic pancreatitis. Acta Gastroenterol. Belg. *23*:396, 1960.
143. Bank, S., et al.: Further observation on calcified medullary bone lesions in chronic pancreatitis. Gastroenterology, *51*:224, 1966.
144. Khademi, M., Lazaro, E. J., and Rickert, R. R.: Selective arteriography in the diagnosis of chronic inflammatory pancreatic disease. Am. J. Roentgenol. Radium Ther. Nucl. Med., *119*:141, 1973.
145. Robbins, A. H., et al.: Endoscopic pancreatography: Analysis of radiologic findings in pancreatitis. Radiology, *11*:293, 1974.
146. Zimmon, D. S., et al.: Endoscopic retrograde cholangiopancreatography in the diagnosis of pancreatic inflammatory disease. Radiology, *113*:287, 1974.
147. Rosch, J., and Bret, J.: Arteriography of the pancreas. Am. J. Roentgenol. Radium Ther. Nucl. Med., *94*:182, 1965.
148. Tucker, P. C., and Webster, P. D.: Traumatic pseudocysts of the pancreas. Arch. Intern. Med., *129*:583, 1972.
149. Michel, J.: Radiologic study of mucoviscidosis of the pancreas. J. Radiol. Electrol., *42*:114, 1961.
150. Tucker, A. S., et al.: Roentgen diagnosis of complications of cystic fibrosis. Am. J. Roentgenol. Radium Ther. Nucl. Med., *89*:1084, 1963.
151. Nice, C. M.: Exocrine gland dysfunction (mucoviscidosis) in adults. Radiology, *81*:828, 1963.
152. Bernard, E., et al.: The bronchial emphysema — peptic ulcer syndrome and role of mucoviscidosis in its pathogenesis. J. Fr. Med. Chir. Thorac., *16*:751, 1962.
153. Marshak, R. H., and Lindner, A. F.: *Radiology of the Small Intestine.* Philadelphia, W. B. Saunders Company, 1975.
154. Holsclaw, D. S., Rocmans, C., and Shnachman, H.: Intussusception in patients with cystic fibrosis. Pediatrics, *48*:51, 1971.
155. Taussig, L. M., Saideno, R. M., and di Sant'Agnese, P. A.: Radiographic abnormalities of the duodenum and small bowel in cystic fibrosis in pancreas (mucoviscidosis). Radiology, *106*:369, 1973.
156. Berk, R. N., and Lee, F. A.: Late gastrointestinal manifestations of cystic fibrosis of the pancreas. Radiology, *106*:377, 1973.
157. Salik, O. J.: Pancreatic carcinoma. Am. J. Roentgenol. Radium Ther. Nucl. Med., *86*:1, 1961.
158. Eaton, S. B., et al.: Comparison of current radiologic approaches to the diagnosis of pancreatic disease. N. Engl. J. Med., *279*:389, 1968.
159. Buranasiri, S., and Baum, S.: The significance of the venous phase of celiac and superior mesenteric arteriography in evaluating pancreatic carcinoma. Radiology, *102*:11, 1972.
160. Daffner, J. E., and Brown, C. H.: Regional enteritis. Ann. Intern. Med., *49*:580, 1958.
161. Marshak, R. H., et al.: Segmental colitis. Radiology, *73*:707, 1959.
162. Hawk, P., et al.: Regional enteritis of the colon. J.A.M.A., *201*:112, 1967.
163. Marshak, R. H., and Lindner, A. E.: Granulomatous colitis. Semin. Roentgenol., *3*:27, 1968.
164. Nelson, S. W.: Some interesting and unusual manifestations of Crohn's disease of the stomach, duodenum, and small intestine. Am. J. Roentgenol. Radium Ther. Nucl. Med., *107*:86, 1969.
165. Schachter, H., Goldstein, M. J., et al.: Ulcerative and granulomatous colitis: Validity of differential diagnostic criteria. Ann. Intern. Med., *72*:841, 1970.
166. Weedon, D. D., Shorter, R. G., et al.: Crohn's disease and cancer. N. Engl. J. Med., *289*:1099, 1973.
167. Gonzalez, G., and Kennedy, T.: Crohn's disease of the stomach. Radiology, *113*:27, 1974.
168. Farman, J., et al.: Crohn's disease of the stomach. Am. J. Roentgenol. Radium Ther. Nucl. Med., *123*:242, 1975.
169. Thompson, W. N., Cockrill, H., and Rice, R. P.: Regional enteritis of the duodenum. Am. J. Roentgenol. Radium Ther. Nucl. Med., *123*:252, 1975.
170. Edling, N. P. G., and Eklof, O.: Roentgenologic study of the course of ulcerative colitis. Acta Radiol., *54*:397, 1960.
171. Wolf, B. S., and Marshak, R. H.: Toxic segmental dilatation of colon in fulminating ulceration colitis. Am. J. Roentgenol. Radium Ther. Nucl. Med., *82*:985, 1959.
172. Hodgson, J. R., and Sauer, W. G.: Roentgenologic features of carcinoma in chronic ulcerative colitis. Am. J. Roentgenol. Radium Ther. Nucl. Med., *86*:91, 1961.

173. Saterapoulos, C., and Gilmore, J. H.: Roentgen diagnosis of acute appendicitis. Radiology, 71:246, 1958.
174. Stein, G. N., Bennett, H. H., and Finklestein, A.: Preoperative diagnosis of Meckel's diverticulum in adults. Am. J. Roentgenol. Radium Ther. Nucl. Med., 79:815, 1958.
175. Devroede, G. J., Taylor, W. F., et al.: Cancer risk and life expectancy of children with ulcerative colitis. N. Engl. J. Med., 285:17, 1972.
176. Krieger, J., Seaman, W. B., and Porter, M. R.: The roentgenologic appearance of sclerosing cholangitis. Radiology, 95:369, 1970.
177. Soter, C. S.: The radiologist and acute appendicitis. Semin. Roentgenol., 8:375, 1973.
178. Ponka, J. L., Brush, B. A., and Fox, J. D.: Differential diagnosis of carcinoma of colon and diverticulitis. J.A.M.A., 172:515, 1960.
179. Marshak, R.: Personal Communication.
180. Beranbaum, S. L., Zausner, J., and Lane, B.: Diverticular disease of the right colon. Am. J. Roentgenol. Radium Ther. Nucl. Med., 115:334, 1972.
181. Stevenson, J. K., Oliver, T. K., et al.: Neonatal necrotizing enterocolitis. J. Pediatr. Surg. 6:28, 1971.
182. Pochaczevsky, R., and Kassner, G.: Necrotizing enterocolitis of infancy. Am. J. Roentgenol. Radium Ther. Nucl. Med., 113:283, 1971.
183. Richmond, J. A., and Mikity, V.: Benign form of necrotizing enterocolitis. Am. J. Roentgenol., 123:301, 1975.
184. Schapiro, R. L., and Newman, A.: Acute enterocolitis. A complication of antibiotic therapy. Radiology, 108:263, 1973.
185. Tully, T. E., and Feinberg, S. B.: Reappearance of antibiotic-induced pseudomembranous enterocolitis. Radiology, 110:563, 1974.
186. Sherbon, K. J.: Radiology in pseudomembranous colitis. Aust. Radiol. 16:66, 1972.
187. Miller, W. T., DePoto, D. W., et al.: Evanescent colitis in young adults. Radiology, 100:71, 1971.
188. Tully, T. E., and Feinberg, S. B.: Those other types of enterocolitis. Am. J. Roentgenol. Radium Ther. Nucl. Med., 121:291, 1974.
189. Barner, J. L.: Colitis cystica profunda. Radiology, 89:435, 1967.
190. Goldberg, H. I., et al.: Colitis cystica profunda, RPC Case of the Month from A.F.I.P. Radiology, 96:447, 1970.
191. Schwartz, S., et al.: Some aspects of vascular disease of the small intestine. Radiology, 84:616, 1965.
192. Lawrason, F. D., et al.: Ulcerative-obstructive lesions of small intestine. J.A.M.A., 191:64, 1965.
193. Schwartz, S. A., et al.: Roentgenologic features of vascular disorders of the intestines. Radiol. Clin. North Am., 2:71, 1964.
194. Carlson, H. C.: Localized nonspecific ulceration of the small intestine. Radiol. Clin. North Am., 7:97, 1969.
195. Wang, C. C., and Reeves, J. D.: Mesenteric vascular disease. Am. J. Roentgenol. Radium Ther. Nucl. Med., 83:895, 1960.
196. Nelson, S. W., and Eggleston, W.: Findings on plain roentgenograms of the abdomen associated with mesenteric vascular occlusion with a possible new sign of mesenteric venous thrombosis. Am. J. Roentgenol. Radium Ther. Nucl. Med., 83:886, 1960.
197. Marshak, R. H., et al.: Segmental infarction of the colon. Am. J. Dig. Dis., 10:86, 1965.
198. Dunbar, J. D., and Nelson, S. W.: Nonangiographic manifestations of intestinal vascular disease. Am. J. Roentgenol. Radium Ther. Nucl. Med., 99:127, 1967.
199. Tomchik, F. S., et al.: The roentgenologic spectrum of bowel infarction. Radiology, 96:249, 1970.
200. Scott, J. R., Miller, W. T., et al.: Acute mesenteric infarction. Am. J. Roentgenol. Radium Ther. Nucl. Med., 113:269, 1971.
201. Smith, S. L., Tutton, R. H., and Ochsner, S. F.: Roentgenologic aspects of intestinal ischemia. Am. J. Roentgenol. Radium Ther. Nucl. Med., 116:249, 1972.
202. Brown, A. R.: Nongangrenous ischemic colitis. Br. J. Surg., 59:463, 1972.
203. Gielandus, L. A., and Lyall, A. D.: Chronic mid-gut ischemia. Clin. Radiol., 14:322, 1963.
204. Baum, S.: Editorial: mesenteric vascular insufficiency. Am. J. Gastroenterol. 45:481, 1966.
205. Cornell, S. H.: Severe stenosis of the celiac artery. Radiology, 99:311, 1971.
206. Myers, M. A., Kaplowitz, N. and Bloom, A. A.: Malabsorption secondary to mesenteric ischemia. Am. J. Roentgenol. Radium Ther. Nucl. Med., 119:352, 1973.
207. Stanley, J. C., and Fry, W. J.: Median arcuate ligament syndrome. Arch. Surg., 103:252, 1971.
208. Wiott, J. F., and Felson, B.: Gas in the portal venous system. Am. J. Roentgenol. Radium Ther. Nucl. Med., 86:920, 1961.
209. Fred, H. L., Mayhall, C. G., and Harle, T. S.: Hepatic portal venous gas. Am. J. Med., 44:557, 1968.
210. Arnon, R. G.: and Fishbein, J. F.: Portal venous gas in pediatric age group. J. Pediatr., 79:255, 1971.
211. Felson, B., and Levin, E. J.: Intramural hematoma of the duodenum. Radiology, 63:823, 1954.
212. Slonin, L.: Duodenal hematoma. Aust. Radiol., 15:236, 1971.
213. Keefe, E. J., Gagliardi, R. A., and Pfister, R. C.: The roentgenographic evaluation of ascites. Am. J. Roentgenol. Radium Ther. Nucl. Med., 101:388, 1967.
214. Makker, S. P., Tucker, A. S., et al.: Nonobstructive hydronephrosis and hydroureter associated with peritonitis. N. Engl. J. Med., 287:535, 1972.

215. Fred, H. L., Eiband, J. M., and Collins, L. C.: Calcifications in intra-abdominal and retroperitoneal metastases. Am. J. Roentgenol. Radium Ther. Nucl. Med., 91:138, 1964.
216. Piro, A. J., et al.: The use of intracavitary contrast media in patients with neoplastic effusions. J.A.M.A., 206:821, 1968.
217. Arnheim, E. E., et al.: Mesenteric cysts in infancy and childhood. Pediatrics, 24:469, 1959.
218. Leonidas, J. C., Kopel, F. B., and Danese, C. A.: Mesenteric cyst associated with protein loss in the gastrointestinal tract. Am. J. Roentgenol. Radium Ther. Nucl. Med., 112:150, 1971.
219. Boyd, D. P., et al.: Carcinoma of the esophagus. N. Engl. J. Med., 258:271, 1958.
220. Bateson, E. M.: Carcinoma of the esophagus. Aust. Radiol., 13:345, 1969.
221. Lawson, T. L., Dodds, W. J., and Sheft, D. J.: Carcinoma of the esophagus simulating varices. Am. J. Roentgenol. Radium Ther. Nucl. Med., 107:83, 1969.
222. Green, A. E., et al.: Leiomyoma of the esophagus. Am. J. Roentgenol. Radium Ther. Nucl. Med., 82:1058, 1959.
223. Olbert, F.: Leiomyoma of the esophagus. Fortschr. Roentgenstr., 113:11, 1970.
224. Gutmann, R. A.: Difficulties of diagnosis between gastritis and cancer. Arch. Mal. Appar. Dig., 49:5, 1960.
225. Mainzer, F., Amberg, J. R., and Margulis, A. R.: Superficial carcinoma of the stomach. Radiology, 93:109, 1969.
226. Marshak, R. H., and Lindner, A. E.: Polypoid lesions of the stomach. Semin. Roentgenol., 6:151, 1971.
227. Watson, A. R., et al.: Benign gastric neoplasms. Tex. Med., 55:890, 1959.
228. Marshak, R. H., and Feldman, F.: Gastric polyps. Am. J. Dig. Dis., 10:909, 1968.
229. Rooney, D. R.: Aberrant pancreatic tissue in stomach. Radiology, 73:241, 1959.
230. Masley, P. M.: Leiomyosarcoma of the stomach. Am. J. Dig. Dis., 4:792, 1959.
231. Berk, R. N., Scher, G. S., and Bode, D. F.: Unusual tumors of the gastrointestinal tract. Am. J. Roentgenol. Radium Ther. Nucl. Med., 113:159, 1971.
232. Phillips, J. C., Lindsay, J. W., and Kendall, J. A.: Gastric leiomyosarcoma. Am. J. Dig. Dis., 15:239, 1970.
233. Redd, B. L.: Lymphosarcoma of the stomach. Am. J. Roentgenol. Radium Ther. Nucl. Med., 82:634, 1959.
234. Bush, R. S., and Ash, C. L.: Primary lymphoma of gastrointestinal tract. Radiology, 92:1349, 1969.
235. Martel, W., et al.: Small bowel tumors. Radiology, 75:368, 1960.
236. Marshak, R. H.: Roentgen findings in lymphosarcoma of small intestine. Am. J. Roentgenol. Radium Ther. Nucl. Med., 86:682, 1961.
237. Keats, T. E., and Sakai, H. Q.: Evaluation of the sources of error in the roentgenologic diagnosis of neoplasm of the small intestine. Gastroenterology, 29:554, 1955.
238. Mellins, H. Z., and Blennerhassett, J. B.: Polypoid and ulcerative lesions in the colon and small intestine. N. Engl. J. Med., 283:749, 1970.
239. Kyriakos, M.: Malignant tumors of the small intestine. J.A.M.A., 229.700, 1974.
240. Cottone, D., and Aquila, N.: Peutz-Jeghers syndrome. Radiol. Med. (Torino), 44:113, 1958.
241. Godard, J. E., Dodds, W. J., et al.: Peutz-Jeghers syndrome. Am. J. Roentgenol. Radium Ther. Nucl. Med., 113:316, 1971.
242. Dodds, W. J., Schulte, W. J., et al.: Peutz-Jeghers and gastrointestinal malignancy. Am. J. Roentgenol. Radium Ther. Nucl. Med., 115:374, 1972.
243. Allcock, J. M.: Clinical and radiological diagnosis of carcinoma of colon. Br. J. Radiol., 31:272, 1958.
244. Messinger, N. H., Bobroff, L. M., and Beneventano, T. C.: Lymphosarcoma of the colon. Am. J. Roentgenol. Radium Ther. Nucl. Med., 117:281, 1973.
245. Meyers, M. A., and McSweeney, J.: Secondary neoplasms of the bowel. Radiology, 105:1, 1972.
246. Spjut, H. J., and Perkins, D. E.: Endometriosis of the sigmoid colon and rectum. Am. J. Roentgenol. Radium Ther. Nucl. Med., 82:1070, 1959.
247. Lilja, B., and Probst, F.: Intestinal endometriosis. Acta Radiol., 4:545, 1966.
248. Theander, G., and Wehlin, L.: The radiology of pelvic endometriosis. Clin. Radiol., 19:19, 1968.
249. Felson, B., and Wiot, J. F.: Some interesting right lower quadrant entities. Radiol. Clin North Am. 7:83, 1969.
250. Weber, H. M.: Roentgenologic demonstration of polypoid lesions and polyposis of the large intestine. Am. J. Roentgenol. Radium Ther. Nucl. Med., 25:377, 1931.
251. Brombart, M.: Pedunculated polyps of the ilio-pelvic colon in the adult. J. Belg. Radiol., 54:65, 1971.
252. McKenney, D. C.: Multiple polyposis: congenital, heredofamilial, malignant. Am. J. Surg., 46:204, 1939.
253. Koehler, P. R., Kyaw, M. M., and Fenlon, J. W.: Diffuse gastrointestinal polyposis with ectodermal changes: Cronkhite-Canada syndrome. Radiology, 103:589, 1972.
254. Diner, W. C.: Cronkhite-Canada syndrome. Radiology, 105:715, 1972.
255. Frye, T. R.: Villous adenoma of the sigmoid colon. Radiology, 73:71, 1959.
256. Turek, R. E., Davis, W. C., et al.: The roentgenographic diagnosis of villous tumors of the colon. Am. J. Roentgenol. Radium Ther. Nucl. Med., 113:349, 1971.
257. Bockus, H. L.: Gastroenterology, 3rd ed. Philadelphia, W. B. Saunders Company, 1975.
258. Grundy, D. J., King, P. A., and Lloyd, G.: Comparative evaluation of preoperative and operative radiology in biliary tract disease. Br. J. Surg., 59:205, 1972.

DISEASES OF THE DIGESTIVE SYSTEM

1126

259. McCort, J. J.: Radiographic signs of acute suppurative cholecystitis. Calif. Med., 90:139, 1959.
260. Weems, H. S., and Walker, L. A.: Radiographic diagnosis of acute cholecystitis and pancreatitis. Radiol. Clin. North Am., 2:89, 1964.
261. Keller, H. L., Ferstl, M., and Rupp, N.: Roentgenographic and clinical findings in emphysematous cholecystitis. Fortschr. Roentgenstr., 115:475, 1971.
262. Drucker, V.: Small-intestinal gallstone ileus. Arch. Surg., 79:22, 1959.
263. Eisenman, J. I., Finck, E. J., and O'Loughlin, B. J.: Gallstone ileus: a review. Am. J. Roengenol., 101:361, 1967.
264. Eaton, S. B., Ferrucci, J. T., et al.: Diagnosis of choledocholithiasis by barium duodenal examination. Radiology, 102:267, 1972.
265. Hayes, M. A., et al.: The developmental basis for bile duct anomalies. Surg. Gynecol. Obstet., 107:447, 1958.
266. Eckert, J. F., and Carvalho, R. S.: Congenital biliary atresia: case of the month. Radiology, 90:600, 1968.
267. Hankamp, L. J.: Congenital choledochal cyst. J. Dis. Child., 97:97, 1959.
268. Hon, S. Y., Collins, L. C., and Wright, R. M.: Choledochal cyst: report of five cases. Clin. Radiol., 20:332, 1969.
269. Rosenfield, N., and Griscom, N. T.: Choledochal cysts: Roentgenologic techniques. Radiology, 114:113, 1975.
270. Khilnani, M. T., et al.: Roentgen features of carcinoma of gallbladder. Radiology, 79:204, 1962.
271. Abrams, R. M., Meng, C., et al.: Angiographic demonstration of carcinoma of the gallbladder. Radiology, 94:277, 1970.
272. Sprayregen, S., and Messinger, N. H.: Carcinoma of the gallbladder: diagnosis and evaluation of regional spread by angiography. Am. J. Roentgenol. Radium Ther. Nucl. Med., 116:382, 1972.
273. Ochsner, S. F., and Ochsner, A.: Benign neoplasms of gallbladder. Ann. Surg., 151:630, 1960.
274. Loitman, B. S., et al.: Papillomas of gallbladder. Am. J. Roentgenol. Radium Ther. Nucl. Med., 88:783, 1962.
275. Jutras, J. A.: Hyperplastic cholecystoses. Am. J. Roentgenol. Radium Ther. Nucl. Med., 83:796, 1960.
276. Jutras, J. A., and Lavesque', H.: Adenomyoma and adenomyomatosis of the gallbladder. Radiol. Clin. North Am., 4:483, 1966.
277. Ochsner, S. F.: Intramural lesions of the gallbladder. Am. J. Roentgenol. Radium Ther. Nucl. Med., 113:1, 1971.
278. Evans, J., and Mujahed, Z.: Roentgenographic aids in diagnosis of neoplasms of liver and extrahepatic ducts. J.A.M.A., 171:7, 1959.
279. Legge, D. A., and Carlson, H. C.: Cholangiographic appearance of primary carcinoma of the bile ducts. Radiology, 102:259, 1972.
280. Albo, R. J., and Obata, W. G.: Radiologic diagnosis of primary sclerosing cholangitis. Radiology, 81:123, 1963.
281. Warren, K. W., et al.: Primary sclerosing cholangitis. Am. J. Surg., 111:23, 1966.
282. Legge, D. A., Carlson, H. G., et al.: Cholangiographic findings in cholangiolitic hepatitis. Am. J. Roentgenol. Radium Ther. Nucl. Med., 113:16, 1971.
283. Mujahed, Z., Glenn, F., and Evans, J. A.: Communicating cavernous ectasia of the intrahepatic ducts (Caroli's disease). Am. J. Roentgenol. Radium Ther. Nucl. Med., 113:21, 1971.
284. Boijsen, E.: Selective hepatic angiography in primary and secondary tumors of the liver. Rev. Int. Hepatol., 15:385, 1965.
285. Foster, S. C., Schneider, B., and Seaman, W. B.: Gas-containing pyogenic intrahepatic abscesses. Radiology, 94:613, 1970.
286. Novy, S. B., Wallace, S., et al.: Pyogenic liver abscess. Am J. Roentgenol. Radium Ther. Nucl. Med., 121:388, 1974.
287. Catinat, J., et al.: On a new case of Budd-Chiari syndrome. Presse Med., 68:1749, 1960.
288. Levander, M., and Pontin, J.: Budd-Chiari's syndrome diagnosed by means of phlebography in a case of retroperitoneal sarcoma. Acta Med. Scand., 163:251, 1959.
289. Pollard, J. J., and Nesebar, R. A.: Abdominal angiography. N. Engl. J. Med., 279:1093, 1968.
290. Kreel, L., Freston, J. W., and Clain, D.: Radiology in the Budd-Chiari syndrome. Br. J. Radiol., 40:755, 1967.
291. Ramsay, G., and Britton, R. C.: Intraparenchymal angiography in the diagnosis of hepatic veno-occlusive diseases. Radiology, 90:716, 1968.
292. Deutsch, V., Rosenthal, T., et al.: Budd-Chiari syndrome. Am. J. Roentgenol. Radium Ther. Nucl. Med., 116:430, 1972.
293. Bergstrand, I.: The localization of portal obstruction by splenoportography. Am. J. Roentgenol. Radium Ther. Nucl. Med., 85:1111, 1961.
294. Dotter, R. J.: Extrahepatic portal obstruction in childhood and its angiographic diagnosis. Am. J. Roentgenol. Radium Ther. Nucl. Med., 112:143, 1971.
295. Schorr, S., and Birnbaum, D.: Raised position of right kidney (in liver disorders). Radiol. Clin. North Am., 28:102, 1959.
296. Piper, D. W.: Radiographic study of portal and hepatic venous systems in portal cirrhosis. Am. J. Dig. Dis., 6:499, 1961.
297. Boijsen, E.: Selective angiography of celiac axis and superior mesenteric artery in cirrhosis of the liver. Rev. Int. Hepatol., 15:2323, 1968.

298. Marshak, R., et al.: Intestinal edema. Am. J. Roentgenol. Radium Ther. Nucl. Med., *101*:379, 1967.
299. Reuter, S. R., and Atkin, T. W.: High dose left gastric angiography for demonstration of esophageal varices. Radiology, *105*:573, 1972.
300. Kessler, R. E., Tice, D. A., and Zimmon, D. S.: Retrograde flow of portal vein blood in patients with cirrhosis. Radiology, *92*:1038, 1969.
301. Morita, M., and Kihara, T.: Intravenous cholecystography and metabolism of meglumine iodipamide in Dubin-Johnson syndrome. Radiology, *99*:57, 1971.
302. Stauffer, J. Q., Lapinski, M. W., et al.: Focal nodular hyperplasia of the liver and intrahepatic hemorrhage in young women on oral contraceptives. Ann. Intern. Med., *83*:301, 1975.
303. Brust, R. W., and Conlon, P. C.: Roentgen manifestations of primary hepatoma. Am. J. Roentgenol. Radium Ther. Nucl. Med., *87*:777, 1962.
304. Yü, C.: Primary carcinoma of the liver (hepatoma). Its diagnosis by selective celiac arteriography. Am. J. Roentgenol. Radium Ther. Nucl. Med., *94*:142, 1967.
305. Kido, C., Sasaki, T., and Kaneko, M.: Angiography of primary liver cancer. Am. J. Roentgenol. Radium Ther. Nucl. Med., *113*:70, 1971.
306. Jewel, K. L.: Primary carcinoma of the liver: Clinical and radiologic manifestations. Am. J. Roentgenol. Radium Ther. Nucl. Med., *113*:84, 1971.
307. Man, B., Kraus, L., and Pikielny, S.: Catheterization of the umbilical vein and its use for hepatography. Clin. Radiol. *32*:350, 1971.
308. Kurtz, R. C., et al.: Esophageal varices secondary to primary and metastatic liver tumors. Arch. Intern. Med., *134*:50, 1974.

13

DISEASES OF NUTRITION

Kwashiorkor

Kwashiorkor results from inadequate protein intake and may cause damage to the autonomic nervous system, leading to alterations in the tone and motility of the entire gastrointestinal tract. Frequently there is ascites due to hypoproteinemia.

On progress meal studies of the small bowel, hypertonicity and hypermotility are often noted. Dilated, hypotonic and hypomotile small bowel loops, especially in the jejunum, are encountered in more severe cases. Areas of hypertonicity and hypotonicity may occur in the same individual. The radiographic pattern is often indistinguishable from the deficiency pattern found in many of the malabsorption syndromes.

On plain films there are usually multiple fluid levels in the small bowel loops and evidence of ascites.

In mild cases the small bowel rapidly returns to normal under treatment, but in more severe cases it may remain abnormal for many months after clinical recovery.

Retarded bone growth with small tubular bones and thinned cortices is often associated.[1, 2]

Rickets and Osteomalacia

The bone changes of osteomalacia due to vitamin D deficiency in adults are discussed under *Osteomalacia,* page 1324.

Failure of calcium deposition in growing bone causes the alterations of bone seen in rickets. Calcium deficiency produces demineralization of many secondary bony trabeculae and prominence of the primary trabeculae, so that the bone appears demineralized and coarse. These changes are most marked in areas of very rapid bone growth.

In the zone of provisional calcification (the metaphyseal end), failure of calcium deposition leads to overgrowth of noncalcified osteoid tissue. The consequent fraying of the metaphyseal end produces a cupped appearance, and the normally sharp, dense metaphyseal line disappears. The increase in uncalcified osteoid tissue leads to widening of the lucent space between the metaphysis and epiphysis (epiphyseal line). This is a characteristic roentgenologic finding.

Excessive osteoid tissue in the anterior rib ends causes thickening of the anterior borders—the rachitic rosary. Bowing of the dimineralized long bones may develop. Softening of the skull may also cause deformity. Fontanelle closure is often delayed.

In severe rickets there may be pseudofractures similar to those seen in osteomalacia in the adult. Thin stripe shadows resembling periosteal calcifications may be seen. These are actually zones of poorly calcified osteoid tissue arising from the periosteum.

Rickets due to renal tubular dystrophy or intestinal malabsorption produces identical roentgenologic findings.

During the healing phase, periosteal new bone formation is frequently seen. There is recalcification of the provisional zone of calcification. The epiphyseal centers regain their normal sharpness of outline and density. Remineralization of the skeleton may take months, and the deformities from bowing and fractures may be the only residual evidence of the disease.[3]

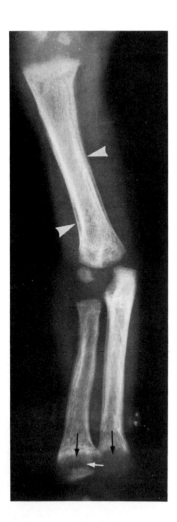

Figure 13–1 **Active Rickets.** Layers of subperiosteal calcification are best seen in the humerus *(arrowheads)* and are due to calcification in subperiosteal osteoid tissue. The typical frayed cupped metaphysis *(black arrows)* and the widened space between the epiphysis and metaphysis *(white arrow)* are prominent signs.

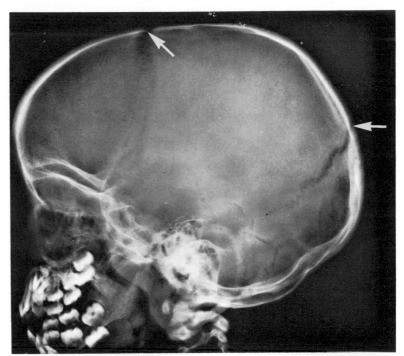

Figure 13–2 **Active Rickets.** In a 2½ year old child, the fontanelles *(arrows)* are still open, a common finding in active rickets.

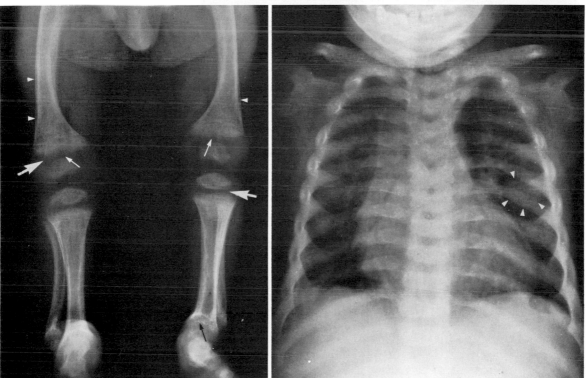

A   B

Figure 13–3 **Advanced Rickets.**

   A, The long bones are demineralized, and the trabeculae are coarsened in a two year old child. The metaphyseal ends are broadened, frayed, and irregular *(small arrows)*. The usually sharp metaphyseal line of density is absent, and the distal tibial metaphyses are cupped *(black arrow)*. There is increased space between the metaphysis and epiphysis *(large arrows)*. The femora are bowed, with thickened cortices medially. Periosteal layering *(arrowheads)* in the femora represents early healing with vitamin D therapy.

   B, Bulbous enlargement of the anterior ends of the ribs, mainly osteoid tissue *(arrowheads)*, is often seen. There is marked osseous demineralization and coarsened trabeculae.

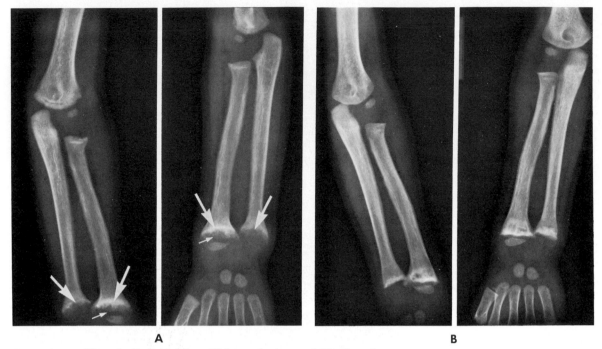

Figure 13-4 **Vitamin D Deficiency Rickets: Active and Healing Stages.**

A, The patient was 2½ years old. Characteristic changes of active rickets are demonstrated in the wrists. The metaphyses are cupped, frayed, broadened, and irregular *(large arrows);* the space between the metaphyses and epiphyses *(small arrows)* is widened—possibly the most diagnostic finding in active rickets. All the bones are demineralized to some extent, and the trabeculae are coarsened; this is seen most clearly on comparison with later films.

B, Six months after vitamin D therapy, the metaphyses are less cupped and frayed, and they are narrower. Although some irregularities persist, the metaphyses will become normal with further growth.

This distance between metaphysis and epiphysis is normal, indicating disappearance of the excess noncalcified osteoid tissue, and the bones have recovered their normal mineral density.

Beriberi

In well-advanced disease, there will be nonspecific cardiac enlargement and pulmonary changes of congestive failure and pleural effusions. Right heart failure is common.

In less severe or earlier cases, cardiac enlargement with increased arterial vasculature and prominent pulmonary arteries—the high output heart—may be seen. This is due to peripheral vasodilatation with a rapid circulation time and increased venous return.

A rapid and dramatic decrease in heart size usually occurs after thiamine therapy.[4]

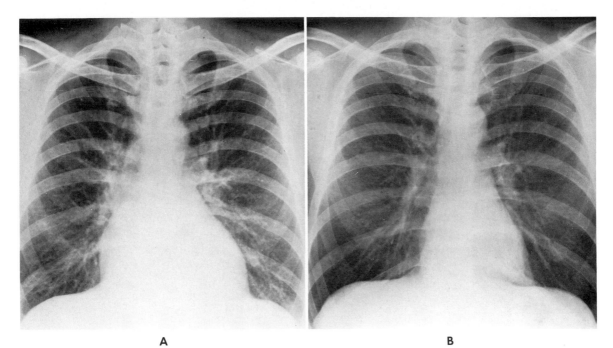

A   B

Figure 13–5   **Beriberi Associated with Chronic Alcoholism.**

A, The heart is moderately enlarged. The pulmonary arterial vasculature is prominent, and extends to the lung periphery *(best seen at the right base in this film).* No congestive failure has occurred.

B, Following prolonged vitamin B₁ therapy, the heart and vasculature have returned to normal proportions.

Scurvy

The fundamental changes are caused by osteoporosis and hemorrhage resulting from vitamin C deficiency. Diffuse demineralization with trabecular loss leads to a ground-glass appearance of bone. The cortices are thinned, and the zone of provisional calcification at the metaphyseal ends remains dense—the white line of scurvy. The prominent cortex of the demineralized epiphysis provides the important ring sign of this disease. Changes around the metaphysis are characteristic: a zone of rarefaction is seen proximal to the dense metaphyseal line, and lateral extension of the zone of provisional calcification gives rise to spur-like projections. Weakening of the submetaphyseal zone may cause fracture and, ultimately, subluxation of the zone of provisional calcification and the epiphysis.

Subperiosteal hemorrhage along the the shafts of the long bones is not uncommon; these hemorrhages calcify during the course of therapy. The bones become normal following adequate treatment.[5]

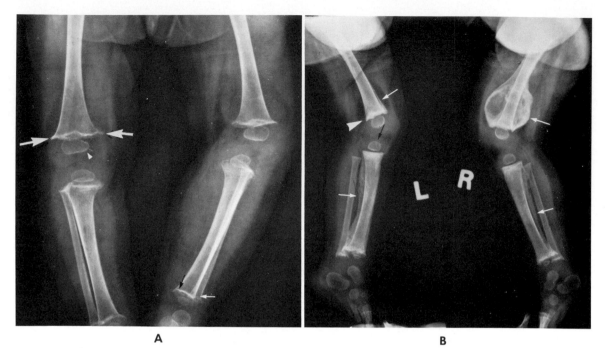

A   B

Figure 13–6 **Active Scurvy: Two Infants.**

   A, The usual roentgenologic findings of active scurvy are demonstrated. All the bones show ground-glass demineralization, with thinned cortices. The white line of scurvy is demonstrated most clearly in the lower left tibia *(black arrow)*. The spur-like extensions of the zone of provisional calcification are present in all the bones *(large white arrows)*. Submetaphyseal rarefaction is best seen in the lower tibia and fibula *(small white arrow)*. The cortical ring around the epiphyses is fairly prominent *(arrowhead)*. No subperiosteal hemorrhages are apparent.

   B, A second infant was undergoing treatment for scurvy, but characteristic bone changes are still present. These include the white line and metaphyseal spurring *(arrowhead)*, calcifying subperiosteal hemorrhages in both femora and tibiae, but most extensive in the right femur *(white arrows)*, ring epiphyses *(black arrow)*, and ground-glass osteoporosis of all the bones.

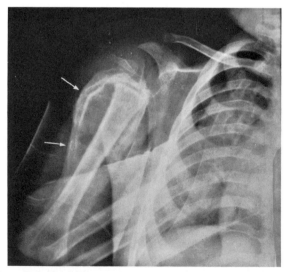

Figure 13–7 **Scurvy: Healing: Calcified Hemorrhage.**   White arrows point out the bowed calcification at the border of a large subperiosteal hemorrhage in the right upper humerus. Other bone changes have regressed with treatment.

Obesity

Layers of subcutaneous fat, readily recognized on radiograms, appear as relatively lucent areas in comparision with muscular and other nonfatty soft tissues.

In the moderately to severely obese person, the diaphragms are usually elevated and the basal pulmonary markings may be accentuated. The heart assumes a transverse position, sometimes simulating cardiomegaly. Prominent pericardial fat pads are frequently noted. The radiographic findings in conditions associated with obesity, such as Cushing's disease and hypothyroidism, are discussed elsewhere. (See text under headings of underlying disorder.)

Pickwickian obesity, which is associated with hypoxia, carbon dioxide retention, and secondary polycythemia, can result in cor pulmonale and pulmonary hypertension. The main pulmonary arteries are dilated, and eventually cardiac enlargement from right ventricular hypertrophy and dilatation can ensue. As the pulmonary hypertension becomes more marked, a disparity between central and peripheral vasculature may be observed.[6]

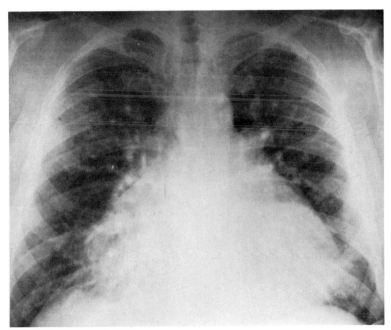

Figure 13–8 **Pickwickian Obesity with Polycythemia.** The heart is considerably enlarged, mainly from right ventricular dilatation. In addition to cor pulmonale there is prominence of the peripheral vessels, especially at the bases, due to the polycythemia and hypervolemia.

REFERENCES

1. Kowalski, R.: Roentgenologic studies of the alimentary tract in kwashiorkor. Am. J. Roentgenol. Radium Ther. Nucl. Med., *100*:100, 1967.
2. Adams, P., and Berridge, F. R.: Effects of kwashiorkor on cortical and trabecular bone. Arch. Dis. Child., 44:705, 1969.
3. Bromer, R. S., and Harvey, R. M.: Roentgen diagnosis of rickets. Radiology, *51*:1, 1948.
4. Reverdy, H. J., Jr.: Beriberi heart disease. Circulation, *19*:275, 1959.
5. Ellenbogen, L. S., et al.: Roentgen findings in diagnosis and management of infantile scurvy. J. Med. Soc. N. J., *48*:73, 1951.
6. Burwell, C. S., et al.: Pickwickian syndrome. Am. J. Med., *21*:811, 1956.

HEMATOLOGIC AND HEMATOPOIETIC DISEASES

THE ANEMIAS

Megaloblastic Anemia

In pernicious anemia, radiographic evidence of gastric atrophy (atrophic gastritis) is seen in about 80 per cent of cases. In megaloblastic anemia due to malabsorption, small bowel changes may be present.

In gastric atrophy the stomach is often long and tubular, and the rugae on the greater curvature are either small or absent, especially when the stomach is distended with barium. The fundus is frequently somewhat narrow and is generally smooth or "bald," owing to the absence of the usually prominent rugal folds. In the partially gas-filled fundus the barium produces a characteristic speckled appearance in the erect position at the barium-air interface in over 75 per cent of cases; the exact cause is unknown.

In the partially barium-filled stomach the longitudinal folds may not appear abnormal, but the transverse folds along the greater curvature are thin, crenated, and regularly patterned, in contrast to the usual heavy irregular folds of a normal stomach. This is best appreciated on erect films.

A greater than normal incidence of gastric polyps occurs in patients with pernicious anemia (over 4 per cent).

In cases of megaloblastic anemia due to intestinal malabsorption, studies of the small intestine may reveal a sprue-like pattern (see p. 978), or may disclose a specific cause of the malabsorption, such as blind intestinal loop, multiple jejunal diverticulosis, or infiltrative disease of the small intestine (e.g., lymphosarcoma, scleroderma, or Whipple's disease). Malabsorption is discussed under *Diseases of Malabsorption,* p. 974).

Roentgen evidence of atrophic gastritis without pernicious anemia is often found in elderly individuals (see *Gastritis*, p. 937). Conversely, the absence of such gastric findings in a patient with a megaloblastic anemia should prompt a search of the small bowel for roentgen evidence of changes associated with malabsorption or other small bowel disease.[1-4]

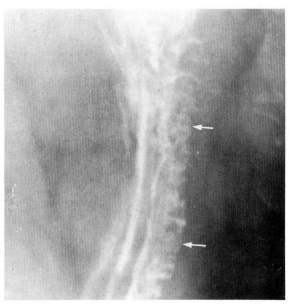

Figure 14–1 **Pernicious Anemia: Atrophic Gastritis.** Erect film of partially filled stomach shows the gastric folds on the midportion of the greater curvature *(arrows)* to be small, thin, and regular, so that the border of the curvature is fairly smooth. Normally the folds on the greater curvature are large, uneven, and irregular.

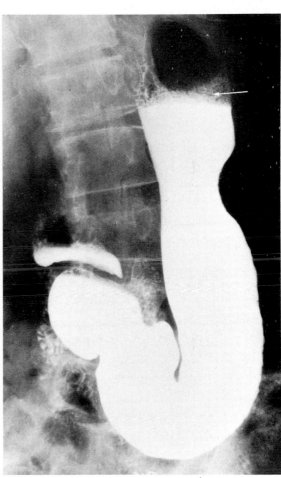

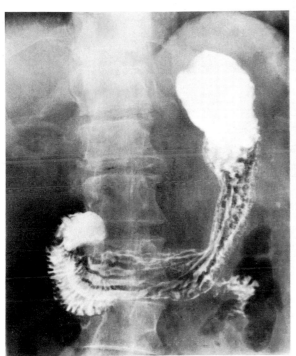

A   B

Figure 14–2 **Pernicious Anemia: Atrophic Gastritis.**

A, The longitudinal folds in the partially distended stomach appear normal, but the transverse folds along the greater curvature are abnormally small, thin, and even, similar to those in the preceding figure. Note the smooth "bald" fundus.

B, After further distention with barium with the patient in erect posture, the stomach appears long, the fundus is narrow, and almost no folds are seen. The speckled appearance at the air-barium interface *(arrow)* is a frequent and characteristic finding in atrophic gastritis. (Courtesy B. F. Vaughn, Perth, W. Australia.)

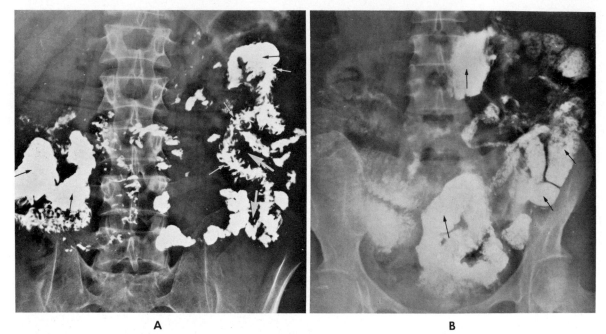

A   B

Figure 14–3 **Megaloblastic Anemia: Malabsorption and Small Bowel Changes in Two Patients.**

Varying degrees of the small bowel malabsorption pattern are illustrated in two patients with non-tropical sprue.

A, Segmentation of the barium column is pronounced; only a few loops are dilated and patternless *(black arrows)*. The mucosal folds are thickened *(small white arrows)* and the space between the loops is widened due to the thickened walls *(large white arrows)*.

B, The dilated and patternless barium collections (moulage) are more pronounced *(arrows)*. Mucosal thickening, segmentation, and thickening of the bowel walls are not prominent.

Aplastic Anemia (Fanconi Syndrome)

The syndrome consists of refractory hypoplastic anemia, often with pancy-topenia, brown pigmentation of the skin, and associated multiple congenital anomalies. It is apparently hereditary and familial. Abnormalities include dwarf-ism, hypogenitalism with retarded bone age, microcephaly, renal anomalies, and skeletal deformities of varying severity.

The most common skeletal abnormalities are an absent or hypoplastic thumb and anomalies of the radial side of the wrist; these occur in the majority of cases. Hypoplasia of one or more of the bones of the hand is seen in almost half the cases. A hypoplastic or absent radius is not uncommon. Minor anomalies of the feet or spine are extremely common. In about one fourth of the cases osteoporosis is present. Renal anomalies are found in about 25 per cent of cases and include aplas-tic, horseshoe, or ectopic kidneys.

In a child or young adult with an aplastic or hypoplastic anemia, the presence of the deformities on the radial side of the hand or wrist, in association with re-tarded bone age, short stature, renal anomalies, or microcephaly occurring either alone or in combination, should suggest the diagnosis of Fanconi anemia.[5-8]

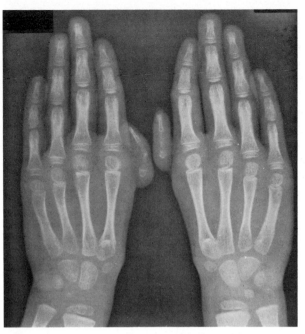

Figure 14–4 **Congenital Aplastic Anemia in a 6½ Year Old Boy.** There are extremely small rudimentary thumbs bilaterally. Skeletal bone age is retarded, as evidenced by the decrease in expected number of ossified carpal bones.

Rudimentary thumbs or anomalies of the radial side of the wrist, and delayed skeletal maturation are among the most frequent abnormalities in children with Fanconi syndrome. (Courtesy Dr. J. H. Juhl, Madison, Wisconsin.)

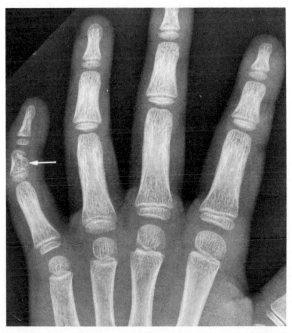

Figure 14–5 **Congenital Aplastic Anemia (Fanconi Syndrome).** The fifth finger is curved, with a deformed and hypoplastic middle phalanx *(arrow)*. The patient's older sister had a similar deformity, as well as aplastic anemia. Neither had pigmented skin.

Myelophthisic Anemia

The cell-forming function of bone marrow can be significantly impaired by space-occupying lesions, encroachment resulting from cortical thickening, or replacement by nonhematopoietic tissue. Both malignant and benign lesions of bone marrow may produce changes in the bones, which occasionally may be characteristic of the underlying disease. Extensive metastases to bone, especially from the breast or prostate, and multiple myeloma are frequent causes of the anemia. Less commonly, myelofibrosis, reticuloendotheliosis, and osteopetrosis can cause replacement of hematopoietic tissue in the marrow. In severe myelophthisic anemia, splenic enlargement from extramedullary hematopoiesis often occurs.

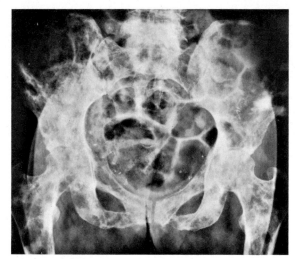

Figure 14–6 **Myelophthisic Anemia: Metastatic Carcinoma from Breast.** The pelvis, lumbar spine, and upper femora are riddled with osteolytic and osteoblastic metastatic lesions.

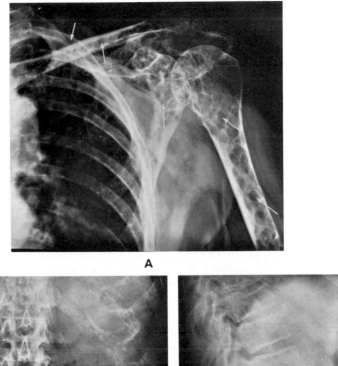

A

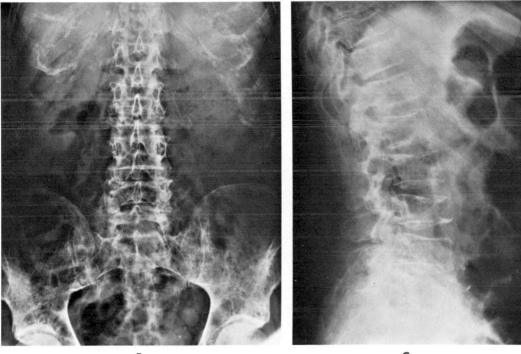

B   C

Figure 14–7 **Myelophthisic Anemia Associated with Widespread Multiple Myeloma.**

A, Extensive osteolytic lesions of various sizes *(arrows)* are seen in the humerus, scapula, ribs, and clavicles.

B, There are similar lesions of the pelvis and sacrum.

C, The lumbar bodies appear greatly demineralized because of extensive medullary myelomatous tissue. Compression fractures have produced deformities of T10 and L3.

Early myelomatous infiltration of the vertebral bodies often gives rise initially to an osteoporotic appearance indistinguishable from that of senile osteoporosis. Later, more characteristic destructive changes are observed.

Replacement of hematopoietic tissue in the skull, pelvis, ribs, vertebrae, and ends of the long bones by myelomatous tissue has resulted in severe myelophthisic anemia.

Iron Deficiency Anemia (Hypochromic Anemia)

No radiographic bone changes are usually seen in iron deficiency anemia occurring in adults. However, with persistent and chronic anemia (less than 5 g. hemoglobin) the picture of a high output heart may develop. Dilatation of the right and, to a lesser extent, the left ventricle may occur, and fullness may develop in the main pulmonary artery segment.

When anemia begins in infancy or childhood and is severe and prolonged, there may be bone changes similar to, but less severe than, those seen in Cooley's anemia or hereditary spherocytosis. Hyperplasia of the marrow causes widening of the skull diploë and thinning of the outer table. Other bones, particularly those in the hand, may show osteoporosis and coarsened trabeculae. The changes may persist into adult life if the anemia continues. Such findings are uncommon except in areas where nutritional anemia is prevalent and untreated.

In the Plummer-Vinson syndrome, one or more anterior webs (sideropenic web) of the upper esophagus are often seen radiographically, usually associated with dysphagia. This syndrome is commonly described in females but can also occur in males. An increased tendency to develop esophageal carcinoma is said to be associated with sideropenic web, but this point is still unresolved. Esophageal webs can also occur in individuals without dysphagia or anemia, and appear to be without significance in these cases. Detection of some webs may require cineradiography, since the constriction may be a transient phenomenon.[8-11]

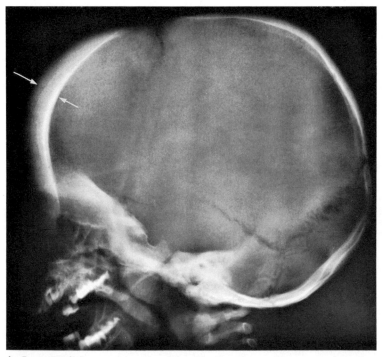

Figure 14–8 **Chronic Iron Deficiency Anemia: The Skull**   The patient was 3 years old. There is a definite increase in the width of the diploetic space *(arrows)*. The external table is thinned and difficult to identify.

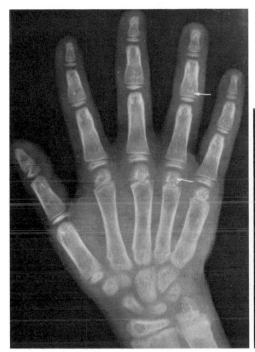

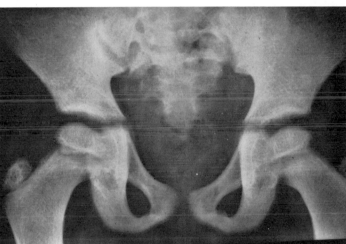

A   B

Figure 14-9   **Chronic Iron Deficiency Anemia: Bone Changes.**

The nutritional anemia of this child had existed since early childhood. The red blood cell count was 2.1 million, and the hemoglobin was 4 g.

A, The bones of the hand are osteoporotic; the marrow cavities are somewhat widened, and the cortices are thinned. The trabeculae are coarsened *(arrows).*

B, There is marked coarsening of the trabeculae throughout the bones of the pelvis and the upper femora.

The bone changes are identical to those seen in severe hemolytic anemia and Cooley's anemia. (Courtesy Dr. M. Aksoy, Istanbul, Turkey.)

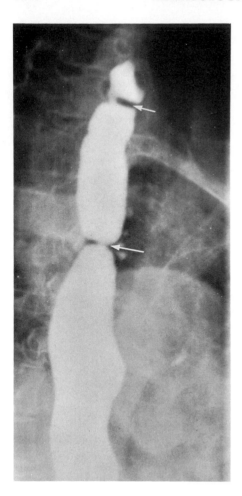

Figure 14–10   **Iron Deficiency Anemia with Sideropenic Webs.** Two thin concentric bands of constriction are seen in the barium-filled esophagus *(arrows)*. The upper web is in the cervical esophagus just below the pharyngoesophageal junction; the lower is in the upper thoracic esophagus. The constricted area is the anterior portion of the esophagus *(upper web)*, whereas in a cricopharyngeal web the constriction is usually in the posterior portion.

Dysphagia is a prominent symptom in patients with sideropenic webs.

HEMOLYTIC DISORDERS

Hereditary Spherocytosis

Bone changes result from hyperplasia of the marrow due to compensatory erythropoietic activity. Changes occur only in severe and prolonged cases of anemia and are consequently less frequent and less severe than the bone changes seen in Cooley's anemia or sickle cell anemia. The most common finding is a widened diploë in the skull. Frequently the trabeculae appear perpendicular and striated, producing the hair-on-end appearance. Changes in the long bones are infrequent. Rarely, in severe cases masses of extramedullary hematopoiesis are seen in the posterior mediastinum.[8, 12]

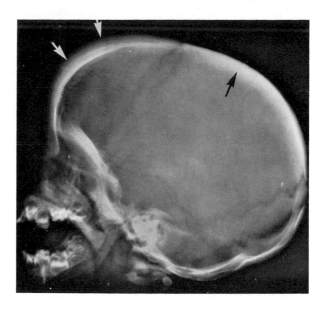

Figure 14-11 **Hereditary Spherocytosis in Infant.** The diploë of the skull is widened, and there are fine perpendicular bony striae in the outer table *(white arrows).* In the parietal area *(black arrow),* thickening of the table is also a reaction to the hyperplastic marrow. These findings are nonspecific and can occur in any severe anemia of infancy or childhood in which there is prolonged compensatory hyperplasia of the bone marrow.

Chronic Hemolytic Anemia with Paroxysmal Nocturnal Hemoglobinuria

Radiographic changes are not seen unless prolonged and severe hemolysis leads to deposition of iron in the kidneys, in which case there is increased density of the renal shadows.[13]

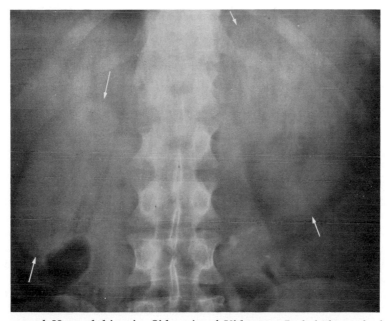

Figure 14-12 **Paroxysmal Hemoglobinuria: Siderosis of Kidneys.** Both kidney shadows are sharp and distinct *(arrows);* even the upper poles are clearly defined. Such increased radiopacity is due to deposits of hemosiderin in the renal tubules. However, density changes are difficult to interpret since they vary with radiographic technique.

Sickle Cell Disease

Most of the roentgen changes in sickle cell disease are the result of chronic anemia or of focal ischemia due to sludging of red cells. Anemia causes bone marrow hyperplasia and often cardiac enlargement. Red cell sludgings can cause ischemia and infarction in various tissues.

In the bones, marrow hyperplasia causes osteoporosis, widening of the medullary cavity, and cortical thinning. The secondary trabeculae are resorbed, and the remaining primary trabeculae are thickened, giving a coarsened texture. The bones, however, often appear dense radiologically owing to the thickened primary trabeculae.

These changes are most striking in growing bones. The appearance of the long bones and skull is similar to but less marked than Cooley's anemia (thalassemia). A characteristic biconcave deformity of the vertebral bodies may be due to nucleus pulposus impressions on softened vertebral bodies and/or to ischemic changes in the vertebral end plates. These vertebral changes persist into adult life, while other bone changes due to marrow hyperplasias tend to disappear.

Infarcts can occur in the metaphyses and diaphyses of long bones. If extensive, there may be lytic changes, often with periosteal reaction, simulating an acute osteomyelitis. In the hands or feet, lytic areas in widened bones with thinned cortex produce the characteristic sickle cell dactylitis. Ischemic aseptic necrosis may appear in the humeral or femoral heads. Characteristic calcifications eventually appear in the medullary infarcted areas. In adults, especially those with SC disease, there may be cortical thickening in the long bones, perhaps an end result of extensive previous cortical infarcts.

Osteomyelitis is a common complication. It is often diaphyseal and is frequently caused by salmonella. It may be superimposed upon a recent infarction or may follow a sicklemic abdominal crisis with focal areas of bowel infarction and subsequent salmonella bacteremia. The inflammatory lytic areas and periosteal reaction may resemble and be indistinguishable from acute bone infarction. Fracture of bones involved by infarction and/or osteomyelitis can occur.

The most frequent urographic finding is blunting of the calices. This occurs in about 75 per cent of cases and is due not to chronic pyelonephritis but to pericaliceal fibrosis secondary to vascular stasis. The cortical tissue is usually not thinned and the renal outline is regular, in contrast to chronic pyelonephritis. In some cases a central type of papillary necrosis occurs, with extension of contrast material from the center of the calix. Some degree of renal enlargement appears in about 35 per cent of cases. A progressive glomerular degeneration can also occur, leading occasionally to uremia. Angiography may reveal focal cortical hypertrophy and/or areas of cortical thinning and medullary hypertrophy. Sometimes, scar formation and an irregularly pruned vascular tree are seen.

During a sickle cell abdominal crisis, there may be dilated small bowel loops, owing to a paralytic ileus.

Gallstone formation, apparently due to repeated episodes of hemolysis, occurs in about half the cases. Splenic enlargement can occur in SC disease, but in SS disease repeated splenic infarctions lead to progressive shrinkage and ultimate autosplenectomy.

Cardiomegaly is the most frequent abnormality seen on the chest film and is probably secondary to severe anemia and elevated cardiac output. The ascending aorta and aortic arch may become prominent. A pneumonia, often pneumococcal, is a common complication and is the most frequent cause of hospitalization. Pulmonary infarction may produce pleural pneumonia, especially at the bases. Repeated episodes of infarction can lead to parenchymal fibrosis. Cor pulmonale and pulmonary hypertension may eventually develop.

All the roentgen changes of SS disease can occur in SC disease and also in sickle cell–beta thalassemia disease, but with decreased frequency and severity.[8, 14–21]

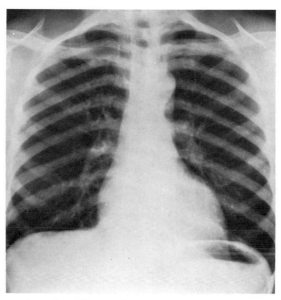

Figure 14–13 **Sickle Cell Anemia: The Ribs.** The ribs have a coarsened trabecular pattern. The anterior ribs may appear as dense as, or denser than, the posterior ribs, a nonspecific but suggestive finding.

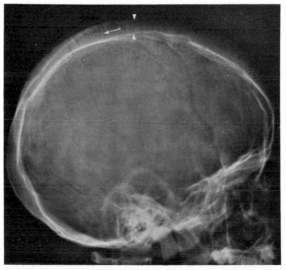

Figure 14–14 **Sickle Cell Anemia: The Skull.** There is increased width of the diploetic space (*arrow*), vertical trabecular striations (*arrowheads*), and thinning of the outer table. These changes, caused by marrow hyperplasia, are nonspecific and are seen in any severe childhood anemia in which there is erythropoietic activity, such as Cooley's anemia, spherocytosis, and severe iron deficiency anemia. These skull changes do not occur in anemia that begins in adult life.

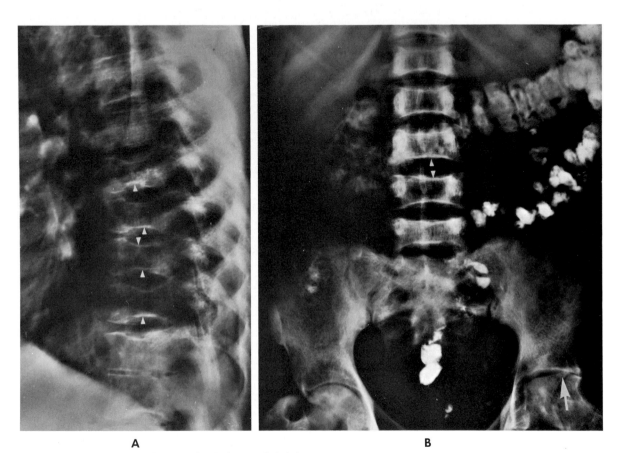

A   B

Figure 14–15   **Sickle Cell Anemia: Spine and Pelvis.**

A, Lateral view demonstrates demineralization of the dorsal bodies and thinning of the end plates. Biconcave deformities *(arrowheads)* are caused by pressure of the nucleus pulposus on the softened bodies. These findings are characteristic.

B, Anteroposterior view of the pelvis and lumbar spine reveals demineralization and trabecular coarsening. There are biconcave deformities of the vertebrae *(arrowheads).*

The articular surface of the left femoral head is irregular and flattened *(arrow),* and there is irregularity of the joint space. These femoral changes are caused by ischemic aseptic necrosis.

Demineralization and trabecular coarsening of bone, deformities of the vertebrae, and changes of aseptic necrosis are all characteristic of sickle cell anemia.

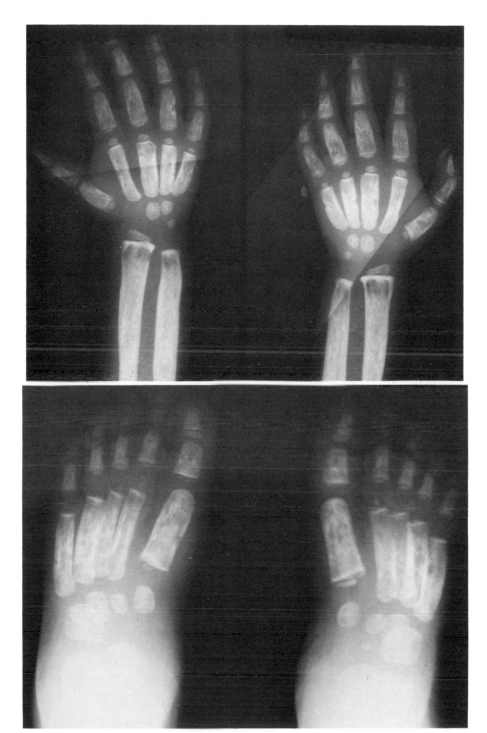

Figure 14–16 **Sickle Cell Dactylitis in a 2 Year Old.** All the long bones of both hands and feet are widened and have thinned cortices. Mottled rarefaction is seen in all the bones, including the bones of the forearms.

The medullary expansion and cortical thinning are due to the excess hematopoietic tissue, but the mottled rarefaction is due to diffuse bone infarction.

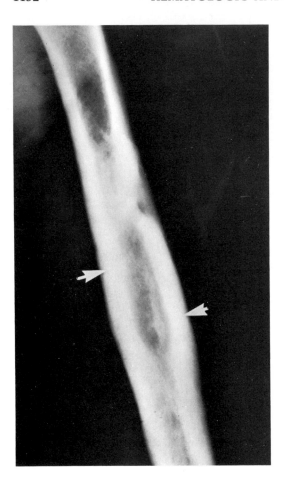

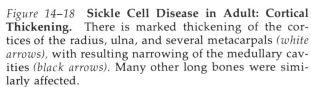

Figure 14–17 **Sickle Cell Anemia: Salmonella Osteo-myelitis.** The humeral shaft is widened, with marked cortical thickening *(arrows)*, and an irregularly narrowed medullary cavity.

The picture is characteristic of chronic osteomyelitis. The causative organism was salmonella; the involvement is diaphyseal, rather than metaphyseal as is usual in ordinary coccal osteopmyelitis.

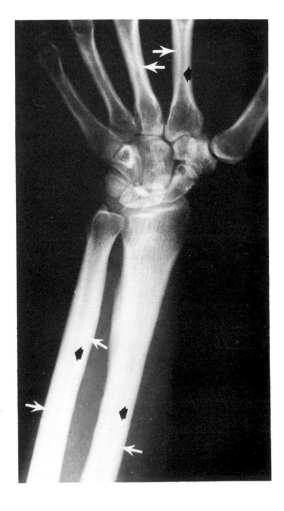

Figure 14–18 **Sickle Cell Disease in Adult: Cortical Thickening.** There is marked thickening of the cortices of the radius, ulna, and several metacarpals *(white arrows)*, with resulting narrowing of the medullary cavities *(black arrows)*. Many other long bones were similarly affected.

The cortical thickening is probably the late result of periosteal bone infarcts during childhood.

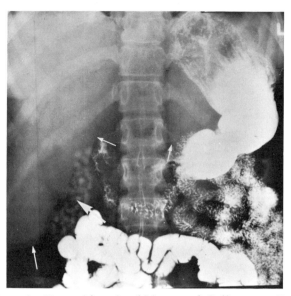

Figure 14–19   **Sickle Cell Anemia: Hemosiderosis of Liver, and Gallstones.**   Repeated and frequent sickle cell hemolytic crises in a young woman have led to deposition of hemosiderin in the liver. These iron deposits have increased the radiographic density of the enlarged liver, causing unusually good visualization of the liver borders *(small arrows).*

Gallstones *(large arrow)* are probably due to repeated hemolysis and increased bilirubin excretion. It is not unusual for young patients with congenital hemolytic anemias to develop gallstones.

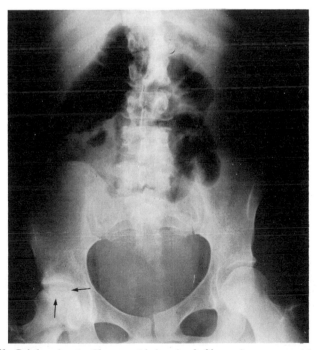

Figure 14–20   **Sickle Cell Crisis: Acute Ileus.**   Abdominal film of a young black male with acute abdominal pain and fever discloses several greatly distended small bowel loops in the upper abdomen. Fluid levels were seen in the erect posture. Ordinarily, such findings are due either to a "sentinal" ileus from an adjacent acute inflammation (pancreatitis, cholecystitis, or appendicitis) or to a mechanical small bowel obstruction. In the case shown here, the associated finding of aseptic necrosis—lucent lines across the femoral head—in the right femoral head *(arrows)* suggests the correct diagnosis of acute ileus associated with a sickle cell crisis.

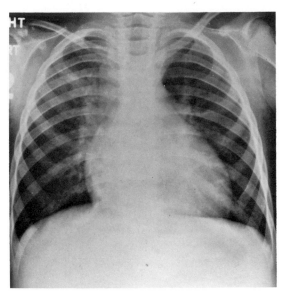

Figure 14–21 **Sickle Cell Anemia: Cardiomegaly.**   There is marked cardiac enlargement with increased hilar vascularity and a prominent pulmonary conus. The anterior ribs are somewhat dense and prominent.

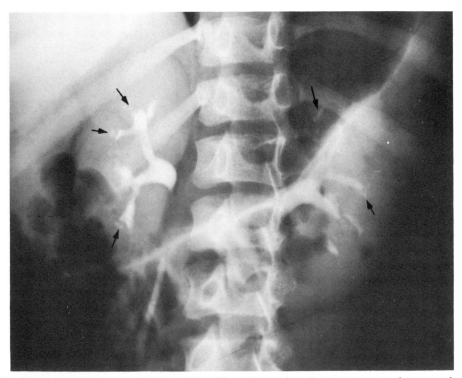

Figure 14–22 **Sickle Cell Disease with Renal Papillary Necrosis.**   Intravenous pyelogram of an 8 year old boy with sickle cell disease reveals irregularities of all the calices, with small collections of contrast material extending from many of the calices *(arrows)*.
    Papillary necrosis is apparently more frequently encountered in SC than in SS disease.

Thalassemia Major (Cooley's Anemia)

Bone changes are caused by erythropoietic hyperplasia of the bone marrow in response to the anemia and are the most marked of all the findings in childhood anemias. The cortices are thinned, the medullary cavities are expanded, and many secondary trabeculae are resorbed, producing osteoporosis. Focal collections of hyperplastic marrow can cause local radiolucencies. Some primary trabeculae are thickened, causing coarsened bone texture. In the long bones a loss of the normal modeling in the shafts leads to a squared-off or even a biconcave appearance.

In the skull the diploë is widened, the outer table is displaced and thinned, and the vertical trabeculations often exhibit a "hair-on-end" appearance. Characteristically there is retarded or absent aeration of the paranasal sinuses and temporal bones secondary to the marrow hyperplasia. A disproportionate overgrowth of the maxilla may lead to a mongoloid type of facies.

The vertebrae are osteoporotic and coarsely trabeculated. The ribs have thinned cortices and may develop a rib-within-a-rib appearance. Bulbous expansion of the most posterior segment of a rib is almost a pathognomonic finding.

Premature fusion of the epiphyses is common and often is only partial, leading to some deformities.

Extramedullary hematopoiesis is common and widespread, leading to hepatomegaly, splenomegaly, and lymph node enlargement. Paravertebral masses of hematopoietic tissue, usually multiple but occasionally solitary, are often seen. These are lobular and well circumscribed masses, usually between T2 and T11.

Complications include hemochromatosis, pericardial and myocardial abnormalities, hyperuricemia, and bilirubin stones.

Thalassemia minor and hemoglobin C, S, H, and E diseases have similar but less-marked roentgen changes.

In infants and children, alterations may be seen in all bones, but only changes in the skull, spine, and pelvis persist into adult life.[8, 22, 23]

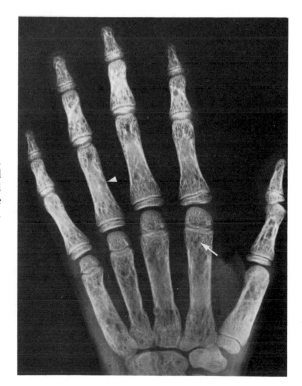

Figure 14–23 **Thalassemia Major: Hand and Wrist.** There is pronounced coarsening of the trabeculae of all bones of the hand and wrist. Osteoporosis *(arrows)* and thinning of the cortices *(arrowhead)* are evident. The abnormal modeling is due to expansion of the shafts. These changes may regress during adolescence.

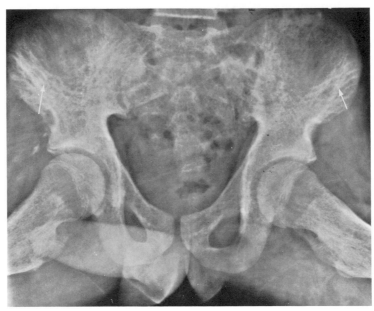

Figure 14–24 **Thalassemia Major: Pelvis.** In a 16 year old boy there is marked coarsening of the trabeculae and osteoporosis *(arrows)* of the entire pelvis. Cortical thinning is pronounced in the ilia but less marked in the upper femora.

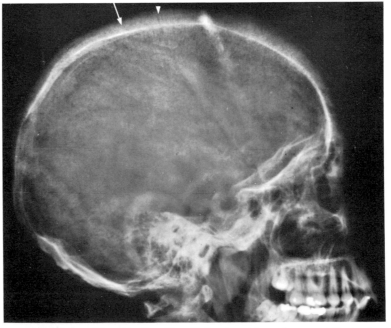

Figure 14–25 **Thalassemia Major: The Skull.** The diploë is widened, especially in the frontal and parietal areas *(arrow)*. Perpendicular bone trabeculae produce striations, and the outer table is considerably thinned *(arrowhead)*.

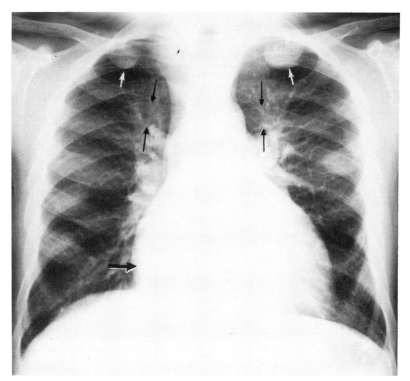

Figure 14–26 **Thalassemia Major: Rib Changes and Extramedullary Hematopoiesis.** The inner aspects of several upper ribs *(small black arrows)* are expanded, owing to local bone marrow hyperactivity. This is a fairly frequent finding in severe thalassemia. The distal ends of the first ribs *(white arrows)* are similarly expanded as a result of marrow activity.

The double density along the lower right cardiac border *(large black arrow)* was due to a mass of extramedullary hematopoiesis in the posterior mediastinum. (See lateral film in Figure 9–187).

Erythroblastosis Fetalis

Transverse bands of diminished density are seen just below the metaphyseal ends of the long bones in about 20 per cent of affected newborns. These changes, however, are nonspecific and are also found in many acute and chronic diseases of infancy.

Fetal hydrops due to erythroblastosis may be suggested by films of the abdomen taken late in pregnancy. The normally distinct fat line between the fetus and the placenta is obliterated by the edematous fetal soft tissues; this does not occur in hydramnios associated with other fetal abnormalities.

Less reliable roentgenologic findings include elevation of the fetal ribs resulting from enlargement of the heart and abdomen, displacement of the fetus from the midline due to enlargement of the fetal abdomen and placenta, abnormal position of the fetal extremities, or evidence of fetal death. These signs are all nonspecific unless associated with obliteration of the fetal fat line.[24, 25]

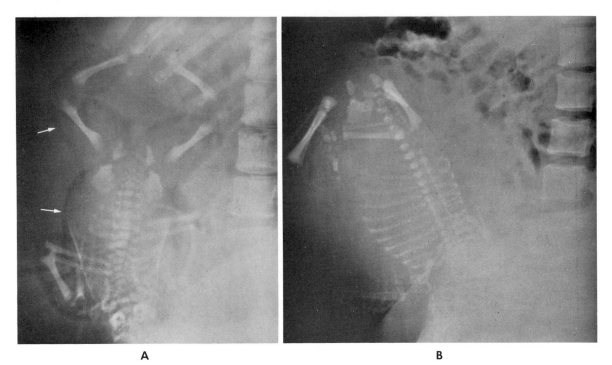

A　　　　　　　　　　　　　　　　　　B

Figure 14–27　**Erythroblastosis Fetalis with Fetal Hydrops in Utero: Absence of Fetal Fat Line.**

A, Lateral film of a normal pregnancy shows a distinct line of fat lucency *(arrows)* between the fetus and placenta. This fetal fat line remains unobliterated in other nonerythroblastotic fetal abnormalities.

B, No fetal fat line is seen in a case of fetal hydrops due to erythroblastosis. The fetal ribs are elevated because of enlargement of the fetal abdomen and heart.

HEMOCHROMATOSIS

Diffuse visceral deposition of iron can result either from increased intestinal absorption or from continued excessive ingestion. The former is usually due to a hereditary defect. The greatest iron concentration appears in the liver and spleen; in the idiopathic hereditary form there may also be sufficient deposition in the skin and pancreas to produce "bronzed diabetes."

Radiographically, the liver and spleen are enlarged; if their iron concentration is high, they may become more radiopaque than normal. Assessment of increased radiopacity of the liver and spleen masses may be difficult because of density variations from different radiographic techniques. If there is a substantial increase in radiodensity, all the borders of the liver and spleen become more distinct, and the upper border of the liver can be identified as a separate line distinct from the diaphragmatic density. Liver cirrhosis and its accompanying radiographic findings of esophageal varices and ascites may occur, but these are late and advanced findings.

Cardiomyopathy is a common complication, leading to cardiac enlargement and congestive failure.

Not infrequently, chondrocalcinosis is seen, especially in the wrists and metacarpophalangeal joints. Acute arthritic episodes may occur, similar to pseudogout. Chronic degenerative joint changes are frequent, with or without chondrocalcinosis.

Almost half of the patients show arthritic changes radiographically. Commonly, the second and third metacarpophalangeal joints are involved, with joint space narrowing, irregularity of articular surfaces, sclerosis, and subarticular cyst formation. Osteophytes are common. Other joints may be involved.

In the acquired form, which is seen most commonly in the Bantus, who ingest large quantities of iron-containing alcoholic beverages, almost 50 per cent of patients also develop a severe osteoporosis of the spine, often with vertebral collapse. The cause of the osteoporosis is uncertain but the condition may be due to hypogonadism secondary to severe liver dysfunction.

Hemochromatosis due to excess iron ingestion is often termed *hemosiderosis*. The latter term, however, would be more accurately limited to local tissue deposits of hemosiderin resulting from hemorrhage, venous congestion, or increased red cell hemolysis such as occurs in idiopathic pulmonary hemosiderosis (see p. 505), Goodpasture's syndrome (see p. 804), the lungs in mitral valvular disease (see Fig. 10–96), the kidneys in paroxysmal hemoglobinuria (see p. 1147), and the liver in sickle cell anemia (see Fig. 14–19).[13, 24-29]

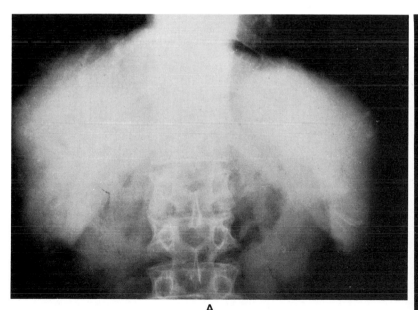

A

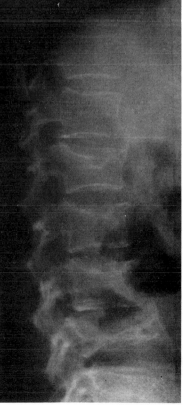

B

Figure 14–28 **Hemochromatosis (Hemosiderosis) and Osteoporosis in a Bantu.**

A, The enlargement and extraordinary density of the liver and spleen are due to diffuse iron deposits.

B, Lateral film of the lumbar spine demonstrates marked osteoporosis and multiple compression fractures of the lumbar bodies.

Up to one half of Bantus who develop hemosiderosis show some degree of spinal osteoporosis. (Courtesy N. Joffe, Johannesburg, South Africa.)

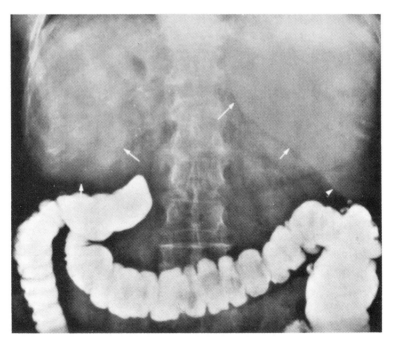

Figure 14–29 **Hemochromatosis: Splenomegaly and Hepatomegaly.** The increased density of the enlarged liver and spleen is evident from the distinct borders *(arrows)* of these organs in contrast to the adjacent soft tissues. Both flexures of the colon are displaced downward.

POLYCYTHEMIA

Primary Polycythemia (Polycythemia Vera)

An increased number of red cells, white cells, and platelets occur in primary polycythemia.

The increased blood volume in this condition can result in increased pulmonary vascularity, manifested by dilated vessels extending to the lung peripheries. In about one fifth of cases the lung fields reveal one or more areas of atelectasis, fibrosis, or focal consolidation, due to recent or old infarctions from intravascular thrombosis. The heart is not enlarged unless systemic hypertension develops. Distended pulmonary vessels without cardiomegaly are somewhat suggestive of primary polycythemia.

Splenomegaly can be detected radiographically in about half the cases. Long-standing polycythemia is sometimes complicated by myelofibrosis; the bones may then become sclerotic.[30]

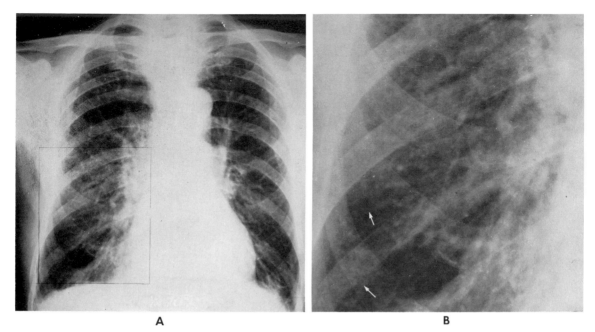

A   B

Figure 14–30 **Primary Polycythemia: Vascular Changes.**

A, There is an increase in the number and width of the vascular shadows from the hila to the periphery. The heart is not enlarged.

B, The extreme vascular distention is more clearly seen in enlarged view of the right lower lung field. The patient's packed red cell volume was 70 per cent. (Courtesy Drs. R. G. Pitman and R. E. Steiner, London, England.)

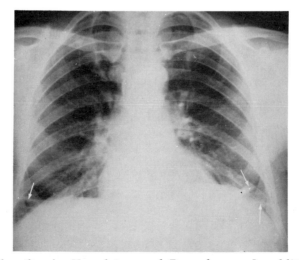

Figure 14–31 **Primary Polycythemia: Vasculature and Parenchyma.** In addition to an increase in the number and width of the vascular shadows (best seen at the bases), there are bands of density in both lower lung fields *(arrows).* These are probably residua of earlier pulmonary infarcts. There is no cardiac enlargement.

Secondary Polycythemia

Secondary polycythemia can occur in chronic anoxic states such as high altitude habitation, chronic lung disease, and congenital cyanotic heart disease. Other conditions that can cause secondary polycythemia include renal cell carcinoma (1 to 4 per cent of cases), hepatoma (up to 10 per cent of cases), cerebellar hemangioblastoma (10 to 20 per cent of cases), renal adenoma or cyst (rarely), and uterine fibroids. Only the red cells are significantly increased in number.

There are no changes in the pulmonary vasculature since the blood volume is not significantly elevated in secondary polycythemia. In children with severe secondary polycythemia due to cyanotic heart disease, the skull may show thickened tables and vertical striations, similar to the changes in Cooley's anemia.[31, 32]

DISEASES OF THE WHITE BLOOD CELLS

Acute Leukemia

In childhood leukemia, which is virtually always acute, bone changes eventually occur in about two thirds of cases. The bone lesions are due to intramedullary leukemic cell infiltration, hemorrhage, or infarction, or a combination of these factors. The most common radiographic lesions are osteolytic areas, radiolucent metaphyseal bands, and diffuse demineralization. Periosteal reaction is somewhat less frequent. Rarely, osteosclerosis is encountered. These lesions may exist alone or in combination.

The osteolytic lesions can occur in any bone but are most often found in the metaphyses of long bones. Initially there are punctate areas of medullary radiolucency, producing a moth-eaten appearance. Subsequent coalescence produces larger irregular areas of confluent destruction that often extend to and involve the cortex. Frequently, periosteal reaction will appear adjacent to these lesions; rarely, periosteal reaction alone is encountered.

Bands of juxtametaphyseal radiolucency are seen in numerous conditions in infancy and are nonspecific, but their occurrence in children over the age of 2 suggests acute leukemia.

Diffuse demineralization, if present, is best demonstrated in the spine. It may be confused with changes due to steroid therapy. Two or more of these roentgen bone changes in a child should suggest acute leukemia.

In adults, there may be some demineralization (steroids?) and occasionally small lytic bone lesions resembling myeloma or metastatic disease.

Although leukemic infiltration of the kidneys is a frequent autopsy finding, urographic changes are relatively uncommon. There may be bilateral renal enlargement with elongations of the calices, simulating polycystic kidney disease. Leukemic infiltration, hemorrhage, and edema cause the renal enlargement.

Abnormalities on chest films occur in almost half the cases, most frequently in acute lymphocytic leukemia. Enlargement of mediastinal and hilar nodes is the most common finding. Variable and nonspecific pulmonary infiltrates due to leukemic deposits or secondary infection are not uncommon.

Moderate hepatosplenomegaly is often apparent on the abdominal films.[33-39]

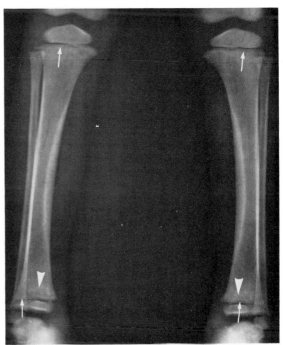

Figure 14-32 **Acute Leukemia: Bone Changes.** Thin submetaphyseal lines of decreased density *(arrows)* can be seen in both tibiae, just below the epiphyseal lines. There is no periosteal reaction or bone destruction, but mottled areas of increased density *(arrowheads)* are apparent in the lower metaphyses. In themselves, lines of decreased density are not specific, but in conjunction with the other metaphyseal changes they definitely suggest acute leukemia. The femora and tibiae are the bones most frequently involved in acute leukemia.

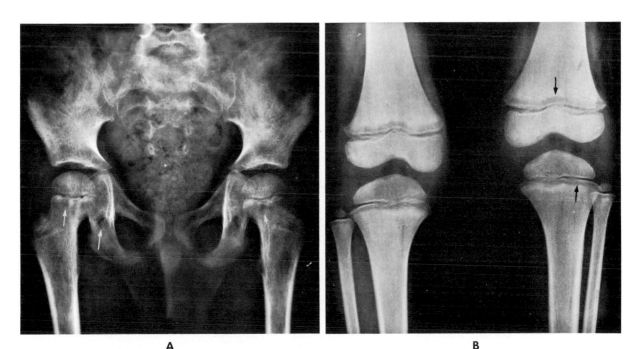

A

B

Figure 14-33 **Acute Leukemia: Bone Destruction and Osteoporosis.**

   A, The pelvis and upper femora are demineralized, and the trabeculae are coarsened. Scattered areas of bone destruction *(arrows)* are seen in the femoral neck and both ischia.

   B, There is a submetaphyseal band of decreased density *(arrows)* in all the bones of the knees.

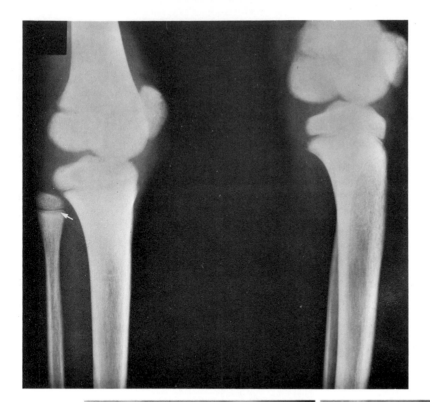

Figure 14–34 **Acute Leukemia: Osteosclerosis.** An osteosclerotic reaction to leukemic bone infiltration is uncommon. In this child there is pronounced density in the upper tibia, lower femur, and metaphysis of the fibula, and a characteristic zone of decreased density just below the metaphysis of the fibula *(arrow)*.

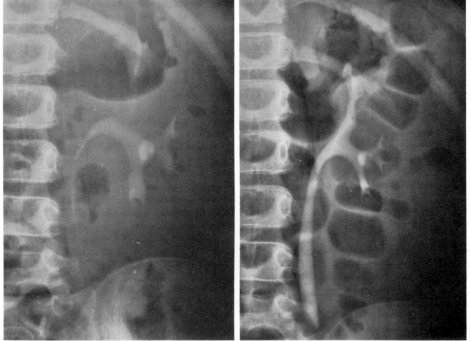

A   B

Figure 14–35 **Subacute Leukemia: Kidney Infiltration.**

A, The left kidney is enlarged and the infundibula are widened and lengthened. The upper infundibulum arises vertically from the renal pelvis and appears stretched.

B, Following chemotherapy, the kidney size is much decreased, and the infundibula and calices now appear normal. The upper infundibulum is now normally curved.

In many cases, bilateral stretching and narrowing of the infundibulum due to leukemic infiltration simulates polycystic disease.

Chronic Leukemia

Splenomegaly, which may be quite marked, is virtually a constant finding in patients with chronic leukemia.

Pulmonary changes are found in about half the cases and are more common in the lymphocytic than in the myelocytic form. Enlarged mediastinal and hilar nodes, pleural effusion, and pulmonary leukemic infiltration are the most frequent findings. Pneumonia, fungal infections, and infarction are fairly common complications, especially in chronic lymphocytic leukemia; often these secondary pulmonary lesions cannot be distinguished from leukemic infiltration. Congestive heart failure resulting from severe anemia is also common. Although leukemic infiltration can involve any organ, bone or gastrointestinal involvement is seldom seen in adults.

The typical bone changes, which are seen in less than 10 per cent of adults, are generalized demineralization, usually in the flat bones in which active marrow persists, local areas of destruction in the flat or long bones, and, occasionally, periosteal new bone formation. These changes often are indicative of passage into the acute leukemic state.

In the gastrointestinal tract there may be local or diffuse infiltration, simulating a malignant primary tumor.

Rarely, the parotid glands are infiltrated with lymphocytes, causing disorganization of the salivary glands—the Mikulicz syndrome.[12, 35, 36, 39]

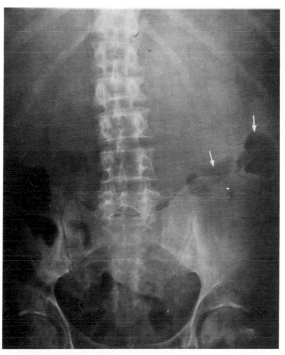

Figure 14–36 **Chronic Myelogenous Leukemia: Splenomegaly.** The greatly enlarged spleen has filled the left upper quadrant and caused depression of the gas-filled splenic flexure of the colon *(arrows)*. The enlarged liver is seen as a homogeneous density filling the right upper quadrant.

Splenic enlargement is usually much more marked in myelogenous leukemia than in lymphocytic leukemia.

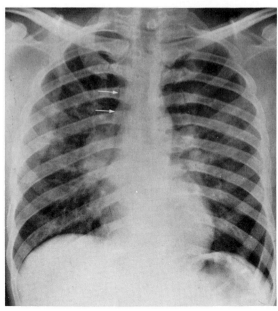

Figure 14–37 **Chronic Lymphocytic Leukemia: Adenopathy and Pulmonary Infiltration.** The large hilar shadows are a manifestation of hilar adenopathy. Right paratracheal nodal enlargement is evident *(arrows),* and leukemic infiltration extends peripherally from both hila. A similar pulmonary picture may be seen in sarcoidosis.

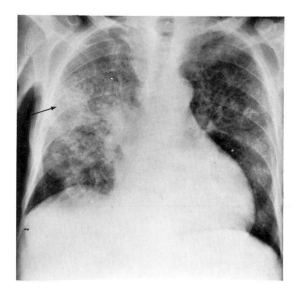

Figure 14–38 **Chronic Myelogenous Leukemia: Cardiomegaly, Vascular Congestion, Leukemic Infiltrates, and Infection.** The heart is greatly enlarged, probably owing to the chronic anemia (high output heart); there is vascular congestion in the upper lobes. The nodular densities scattered throughout the right lung were leukemic infiltrates. The more homogeneous density *(arrow)* was superimposed pneumonitis, which cleared with antibiotic therapy. The right hilar shadow is enlarged from adenopathy.

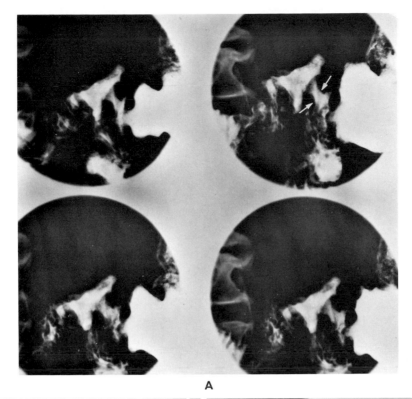

A

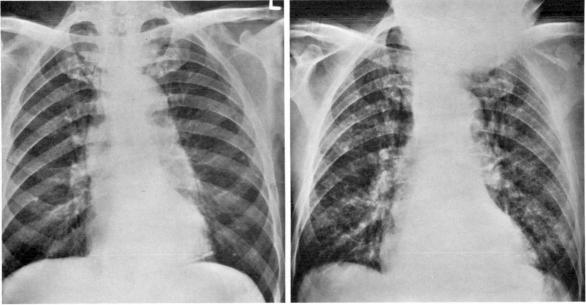

B   C

Figure 14–39   **Chronic Myelocytic Leukemia: Gastric and Pulmonary Lesions.**

The patient was a 56 year old man who had had an acute gastric hemorrhage.

A, There is a persistent area of infiltration, narrowing, and mucosal distortion *(arrows)* in the gastric antrum. The lesion was thought to be a malignant tumor but proved to be a leukemic infiltration.

B, In a film of the chest made at the same time there is an arteriosclerotic uncoiled aorta but there is no adenopathy or infiltration.

C, One and one half years later the lung fields show diffuse leukemic infiltration. The heart is enlarged owing to persistent anemia.

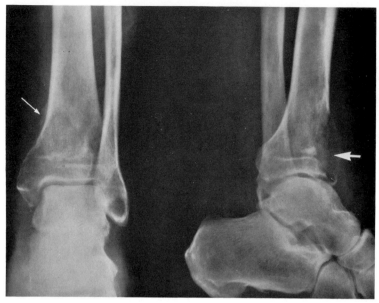

Figure 14–40 **Chronic Lymphocytic Leukemia: Bone Destruction.**   Extensive osteolytic process involves the anterior aspect of the lower tibia *(large arrow)*. There is a small area of periosteal new bone formation on the medial side of the tibia *(small arrow)*. The most common finding in the flat bones in chronic leukemia is diffuse demineralization.

Myelofibrosis with Myeloid Metaplasia (Agnogenic Myeloid Metaplasia)

A pronounced splenomegaly is a virtually constant finding in this disorder.

Osteosclerosis occurs in about half the cases. The spine, ribs, and pelvis are the most common sites, but the proximal long bones are frequently affected. The distal extremities and skull are sometimes also involved. The osteosclerosis is due to thickened dense trabeculae, and may be diffuse and homogeneous or focal and spotty. The latter may give rise to a mottled moth-eaten appearance with the uninvolved portions appearing *relatively* osteolytic. Endosteal cortical thickening can occur in the long bones and may narrow the medullary cavity.

In some cases, one or more tumor-like masses may be seen in the posterior mediastinum; these are extramedullary hematopoietic masses.

Osteosclerosis can occur in many other conditions, but in an adult with marked splenomegaly, osteosclerosis is strongly suggestive of myelofibrosis with myeloid metaplasia.[40-42]

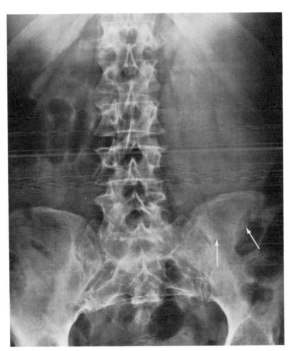

Figure 14–41 **Myelofibrosis without Osteosclerosis.**   The spleen is enormous, extending below the iliac crest *(arrows)*. No bony changes are detectable in the pelvis or lumbar spine, although clinical myelofibrosis had existed for 12 years. The bones appear normal in about half the cases of myelofibrosis.

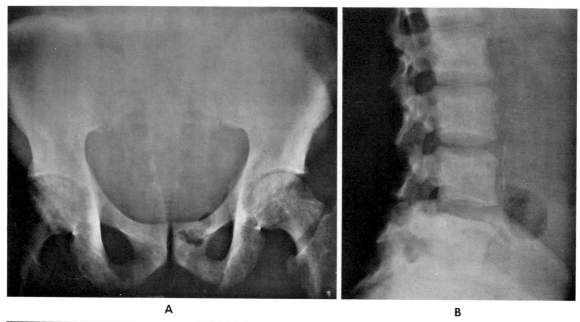

A

B

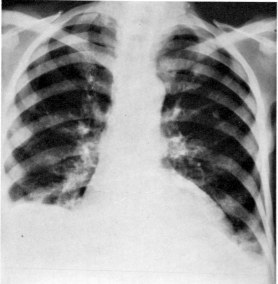

C

Figure 14–42 **Myelofibrosis with Osteosclerosis.**

A, The entire pelvis has an increased density. In the pubic and ischial bones the sclerosis is somewhat patchy, giving a mottled appearance to these bones.

B, The diffuse increased density of the lumbar vertebrae is pronounced.

C, There is homogeneous increased density of the ribs and clavicle. Cardiomegaly is a result of the chronic anemia. Elevation of the right diaphragm and the horizontal densities above the left diaphragm are caused by hepatomegaly and splenomegaly.

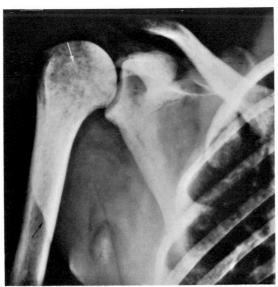

Figure 14–43 **Myelofibrosis: Shoulder Girdle Sclerosis.** Spotty sclerosis of the head of the humerus *(white arrow)* produces a mottled appearance; the increased density in the upper shaft is diffusely homogeneous. The apparent sharp transition *(black arrow)* to normal density is due to overlying soft tissue folds. The scapula, clavicle, and ribs are uniformly dense.

LYMPHORETICULAR NEOPLASMS

Lymphangiography

Lymphangiography is utilized most often to demonstrate enlargement, neoplastic infiltration, or displacement of inguinal and para-aortic retroperitoneal nodes. The lymphomatous diseases (Hodgkin's disease and lymphosarcoma) may produce characteristic foamy enlarged nodes. Metastatic disease from pelvic organs or testicle may cause defects in the opacified nodes. These defects are more significant when found in enlarged nodes, since incomplete opacification of normal nodes may simulate metastatic defects. Lymphatic obstruction and collateral vessel filling may sometimes be seen in metastatic disease. Lymphangiography is extensively employed for staging Hodgkin's disease prior to therapy.

Helpful information can be obtained from lymphangiography in patients with chylothorax, chyluria, or lymphatic obstruction.[43]

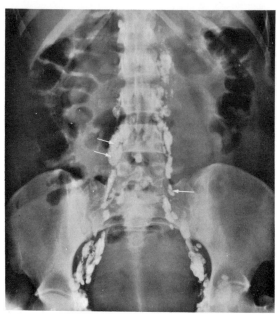

Figure 14–44 **Normal Bilateral Lymphangiogram.**   The chain of iliac and retroperitoneal lymph nodes is clearly demonstrated following bilateral injection directly into a lymphatic vessel on the dorsum of each foot. There is normal variation in the size of the nodules *(arrows)*. Normal nodes are fairly homogeneous and have a smooth outline.

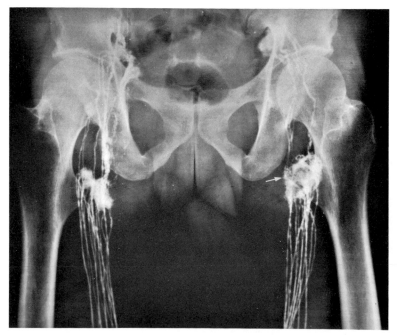

Figure 14–45 **Bilateral Lymphangiogram: Metastatic Malignant Lesion in the Inguinal Nodes.**   In a large node *(arrow)* in the left inguinal area there are multiple filling defects from invasion by malignant tissue masses. The nodes in the right inguinal area are somewhat irregular, but no filling defects can be demonstrated. A squamous cell carcinoma of the skin was the primary lesion. (Courtesy Dr. Burton Schaeffer, Philadelphia, Pennsylvania.)

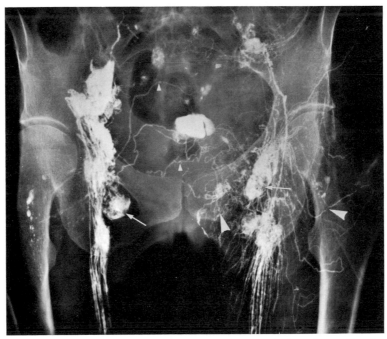

Figure 14-46 **Bilateral Lymphangiogram: Metastatic Malignant Lesion from Carcinoma of the Cervix.** Many of the inguinal and iliac nodes are not opacified because they have been replaced entirely by malignant tissue. Some of the opacified nodes contain filling defects as a result of malignant involvement *(arrows)*. There is virtually no lymphatic opacification above the pelvis, indicating obstruction of these channels. Abnormal opacification of many collateral channels *(large arrowheads)* and lymphatics communicating across the midline *(small arrowheads)* is a consequence of complete obstruction above.

Filling defects in a lymph node that appears normal otherwise do not necessarily signify nodal infiltration by disease; such defects may occur because of incomplete filling of a normal node. Defects in an enlarged node or evidence of lymphatic obstruction is a far more significant finding.

Figure 14-47 **Bilateral Lymphangiogram: Hodgkin's Disease.** Greatly enlarged nodes in which there is scanty reticular stippling of opaque material are demonstrated in the inguinal and iliac areas bilaterally *(arrows)*. The appearance is characteristic of Hodgkin's disease and other lymphoblastomas but is rarely found in nodal enlargement from other causes.

Lymphangiography is particularly useful in uncovering unsuspected involvement of the retroperitoneal nodes, particularly in the lymphoblastomatous diseases. (Courtesy Dr. Burton Schaeffer, Philadelphia, Pennsylvania.)

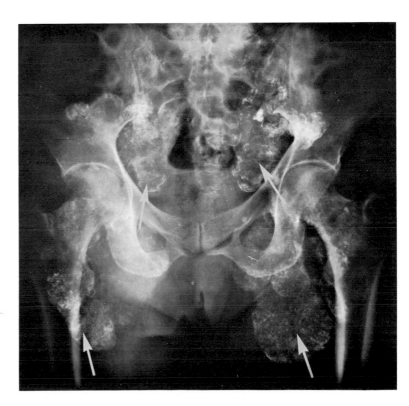

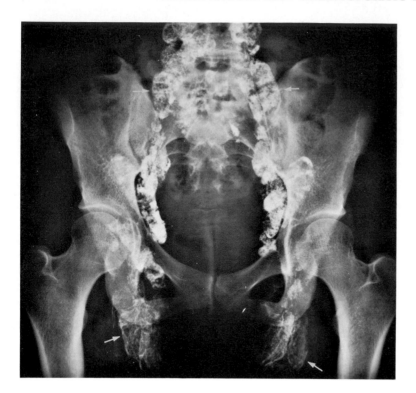

Figure 14–48 **Bilateral Lymphangiogram: Enlarged Inguinal Nodes in Sarcoid Resembling Hodgkin's Disease.** The inguinal nodes on both sides are moderately enlarged and have the stippled reticular pattern *(arrows)* that is ordinarily considered characteristic of Hodgkin's disease. The appearance is characteristic of lymphoblastomatous involvement, but is sometimes seen in other conditions with enlarged nodes. (Courtesy Dr. Burton Schaeffer, Philadelphia, Pennsylvania.)

Lymphosarcoma

Lymphosarcoma can occur in almost any tissue or organ, either as a primary or a metastatic lesion. Multiple organ involvement is usual, suggesting multicentric origins. Radiographic findings are most frequent in the chest, the gastrointestinal tract, and the skeleton.

In the chest there may be lymph node or parenchymal involvement, or both. The hilar and mediastinal nodes are enlarged, usually bilaterally, with fairly sharp regular margins. The parenchymal lesions are variable; patchy ill-defined infiltrates, scattered areas of consolidation, or nodular metastatic-like lesions can occur either alone or in combination. Pleural involvement and effusion are fairly frequent.

The rare primary lymphosarcoma of the lung often presents as an alveolar parenchymal density, simulating a chronic pneumonia or a bronchogenic carcinoma. Associated mediastinal nodes or pleural effusion is rare.

Involvement of the gastrointestinal tract occurs in about 10 per cent of cases. Gastric lymphosarcoma usually appears as an infiltrating or polypoid mass that is indistinguishable from carcinoma although it may be more diffuse and often affects younger individuals than does carcinoma. Less often, infiltration of the gastric submucosa produces the appearance of greatly enlarged folds and thumbprint defects, a more suggestive finding. (See p. 1059.)

In the small bowel, nodular intraluminal masses, diffuse submucosal infiltration, and mesenteric involvement are seen. Diffuse thickening of the wall and valvulae with scattered nodular lesions are characteristic. Dilated loops and occasionally fistulous formation can occur. Sometimes a segment of the bowel may appear almost aneurysmally dilated owing to diffuse tumor invasion. In the lymphatic-rich ileum, lymphosarcomatous involvement may simulate the roentgen picture of sprue. Unlike Hodgkin's disease of the small bowel, lymphosarcoma rarely leads to fibrosis, narrowing, and small bowel obstruction.

In the colon, lymphosarcoma is usually a polypoid or infiltrating mass indistinguishable from carcinoma, although longer segments tend to be involved by lymphosarcoma. A rarer, diffuse nodular form may simulate polyposis of the colon. (See p. 1074.)

Bone involvement occurs in about 10 per cent of cases, most often affecting the skull, spine, pelvis, and bones of the proximal limbs. The hematogenous lesions produce a mottled medullary destruction; cortical involvement is late and infrequent. Occasionally a diffuse medullary sclerosis may occur, especially in one or more vertebral bodies. This type of dense vertebral body is more common in Hodgkin's disease. In a bone involved by extension of a soft tissue lesion, there is usually cortical and adjacent trabecular destruction.

Retroperitoneal lymphosarcomatous mass or nodes can displace the kidneys or ureters and may obliterate one or both psoas shadows. Retroperitoneal node involvement is usually best demonstrated by abdominal lymphangiography. Infiltration of the renal parenchyma can produce enlargement of one or both kidneys and distortion or displacement of the calices, an appearance that sometimes strongly resembles polycystic kidneys.

A moderate splenomegaly is often found in systemic lymphosarcoma.

Lymphosarcoma, Hodgkin's disease, and reticulum cell sarcoma have almost indistinguishable roentgen findings.[39, 44-50]

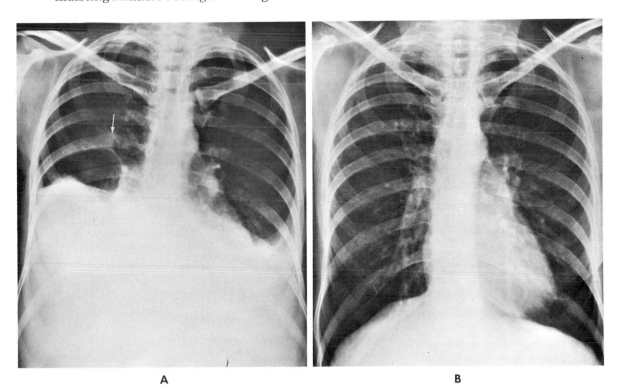

A   B

Figure 14–49   **Lymphosarcoma with Pleural Effusion.**

A, Bilateral effusions at the bases have obscured the lower lung fields. On the right the fluid is infrapulmonic, simulating an elevated right diaphragm. A patch of lymphomatous infiltration is seen adjacent to the right hilar area *(arrow)*. No mediastinal or hilar adenopathy is apparent. Hepatomegaly and splenomegaly were also present.

B, After a course of therapy, the effusions and infiltrations have cleared completely. The chest film is now normal.

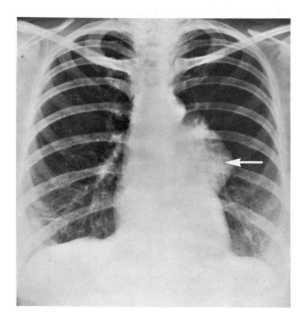

Figure 14–50 **Lymphosarcoma with a Mass of Hilar Nodes.** A large lobulated circumscribed density *(arrow)* occupies the left hilum. In lateral view the density was seen also in the hilar area. There were no other chest findings. In an older patient, such findings would suggest bronchogenic carcinoma.

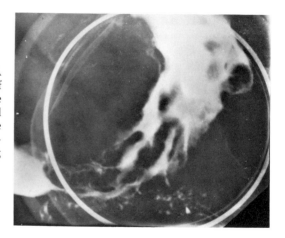

Figure 14–51 **Primary Lymphosarcoma of Stomach.** A film made with compression reveals extensive defects of the lower two thirds of the stomach. The defects resemble giant gastric folds; however, the rigidity of the gastric wall suggests an infiltrative process. Although an appearance simulating enlarged folds may be seen in gastric lymphosarcoma, more often the finding is that of an infiltrating mass which is indistinguishable from carcinoma.

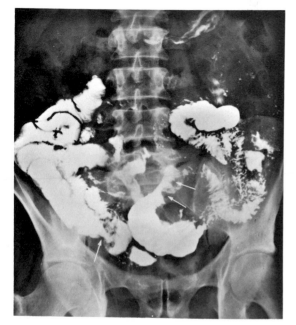

Figure 14–52 **Nodular Lymphosarcoma of Small Intestine.** Multiple nodular defects *(arrows)* are seen in the ileum, but there is no evidence of obstruction. There is local dilatation of the pelvic loop of ileum. The walls of the small bowel are not thickened. When multiple nodules are found, especially in the ileum, lymphosarcoma should be considered.

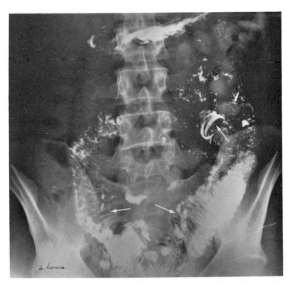

Figure 14–53 **Infiltrative Lymphosarcoma of Small Intestine.** The ileum is moderately dilated, and the mucosal folds are considerably thickened and prominent *(lower arrows)*. This thickening due to submucosal infiltration is also seen in other diseases, particularly regional ileitis; however, there is a single large nodular defect *(upper arrow)* due to a lymphosarcomatous mass that has intussuscepted. The combination of nodules and submucosal infiltration in the small bowel suggests lymphoblastomatous involvement.

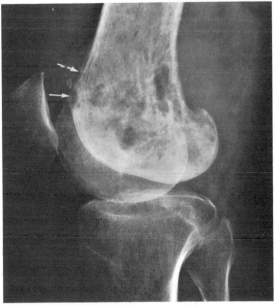

Figure 14–54 **Lymphosarcoma Involving Lower Femur.** There are patchy areas of destruction separated by normal or thickened trabeculae. The involvement is primarily medullary, but it extends to the cortex anteriorly *(lower arrow)*. A small segment of periosteal proliferation is seen just above the area of destroyed cortex *(upper arrow)*. These changes are typical. Rarely, a soft tissue mass may develop, but only after the lesion has extended well beyond the cortex. When the bone is invaded by an adjacent soft tissue lymphomatous mass, cortical destruction is the dominant finding.

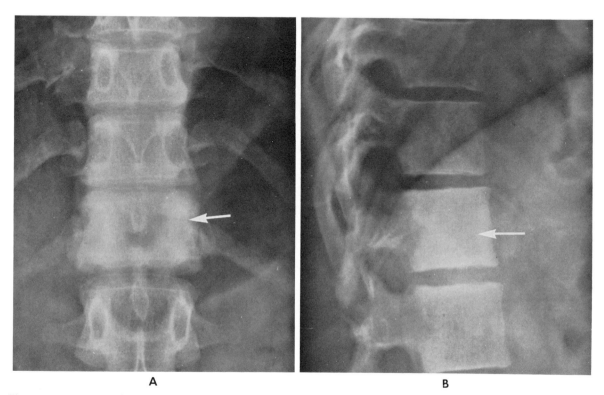

A   B

Figure 14–55 **Lymphosarcoma: Osteosclerotic Vertebral Body.**

A, In anteroposterior view there is generalized increased density of the twelfth dorsal body; the outline of the pedicles *(arrow)* is partially obscured by the sclerosis. There is a slight but definite increase in the width of the twelfth dorsal body (compare with those above and below it).

B, In lateral view the vertebra *(arrow)* appears dense, but is regular.

Single or multiple sclerotic, slightly expanded vertebrae are not uncommon in the lymphomatous diseases; they occcur more frequently in Hodgkin's disease than in lymphosarcoma. A solitary dense vertebra found in an older person is most often due to Paget's disease. The increased bone density in lymphoma results from overgrowth of cancellous bone secondary to deposition of neoplastic tissue in the marrow, whereas in Paget's involvement there is cortical thickening at the vertebral margins.

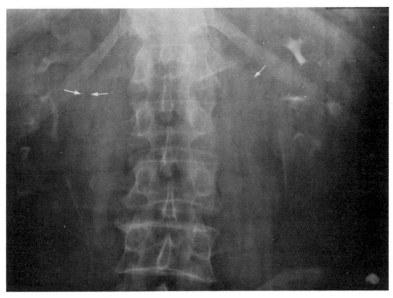

Figure 14–56 **Retroperitoneal Lymphosarcomatous Masses.** Abdominal film made during intravenous urography demonstrates bilateral bulging of the upper psoas muscle shadows *(arrows)*, which have been infiltrated by the lymphosarcoma. Normally the upper psoas line is virtually contiguous with the bony spine. Both kidneys are displaced laterally, especially on the left. The left kidney has also been rotated to a more vertical axis owing to lateral displacement of its upper pole by the tumor. Normally the angle of the kidneys is such that both upper poles are closer to the midline than are the lower poles. There appears to be no invasion or alteration of function in the kidneys.

Lymphangiography is the preferred procedure for demonstrating retroperitoneal nodes early in the disease. The kidneys may be displaced by any large retroperitoneal mass.

Reticulum Cell Sarcoma

The same tissues and organs are affected as in lymphosarcoma, producing similar changes roentgenologically. However, reticulum cell sarcoma occurs in older persons and is quite rare in children and young adults.

Generally pulmonary lesions are indistinguishable from those of lymphoma (see p. 1175). However, the nodular parenchymal lesions tend to be more sharply defined than in lymphosarcoma.

Primary reticulum cell sarcoma of bone is a distinct entity and is discussed on page 1400.[39]

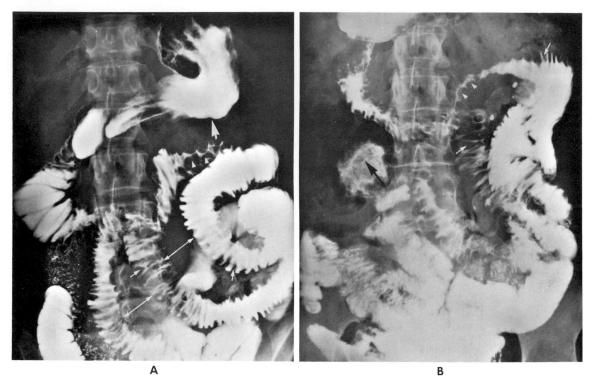

A   B

Figure 14–57 **Reticulum Cell Sarcoma of Small Intestine.** In progress meal study, *A* is a one-hour film, and *B* is a two-hour film. Extreme thickening of the jejunal walls is evidenced by the marked increase in the space *(double-headed arrows)* between the barium-filled loops. Prominence of the folds *(small arrows)* is due to submucosal infiltration. A number of submucosal tumor masses are seen at the duodenojejunal junction *(small arrowheads)*; this loop was rigid and fixed, and thickening of the wall caused upward displacement of the stomach *(large white arrow)*. One segment is dilated *(black arrow)* and contains diffuse filling defects. There was no obstruction, and transit time was not delayed. The ileal loops were slightly dilated but appeared normal otherwise.

The patient was a 50 year old woman from whom a solitary reticulum cell sarcoma of the breast had been removed one year previously. There were no peripheral nodes or mediastinal masses.

Although extensive infiltration of the bowel walls and mucosa may be found in other diseases, such as Whipple's disease, the finding of nodular defects, local areas of dilatation, and fixation of loops is characteristic of lymphosarcoma or reticulum cell sarcoma.

African Lymphoma (Burkitt's Tumor)

This poorly differentiated lymphosarcoma is the most common childhood tumor in Africa and New Guinea. The maxillomandibular region is the most frequent site (over 70 per cent), but usually there are also widespread visceral lesions, often symmetric, suggesting multicentric origin. The lung fields and peripheral nodes are usually spared. Untreated, the disease is rapidly fatal.

The typical roentgen manifestations are intramedullary lesions of one or both maxillary bones. Progressive lytic destruction and early invasion of the antra are common. Soft tissue masses over the affected bone appear rapidly, sometimes accompanied by perpendicular periosteal spicules.

Long bones are less frequently affected. Involvement is characterized by ill-defined medullary lytic areas in or near the metaphyses, frequently accompanied by periosteal reaction of the "onion skin" or the perpendicular "sunburst" type, mimicking osteogenic sarcoma, Ewing's sarcoma, metastatic neuroblastoma, or bone leukemia.

Kidney involvement may be bilateral, and multiple lymphomatous masses may simulate polycystic kidney disease. Extrarenal retroperitoneal masses may obliterate a psoas shadow and displace an upper ureter.

Chest involvement is quite uncommon. Well-defined parenchymal masses and pleural effusion may appear.

Although the jaws are usually the most common site of involvement in African lymphoma, in the American form of Burkitt's tumor, the abdomen is more often the affected primary site.[39, 51-54]

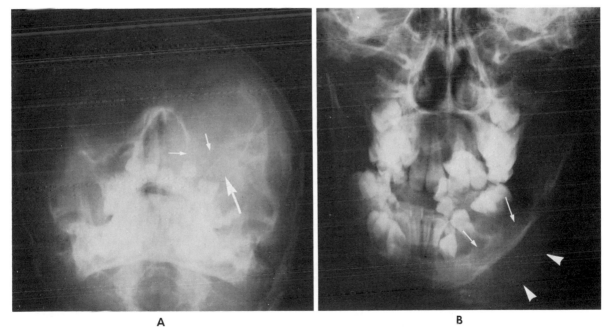

A   B

Figure 14–58   **African Lymphoma (Burkitt's Tumor): Two Patients.**

A, The left antrum is obliterated *(large arrow),* and its lateral and superior walls *(small arrows)* show loss of bone. The haze overlying the left orbit, nasal cavity, and entire maxillary area is due to the large overlying soft tissue mass. The lymphoma has invaded the left antrum and left orbit. The patient was a 5 year old girl with proptosis of one month's duration.

B, In another child there is destruction of the alveolar margin of the left mandible *(small arrows)* and a soft tissue mass *(arrowheads).*

Coalescing osteolytic lesions and a soft tissue mass, most often in the maxillary region, are the most common and most characteristic radiographic findings in Burkitt's lymphoma. (Courtesy Dr. D. J. Bassett, Australia.)

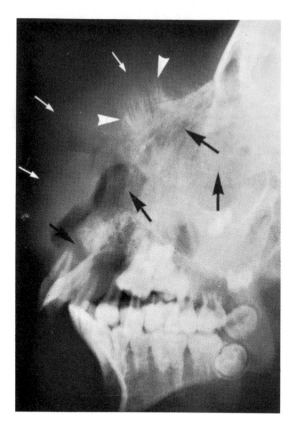

Figure 14-59 **African Lymphoma (Burkitt's Tumor) of the Maxilla: Periosteal Spiculation.** Lateral view of facial bones of a child reveals extensive destruction of the alveolar ridge, maxilla, and orbit *(black arrows)*, with obliteration of all bony landmarks. Fine perpendicular periosteal spicules *(arrowheads)* are projecting into the large overlying soft tissue mass *(white arrows)*. (Courtesy Dr. W. P. Cockshott, Hamilton, Ontario.)

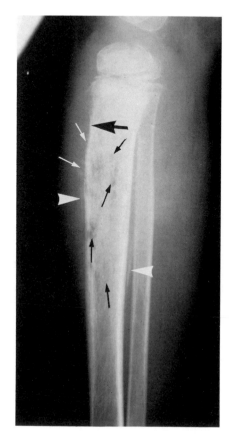

Figure 14-60 **African Lymphomia (Burkitt's Tumor) Involving Tibia.** There are numerous irregular lytic medullary areas *(small black arrows)* and cortical destruction *(large black arrow).* Excluding the epiphysis, the entire upper half of the tibia is involved. There is periosteal reaction of both the layering type *(arrowheads)* and the perpendicular spicule type *(white arrows)*. Soft tissue swelling overlies the lesion.

Radiographically the appearance closely simulates Ewing's sarcoma. (Courtesy Dr. W. P. Cockshott, Hamilton, Ontario.)

Follicular Lymphoma (Brill-Symmers Disease)

The ordinary manifestations of this disease are enlarged lymph nodes, which produce no radiographic findings. Lymphography reveals nonspecific nodal defects, stippling or hypertrophy, but the study may be useful for demonstrating unrecognized involvement of abdominal nodes.

Occasional involvement of mediastinal nodes may produce a lobulated mediastinal shadow, indistinguishable from that occurring in lymphosarcoma or Hodgkin's disease. Regression following radiation therapy is unusually rapid and may be permanent.

Many authors believe this to be a more benign form of lymphosarcoma or reticular cell sarcoma rather than a distinct entity.[39, 55]

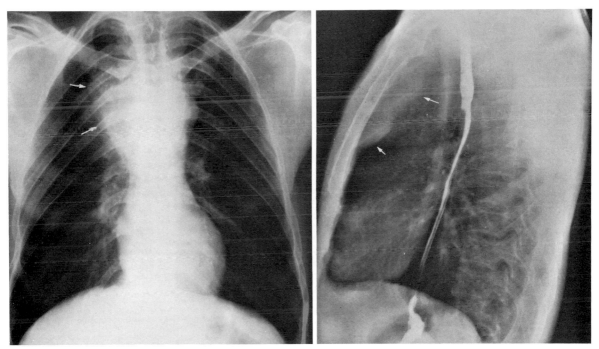

Figure 14–61 **Giant Follicular Lymphoma of Anterior Mediastinum.** The lobulated mass in the right upper anterior mediastinum *(arrows)* represents an aggregation of enlarged nodes. No parenchymal involvement is evident.

Mycosis Fungoides

This invariably fatal disease is considered to be a lymphoma of the skin. Most cases eventuate in visceral lymphomatosis, with pulmonary involvement a prominent feature. Radiographically there may be enlargement of the hilar nodes and reticular nodular lymphomatous infiltrates in the later stages of the disease. Alveolar lymphomatous densities also may appear, simulating pneumonias. Moderate splenomegaly is often present.

Lymphangiography will disclose abnormal femoral, iliac, and periaortic lymph nodes in most patients with mycosis fungoides; in about 25 per cent of patients, these show the characteristic changes of lymphomatous nodes (see Fig. 14–47). Lymphographic findings correlate fairly well with the clinical stage of the disease.[56, 57]

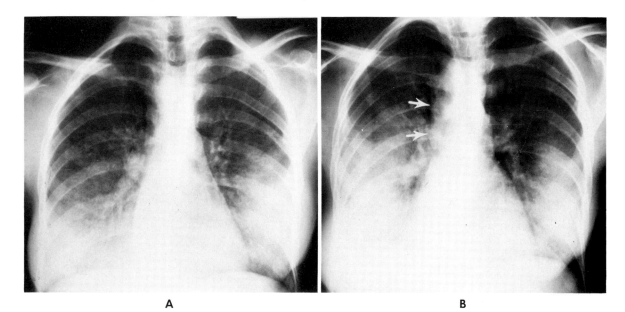

A   B

Figure 14–62 **Mycosis Fungoides with Pulmonary Lymphomatosis.**

A, An 18 year old girl with known mycosis fungoides, whose chest film was normal six weeks prior to hospitalization, had developed fever, cough, and malaise.

There are diffuse, bilateral, confluent alveolar densities in both lower lung fields, with ill defined borders. Bilateral pneumonia was suspected.

B, A week later, the basal alveolar densities have increased, particularly on the right. In addition, there appears to be a lobulated widening of the right mediastinum *(arrows).* Open biopsy of the lung revealed diffuse alveolar lymphosarcoma.

Most patients with mycosis fungoides eventually develop visceral lymphosarcoma, most often in the lungs and hilar nodes.

Hodgkin's Disease

Almost any tissue or organ can be affected, but roentgenologic manifestations are most common in the chest, bones, and abdomen. Hilar or mediastinal nodal enlargement can be demonstrated at some time during the course of the disease in more than half the cases. Mediastinal nodal enlargement nearly always precedes hilar involvement, the masses in many cases being bilateral and only rarely displacing adjacent structures. Calcification of the mediastinal mass or nodes occasionally develops, usually the result of radiation therapy.

The lung parenchyma may be involved in from 6 to 30 per cent of cases although this involvement usually occurs late in the disease. Generally, linear densities extend from the enlarged hilum; these probably represent lymphatic spread. Discrete lesions, resembling pneumonic patches or metastatic nodules, are considerably less common, constituting about 10 per cent of the lung lesions; occasionally they undergo necrosis and cavitation. Many of these nodules show fine infiltrations radiating into the periphery. Pleural effusion occurs in up to one fourth of cases but develops late in the course of disease and usually accompanies parenchymal involvement. Other thoracic complications include vena cava obstruction, pericardial effusion, and cardiac involvement. Tracheal and bronchial compression usually do not occur.

Detectable bone lesions are present in about 10 or 20 per cent of cases, the spine being the site in half of these. The pelvis, sternum, ribs, long bones, and skull are less frequently involved. Bone changes may result from direct invasion from adjacent diseased nodes or from hematogenous spread. In direct invasion, the periosteum is first involved, and the disease then spreads through the medullary spaces and destroys the marrow by lysis of the trabeculae. Occasionally, osteosclerosis may develop. In the hematogenous form there are sclerotic or a combination of sclerotic and lytic lesions. Vertebral lesions are generally sclerotic, giving rise to the so-called ivory vertebrae, a characteristic finding. In the spine, the anterior margins of the affected vertebral bodies may be eroded by pressure invasion of adjacent nodes. Almost one half of patients will have associated paravertebral soft tissue masses.

Hepatomegaly and splenomegaly are often present. Retroperitoneal masses (see *Lymphosarcoma*, p. 1174) may produce obliteration and distortion of the psoas shadows and may cause displacement of the ureter, kidney, or vena cava. Lymphangiography is helpful in determining the size and location of pelvic and retroperitoneal nodes and is employed for staging of the disease prior to therapy.

Gastrointestinal involvement occurs in about 5 to 6 per cent of cases, usually in the stomach or small bowel. Esophageal and colon lesions are extremely rare.

About half the gastrointestinal lesions occur in the stomach. There may be one or more ulcerations in a poorly distensible segment, wall infiltrations, or thickened infiltrated folds alone or in combination. Distinction from a scirrhous carcinoma is usually impossible; thickened folds alone may simulate lymphosarcoma.

Involvement of the small bowel may be diffuse or segmental. Submucosal nodules and irregularly thickened walls and mucosa are characteristic. The appearance is quite similar to lymphosarcoma; however, persistent areas of narrowing are not unusual in Hodgkin's involvement but are rare in lymphosarcoma.

Both common and uncommon bacterial and fungal infections may complicate Hodgkin's disease because of disturbance of the immune mechanism by the disease itself and from administered steroids.[39, 58-61]

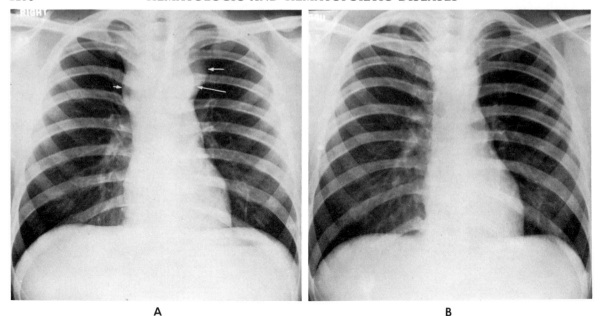

A   **B**

Figure 14–63   **Hodgkin's Disease: Mediastinal Adenopathy.**

A, There are multiple masses *(arrows)* of enlarged nodes on both sides of the superior mediastinum (paratracheal nodes), as well as widening of the mediastinum in the hilar areas: however, there are no obvious hilar nodes. Neither the trachea nor the esophagus is displaced.

B, Following radiotherapy, the mid and upper mediastinum have returned to normal size and contour. The mediastinal masses have disappeared.

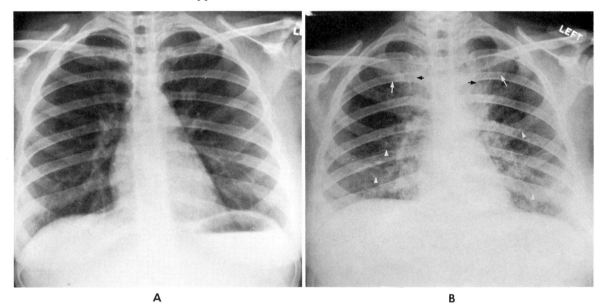

A   **B**

Figure 14–64   **Hodgkin's Disease: Fulminating Lymphatic Spread.**

The patient was a 14 year old girl.

A, Posteroanterior view is negative; a cervical node biopsy had disclosed Hodgkin's disease.

B, Four months later, the patient developed progressive dyspnea; there are densities on both sides of the superior mediastinum *(black arrows),* without distinct borders. Infiltrates extend to both lung fields *(white arrows).*

These findings were due to rapid growth of the mediastinal nodes, with lymphatic extension into the upper lung parenchyma.

Extensive infiltration throughout the lung fields *(arrowheads)* probably represents lymphatic spread from the hilar nodes.

The extraordinarily rapid growth of the mediastinal nodes and lymphatic spread from the nodes into the parenchyma are responsible for the indistinct borders of these nodes.

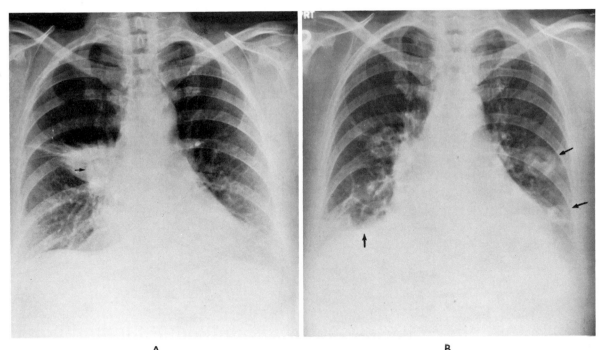

A   B

Figure 14–65 **Hodgkin's Disease: Progressive Parenchymal Lung Involvement.**

A, There is parenchymal infiltration extending from an enlarged right hilar node *(arrow)* almost to the lateral border of the lung; the infiltration is probably via the lymphatic channels.

B, Many months later, when the patient no longer responded to therapy, there were nodular masses with cavitation in the left chest *(arrows)* and diffuse infiltration and fluid at the right base *(arrow).* The right hilar mass is still evident, but the parenchyma has cleared to some extent.

Nodular pulmonary masses are a late finding in Hodgkin's disease; cavitation is unusual.

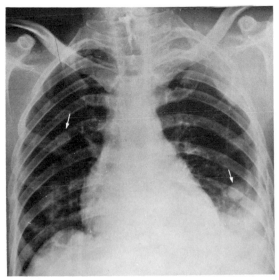

Figure 14–66 **Hodgkin's Disease: Late Findings.** In addition to nodular parenchymal lesions *(arrows),* there is extensive pleural reaction along the entire left lateral chest wall and left base. The enlarged cardiac silhouette was due to pericardial effusion.

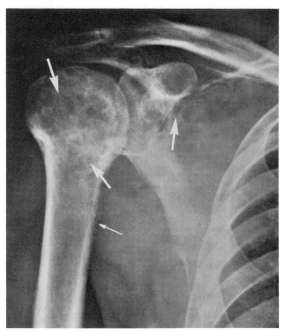

Figure 14–67 **Hodgkin's Disease: Bone Involvement.**   Diffuse lytic mottling with areas of sclerosis *(large arrows)* in the head and neck of the humerus and the upper portions of the scapula is characteristic of hematogenous medullary bone involvement from Hodgkin's disease. In the upper portion of the shaft the disease has extended to the cortex, producing some cortical irregularity and periosteal reaction *(small arrow)*.

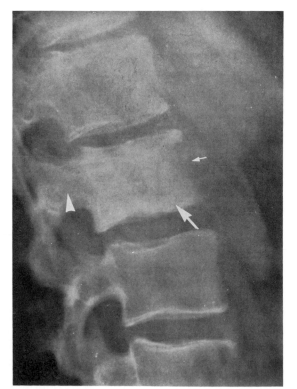

Figure 14–68 **Hodgkin's Disease: Sclerotic Vertebra.** An overall increased density of a vertebral body *(large arrow)* is the most frequently seen roentgenologic change in Hodgkin's disease of the vertebrae. The sclerotic process also involves the pedicles *(arrowhead)*. The lytic area in the anterior aspect of this body *(small arrow)* was due to a complicating staphylococcal osteomyelitis of the vertebral body. It is not uncommon for bacterial and fungal infections to develop during prolonged steroid therapy.

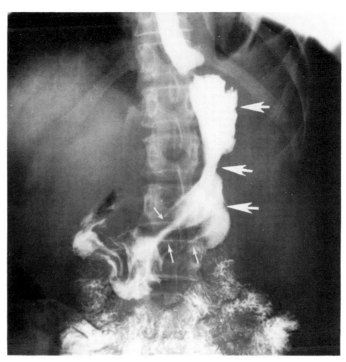

Figure 14–69 **Hodgkin's Disease of the Stomach.** The stomach is displaced medially by an enlarged spleen. The gastric fundus is narrowed, and the greater curvature is rigid, irregular, and infiltrated *(large arrows)*. The folds in the midstomach are infiltrated and greatly thickened *(small arrows)*, and are quite similar to the classic findings of lymphosarcoma. No ulcerations are seen.

The principal radiographic findings in Hodgkin's disease of the stomach are one or more ulcerations in a poorly distensible area, wall infiltration, and thickened infiltrated folds, either alone or in combination. Involvement is often more extensive than that seen in carcinoma; however, most often the changes are indistinguishable from those of scirrhous carcinoma.

INFECTIOUS MONONUCLEOSIS

Roentgenologic evidence of hilar or mediastinal node enlargement is found in about 10 per cent of cases. It is minimal and easily overlooked, and may be unilateral. Frequently this enlargement is recognized only with serial films demonstrating changes in hilar size.

In about 10 per cent of cases there are minimal parenchymal lung infiltrates that are usually patchy and nonspecific. Splenic enlargement can be demonstrated roentgenographically in only a limited number of cases.

A few cases of transient periosteal reaction with bone and limb pain have been reported.[62, 63]

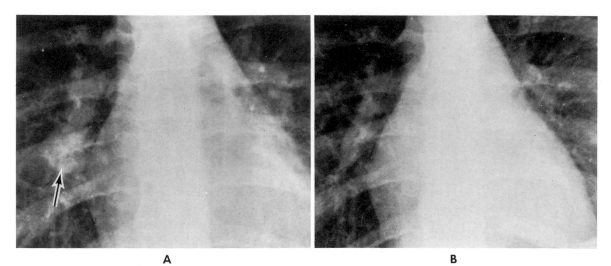

A   B

Figure 14–70   **Infectious Mononucleosis: Hilar Node Enlargement.**

   A, During the height of the illness, the right hilar shadow is somewhat enlarged, particularly its lower portion *(arrow).* The left hilum appears normal in size.

   B, Film made when the patient was not ill shows the marked decrease of the right hilar shadow. The left hilum, which did not appear enlarged on the prior film, is also considerably smaller.

   Mild to moderate hilar node enlargement in infectious mononucleosis is probably more common than supposed but can often be recognized only in retrospect, when compared with films made before or after the illness.

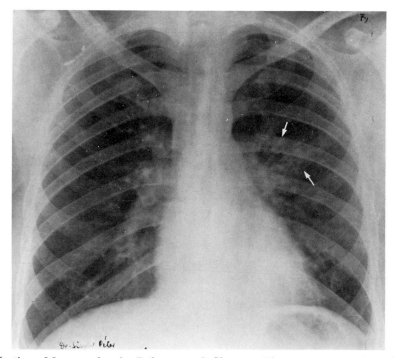

Figure 14–71   **Infectious Mononucleosis: Pulmonary Infiltrate.**   There is a parenchymal infiltrate *(arrows)* in the left lung adjacent to the hilum. Both hilar shadows are prominent, due to minimal nodal enlargement.

   Such infiltrates are uncommon and have no distinguishing characteristics.

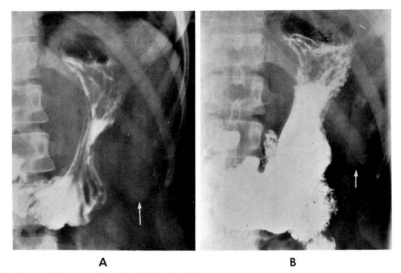

Figure 14–72 **Infectious Mononucleosis: Splenic Enlargement.**

A, The tip of the enlarged spleen *(arrow)* extends below the twelfth rib. The spleen is abnormally wide and long, and has produced a smooth indentation on the greater curvature of the barium-filled stomach; further enlargement might cause displacement toward the spine.

Splenomegaly from any cause can give rise to these findings. Depression of the splenic flexure of the colon is usually observed also.

B, Three weeks later the spleen is considerably smaller; the tip is higher *(arrow),* and the gastric indentation is less pronounced. (Courtesy Dr. A. Bogsch, Budapest, Hungary.)

EOSINOPHILIC GRANULOMA AND RELATED SYNDROMES (HISTIOCYTOSIS X)

Eosinophilic granuloma, Hand-Schüller-Christian disease, and Letterer-Siwe disease were formerly considered to be variants of a single entity, histiocytosis X. Currently, however, Hand-Schüller-Christian disease is considered to be multifocal eosinophilic granuloma, while Letterer-Siwe disease is possibly an unusual form of malignant lymphoma (histiocytic lymphoma). Eosinophilic granuloma usually appears as a solitary bone lesion. Hand-Schüller-Christian disease is the chronic disseminated form, affecting multiple bones and other tissues. Letterer-Siwe disease is the acute disseminated form, which occurs in children usually under three. Infrequently, histiocytosis X diffusely involves the lungs.

The skull, femur, and spine are the most common sites of skeletal lesions. These originate in the medullary cavity and are entirely lytic. Although usually sharply defined, more rapidly growing lesions may have hazy borders. The lesions in flat bones show no periosteal reaction, but in long bones, especially in children, extension into the cortex with periosteal new bone formation is not rare. This radiographic appearance may suggest a malignant bone lesion, but there is no associated soft tissue mass. In the skull, there is a predilection for the anterior half of the base. One or both tables may be eroded. Multiple large coalescent lesions produce the "geographic skull." Rarely, a small bony sequestrum remains in a lytic area. Lesions in other flat bones show rather sharply demarcated lytic medullary defects. Vertebral involvement may result in collapse and flattening of a vertebral body — vertebra plana — a highly suggestive finding in children. Occasionally diffuse marrow involvement may cause generalized osteoporosis without focal lytic lesions.

Pulmonary histiocytosis, although uncommon, produces changes that are often highly suggestive of the diagnosis. A fine reticular lung pattern is the earliest finding. Later, miliary nodules appear, followed by eventual diffuse fibrosis. Diffuse areas of interstitial emphysema become apparent. The small nodules on a background of diffuse fibrosis accompanied by diffuse lucent areas of emphysema constitute the characteristic honeycomb lung (see also *Honeycomb Lung*, p. 487). Pneumothorax from rupture of a subpleural emphysematous bleb is a fairly common complication. Hilar adenopathy does not occur.[64-70]

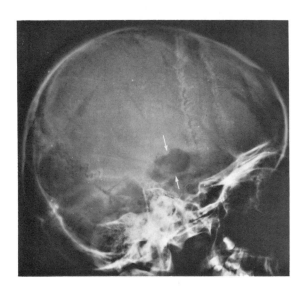

Figure 14–73 **Eosinophilic Granuloma of Skull.** A circumscribed osteolytic area without marginal sclerosis is demonstrated in the temporal bone *(arrows)*. This solitary lesion is typical of an eosinophilic granuloma, and the skull is the most common site.

Figure 14–74 **Solitary Eosinophilic Granuloma of Rib.** An osteolytic lesion *(arrows)* has the characteristic circumscribed border, with no sclerosis or bone expansion.

Such solitary eosinophilic granulomas occur mainly in the flat bones; the skull, ribs and pelvis are the usual sites.

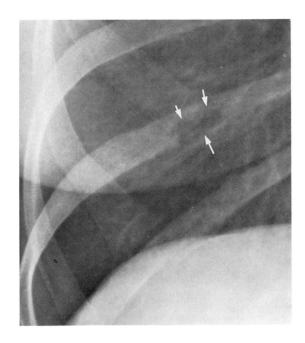

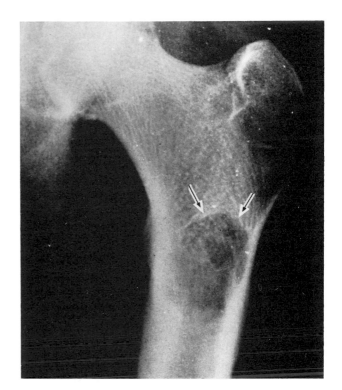

Figure 14–75 **Solitary Eosinophilic Granuloma of Femur.** The lesion demonstrates the characteristic features of bone histiocytosis: it is lytic, entirely in the medullary cavity, sharply marginated *(arrows),* and shows no marginal sclerosis.

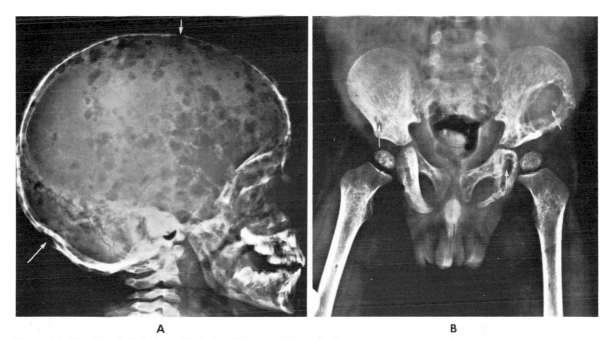

A   B

Figure 14–76 **Hand-Schüller-Christian Disease: Bone Lesions.**

A, There are numerous lytic lesions, sharply marginated and of varying size. The greater involvement of the anterior half and periorbital region of the skull is a common finding. The lesions all originate in the diploë, but as they enlarge they may cause erosion of either table *(arrows).*

B, Similar lesions are present in the pelvis *(arrows).* There is a huge lytic area in the left ilium and smaller lesions in the right ilium and ischial bones. The coarsened trabeculae and demineralization throughout the pelvis result from diffuse histiocytic infiltration of the marrow. (Courtesy J. DeWitte, Gent, Belgium.)

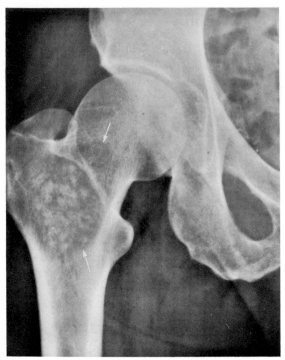

Figure 14–77 **Hand-Schüller-Christian Disease.** There is a large osteolytic lesion with sharply margin-ated borders *(arrows)*, within which are numerous small irregular bony sequestra.

Other bone lesions in this patient showed similar sequestra.

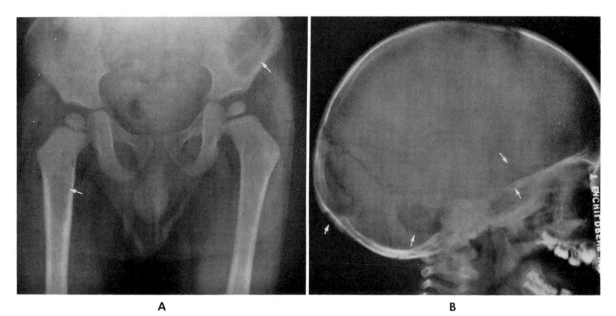

A   B

Figure 14–78 **Letterer-Siwe Disease: Skeletal Lesions.**

The patient was 2 years old.

A, The lesion in the right upper femur *(arrow)* is medullary and lytic and has a sharp border; it has caused scalloping of the endosteum. The lesion in the left ilium *(arrow)* is more regular in outline.

B, The skull lesions *(arrows)* are characteristically lytic with sharp borders. These borders are less sharp in rapidly growing lesions.

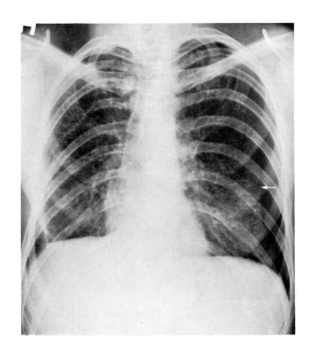

Figure 14–79 **Pulmonary Histiocytosis X: Honeycomb Lung.** There is a diffuse reticular and nodular infiltration of both lungs, with small cyst-like areas of emphysema between the densities—characteristics of honeycomb lung. Many disorders that cause diffuse pulmonary fibrosis may give rise to a similar appearance.

The pneumothorax on the left *(arrow)* is due to rupture in a subpleural emphysematous area and is a fairly common complication of honeycomb lung.

The sixth rib on the right was resected during unrelated earlier surgery. (Courtesy Dr. William Weiss, Philadelphia, Pennsylvania.)

LIPID STORAGE DISORDERS

Gaucher's Disease

This metabolic disorder is characterized by abnormal lipid accumulations (glucocerebrosides) in reticuloendothelial cells (Gaucher cells) of the spleen, liver, and bone marrow.

In addition to hepatosplenomegaly, the most frequent radiographic changes are in the skeletal system. The femora, shoulders, spine, and pelvis are most often involved. Skull lesions are infrequent.

Expansion, demineralization, and cortical thinning of the long bones are common early in the disease. Pathologic fractures often occur. Flaring of the lower femora due to marrow infiltration causes abnormal modeling and produces the Erlenmeyer-flask appearance. Aseptic necrosis may develop in the femoral head and, less often, in the humeral head. A generalized osteoporosis is not infrequent.

Other frequent bone lesions include sharply circumscribed radiolucent defects, scalloping of the endosteal cortex, and coarsened trabeculae between lytic lesions. Solid or lace-like periosteal reaction often occurs.

In the spine, general osteoporosis may occur, often with collapse of one or more vertebrae. Occasionally, focal areas of osteosclerosis are seen, simulating osteoblastic metastases.

Marginal sclerosis of the sacroiliac joints and occasionally actual joint obliteration can occur.

Involvement of the liver may lead to angiographic changes similar to those seen in cirrhosis.

Pulmonary infiltrates are seen only in children and usually appear as diffuse miliary lesions similar to the changes in Niemann-Pick disease.[71-73]

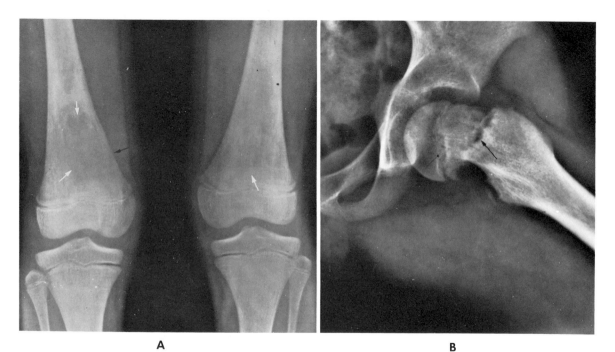

A   B

Figure 14–80 **Gaucher's Disease.**

The patient was an 11 year old boy.

A, In both lower femora (metaphyses) there is an irregular area of osteoporosis *(white arrows);* it is more marked in the right femur. Widening of the lower femora gives rise to the Erlenmeyer flask appearance. The cortices are very much thinned *(black arrow).*

B, There is a pathologic fracture of the femoral neck *(arrow),* associated with a bone lesion that extends down to the intertrochanteric region.

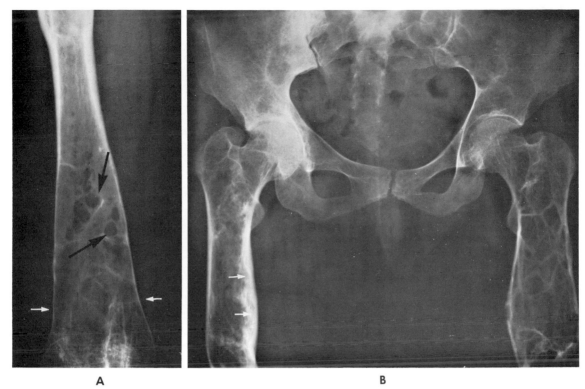

A   B

Figure 14–81 **Gaucher's Disease.**

There is extensive involvement of both femora in a 38 year old man.

A, The lower femur has an Erlenmeyer flask appearance, with generalized osteoporosis and cortical thinning *(white arrows).* Multiple smaller areas of lysis *(black arrows)* are scattered within the lower femur. Sclerosis and deformity from an old healed fracture are evident in the upper shaft.

B, Extensive involvement of the upper femora has resulted in widening, osteoporosis, cortical thinning, and localized lytic areas, most marked in the left femur. Scalloping of the inner cortex of the right femur *(arrows)* is due to expansion of the lesions.

Figure 14–82 **Gaucher's Disease: Splenoportogram.** The intrahepatic portal vessels appear bare because normal arborization of the small peripheral vessels is lacking *(arrows).* The portal vein is well opacified *(arrowhead).*

The portal vasculature often has a similar appearance in liver cirrhosis. Apparently, in liver involvement by Gaucher's disease, as in cirrhosis, the smaller portal vessels are obliterated.

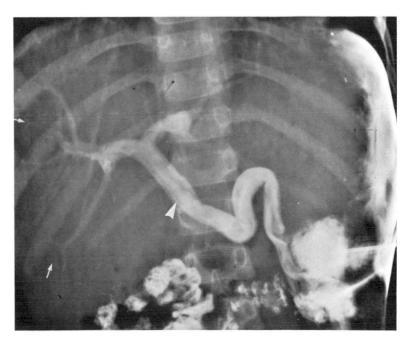

Niemann-Pick Disease

This disorder is characterized by deposition of sphingomyelin in various tissues. Hepatomegaly and splenomegaly are present in all cases and are the only radiographic findings in the rare individual who survives until adolescence.

Nearly all other cases show fine nodular diffuse pulmonary infiltrates, with linear strands, which persist unchanged throughout the abbreviated lifespan of the patient. Osteoporosis and coxa valga occur in most patients, often with modeling defects, which give the Erlenmeyer-flask appearance to the lower femora and upper tibia. Unlike Gaucher's disease, lytic lesions do not occur. In about one third of cases, there is widening of the metacarpals, with thin cortices and coarse trabeculations.

Hepatosplenomegaly, persistent small nodular pulmonary infiltrates, and osteoporosis in an infant are highly suggestive of the diagnosis of Niemann-Pick disease.

In *Wolman's disease* (familial cholesterolosis), a xanthomatous disorder that resembles Niemann-Pick disease clinically, there is enlargement and calcification of the adrenal glands.[74-77]

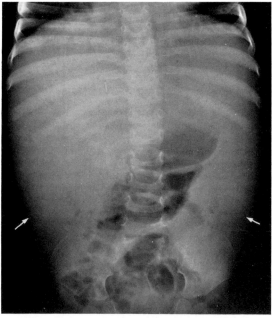

Figure 14–83 **Niemann-Pick Disease: Splenohepatomegaly.** The liver and spleen of this young patient are greatly enlarged, filling the entire upper abdomen and extending almost to the iliac crests *(arrows)*. Enlargement has caused the flanks to bulge.

Marked hepatomegaly and splenomegaly are invariably present in Niemann-Pick disease.

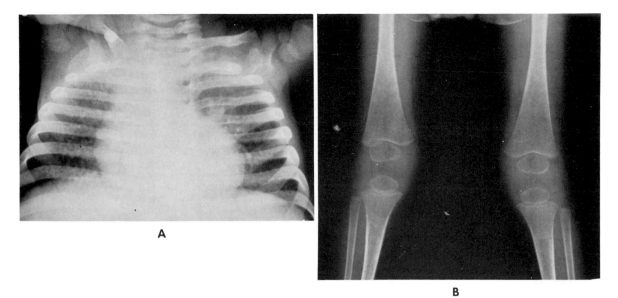

Figure 14–84 **Niemann-Pick Disease: Changes in Lung and Bone.**

A, Fine nodular infiltrations are diffusely scattered throughout both lung fields. These nodular lesions remain unchanged over extended periods of time.

B, The long bones of the lower extremities are diffusely demineralized, with thinned cortices. The metaphyses are widened, giving an Erlenmeyer flask appearance to the lower femora, similar to Gaucher's disease. (Courtesy Dr. H. L. Gildenhorn, Duarte, California.)

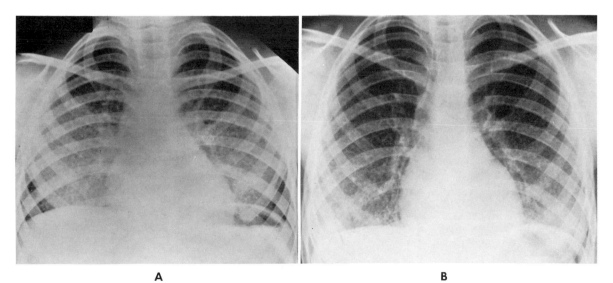

Figure 14–85 **Niemann-Pick Disease: Persistent Infiltrates.**

A, Diffuse fine nodulation throughout the lung fields.

B, Eight years later the pulmonary infiltrates persist, with no apparent change. (Courtesy W. I. Forsythe, Belfast, Ireland.)

PLASMA CELL DYSCRASIAS

Multiple Myeloma

This disease most often affects individuals above age 50.

The lesions arise in the bone marrow as discrete enlarging masses or as diffuse neoplastic infiltrations, or as both. In earlier stages the bone changes are not detected, but eventually bone lesions can be seen radiographically in about 90 per cent of patients with multiple myeloma. Involvement is most frequent in the marrow-rich flat bones of the axial skeleton, which include the skull, spine, pelvis, ribs, clavicles, and scapulae. Long bone involvement is most often seen in the upper humeri and upper femora, but it can be widespread.

Diffuse destruction of the bony trabeculae may cause changes indistinguishable from ordinary osteoporosis. More massive and discrete lesions will produce lytic areas, with either sharp or indefinite margins. Extension to the cortex will cause scalloped erosions of the endosteum. Bone expansion can occur, and the lesions may break through the cortex and periosteum to form soft tissue masses. Pathologic fractures occur in about half the cases. The distribution and appearance of the bone lesions are often indistinguishable from metastatic malignancy.

In the skull, the lesions are usually sharply demarcated punched-out lytic areas. In the spine and pelvis, myelomatous osteoporosis and compression fractures of the vertebral bodies are readily mistaken for senile osteoporosis. Destructive spine lesions will usually be limited to the vertebral body, sparing the pedicle, in contrast to metastatic malignancy. This may be a helpful finding for distinguishing the two conditions. Rib involvement is often associated with an extrapleural soft tissue mass; this is a less frequent occurrence in ordinary rib metastasis. Contiguous lytic areas with bone expansion may simulate osteitis fibrosa cystica or even fibrous dysplasia.

Osteoblastic bone lesions, although extremely rare in myeloma, can occur as either focal areas or diffuse sclerosis.

Complicating respiratory infections, especially pneumonia, are frequent, apparently because of the immunologic disturbance associated with abnormal globulins. Occasionally, nephrocalcinosis may develop as a result of prolonged hypercalcinuria. Renal shutdown following intravenous pyelography has been reported.

From 10 to 20 per cent of patients develop amyloidosis, often involving the gastrointestinal tract, kidneys, and joints (see *Amyloid Disease,* p. 1208).[12, 78, 79]

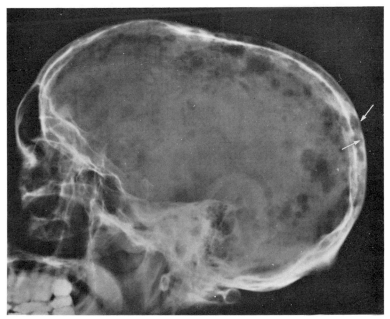

Figure 14–86 **Multiple Myeloma: Skull Lesions.** There are numerous sharply marginated lytic areas of various sizes and shapes throughout the bones of the skull. All are in the medullary portion of the bones and cause scalloping and thinning of the external table *(arrows)*. Often these lesions cannot be distinguished from metastatic malignant lesions, although in the latter the margins may not be as sharply defined.

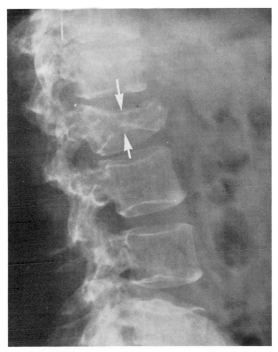

Figure 14–87 **Multiple Myeloma: Lumbar Spine.** There are no clear-cut lytic areas, but the lumbar bodies are osteoporotic. A compression fracture *(arrows)* of L2 demonstrates a still intact cortex. This radiographic appearance is very common in multiple myeloma and can easily be mistaken for senile osteoporosis, in which compression fractures are also common.

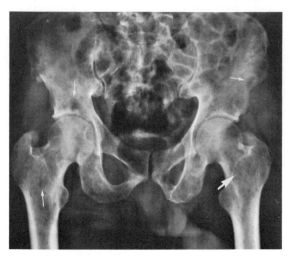

Figure 14–88 **Multiple Myeloma: Diffuse Lesions of the Pelvis and Upper Femora.** There are diffuse lesions throughout the pelvis and upper femora. The larger lesions *(small arrows)* and smaller lesions *(large arrow)* are not punched-out and have rather fuzzy borders.

When marrow infiltration is even and diffuse, there may be no discernible radiographic areas of lysis, and the bones will appear slightly demineralized or normal.

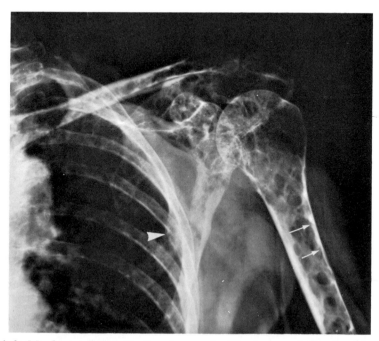

Figure 14–89 **Multiple Myeloma: Extensive Involvement.** The bones of the shoulder girdle and ribs are extensively involved. In the humerus the lesions overlap; they are sharp round lytic areas of various sizes. There is extensive erosive scalloping of the internal cortex *(small arrows)* in all the involved bones.

The extrapleural soft tissue density *(arrowhead)* is from a rib lesion. Rib lesions with extrapleural soft tissue masses are commonly seen in multiple myeloma.

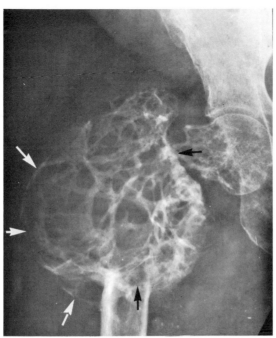

Figure 14-90   **Multiple Myeloma: Expansile Bone Lesions.**   There is marked cystic expansion of the upper femur. A lacy network of bony septa and a thin expanded cortex *(white arrows)* create an appearance similar to that of osteitis fibrosa cystica. There are pathologic features above and below the expanded area *(black arrows)* and involvement beyond the fractures. It is unusual for this degree of expansion to occur in the long bones.

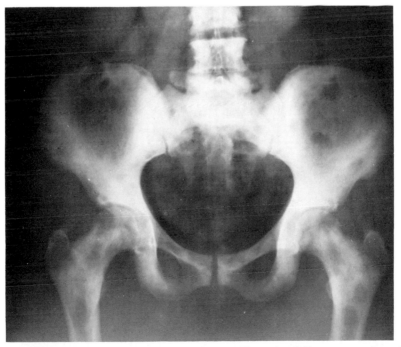

Figure 14-91   **Multiple Myeloma: Osteosclerotic Lesions.**   There is diffuse osteosclerosis in the lumbar bodies and pedicles and upper pelvis and sacrum. More discrete osteoblastic lesions are present in the upper femora and pubic-ischial bones.

　　These bone changes are indistinguishable from those of osteoblastic metastasis.

　　Osteosclerotic changes in multiple myeloma are extremely uncommon. (Courtesy Drs. P. D. T. Clarisse and T. W. Staple, St. Louis, Missouri.)

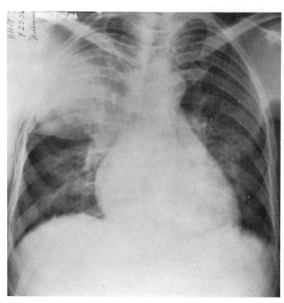

Figure 14–92 **Multiple Myeloma: Lobar Pneumonia.** There is homogeneous consolidation of the base of the right upper lobe. The incidence of pulmonary and other infections is high in myeloma because of abnormal proteins that diminish the immunologic response. The heart is enlarged due to chronic anemia.

Macroglobulinemia of Waldenström

In this rare disease, malignant lymphoplasmacytic cells are deposited in many tissues, particularly the reticuloendothelial structures. Anemia, elevation of serum globulins and macroglobulins, and increased viscosity of the blood are usually present. The disease affects older individuals; 80 per cent of the patients are over 50 years of age. The clinical course is protracted to five years or more.

Radiographic findings are inconstant but can occur in the chest, small bowel, abdomen, and bones. Hepatosplenomegaly is the most common and often the only radiographic finding.

Chronic pleural effusions and neoplastic parenchymal infiltrates are the most common chest lesions; these findings are nonspecific and may persist for long periods without much change—a confusing radiographic picture. Occasionally there may be mediastinal masses, usually neoplastic but sometimes due to extramedullary hematopoiesis. Because of the immunologic abnormalities, recurrent pneumonias are not uncommon. Hyperviscosity of the blood can lead to cardiomegaly and even pulmonary edema.

Small bowel studies may reveal thickened folds and walls; this infiltrative pattern is similar to that of other lymphomatous diseases. Hepatosplenomegaly is sometimes apparent on the abdominal film.

Osteoporosis, sometimes severe, may be present but cannot be distinguished from senile osteoporosis. Punched-out bone lesions indistinguishable from multiple myeloma can occur but are unusual.[80-83]

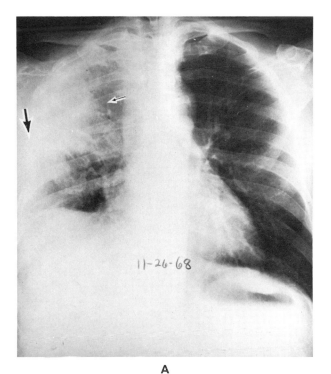

A

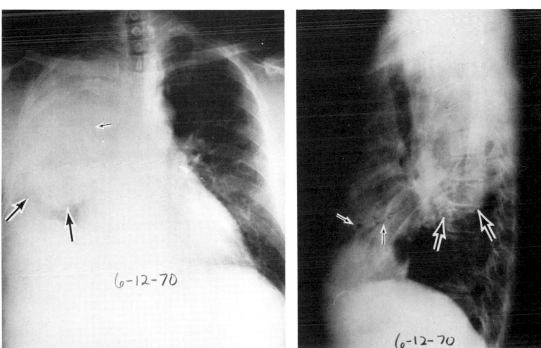

B

Figure 14–93 **Macroglobulinemia of Waldenström: Chronic and Progressive Pulmonary and Pleural Involvement.**

A, A chest film made in 1968 shows extensive pleural density on the right *(large arrow)* and associated alveolar consolidation as evidenced by the air bronchogram *(small arrow).* The left lung is normal.

B, Posteroanterior and lateral films made one and a half years later show a large loculated pleural collection *(large arrows)* and persistent parenchymal consolidation with air bronchograms *(small arrows).*

Illustration continued on the following page

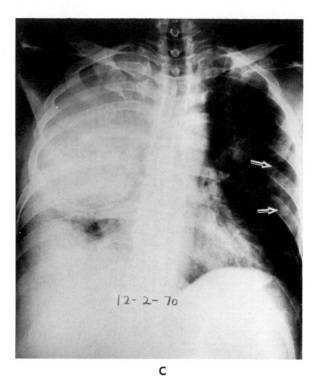

C

Figure 14–93   (Continued)

C, Six months later the right chest is unchanged, but new nodular infiltrates have appeared in the left lung *(arrows)*.

Persistent and progressive pleural and pulmonary lesions are frequently found in Waldenström's macroglobulinemia. The parenchymal densities are tumor infiltrates. Osteoporosis, commonly found in this condition, was not present in this patient.

Solitary Myeloma

A single myelomatous lesion without roentgenologic or clinical evidence of other marrow involvement can originate in the flat bones, especially the pelvis. Localized growth produces lytic defects, usually in the form of a single well-defined lesion. Occasionally, multiple contiguous cyst-like defects are seen, but these are difficult to diagnose radiographically. In many cases the localized lesion is the first manifestation of a generalized myelomatosis. In the spine, solitary myeloma may present as vertebra plana—a collapsed and flattened vertebral body.[12]

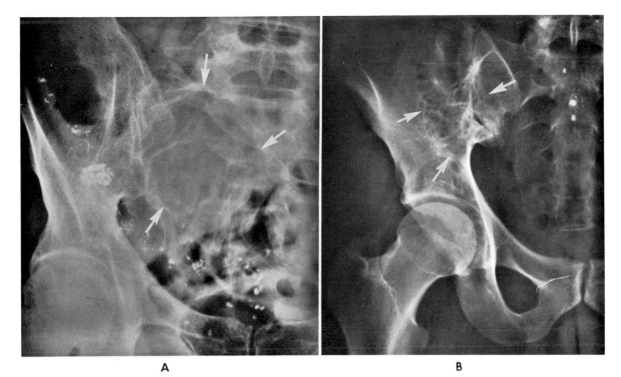

A   B

Figure 14-94   **Solitary Myeloma of the Pelvis: Two Patients.**

A, In the right side of the sacrum there is a large, expansile, lytic lesion *(arrows)* that has distinct borders. No other skeletal lesions were found.

B, A collection of multiple contiguous cyst-like areas *(arrows)* in the right ilium proved to be a solitary lobulated myeloma. This roentgenographic appearance is similar to that of the femoral lesion in Figure 14–90. A benign multilocular cyst or osteitis fibrosa cystica may have a similar radiographic appearance.

Extramedullary Plasmacytoma

Extramedullary plasma cell tumors are the least frequent form of myelomatosis. The lesions may be single or multiple, and any tissue may be involved. The upper respiratory tract is the most common site; associated enlarged regional nodes are found in about 20 per cent of cases. Mediastinal and hilar nodes can also occur but are infrequent.

Gastrointestinal plasma cell lesions have been reported in virtually every portion of the digestive tract except the esophagus; the stomach is the most frequent site. Radiographically these appear as nonspecific filling defects or as infiltrating and constricting lesions.

Only about 25 per cent of the extraosseous tumors precede or accompany bone defects. However, positive bone marrow biopsies are found in a higher percentage of cases.[84-86]

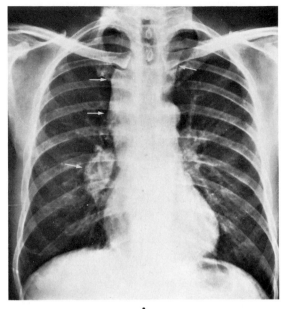

A

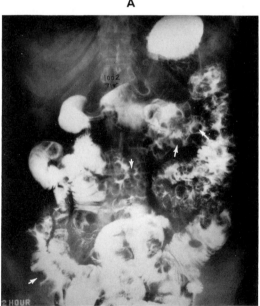

B

Figure 14–95 **Extramedullary Plasmacytomas: Two Patients.**

A, Lobulated masses *(arrows),* producing irregular widening of the superior mediastinum, and the right hilar mass *(arrow)* were due to plasmacytomas involving lymph nodes.

Diffuse plasma cell infiltration of the bone marrow and a solitary myelomatous bone lesion were also present.

B, In another patient, a huge number of rounded masses, a few of which are indicated by arrows, are diffusely scattered throughout the entire small bowel. These proved to be plasmacytomas. No bone lesions were present.

Amyloid Disease

Radiographic changes in the respiratory, gastrointestinal, and cardiovascular system can be seen in both primary and secondary amyloidosis; renal involvement occurs in most cases but there may be no radiographic findings. Rarely, soft tissue and bone lesions are seen.

The primary form is often heredofamilial. The secondary form may accompany the plasma cell dyscrasias, or complicate various neoplastic or chronic inflammatory diseases. Rheumatoid arthritis and other collagen vascular diseases are frequent precursors of amyloid disease.

Respiratory amyloid deposition is seen in only a small percentage of patients with amyloid disease. There may be diffuse infiltration of the trachea and bronchi, infiltration of the alveoli, inconspicuous stippling, or even a widespread reticular nodular pattern in the lung fields. Rarely, there are tumor-like masses that can produce atelectasis. The paranasal sinuses may also be involved and produce a picture similar to that of a mucocele. All of the above lesions are nonspecific and can mimic many other conditions.

In the stomach the submucosal deposition of amyloid can cause pyloric narrowing and, rarely, ulceration. In the small intestine there may be thickened walls with thickened folds. Malabsorption can result. In the colon a roentgen picture similar to that of ulcerative colitis may be seen. The intestinal tract is affected in less than 6 per cent of cases, usually in primary amyloid disease.

Deposition of amyloid in the myocardium may produce cardiomegaly and eventual decompensation. Hepatomegaly and splenomegaly are found in over half the patients. The kidneys, although eventually involved in most cases, may appear normal or slightly enlarged; occasionally they are even reduced in size. No specific urographic changes occur. Renal failure or a nephrotic syndrome may accompany the renal enlargement, a combination of findings that is somewhat suggestive of amyloid disease.

The bone lesions may be nonspecific medullary lytic areas, or may appear as periarticular erosions from adjacent soft tissue amyloid deposits, somewhat similar to gouty arthritis.

Secondary amyloid disease is far more common than the primary type.[87-91]

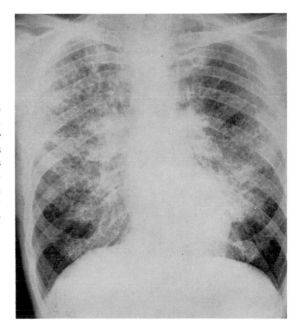

Figure 14-96 **Secondary Amyloidosis of Lung: Lymphoma.** In a man 50 years of age, widespread infiltration radiates from both hilar areas and has a nodular and reticular appearance. The prominent hilar shadows are due to enlargement of the nodes. Both the nodes and the infiltrates consisted of deposits of amyloid, although radiologically it is impossible to distinguish these deposits from those of other disseminated diseases. (Courtesy Drs. C. Wang and L. Robbins, Boston, Massachusetts.)

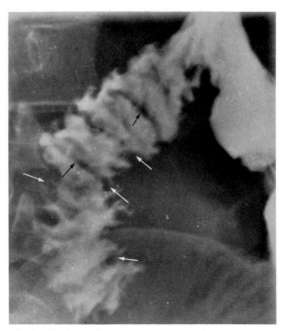

Figure 14–97 **Amyloidosis of Small Intestine in Patient with Multiple Myeloma.** Enlarged view of duodenal loop demonstrates irregular walls (*white arrows*) and extensive thickening of the folds (*black arrows*), caused by submucosal amyloid infiltration.

Intestinal tract involvement may be widespread and diffuse, but occasionally a localized mass of amyloid simulates a gastric or small bowel tumor. (Courtesy Dr. C. Wang, Boston, Massachusetts.)

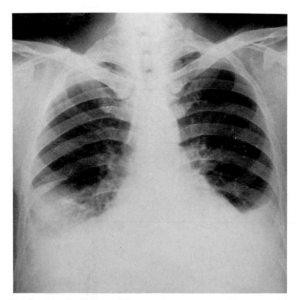

Figure 14–98 **Primary Amyloidosis of Heart.** The patient was a 49 year old man. The heart is enlarged. There are bilateral basal pleural effusions from cardiac decompensation. The appearance is nonspecific and is similar to that of all the myocardiopathies. Cardiomegaly caused by deposition of amyloid occurs more frequently in the primary form of amyloidosis. (Courtesy Dr. C. Wang, Boston, Massachusetts.)

Heavy Chain Disease

Heavy chain disease involving the IgG proteins is a rare condition resembling lymphoma, with lymphadenopathy, splenomegaly, and hepatomegaly, but without bone lesions. In addition to radiographic evidence of hepatosplenomegaly, pulmonary infections often occur, especially in the terminal stages of the disease.

Mediterranean lymphoma, an IgA protein disturbance, is characterized by severe chronic diarrhea, abdominal pain, and malabsorption. It occurs primarily in young individuals of Jewish or Arab descent. Radiographically, the small bowel is involved, usually showing dilatation of the second and third portions of the duodenum and thickening of the walls of the jejunum and ileum. Small bowel masses are occasionally seen, and the radiographic picture is quite similar to ordinary lymphosarcoma. Osteoporosis due to diffuse marrow involvement is sometimes seen, but focal lytic bone lesions do not occur.[92, 93]

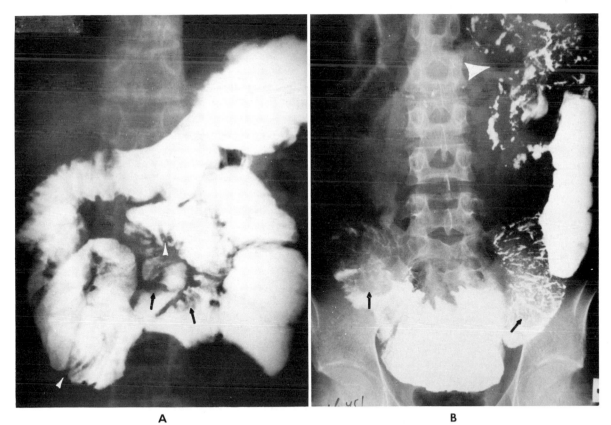

A   B

Figure 14–99 **Mediterranean Lymphoma: IgA Heavy Chain Disease.** Small bowel study in a 20 year old Israeli with a five-year history of watery diarrhea reveals dilatation of the duodenum and jejunum (*A*) and ileum (*B*). The mucosal folds are thickened (*small white arrowheads*), and filling defects are scattered throughout (*black arrows*). Flocculation is also present (*large arrowhead*), and transit time was prolonged.

The intestinal appearance may resemble the malabsorption pattern of sprue, but the nodules are suggestive of lymphosarcoma.

The diagnosis of IgA heavy chain disease with lymphoma was made by blood protein studies and small bowel biopsy. (Courtesy Dr. A. Zlotnick, Jerusalem, Israel.)

DISEASES OF THE SPLEEN

Chronic Congestive Splenomegaly

This syndrome is characterized by marked splenomegaly and portal hypertension. Anemia, leukopenia, and moderate thrombocytopenia are consistently associated.

An enlarged soft tissue mass in the left upper quadrant is readily demonstrated. Even when the splenic borders are not distinct, displacement of the stomach toward the midline or downward displacement of the splenic flexure strongly suggests splenomegaly.

Splenic vein occlusion, usually caused by thrombosis, is a prominent cause of congestive splenomegaly, and esophageal varices frequently develop. Demonstration of the occlusion and opacification of anastomotic venous channels can be obtained in the venous phase of selective splenic or celiac arteriography or after direct percutaneous injection of contrast material into the spleen. Varicosities of the lower esophagus and of the gastric fundus may also be opacified.

Other causes of congestive splenomegaly include portal vein occlusion (usually thrombotic) and intrahepatic obstruction such as occurs in cirrhosis, schistosomiasis, and so forth.

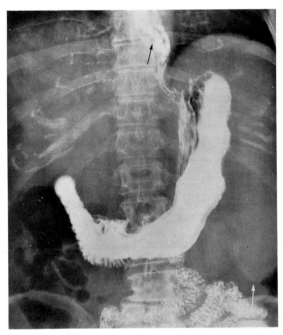

Figure 14–100 **Congestive Splenomegaly.** The tip of the enlarged spleen *(white arrow)* is almost at the iliac crest; the splenic flexure is depressed; the stomach is indented and displaced toward the midline. Varices presenting as multiple small filling defects can be seen *(black arrow)* in the lower end of the barium-filled esophagus.

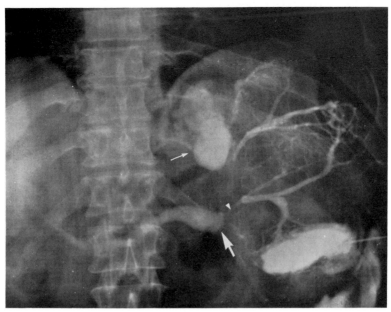

Figure 14-101 **Splenic Vein Thrombosis: Splenoportogram.** The opaque material that has been injected into the spleen cannot enter the occluded splenic veins and therefore passes through the collateral vessels into varices (*small arrow*) in the gastric fundus and then into the distal splenic and portal vein (*large arrow*). The sharp cutoff of the splenic vein distal to the thrombus is clearly depicted (*arrowhead*). The patient's spleen was greatly enlarged, and he experienced hematemesis as a result of the varices.

Splenic Cysts

Splenic cysts are quite rare and extremely variable in size, sometimes attaining massive proportions. Less than 10 per cent of these cysts calcify. The hydatid (echinococcus) cyst is the most common. It calcifies more frequently than nonparasitic cysts, and exhibits a trabeculated and sometimes double rim of calcification. Ring densities of fleck-like calcific deposits may be seen in a small percentage of nonparasitic cysts.

Larger cysts may produce a soft tissue shadow in the left upper quadrant. They may displace the stomach medially and the splenic flexure and the left kidney downward, findings indicative of splenic enlargement.

Small noncalcified cysts cannot usually be seen on plain films. Selective splenic artery opacification may demonstrate an avascular area and displaced vessels, suggesting the correct diagnosis; it may also distinguish the cyst from lymphomatous tumor mass.[94, 95]

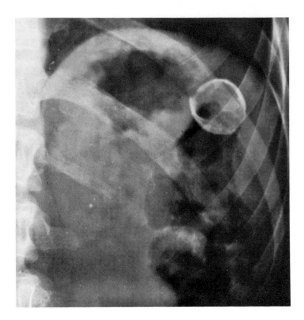

Figure 14–102 **Calcified Simple Splenic Cyst.** The round dense ring calcification in the left upper quadrant was a simple cyst projecting from the hilum of the spleen.

Rupture of the Spleen

Rupture of the spleen is usually due to trauma; rarely, a diseased spleen may rupture spontaneously. A history of trauma and roentgenologic demonstration of an enlarged splenic mass are the cardinal diagnostic features.

A massive tear produces extensive intra-abdominal hemorrhage with immediate severe clinical signs and symptoms. Roentgenologically, the abdominal film may be hazy; the distance between the bowel loops may be increased, together with other roentgen signs of intraperitoneal fluid.

Most often the tear is less massive, and the spleen becomes swollen from edema and parenchymal hemorrhage; a subcapsular hematoma usually develops. The radiographic outlines of the spleen usually are lost, but the enlarged splenic area is recognized by the medial displacement of the gastric gas bubble or of the barium-filled stomach. The gas shadows of the splenic flexure of the colon may be displaced downward. The left kidney may be depressed. Movements of the left diaphragm are usually limited. Fracture of one or more of the lower left ribs will corroborate the diagnosis, but this occurs in only about a fourth of the patients.

Indentations and serrations of the greater curvature of the displaced stomach may occur if the edema and hemorrhage have extended into the gastrolienal ligament. The left psoas shadow is partially or completely obliterated in about half the cases. The descending colon may be displaced mesially by blood, thus increasing the distance between colon and peritoneal fat lines.

In more chronic cases the bleeding remains confined to the spleen and subcapsular area. Progressive enlargement of the splenic area on serial films, in conjunction with a history of trauma, will suggest the diagnosis.

These roentgenographic findings, although indirect, are generally sufficient for diagnosis in clinically suspected cases. In equivocal cases, celiac or splenic angiography usually will be definitive and diagnostic. Extravasation of contrast material into the spleen, amputation of a major splenic artery, and premature visualization of the splenic vein are conclusive findings. Other confirmatory findings include defects or deficiencies in the splenogram of an enlarged spleen. In less severe cases, there may be a mass defect due to an intrasplenic hematoma, small arteriovenous aneurysms, or small defects in the splenogram corresponding to avascular areas.[96-98]

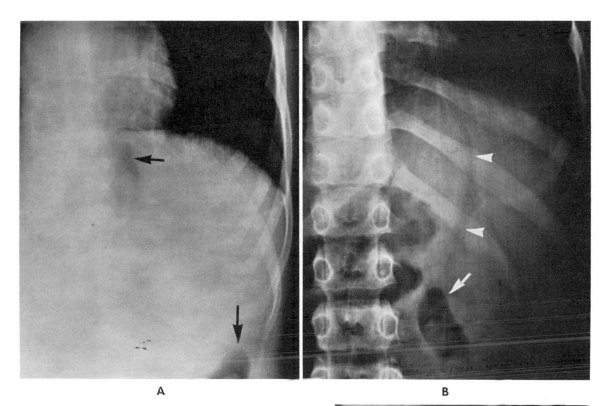

A   B

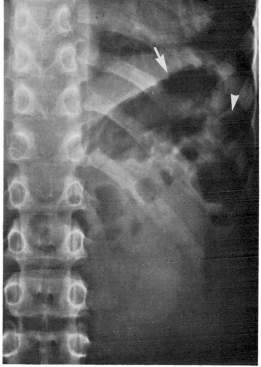

Figure 14–103 **Traumatic Rupture of Spleen.**

A, Erect view of the left upper quadrant shows displacement of the gastric air bubble toward the spine (*upper arrow*). There is also evidence of soft tissue indentation on the gas shadow. The gas-filled splenic flexure of the colon is displaced downward (*lower arrow*). A soft tissue density fills the left upper quadrant, but splenic borders cannot be seen.

B, Recumbent view demonstrates pressure and displacement of the gastric air shadow (*arrowheads*) and depression of the splenic flexure (*arrow*). The finding of splenic enlargement following trauma clearly suggests rupture of the spleen.

C, Following surgical removal of the ruptured spleen, the gas-filled stomach (*arrow*) and splenic flexure (*arrowhead*) have returned to normal position.

C

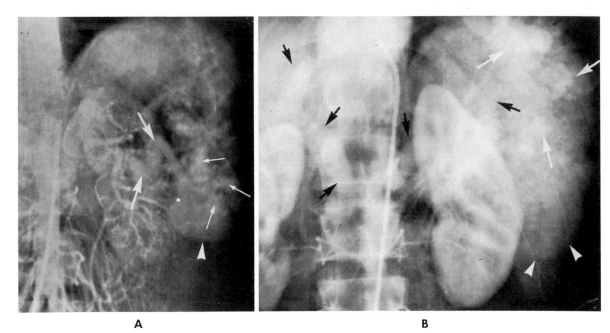

A   B

Figure 14–104   **Laceration of Spleen: Arteriographic Findings in Two Patients.**

A, Film made at 2½ seconds of an aortogram reveals enlargement of the splenic shadow (*arrowhead*), pools of extravasated opaque material within the spleen (*small arrows*), and early filling of the splenic vein (*large arrows*).

B, Aortogram (3 seconds) of another patient discloses similar findings: extravasation within the spleen (*white arrows*), early opacification of the splenic and portal veins (*black arrows*), and enlargement of the splenic shadows (*arrowheads*).

When clinical and routine radiographic findings are equivocal, arteriography may make a definitive diagnosis. Extravasation of the contrast material into an enlarged spleen, and early vein opacification are characteristic and conclusive findings. (Courtesy Dr. Leon Love, Chicago, Illinois.)

Splenic Artery Aneurysm

Calcification of the aneurysmal wall is frequent and may be the only radiographic finding. Since most splenic artery aneurysms are of atherosclerotic origin, there may be associated calcification of a portion of the artery close to the aneurysmal calcification, a valuable diagnostic clue. A large aneurysm can compress the splenic vein and produce congestive splenomegaly.

Definitive diagnosis is made by opacification of the aneursymal cavity during aortic or selective splenic arteriography.[99]

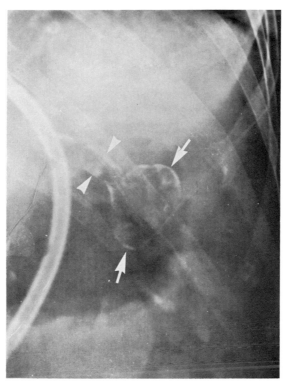

Figure 14–105 **Splenic Artery Aneurysm.** Shell calcification in the left upper quadrant (*arrows*) is in the wall of an aneurysm. The segment of splenic artery from which the aneurysm arises is also calcified (*arrowheads*).

Ring calcifications in the left upper quadrant, especially in older persons, are usually of vascular origin. Positive identification of a suspected aneurysm requires celiac or abdominal aortography.

HEMORRHAGIC DISORDERS

Hemophilia

The most frequent radiographic changes are encountered in the joints and periarticular bones of children, most often in the knees, elbows, and ankles. These changes are due to intra-articular hemorrhage, which may occur without significant trauma. One or more joints may be affected.

Acute and subacute hemarthrosis may produce increased soft tissue density of the distended joint. In more chronic cases, deposition of hemosiderin may lead to increased opacity of the periarticular soft tissues. Chronic recurrent hemorrhage into a joint will cause erosion of the cartilages and periarticular bones; eventually the joint space becomes narrowed and irregular. Periarticular osteoporosis usually occurs, and the entire epiphysis may show coarsened trabeculae. Cyst-like areas of lysis—often quite large—may form in the periarticular bones. Presumably these are pressure erosions from intra-articular collections of blood. In an involved knee the intercondylar notch may be widened and the inferior border of the patella may become squared. Secondary osteoarthritis with osteophyte formation can develop in a chronically affected joint. In some cases the roentgen changes can simulate rheumatoid arthritis or tuberculosis.

Infrequently, minor trauma can cause subperiosteal or intraosseous hemorrhage. The former may result in periosteal elevation and layering while intraosseous hemorrhage can cause lytic changes in the bone that may resemble a malignant bone tumor or an osteomyelitis. Often, a soft tissue component is present. Radiation has been employed to prevent continued bleeding and massive bone destruction.

Abnormalities of the urinary tracts are surprisingly frequent. Obstructive uropathy, apparently secondary to ureteral obstruction from retroperitoneal hemorrhage and subsequent fibrosis, occurs in about one third of hemophiliacs. Other abnormalities are intrarenal hematoma and a mild form of papillary necrosis.

Occasionally, submucosal bleeding into the small bowel wall will cause swollen mucosa, thickening of the bowel wall, and thumbprinting defects in the barium column. These changes are reversible.[100-105]

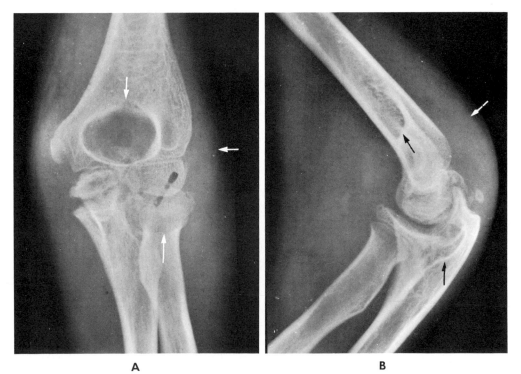

A   B

Figure 14–106 **Hemophilia: Hemarthrosis and Bone Changes.** Anteroposterior (*A*) and lateral (*B*) views of the elbow disclose distended soft tissues (*arrows outside bone*) due to blood accumulation within the joint.
The large cystic areas in the lower humerus and upper ulna (*arrows in bone*) are the result of previous hemorrhages within the joint. The joint spaces are still well preserved.

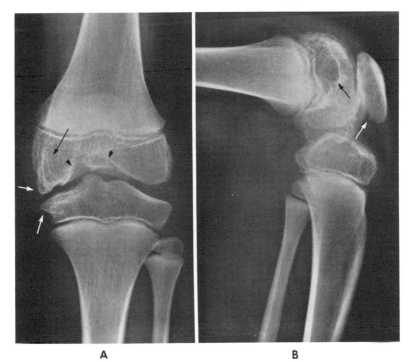

A   **B**

Figure 14–107 **Hemophilic Knee in Young Boy.**

   A, In anteroposterior view there is osteophyte formation at the medial articular edge of the femur and tibia (*white arrows*). The medial half of the joint is irregularly narrowed, and the intercondylar notch is widened (*black arrowheads*). Note coarsened longitudinal trabeculae in the femoral epiphysis (*black arrow*). This type of osteoporosis is characteristic in hemophilic arthropathy, and when associated with the widened intercondylar notch it strongly suggests the diagnosis. No cystic areas are recognizable.

   B, Lateral view reveals a cyst (*black arrow*) in the femoral epiphysis. The undersurface of the patella shows some erosion (*white arrow*).

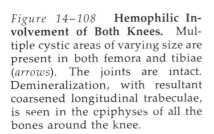

Figure 14–108 **Hemophilic Involvement of Both Knees.** Multiple cystic areas of varying size are present in both femora and tibiae (*arrows*). The joints are intact. Demineralization, with resultant coarsened longitudinal trabeculae, is seen in the epiphyses of all the bones around the knee.

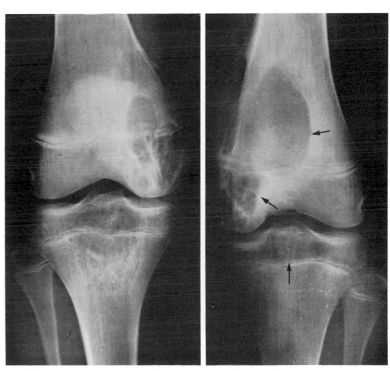

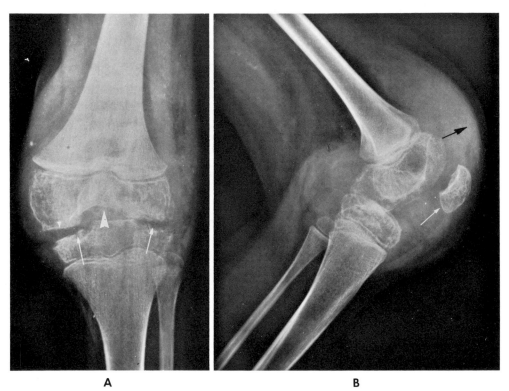

A   B

Figure 14–109   **Hemophilia: Characteristic Bone and Periarticular Changes.**

The patient was a young man with severe hemophilia.

A, In anteroposterior view there is considerable, rather dense soft tissue swelling around the knee. The femoral and tibial epiphyses are severely osteoporotic. The articular margins of the tibia and femur are irregular (*arrows*), and the joint spaces are narrowed and uneven. The medial articular edge of the femur (*small arrowhead*) has a characteristic squared-off appearance. The condylar notch is broadened (*large arrowhead*). No clearly defined cystic areas are seen in the bones.

B, In lateral view the anterior soft tissue swelling (*black arrow*) is prominent and unusually dense, probably owing to hemosiderin deposits. The undersurface of the patella (*white arrow*) also appears to be squared off.

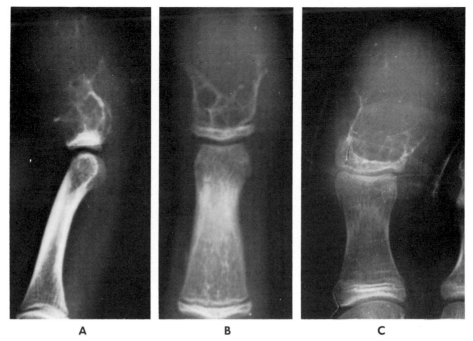

A   B   C

Figure 14-110   **Hemophilia: Bone Destruction: Intraosseous Hemorrhage.**

A and *B,* There is complete destruction of the distal end of the phalanx, with cystic expansion of the proximal portion of the bone. Only the epiphysis is uninvolved. There is considerable soft tissue swelling as the hemorrhage extends into the surrounding tissues.

C, Similar involvement is evident in the distal phalanx of the thumb. This type of osseous destruction, unrelated to a joint, is probably a result of intraosseous hemorrhage. Such hemorrhage in hemophilia is far less common than intra-articular bleeding. (Courtesy G. Stiris, Oslo, Norway.)

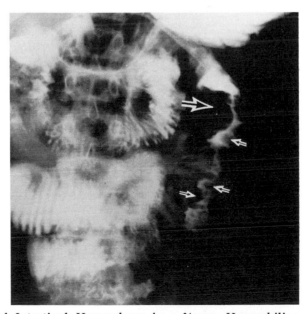

Figure 14-111   **Intramural Intestinal Hemorrhage in a Young Hemophiliac.**   One jejunal segment is irregularly narrowed and shows extensive thumbprinting (*small arrows*) and a large pseudotumor defect (*large arrow*), changes characteristic of intramural submucosal hemorrhage. The apparent separation of this loop from the rest of the small bowel is due to hemorrhagic and edematous thickening of its wall.

Abdominal pain and intestinal bleeding accompanied these radiographic findings. The bowel returned to a normal appearance after resorption of the blood.

Henoch-Schönlein Purpura

There are no radiologic findings in this condition except during an attack of acute abdominal pain. The symptoms are due to submucosal hemorrhage and edema in the small bowel, and may simulate an acute surgical abdomen. Barium studies of the small bowel disclose separation of the loops due to edematous thickening of the walls. The mucosal folds are thickened, and areas of polypoid defects (thumbprinting) due to local submucosal hemorrhages may be present. The roentgen findings resemble those of other infiltrative small bowel diseases such as Whipple's disease, amyloidosis, and lymphoma, but the clinical picture is more specific. At times, the roentgen picture is indistinguishable from ischemic bowel disease. In children the acute abdominal episode may precede the cutaneous and joint manifestations.

Clinical recovery is marked by return of the small bowel to a normal appearance (within one to four weeks).

The joint symptoms of Henoch-Schönlein purpura are not associated with radiographic changes.[106, 107]

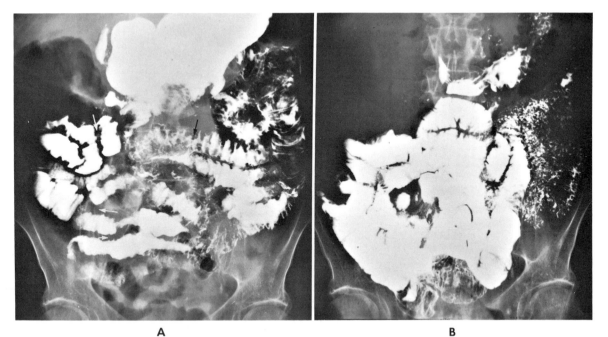

A   B

Figure 14–112 **Submucosal Hemorrhage into Small Intestine During Exacerbation of Anaphylactoid Purpura.**

A, The small bowel pattern is grossly distorted, with thickening of the walls as demonstrated by the increased space between the loops (*white arrows*) and thickened mucosal folds and thumbprinting (*black arrow*) throughout the loops. There is no dilatation or segmentation such as is seen in the deficiency pattern of sprue.

B, One week later the small bowel has a normal appearance.

Hereditary Hemorrhagic Telangiectasia
(Osler-Weber-Rendu Disease)

Although telangiectasia and arteriovenous malformations may occur in any organ or tissue, the most significant findings are seen in the lungs, in the gastrointestinal tract, and, rarely, intracerebrally. The gastrointestinal and cerebral lesions usually cannot be demonstrated by routine studies, but may be uncovered by arteriography.

Pulmonary arteriovenous malformations occur in almost 10 per cent of cases; conversely, about half of all patients with pulmonary arteriovenous fistula or malformations prove to have hereditary hemorrhagic telangiectasia. A well-demarcated parenchymal area of increased density, either saccular or circinate, can be seen communicating with the hilum through enlarged feeding vessels. Planigraphy is often needed to demonstrate the afferent and efferent vessels. On fluoroscopy the feeding vessels and mass may decrease in size during the Valsalva maneuver and increase in size with the Müller maneuver. Definitive diagnosis can be made only with contrast pulmonary angiography, which frequently demonstrates other smaller unsuspected arteriovenous malformations. Similarly, gastrointestinal malformations or telangiectasia may be demonstrated by selective or subselective arteriography.[108, 109]

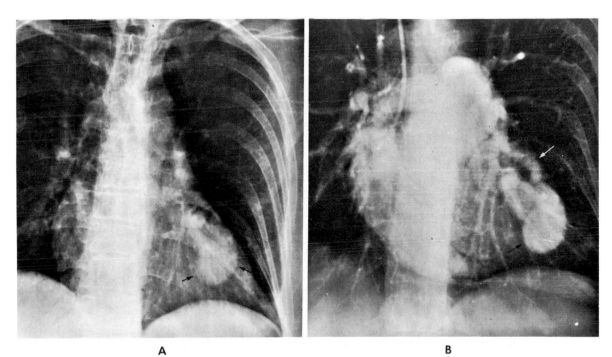

A **B**

Figure 14–113 **Hereditary Hemorrhagic Telangiectasia: Pulmonary Arteriovenous Aneurysm.**

A, There is an oval density behind the heart shadow (*arrows*). Although no connecting vessels could be demonstrated on the plain film, an arteriovenous aneurysm was suspected because of areas of telangiectasia on the lips and hands.

B, Film made during angiocardiography demonstrates opacification of an arteriovenous fistula (*black arrows*) and a definite feeding artery (*white arrow*).

REFERENCES

1. Laws, J. W., and Pitman, R. G.: Radiologic features of primary pernicious anemia. Br. J. Radiol., *33*:229, 1969.
2. Joske, R. A., and Vaughn, M. B.: Radiologic findings in atrophic gastritis and gastric atrophy. Gastroenterology, *42*:7, 1962.
3. Vaughn, B. F., and Pitney, W. R.: Radiographic findings in megaloblastic anemia. J. Coll. Radiol. Austral., *5*:77, 1961.
4. Martin, J. F., et al.: Roentgenographic signs in atrophic gastritis. Am. J. Roentgenol., Radium Ther. Nucl. Med., *94*:343, 1965.
5. McKay, E.: Congenital hypoplastic anemia. Arch. Dis. Child., *37*:663, 1962.
6. Dawson, J. P.: Pancytopenia with multiple congenital anomalies. Pediatrics, *15*:325, 1955.
7. Juhl, J. H., Wesenberg, R. L., and Gwinn, J. L.: Roentgen findings in Fanconi anemia. Radiology, *89*:646, 1967.
8. Moseley, J. E.: Skeletal changes in the anemias. Semin. Roentgenol., *9*:169, 1974.
9. Moseley, J. E.: Chronic iron deficiency anemia. Am. J. Roentgenol. Radium Ther. Nucl. Med., *85*:649, 1961.
10. Aksoy, M., Necdet, C., and Sakir, E.: Roentgenographic bone changes in chronic iron deficiency anemia. Blood, *27*:677, 1966.
11. Seeman, W. B.: Significance of webs in the hypopharynx and upper esophagus. Radiology, *89*:32, 1967.
12. Moseley, J. E.: *Bone Changes in Hematologic Disorders.* New York, Grune & Stratton, Inc., 1963.
13. Millard, D. G.: Renal siderosis. Radiology, *79*:290, 1962.
14. Golding, J. S. R., et al.: Bone changes in sickle cell anemia. J. Bone Joint Surg., *41B*:711, 1959.
15. Marquis, J. B., and Khazem, B.: Sickle cell disease in children: renal roentgenographic changes. Radiology, *98*:47, 1971.
16. Walker, R. R., Alexander, F., et al.: Glomerular lesions in sickle cell nephropathy. J.A.M.A., *215*:437, 1971.
17. Khademi, M., and Marquis, J. R.: Renal angiography in sickle cell disease. Radiology, *107*:41, 1973.
18. Bohrer, S. P.: Fracture complicating bone infarcts and/or osteomyelitis in sickle cell disease. Clin. Radiol., *22*:83, 1971.
19. Reynolds, J., Pritchard, J. A., et al.: Roentgenographic and clinical appraisal of sickle beta-thalassemia disease. Am. J. Roentgenol. Radium Ther. Nucl. Med., *118*:378, 1973.
20. Eckert, D. E., et al.: The incidence and manifestations of urographic papillary abnormalities in patients with S hemoglobinopathies. Radiology, *113*:59, 1974.
21. Schumacher, H. R., Andrews, R., and McLauglin, G.: Arthropathy in sickle cell disease. Ann. Intern. Med., *78*:203, 1973.
22. Caffey, J.: Cooley's anemia. Am. J. Roentgenol. Radium Ther. Nucl. Med., *78*:381, 1957.
23. Korsten, J., et al.: Extramedullary hematopoiesis in patients with thalassemia anemia. Radiology, *95*:257, 1970.
24. Bishop, P. A.: Fetal hydrops. Am. J. Roentgenol. Radium Ther. Nucl. Med., *86*:415, 1961.
25. Savignac, E. M.: Prenatal diagnosis of fetal hydrops. Am. J. Roentgenol. Radium Ther. Nucl. Med., *80*:673, 1958.
26. Atkins, C. J., McIvor, J., et al.: Chondrocalcinosis and arthropathy. Studies in hemochromatosis and idiopathic chondrocalcinosis. Q. J. Med., *39*:71, 1970
27. Easley, R. M., Schreiner, B. F., and Yu, P. N.: Reversible cardiomyopathy associated with hemochromatosis. N. Engl. J. Med., *287*:866, 1972.
28. Gordon, D. A., Clarke, P. V., and Ogryzlo, M. A.: The chondrocalcific arthropathy of iron overload. Arch. Intern. Med., *134*:21, 1974.
29. Ross, D., and Wood, B.: Osteoarthropathy in idiopathic hemochromatosis. Am. J. Roentgenol. Radium Ther. Nucl. Med., *109*:575, 1970.
30. Pitman, R. G., et al.: Radiologic appearance of chest in polycythemia. Clin. Radiol., *12*:276, 1961.
31. Powell, J. W., et al.: Skull roentgenogram in iron deficiency anemia and in secondary polycythemia. Am. J. Roentgenol. Radium Ther. Nucl. Med., *95*:143, 1965.
32. Janower, M. L., et al.: The radiologist in diagnosis of non-endocrine endocrinology. Radiology, *86*:746, 1966.
33. Hilbush, T. F., et al.: Acute leukemia: skeletal manifestations in children. Arch. Intern. Med., *104*:741, 1959.
34. Willson, J. K. V.: Bone lesions of childhood leukemia. Radiology, *72*:672, 1959.
35. Klatte, E. C., et al.: Pulmonary complications of leukemia. Am. J. Roentgenol. Radium Ther. Nucl. Med., *89*:598, 1963.
36. Green, R. A., and Nichols, N. J.: Pulmonary involvement in leukemia. Am. Rev. Resp. Dis., *80*:833, 1959.
37. Simmons, C. R., Harle, T. S., and Singleton, E. B.: The osseous manifestations of leukemia in children. Radiol. Clin. North Am., *6*:115, 1968.
38. Nixon, G. W., and Gwinn, J. L.: The roentgen manifestations of leukemia in infancy. Radiology, *107*:603, 1973.

39. Pear, B. L.: Skeletal manifestations of the lymphomas and leukemias. Semin. Roentgenol., 9:229, 1974.
40. Mezaros, W. T., and Sisson, M.: Myelofibrosis. Radiology, 77:958, 1961.
41. Kempf, F., et al.: Bone lesions in chronic adult erythroblastosis. J. Radiol. Electrol. Med. Nucl., 44:27, 1963.
42. Pettigrew, J. D., and Ward, H. P.: Correlation of radiologic, histologic and clinical findings in agnogenic myeloid metaplasia. Radiology, 93:541, 1969.
43. Maier, J. G., and Schanber, D. T.: The role of lymphangiography in the diagnosis and treatment of malignant testicular tumors. Am. J. Roentgenol. Radium Ther. Nucl. Med., 114:482, 1972.
44. Kress, M. B., and Brantigon, O. C.: Primary lymphosarcoma of lung. Ann. Intern. Med., 55:582, 1961.
45. Hall, E. R., and Blades, B.: Primary lymphosarcoma of lungs. Dis. Chest, 36:1, 1959.
46. Marshak, R. H., Wolf, B., et al.: Lymphosarcoma of small bowel. Am. J. Roentgenol. Radium Ther. Nucl. Med., 86:682, 1961.
47. Keats, T. E., and Teats, C. D.: Roentgen manifestations of thoracic reticulum cell sarcoma. Radiol. Clin. North Am., 6:143, 1968.
48. Wychulas, A. R.: Malignant lymphoma of the colon. Arch. Surg., 93:215, 1966.
49. Schey, W. L., White, H., et al.: Lymphosarcoma in children. Am. J. Roentgenol. Radium Ther. Nucl. Med., 117:59, 1973.
50. Norfray, J., Calenoff, L., and Zanon, B.: Aneurysmal lymphoma of the small intestine. Am. J. Roentgenol. Radium Ther. Nucl. Med., 119:335, 1973.
51. Bassett, D. J.: Burkitt's tumor. Aust. Radiol., 10:319, 1966.
52. Cockshott, W. P.: Radiologic aspects of Burkitt's tumor. Br. J. Radiol., 38:176, 1965.
53. Stutz, A. J., et al.: Burkitt's lymphoma: role of radiotherapy. Radiology, 104:379, 1972.
54. Whittaker, L. R.: Burkitt's lymphoma. Clin. Radiol., 24:339, 1973.
55. Picard, J. D., et al.: A clinical and lymphographic study of Brill-Symmers disease. Ann. Radiol., 9:685, 1966.
56. Bleufarb, S. M., and Steinberg, H. S.: Pulmonary manifestations of mycosis fungoides. Ann. Intern. Med., 36:625, 1952.
57. Escovitz, E. S., Soulen, R. L., et al.: Mycosis fungoides: a lymphographic assessment. Radiology, 112:23, 1974.
58. Fisher, A. M. H., et al.: Hodgkin's disease: a radiologic survey. Clin. Radiol., 13:115, 1962.
59. Hoskins, E. O.: Unusual radiological manifestations of Hodgkin's disease. Proc. R. Soc. Med., 60:729, 1967.
60. Buraczewski, J., Dzivkowa, J., and Zomer, J.: Calcification in lymphogranulomatosis. Fortschr. Roentgenstr., 117:28, 1972.
61. Bloch, C.: Roentgen features of Hodgkin's disease of the stomach. Am. J. Roentgenol. Radium Ther. Nucl. Med., 99:175, 1967.
62. Waterhouse, B. E., and Lapidus, P. H.: Infectious mononucleosis associated with a mass in the anterior mediastinum. N. Engl. J. Med., 277:1137, 1967.
63. Burrows, F. G. O.: Transient periosteal reaction in illness diagnosed as infectious mononucleosis. Radiology, 98:291, 1971.
64. DeWitte, J.: Reticuloendotheliosis. J. Belge Radiol., 40:269, 1957.
65. Green, A. E., and Flaherty, R. A.: Histiocytosis X. Radiology, 75:572, 1960.
66. Teplick, J. G., and Broder, H.: Eosinophilic granuloma of bone. Am. J. Roentgenol. Radium Ther. Nucl. Med., 78:502, 1957.
67. Westling, P., et al.: Systemic reticuloendothelial granuloma. Acta Radiol., 149 (supplement):1, 1957.
68. Takahashi, M., et al.: The variable roentgenographic appearance of idiopathic histiocytosis. Clin. Radiol., 17:48, 1966.
69. Ennis, J. J., Whitehouse, G., et al.: Radiology of the bone changes in histiocytosis X. Clin. Radiol., 24:212, 1973.
70. Cheyne, C.: Histiocytosis X. J. Bone Joint Surg., 53:366, 1971.
71. Levin, B.: Gaucher's disease Am. J. Roentgenol. Radium Ther. Nucl. Med., 85:685, 1961.
72. Amstutz, H. C., and Carey, E. J.: Skeletal manifestations and treatment of Gaucher's disease. Review of twenty cases. J. Bone Joint Surg., 48:670, 1966.
73. Greenfield, G. B.: Bone changes in chronic adult Gaucher's disease. Am. J. Roentgenol. Radium Ther. Nucl. Med., 110:800, 1970.
74. Forsythe, W. I., et al.: Three cases of Niemann Pick's disease in children. Arch. Dis. Child., 34:406, 1959.
75. Gildenhorn, H. L., and Amromin, G. D.: Niemann-Pick disease. Am. J. Roentgenol. Radium Ther. Nucl. Med., 85:680, 1961.
76. Lachman, R., Crocker, A., et al.: Radiologic findings in Niemann-Pick disease. Radiology, 108:659, 1973.
77. Queloz, J. M., Capitanio, M. A., and Kirkpatrick, J. A.: Wolman's disease. Radiology, 104:357, 1972.
78. Clarisse, P. D., and Staple, T. W.: Diffuse sclerosis in multiple myeloma. Radiology, 99:327, 1971.
79. Gompels, B. M., Votaw, M. L., and Martel, W.: Correlation of radiologic manifestations of multiple myeloma with immunoglobulin abnormalities. Radiology, 104:509, 1972.

80. Lemenager, J., et al.: Macroglobulinemia of Waldenström with mediastinal localization. J. Fr. Med. Chir. Thorac., *17*:625, 1963.
81. Benner, R. R., Nelson, D. A., and Lozner, E. L.: Roentgenologic manifestations of primary macroglobulinemia. Am. J. Roentgenol. Radium Ther. Nucl. Med., *113*:499, 1971.
82. Neiman, H. L., Wolson, A. H., and Berenson, J. E.: Pulmonary and plural manifestations of Waldenstrom's macroglobulinemia. Radiology, *107*:301, 1973.
83. Vermess, M., Pearson, K. D., et al.: Osseous manifestations of Waldenstrom's macroglobulinemia. Radiology, *102*:497, 1972.
84. Gilroy, J. A., and Adams, A. B.: Extraosseous infiltration in multiple myeloma. Radiology, *73*:406, 1959.
85. Ennuyer, A., et al.: Plasmacytoma of the upper respiratory–digestive system. Bull. Assoc. Fr. Cancer, *50*:53, 1963.
86. Oberkircher, P. E., Miller, W. T., and Arger, P. H.: Non-osseous presentation of plasma cell myeloma. Radiology, *104*:515, 1972.
87. Wang, C. C., and Robbins, L. L.: Amyloid disease. Radiology, *66*:489, 1956.
88. Brown, J.: Primary amyloidosis. Clin. Radiol., *15*:358, 1964.
89. Pear, B. L.: Radiographic manifestations of amyloidosis. Am. J. Roentgenol. Radium Ther. Nucl. Med., *111*:821, 1971.
90. Gordonson, J. S., et al.: Pulmonary amyloidosis. J. Can. Assoc. Radiol., *23*:269, 1972.
91. Legge, D. A., Carlson, H. C., and Wollaeger, E. E.: Amyloidosis involving the gastrointestinal tract. Am. J. Roentgenol. Radium Ther. Nucl. Med., *110*:406, 1970.
92. Selegman, M., Danon, F., et al.: Alpha chain disease: a new immunoglobulin. Science, *162*:1396, 1968.
93. Zlotnick, A., and Levy, M.: Alpha heavy chain disease: a variant of Mediterranean lymphoma. Arch. Intern. Med., *128*:432, 1971.
94. Forde, W. J., and Finby, N.: Splenic cysts. Clin. Radiol., *12*:49, 1961.
95. Bron, K. M., and Hoffman, W. J.: Preoperative diagnosis of splenic cysts. Arch. Surg., *102*:459, 1971.
96. Schwartz, S. S., et al.: Traumatic rupture of spleen in children: roentgen findings. Am. J. Roentgenol. Radium Ther. Nucl. Med., *82*:505, 1960.
97. Love, L., Greenfield, G. B., et al.: Arteriography of splenic trauma. Radiology, *91*:96, 1968.
98. Brindle, M. J.: Arteriography and minor splenic injury. Clin. Radiol., *23*:174, 1972.
99. Steinberg, I., et al.: Aneurysm of splenic, hepatic and renal arteries. Am. J. Roentgenol. Radium Ther. Nucl. Med., *86*:1108, 1961.
100. Stiris, G.: Bone and joint changes in hemophiliacs. Acta Radiol., *49*:269, 1958.
101. Baldero, J. L., and Kemp, H. S.: The early bone and joint changes in hemophilia and similar blood dyscrasias. Br. J. Radiol., *39*:172, 1966.
102. Grossman, H., et al.: Reversible gastrointestinal signs of hemorrhage and edema in the pediatric age group. Radiology, *84*:33, 1965.
103. Brant, E. E., and Jordan, H. H.: Radiologic aspects of hemophilic pseudo tumors in bone. Am. J. Roentgenol. Radium Ther. Nucl. Med., *115*:525, 1972.
104. Beck, P., and Evans, K. T.: Renal abnormalities in patients with hemophilia and Christmas disease. Clin. Radiol., *23*:349, 1972.
105. Salerno, N. R., Menges, J. F., and Borns, P. F.: Arthrograms in hemophilia. Radiology, *102*:135, 1972.
106. Grossman, H., et al.: Abdominal pain in Schönlein-Henoch syndrome. Correlation with small bowel barium roentgen study. Am. J. Dis. Child., *108*:67, 1964.
107. Grossman, H., Berdon, W. E., and Baker, D. H.: Reversible gastrointestinal signs of hemorrhage and edema in the pediatric age group. Radiology, *84*:33, 1965.
108. Moyer, J. H., et al.: Pulmonary arteriovenous fistulas. Am. J. Med., *32*:417, 1962.
109. Chandler, D.: Pulmonary and cerebral arteriovenous fistula with Osler's disease. Arch. Intern. Med., *116*:277, 1965.

DISEASES OF METABOLISM

FLUID AND ELECTROLYTE BALANCE

Hypokalemia

The depletion of blood and intracellular potassium ion can lead to abdominal distention and a radiographic picture of adynamic ileus. Hypokalemia is most often encountered in the postoperative period but can also occur in diabetic acidosis, after large intravenous infusions of fluid without potassium, after vomiting and diarrhea, and in other conditions associated with potassium loss.

Radiographically the small and large bowel loops are diffusely distended; often, colonic distention predominates. Fluid levels are not abundant, and there is no thickening of the bowel wall.

The distention usually disappears promptly and dramatically after potassium ions have been restored.[1]

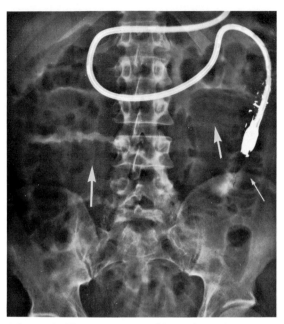

Figure 15–1 **Hypokalemia: Adynamic Ileus.** Loops of large bowel (*large arrows*) and small bowel (*small arrow*) are distended. The rectum contains gas, a finding that usually rules out mechanical obstruction. Fluid levels are absent. The distended loops are close together, whereas in adynamic ileus due to peritonitis they are separated by peritoneal exudate and edema of the bowel walls.

Distended small and large bowel loops, relatively few fluid levels, and a normal space between loops are characteristic of noninflammatory adynamic ileus.

DISORDERS OF CARBOHYDRATE METABOLISM

Diabetes Mellitus

Most of the roentgen findings are nonspecific and are due to neurogenic, infectious, or metabolic complications.

In longstanding diabetes there is an uncommonly high incidence of Mönckeberg's sclerosis of the smaller and middle-size arteries of the extremities. Diffuse calcification of the walls of long segments of a vessel should arouse suspicion of diabetes, particularly in an individual under age 60. Atherosclerosis and ischemic disease are also much more frequent in diabetics.

Increased susceptiblity to infection is often manifested by osteomyelitis of the distal bones of the feet. This is usually a completely lytic process with no periosteal reaction. Often there is a combination of neuropathy, chronic trauma, and infection in these bones, giving rise to juxta-articular bone defects, cortical and endosteal lysis, pencil-like deformities, fragmentation, and even apparent loss of an entire bone. Dramatic reconstitution of bone may occur with control of infection.

In the proximal bones and joints of the feet a Charcot degeneration may take place, with fragmentation, bone loss, and even soft tissue debris, although the latter is less common than in the luetic Charcot joint.

Neurogenic disturbances of the gastrointestinal tract are frequently encountered radiographically. Esophageal dysfunction, usually asymptomatic, is manifested by decreased primary peristalsis, by tertiary contraction waves, and by delayed emptying, particularly in the recumbent position. Delay in gastric emptying and decreased peristaltic activity are frequently noted in asymptomatic diabetics. Small bowel stasis and puddling appear in young diabetics with nocturnal diarrhea. Constipation, a common symptom, may be accompanied by a neurogenically dilated colon; in severe cases a toxic megacolon may be seen. During cholecystography, the gallbladder may appear enlarged; poor contraction may occur with a fatty meal.

In diabetic acidosis there is often severe gastric dilatation and atony, with associated nausea and vomiting adding to the electrolyte imbalance.

Bladder disturbances are common owing to a neurogenically enlarged and atonic bladder that does not empty completely.

Ordinary and unusual infections occur with abnormally high frequency in diabetics. Acute and chronic pyelonephritis (p. 810), renal papillary necrosis (p. 825), and cystitis are relatively frequent. In cystitis emphysematosa due to *E. coli,* collections of submucosal gas surround the bladder. These may rupture into the lumen, producing a gas-filled bladder and pneumaturia (p. 863). An unusual form of cholecystitis, cholecystitis emphysematosa, is found almost exclusively in diabetics and is characterized by an air-filled but nonfunctioning gallbladder (p. 1084). Mucormycosis, especially in the sinuses and lungs, occurs almost uniquely in uncontrolled diabetes.

Involvement of the renal glomeruli and arterioles (Kimmelstiel-Wilson syndrome) occurs in chronic diabetics and may eventuate in a nephrotic syndrome or in chronic renal failure. Renal arteriographic findings may be indistinguishable from the changes of chronic nephritis.[2-6]

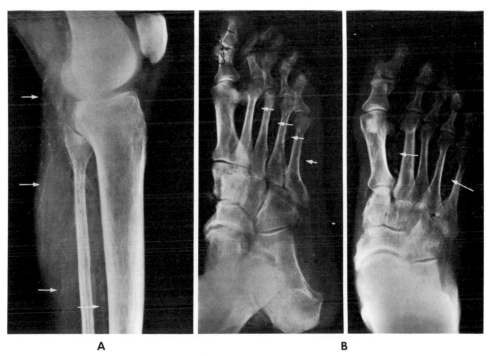

A   B

Figure 15-2 **Diabetes Mellitus: Extensive Arterial Medial Sclerosis with Calcification.**

A, In a 54 year old diabetic, extensive calcification outlines many of the smaller and more tortuous arteries almost in their entirety *(arrows).*

B, The interosseous arteries are calcified throughout their length. Note the tortuosity of most of these vessels *(arrows).*

Medial calcification is not uncommon in the nondiabetic, but it occurs earlier and more extensively in the diabetic. It is also frequently seen in the patient with chronic renal failure who is on maintenance dialysis.

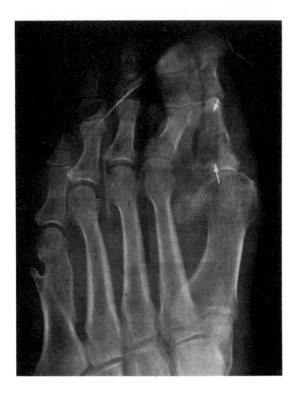

Figure 15–3 **Diabetic Osteomyelitis of Great Toe.** An extensive lytic osteomyelitis *(arrows)* has destroyed much of the shaft of the proximal phalanx, including the cortex. Osteomyelitis of the toes is a fairly frequent complication of diabetes. The absence of periosteal reaction is characteristic and is probably related to the impaired blood supply in the extremities.

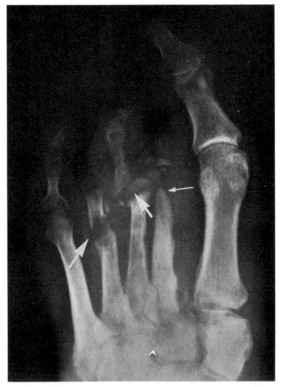

Figure 15–4 **Diabetes Mellitus: Extensive Neurotropic Changes in Foot.** In the metatarsophalangeal area there is periarticular bone destruction *(large arrows)*, fragmentation, and a pointed tapering of the second metatarsal head *(small arrow)*. The latter is a characteristic neurotropic finding.

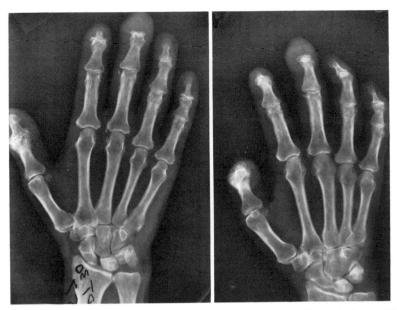

Figure 15-5 **Diabetes Mellitus: Neurotropic Changes in Finger Tips.**   There is loss of both bone and soft tissue substance at the distal ends of the index and middle fingers. Almost the entire distal phalanx of the middle finger has been resorbed. Such changes are also seen in leprosy and in prolonged ischemia associated with Raynaud's phenomenon.

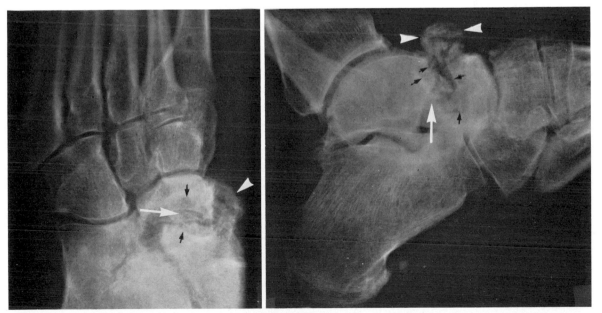

Figure 15-6 **Diabetes Mellitus: Neurotropic (Charcot) Joint in Foot.**   This male diabetic had local swelling of the dorsum of the foot, but no pain.

The talonavicular joint is greatly disorganized. Sharply marginated articular bone loss is seen in both bones *(black arrows)*, and the joint space is irregularly widened *(white arrows)*. Soft tissue calcifications *(arrowheads)* are seen on the dorsolateral aspect. The adjacent bones are not demineralized; the navicular bone is actually somewhat sclerotic.

Sharp articular lysis, joint disorganization, soft tissue calcification, and absence of demineralization are characteristic features of a Charcot joint.

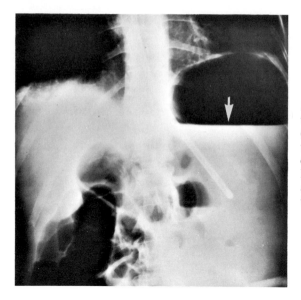

Figure 15–7 **Diabetic Acidosis: Gastric Atony.** Erect view demonstrates accumulation of air and fluid (*arrow*) in the dilated stomach of a young patient who was acidotic. The gastric dilatation was probably a consequence of toxicity and electrolyte imbalance. Neurogenic gastric atonicity is common in diabetes, and is associated with a marked delay in gastric emptying and episodes of vomiting.

Hyperinsulinism

Insulinoma

When an insulin-producing beta cell tumor of the pancreas is clinically suspected, selective celiac and mesenteric arteriography may be able to uncover and localize the tumor prior to surgery. The location of the insulinoma may be determined in a significant percentage of cases by this method.

Angiographically there is usually a small area in which the smaller arteries are somewhat displaced followed by a well-circumscribed, rounded, homogenous capillary blush. There is no large vessel displacement, tortuosity, or arteriovenous shunts. This picture is characteristic but not pathognomonic.[7-10]

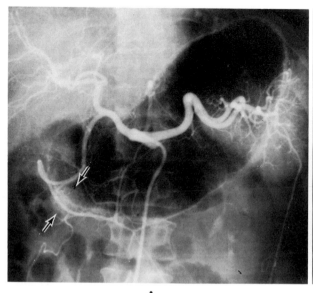
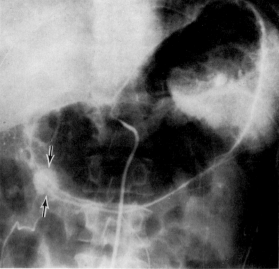

A   B

Figure 15–8 **Insulinoma: Selective Celiac Arteriogram.**

A, A 2 cm. nodule in the head of the pancreas is homogeneously opacified (*arrows*) during the arterial phase. Note the numerous feeding vessels arising from the superior pancreatoduodenal artery.

B, Tumor opacification (*arrows*) persists during the late capillary and venous phase. (Courtesy Dr. H. Y. Epstein, New York City, New York.)

Glycogen Storage Disease (GSD)

There are a number of glycogen storage diseases, each with a different enzyme deficit and a specific eponym.

In *von Gierke's disease* (GSD type I), hepatomegaly is a constant finding. Osteoporosis is present in all patients. Retarded bone development is frequent. Surviving adults often show gouty bone changes associated with hyperuricemia.

Cardiac involvement is the most prominent radiographic finding in infants with *Pompe's disease* (GSD type II), which is the generalized form of glycogen storage disease. The heart is greatly enlarged and globular, but the pulmonary vasculature remains normal until failure ensues. The appearance is indistinguishable from that of endocardial fibroelastosis, rhabdomyoma of the heart, anomalous origin of a coronary artery, and idiopathic hypertrophy. Biopsy is necessary for diagnosis. Angiocardiography demonstrates enlargement of the ventricular chambers and thickening of their walls; emptying is sluggish. Congenital intracardiac defects are rarely associated.[11-13]

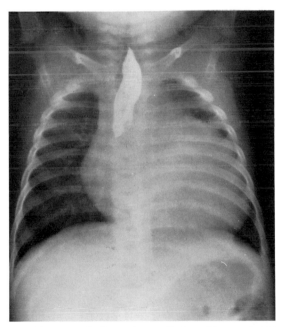

Figure 15–9 **Glycogen Storage Disease of Heart in an Infant (Pompe's Disease).** The heart is greatly enlarged and globular; the left border extends to the chest wall. The pulmonary vasculature is not prominent. Barium is outlined in the upper esophagus. The cardiac enlargement is nonspecific—indistinguishable from the other cardiopathies.

Primary Hyperoxaluria and Oxalosis

Increased urinary excretion of oxalic and glycolic acids occurs in primary hyperoxaluria and can lead to deposition of calcium oxalate in the renal parenchyma, and to renal calculi. Radiographically the nephrocalcinosis and renal calculi are indistinguishable from the picture of renal tubular acidosis. The parenchymal calcifications are irregular, quite dense, and vary in size from punctate areas to large stones, which often enter the collecting system. Progressive calcification, secondary pyelonephritis, and obstructive uropathy can lead to renal failure.

When hyperoxaluria is associated with oxalate deposits in extrarenal tissues, the condition is termed *oxalosis*. In the bone marrow the crystal deposits can cause osteoporosis of varying degrees and even pathologic fractures. Sometimes the rarefaction is limited to metaphyseal and subperiosteal areas, producing a striking roentgen picture. If secondary hyperparathyroidism results from renal damage, it may dominate or alter the bone changes.

There may also be renal calcifications and oxalate calculi in acquired hyperoxaluria, which develops in some cases of ileal resection, chronic inflammatory bowel disease as regional enteritis, malabsorption or cirrhosis.[14-17]

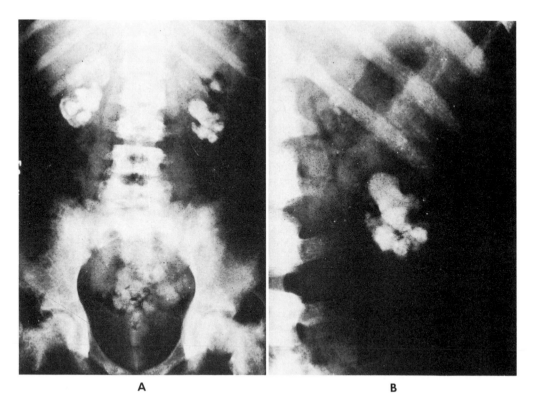

A   B

Figure 15–10 **Oxalosis: Renal and Osseous Findings.**

Renal calculi and hydronephrosis were discovered in a patient five years of age.

A, Abdominal film made at age 15 shows large stag-horn calculi in both kidneys. Fine calcifications are scattered throughout the renal parenchyma. There was bilateral hydronephrosis; the nonprotein nitrogen and serum phosphorus were considerably elevated. The bones are dense.

B, Enlarged view of the left kidney reveals the scattered parenchymal calcifications (nephrocalcinosis) peripheral to the calculi.

Legend continued on the opposite page

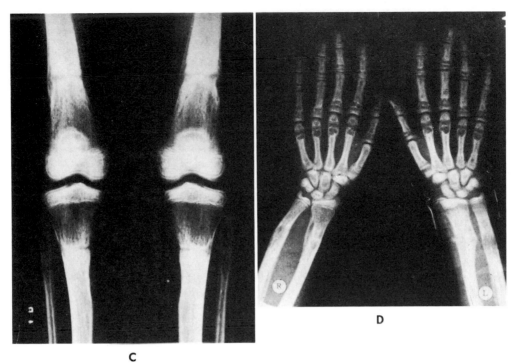

Figure 15–10 (Continued)

C, The femora and tibiae demonstrate extensive metaphyseal demineralization bounded by transverse lucent lines. Lines of subperiosteal demineralization are shown around the articular surfaces.

D, Similar areas of demineralization are evident in the bones of the hands, wrists, and forearms. The changes in the right radius resemble those of localized osteitis fibrosa cystica. There is a healing fracture of the left radius.

The increased density of many of the bones may be due to osteosclerosis, which is often seen in secondary renal hyperparathyroidism. (Courtesy Dr. H. G. Dunn, Vancouver, British Columbia.)

DISORDERS OF LIPID METABOLISM

Familial Hyperlipemia (Hyperglyceridemia)

In familial hyperlipemia with hyperglyceridemia and hypercholesterolemia, soft tissue xanthomatous lesions are frequently encountered; in rare cases similar deposits may involve multiple bones.

The osseous xanthomas produce multiple osteolytic areas, which strongly resemble the much more common lesions of multiple myeloma or metastatic malignancy.

The bone lesions apparently do not disappear or improve even after prolonged lowering of the serum lipids by therapy. There are no symptoms from the bone involvement, although in one case pathologic fractures occurred apparently because senile osteoporosis was associated.[18]

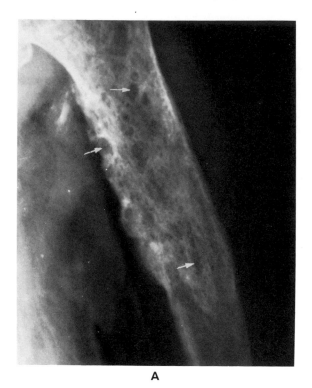

A

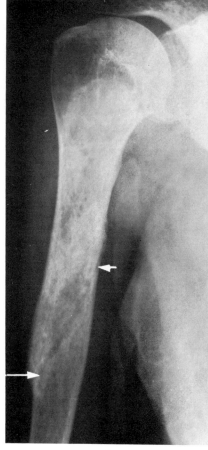

B

Figure 15–11 **Familial Hyperlipemia: Osseous Xanthomatosis.**

A, The upper half of the left humerus of a 66 year old woman is diffusely riddled with lytic areas *(arrows)* of varying size.

B, Similar but less prominent lesions involve the upper half of the right humerus. A pathologic fracture *(arrows),* now healing, led to the bone survey.

Both femora showed similar involvement.

Biopsy confirmed the xanthomatous nature of the lesions. The roentgen lesions resemble multiple myeloma or metastatic malignancy. (Courtesy Dr. R. P. Palmer, Oklahoma City, Oklahoma.)

Lipoatrophic Diabetes Mellitus and Generalized Lipodystrophy

In both the congenital and the acquired forms of this rare condition the total or near-total absence of subcutaneous fat can be readily recognized on radiograms of the extremities. Endosteal cortical thickening and a generalized increase in bone density occur in most cases. Although the cause of cortical thickening is not understood, it is thought to be related to the almost complete absence of marrow fat. Skeletal maturation and bone age are advanced, especially in the congenital cases.

Other less frequent and nonspecific roentgen findings in the congenital form include increased muscular masses, liver enlargement, esophageal varices, and cardiomegaly. The diabetes is insulin-resistant, but not associated with ketosis.

The acquired form begins in adult life and is usually not associated with abnormalities of carbohydrate metabolism (progressive lipodystrophy).[19, 20]

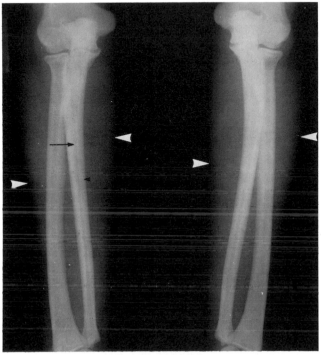

Figure 15-12 **Lipoatrophic Diabetes Mellitus: Both Forearms.** There is complete absence of both subcutaneous fat *(white arrowheads)* and intermuscular fatty layers. The muscle mass is homogeneous.

The somewhat slender radii and ulnae show increased density due to endosteal cortical thickening *(black arrowhead),* which has greatly narrowed the medullary cavity *(arrow).*

These changes of lipoatrophic diabetes (generalized lipodystrophy) occur throughout the body, in contrast to the more common partial or progressive lipodystrophy. The latter is most often seen in women and usually involves only the upper half of the body. (Courtesy Dr. R. H. Gold, San Francisco, California.)

Abetalipoproteinemia

This rare hereditary disease is manifested by severe malabsorption of fats, neurologic deterioration with ataxia, and a progressive pigmentary retinal degeneration.

Small bowel studies will disclose thickening of the intestinal folds, most marked in the duodenum and jejunum. The radiographic appearance strongly resembles the changes of Whipple's disease. (See Fig. 12–126.)[21]

Lipoma

Lipomas are found most frequently in the subcutaneous tissues but can also occur in many other tissues or organs including the submucosa of the colon and the subpleural space. Large lipomas are often lobulated.

Since fat is less radiopaque than normal body tissues, lipomas can often be recognized radiographically as areas of relative radiolucency in the soft tissues. Occasionally larger lipomas in the limbs can bow or erode an adjacent bone. Rarely a parosteal lipoma can cause irregular hyperostoses of a bone. These project into the lucent lipomatous mass, a characteristic finding.

In the colon, lipoma is usually a solitary submucosal lesion, presenting as a smooth, rounded, fairly large filling defect in the barium column. On air-contrast studies it may occasionally appear less dense than other similar-size masses. A tap water enema may be diagnostic, if the tumor appears lucent relative to the water density. The lipoma is the second most frequent benign lesion of the colon. Almost 50 per cent occur in the cecum or ascending colon.

Subpleural lipomas are often lobulated and are visualized by contrast with the lucent lung fields. These lesions appear less dense than other masses and tend to change shape during respiration.[22-25]

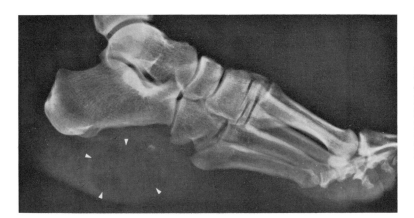

Figure 15–13 **Soft Tissue Lipoma of Heel.** A circumscribed radiolucent mass *(arrowheads)* extends from just below the os calcis to the bottom of the heel. This lipoma has caused the soft tissues of the heel to bulge.

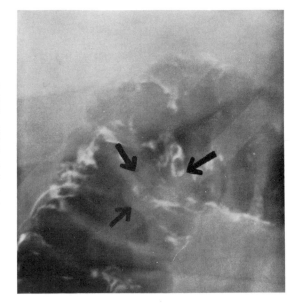

Figure 15–14 **Submucosal Lipoma in Hepatic Flexure of Colon.** Spot view of the air-filled colon following barium enema demonstrates a lobulated mass *(arrows)* projecting into the air column. The rather faint opacity, the absence of a stalk, and the lack of a coating of barium suggest the diagnosis of lipoma, as opposed to adenomatous polyp, which often has a stalk, is much denser in contrast to air, and usually becomes partially coated with barium. A water enema would have disclosed the relative lucency of the lesion to water density.

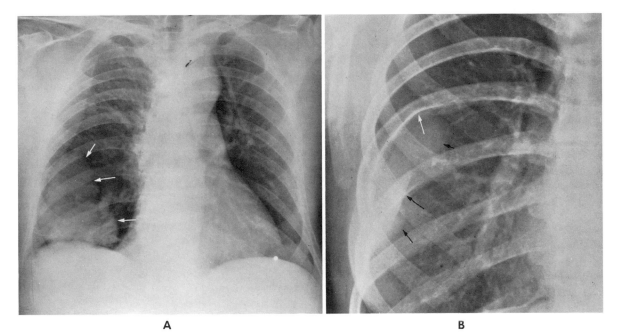

A   B

Figure 15-15   **Subpleural Lipomas: Two Patients.**

A, The lobulated mass in the right lower chest *(arrows)* is considerably less dense than are most solid masses. The mass lies against the chest wall.

B, In another patient the lipoma is lobulated *(black arrows)* and less dense than the usual solid mass. Its subpleural location is evident from the elevation and erosive narrowing of the sixth rib *(white arrow),* with widening of the interspace.

Because these lipomas arise extrapleurally, they do not cause pleural effusion.

Pelvic Lipomatosis

This benign condition of unknown origin is characterized by fat deposition in the extraperitoneal soft tissues around the urinary bladder, rectum, and prostate gland. The disease is apparently limited to males.

Radiographically the fat deposits appear as lucencies in the pelvis, but these may be difficult to appreciate unless overlying bowel gas is minimal or absent. The contrast-filled bladder is elevated and elongated into a tear-shaped configuration, and appears to be rising out of the pelvis. A tear-shaped bladder can also result from other extraperitoneal pelvic masses such as neoplasm or post-traumatic blood collections. However, the association of pelvic lucencies with an elevated, elongated bladder is diagnostic of pelvic lipomatosis. The distal ureters may be deviated laterally or medially. Commonly, a ureter is compressed, sometimes causing hydronephrosis. Usually the barium enema study will also show elevation of the sigmoid colon.[26-28]

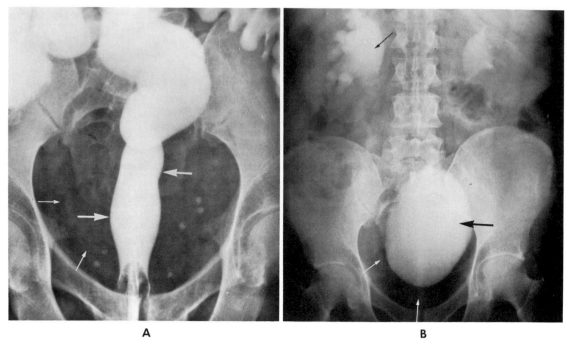

A   B

Figure 15–16 **Pelvic and Perivesical Lipomatosis.**

A, The rectum is narrowed, straightened, and elevated *(large arrows)* by a diffuse pelvic mass. The areas of decreased density *(small arrows)* in the pelvis represent fatty deposits.

B, Pyelographic study indicates that the bladder *(large black arrow)* is elevated and displaced to the left by a perivesicular mass *(white arrows).* Areas of lucency are seen in the soft tissues to the right and below the bladder. The lipomatous mass has also obstructed the lower right ureter, producing hydronephrosis of the right kidney *(small black arrow).*

INBORN ERRORS OF AMINO ACID METABOLISM

Gout

The urate deposits occur most often in the joint and ear cartilages, but bone, tendon, and bursal involvement is also frequent. Radiographic changes develop only after repeated attacks, and negative findings do not rule out the disorder. In many cases only a single joint is originally affected—most often the first metatarsophalangeal joint—but other joints, especially of the hands and feet, are often involved.

Sodium urate crystals are not radiopaque, and their deposition into joint synovia produces only joint and periarticular swelling. The earliest bone changes are small, sharply marginated, juxta-articular lytic areas; later, subarticular cystic areas appear. The cysts are round or oval, have a sclerotic margin, and may be up to 3 cm. in size although they are usually much smaller. Overhanging edges are characteristic of these cyst-like lesions. Calcium may be deposited in the urate collections, producing radiopaque tophaceous periarticular masses. In advanced disease, articular lysis and erosion may become quite extensive. Joint space narrowing eventually occurs, and the roentgen picture may resemble rheumatoid or degenerative arthritis, but without striking osteoporosis. Other findings may include calcification of the menisci or articular cartilages of the knee, calcified deposits in the ear, and bursal swelling, especially of the olecranon, with or without calcification.

Involvement of the sacroiliac joints, once thought to be extremely rare, occurs in up to 15 per cent of cases. Irregularities of the articular margins, cysts with sclerotic rims, and focal osteoporosis may be seen. Unilateral involvement is more common.

Periarticular destruction with discernible tophi is virtually diagnostic of gout, although in about half the cases tophi are not seen.

Renal involvement is frequent, but there are usually no significant pyelographic findings unless uric acid calculi are formed.[29-32]

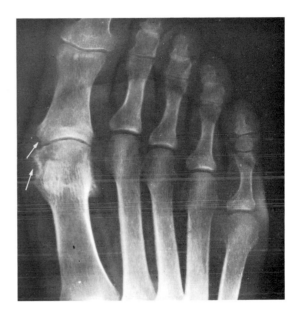

Figure 15–17 **Gout: Early Manifestations in Great Toe.** There is erosion of bone *(arrows)* on the medial aspect of the metatarsal and proximal phalanges adjacent to the first metatarsophalangeal joint. There is no soft tissue swelling, and tophi have not appeared.

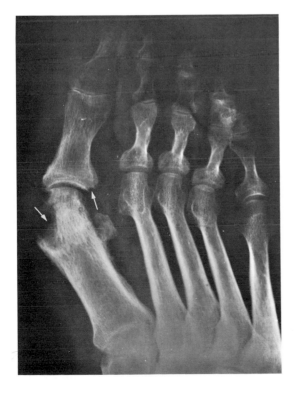

Figure 15–18 **Gout: Advanced Disease in Great Toe.** The articular surface and subarticular bone on the medial side of the first metatarsal have been destroyed *(left arrow),* and there is a small articular punched-out defect on the lateral side of the proximal phalanx *(right arrow).* Note the overhanging edge of the cystic lesion. No tophi, soft tissue swelling, or joint narrowing is present. The bones are well mineralized, since use of the foot is unimpaired between attacks.

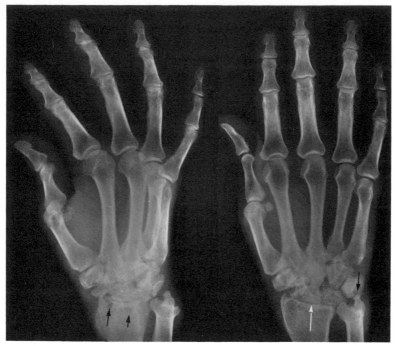

Figure 15–19 **Advanced Gouty Arthritis of Wrist.**   The radiocarpal joint space *(white arrow)* and the carpal joint spaces are narrowed. Punched out areas are demonstrated in the subarticular portion of the radius and in the carpal bones *(black arrows)*. The picture resembles rheumatoid arthritis, and in the absence of tophi a positive diagnosis of gout cannot be made; however, there is less bone demineralization than is usually seen in rheumatoid disease.

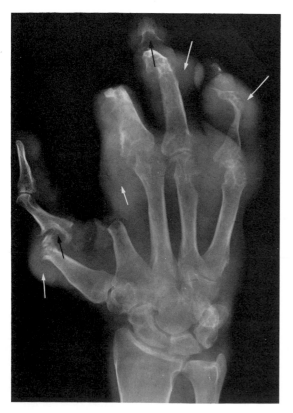

Figure 15–20 **Far-Advanced   Tophaceous   Gout.** Severe bone destruction around all the metacarpophalangeal joints and smaller joints *(black arrows)* has necessitated amputation of the index finger and part of the middle finger. Large, moderately opaque soft tissue swellings around all these joints *(white arrows)* represent noncalcified tophi. Such tophi frequently develop in the ear cartilages. The bones are moderately demineralized.

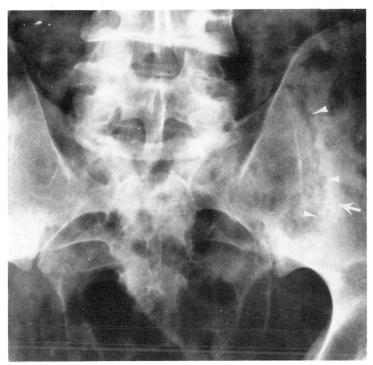

Figure 15–21 **Gout: Sacroiliac Involvement.** The left sacroiliac joint is narrowed and irregular, with marginal erosions *(arrowheads)* and sclerosis *(arrow)*. The other sacroiliac joint was only minimally involved.

Sacroiliac involvement in gout, although uncommon, eventually occurs in up to 15 per cent of untreated cases. The radiographic appearance is nonspecific.

Ochronosis and Alcaptonuria

Deposition of homogentisic acid in connective tissue and cartilage can cause degeneration or calcification, or both, of these structures. This deposition is responsible for many of the clinical and radiologic changes.

Progressive degenerative joint disease, especially of the knees, shoulders, hips, and spine, is the most common radiographic finding. The peripheral joint changes are similar to ordinary osteoarthritis, exhibiting thinning of the joint space, sclerosis of the articular margins, spur formation, and joint mice. Osteoporosis is frequent. Meniscal calcification in the knees is not uncommon. In the spine, changes begin in middle age and consist of thinning of the intervertebral discs, osteoporosis, and narrowing and ankylosis of the apophyseal joints. Calcium is eventually deposited in the discs, a striking and almost pathognomonic finding. The disc degeneration begins in the lumbar area with progressive ascending involvement.

Calcification of the cartilages of the ears is a highly suggestive finding. Para-articular calcifications and ossification of tendon insertions are not uncommon. Renal calculi occur in about 60 per cent of cases.

Although most of the radiologic changes are nonspecific, ankylosing spondylitis with calcified intervertebral discs, peripheral osteoarthritis, and extensive calcification of the ear cartilages are a highly suggestive combination of findings.[33-37]

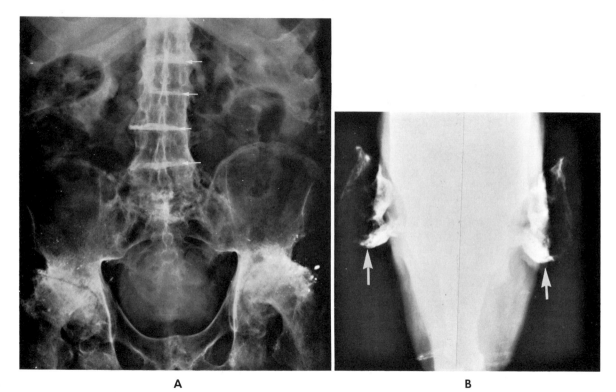

A   B

Figure 15–22   **Ochronosis and Alcaptonuria: 63 Year Old Woman.**

   A, The intervertebral disc spaces are all greatly narrowed and extensively calcified *(arrows).* All the bones are demineralized. There are advanced degenerative changes in both hips, with deformities of the femoral heads, near-complete loss of joint spaces, articular sclerosis, and periarticular calcifications.

   B, There is extensive dense calcification of the cartilages in both ears *(arrows).*

Legend continued on the opposite page

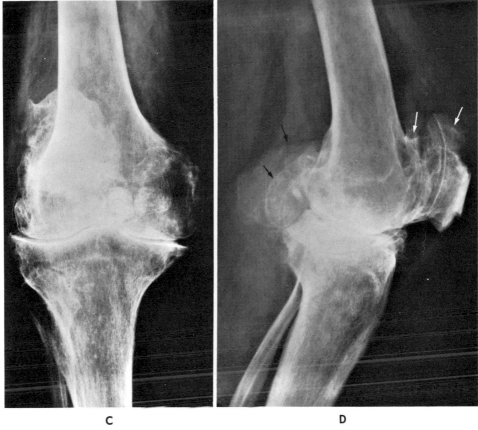

C   D

Figure 15–22 (Continued)

C and D, Far-advanced degenerative arthritis is seen in the knee, with characteristic greatly narrowed joint spaces, sclerosis of the articular surfaces, and pronounced spur formation and bony overgrowth *(white arrows)*. Soft tissue calcification *(black arrows)* is seen behind the joint.

Virtually all the radiologic changes of ochronosis are illustrated in this patient: degenerative arthritis of the knees and hips, osteoporosis, soft tissue calcifications, thinning and calcification of the intervertebral discs, and calcification of the cartilages in both ears (Courtesy Dr. M. M. Thompson, Toledo, Ohio.)

Phenylketonuria

In 30 to 50 per cent of affected infants and children, characteristic changes are found in the metaphyses of long bones, particularly in the wrist. A high incidence of these roentgen changes is noted in infants who have been treated with a low phenylalanine diet.

The metaphysis is cupped, and dense calcific vertical spicules extend from the metaphysis into the epiphyseal cartilage. Often the metaphyseal border is sclerotic. With further growth the spicules are incorporated into the spongiosa as vertical striations. Osteoporosis and delayed skeletal maturation are also frequent. Similar but less marked changes are seen in homocystinuria. The characteristic spicules will differentiate the roentgen picture from that of rickets.

Brain atrophy is common in untreated or well-advanced cases of phenylketonuria and is evidenced by dilated ventricles and dilated subarachnoid pathways on the CT scan or pneumoencephalogram.[38-40]

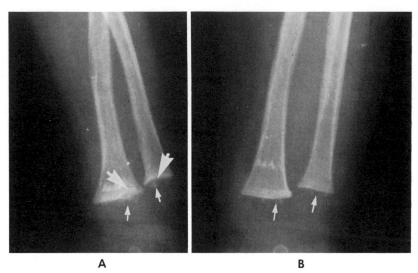

A   **B**

Figure 15–23 **Phenylketonuria: Bone Changes in Two Infants.**

A, There is cupping of the distal ulnar metaphysis and slight cupping of the medial aspect of the radial metaphysis *(large arrows).* Small calcifications are seen in the area of the metaphyseal cartilages *(small arrows).* The metaphyseal border is sclerotic. The bones are slightly demineralized.

B, In the second infant the ulnar metaphysis is slightly cupped, but the radial metaphysis is of normal shape. Fine stippled calcifications are noted in the metaphyseal cartilage area *(arrows).* Demineralization of the bones is minimal. Notice the vertical striations in the distal radius. (Courtesy Dr. D. G. Germann, Kansas City, Kansas.)

Hyperaminoacidurias

Hyperammonemia (Familial Protein Intolerance)

Severe metabolic abnormalities of the urea cycle (argininosuccinicaciduria, hyperammonemia without hyperaminoaciduria, and citrullinemia) produce elevation of blood ammonia and are associated with mental retardation. Osteoporosis is common, and recurrence fractures often occur.

On the CT scan or pneumoencephalogram there are dilated ventricles and dilated subarachnoid sulci due to brain atrophy. Hyperammonemia should be considered in otherwise unexplained cerebral atrophy in children.[41, 42]

Homocystinuria

Skeletal changes are the most common roentgenologic findings in homocystinuria. An almost constant radiographic finding is osteoporosis of the spine, often with biconcave deformities of the vertebrae. Osteoporosis of the long bones occurs in about 75 per cent of cases and may lead to bowing or fractures.

In most affected children, focal calcifications are found in the wrist, either in the epiphyseal cartilage or within the bony epiphysis. Metaphyseal cuffing and some widening of the epiphyseal line occur in about half of these children. These findings are strikingly similar to those seen in phenylketonuria (see Fig. 15–23).

Long thin tubular bones, especially in the hand (arachnodactyly), similar to the bones in Marfan's syndrome appear in about one third of cases. Often the clinical picture is indistinguishable from that of Marfan's syndrome. In the latter, however, osteoporosis of the spine is extremely rare.

Other roentgen findings in homocystinuria include scoliosis, enlarged carpal bones, delayed ossification, microencephaly, and anterior projection and angulation of the xiphisternal prominence (pectus carinatum). Premature vascular calcification is frequent. Occlusive vascular disease is the principal cause of death and may be secondary to minor vascular trauma; angiography therefore should be avoided.[43, 44]

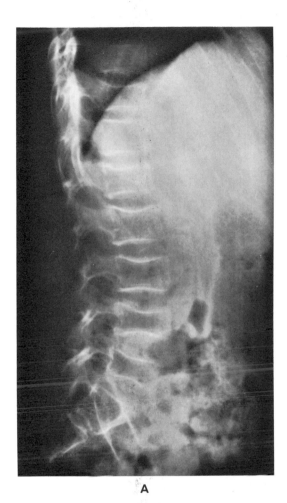

A

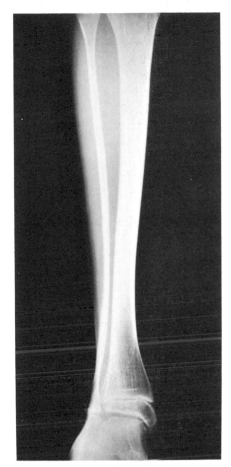

B

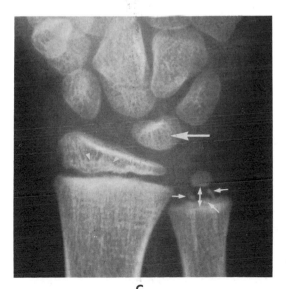

C

Figure 15–24   **Homocystinuria: Characteristic Changes.**

A, The lumbar and lower dorsal vertebrae are markedly osteoporotic and have secondary biconcave deformities (11 year old girl).

B, The tibia and fibula are long and slender, with moderate bowing (12 year old boy).

These changes are similar to osteogenesis imperfecta tarda. Fractures may also occur in these thin bones.

C, There are calcified spicules (*small arrows*) in the ulnar epiphyseal cartilage (note similarity to Fig. 15–23, *Phenylketonuria*). The metaphysis is somewhat cupped, and the epiphyseal line is considerably widened (*double-headed arrow*). There are spicules (*arrowheads*) buried in the radial epiphysis. Ossification of all bones, particularly the lunate (*large arrow*), is retarded (9 year old boy).

Cystinuria

Cystinuria occurs in several of the many hyperaminoaciduric syndromes. Because of the low solubility of cystine, recurrent formation of calculi, often beginning in childhood, is the predominant clinical problem.

The pure cystine calculus is not radiopaque, but calcium salts are usually eventually deposited. In some children a syndrome of growth failure and intestinal malabsorption is associated with cystinuria.[45]

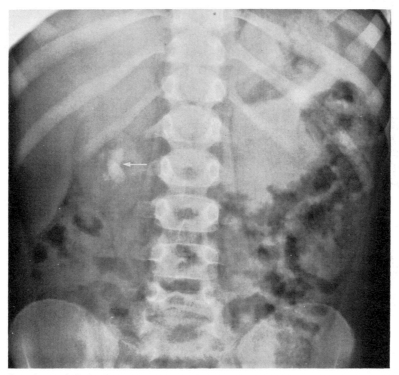

Figure 15–25 **Cystinuria and Calculus.**   There is a large opaque calculus in the right kidney *(arrow)* of a four year old boy. Pure cystine stones are not radiopaque, but calcium salts are generally deposited within the stone as it enlarges.

Fanconi Syndrome

This syndrome has a multiplicity of causes, some inherited and others acquired. Dysfunction of the proximal renal tubules results in generalized hyperaciduria, glycosuria, and hyperphosphaturia. The continuing phosphate loss causes rickets in children and osteomalacia in adults; both disorders have characteristic radiographic findings (see *Rickets and Osteomalacia*, p. 1129, and *Osteomalacia*, p. 1324). In less severe cases of Fanconi syndrome, cortical thickening and bone sclerosis may appear, but the mechanism is unclear. If renal failure occurs (as in cystinosis), the bone changes of secondary hyperparathyroidism may develop.[46, 47]

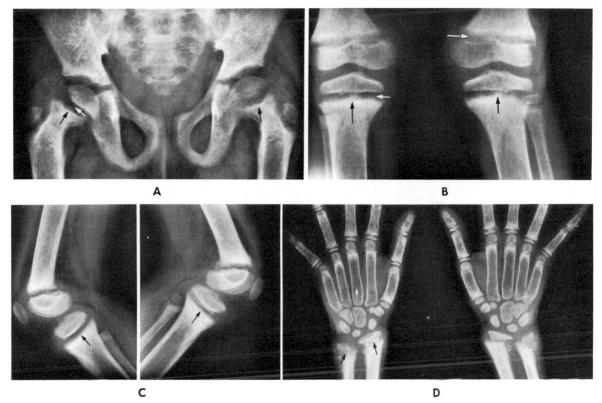

Figure 15–26 **Fanconi Syndrome: Renal Rickets.**

A, B, and *C,* There are typical rachitic changes in the hip and knee joints. The zones of provisional calcification (metaphyseal lines) *(black arrows)* are frayed, irregular, and without a sharp dense border. The distance between epiphysis and metaphysis is greatly widened *(white arrows)*. Demineralization and coarsened trabeculae are evident in the pelvis and femora.

D, There is pronounced osteomalacic demineralization in the carpal bones *(white arrow)*. The shafts are widened and have very coarse trabeculae and thin cortices. There is post-traumatic subluxation of the epiphyses of both forearms *(black arrows)*, a not infrequent complication of rachitic epiphyses.

The roentgenologic picture of renal rickets, whether due to hypophosphatemia, cystinosis, or renal tubular acidosis, is quite similar.

Congenital Hyperuricosuria (Lesch-Nyhan Syndrome)

This syndrome consists of cerebral palsy, mental retardation, growth retardation, hyperuricemia, hyperuricosuria, and self-destructive biting.

The radiographic findings are those of delayed skeletal maturation, bilateral coxa valga and hip subluxations, urinary tract calculi, and changes secondary to the self-inflicted bite wounds. In the older patient the changes of gout may be seen.[48, 49]

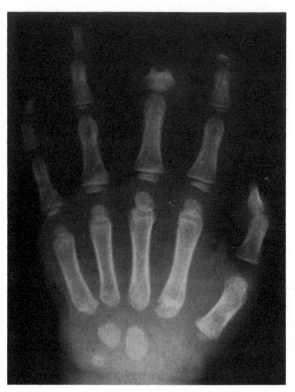

Figure 15–27 **Congenital Hyperuricosuria: The Hand.** Film of the hand of a 5¼ year old boy with congenital hyperuricosuria shows amputation of the index and middle fingers from self-inflicted bite. The bone age is that of a 3 year old.

Traumatic amputation of fingers can also occur in children with familial dysautonomia, congenital indifference to pain, or psychotic states. It may also result from frostbite. (Courtesy Drs. M. H. Becker and J. K. Wallin, New York, New York.)

REFERENCES

1. Lowman, R. M.: The potassium depletion states and postoperative ileus (Editorial). Radiology, *98*:691, 1971.
2. Beck, R. E.: Roentgen findings in complications of diabetes mellitus. Am. J. Roentgenol. Radium Ther. Nucl. Med., *82*:887, 1959.
3. Jacobs, J. E.: Neuropathic (Charcot) joints occurring in diabetes mellitus. J. Bone Joint Surg., *40A*:1043, 1958.
4. Pogonowska, M. J., Collins, M. C., and Dobson, H. L.: Diabetic osteopathy. Radiology, *89*:265, 1967.
5. Katz, L. A., and Spiro, H. M.: Gastrointestinal manifestations of diabetes. N. Engl. J. Med., *275*:1350, 1966.
6. Clouse, M. E., and Gramm, H. F., et al.: Diabetic osteoarthropathy. Am. J. Roentgenol. Radium Ther. Nucl. Med., *121*:22, 1974.
7. Epstein, H. Y., et al.: Angiographic localization of insulinomas. Ann. Surg., *169*:349, 1969.
8. Davies, E. R.: Radiologic and scintographic investigation of spontaneous hypoglycemia. Clin. Radiol., *24*:177, 1973.
9. Robins, J. M., Bookstein, J. J., et al.: Selective angiography in localizing islet-cell tumors of the pancreas. Radiology, *106*:525, 1973.
10. Deininger, H. K.: Radiologic diagnosis of insulinoma. Radiologe, *14*:173, 1974.
11. Martin, J. F., and Bonte, F. J.: Glycogen disease. Am. J. Roentgenol. Radium Ther. Nucl. Med., *66*:922, 1951.
12. Nihill, M. R., Wilson, D. S., and Hugh-Jones, K.: Generalized glycogenosis type II (Pompe's disease). Arch. Dis. Child., *45*:122, 1970.
13. Preger, L., et al.: Roentgenographic skeletal changes in the glycogen storage diseases. Am. J. Roentgenol. Radium Ther. Nucl. Med., *107*:840, 1969.

14. Dunn, H. G.: Oxalosis. Am. J. Dis. Child., *90*:58, 1955.
15. Weber, A. L.: Primary hyperoxaluria. Am. J. Roentgenol. Radium Ther. Nucl. Med., *100*:155, 1967.
16. Smith, L. H., Fromm, H., and Hofmann, A. F.: Acquired hyperoxaluria, nephrolithiasis and intestinal disease. N. Engl. J. Med., *286*:1371, 1972.
17. Micarsen, G., and Radkowski, M. A.: Calcium oxalosis. Radiology, *113*:165, 1974.
18. Brusco, O. J., Howard, R. P., Jarman, J. B., and Furman, R. H.: Osseous xanthomatosis and pathologic fractures in familial hyperlipemia. Am. J. Med., *40*:477, 1966.
19. Gold, R. H., and Steinbach, H. L.: Lipoatrophy diabetes mellitus: roentgen findings in two brothers with congenital disease. Am. J. Roentgenol. Radium Ther. Nucl. Med., *101*:884, 1967.
20. Fairney, A., Lewis, G., and Cottom, D.: Total lipodystrophy. Arch. Dis. Child., *44*:368, 1969.
21. Weinstein, M. A., Pearson, K. D., and Agus, S. G.: Abetalipoproteinemia. Radiology, *108*:269, 1973.
22. Marshak, R. H., and Gerson, A.: Lipoma of colon. Am. J. Dig. Dis., *4*:628, 1959.
23. Ten Eyck, E. A.: Subpleural lipoma. Radiology, *74*:295, 1960.
24. Gramiak, R., and Rorener, H. J.: Roentgen diagnostic observation in subpleural lipoma. Am. J. Roentgenol. Radium Ther. Nucl. Med., *98*:465, 1966.
25. Jacobs, P.: Parosteal lipoma with hyperostoses. Clin. Radiol., *23*:196, 1972.
26. Becker, J. A., Weiss, R. M., et al.: Pelvic lipomatosis. Arch. Surg., *100*:94, 1970.
27. Schiff, M., and Lytton, B.: Pelvic lipomatosis. Arch. Surg., *100*:94, 1970.
28. Moss, A. A., Clark, R. E., et al.: Pelvic lipomatosis: a roentgenographic diagnosis. Am. J. Roentgenol. Radium Ther. Nucl. Med., *115*:411, 1972.
29. Brailsford, J. F.: The radiology of gout. Br. J. Radiol., *32*:472, 1959.
30. Dodds, W. I., and Steinbach, H. L.: Gout associated with calcification of cartilage. N. Engl. J. Med., *275*:745, 1966.
31. Wright, S. T.: Unusual manifestations of gout. Aust. Radiol., *10*:365, 1966.
32. Alarcon-Segovia, D., Cetina, J. A., and Diaz-Jouanen, E.: Sacroiliac joints in primary gout. Am. J. Roentgenol. Radium Ther. Nucl. Med., *118*:438, 1973.
33. Thompson, M. M.: Ochronosis. Am. J. Roentgenol. Radium Ther. Nucl. Med., *78*:46, 1957.
34. Kolář, J., and Křižek, V.: Roentgen signs of alkaptonuric ochronosis. Fortschr. Roentgenstr., *109*:203, 1968.
35. Ward, F. R., and Engelbrecht, P. J.: Alcaptonuria and ochronosis. Clin. Radiol., *14*:170, 1963.
36. Detenbeck, L. C., Young, H. H., and Underdahl, L. O.: Ochronotic arthropathy. Arch. Surg., *100*:215, 1970.
37. Laskar, F. H., and Sargison, K. D.: Ochronotic arthropathy. J. Bone Joint Surg., *52*:653, 1970.
38. Murdock, M. M., and Holman, G. H.: Roentgenologic bone changes in phenylketonuria. Am. J. Dis. Child., *107*:523, 1964.
39. Fisch, R. O., et al.: Growth and bone characteristics of phenylketonurics. Am. J. Dis. Child., *112*:3, 1966.
40. Holt, J. F., and Allen, R. J.: Radiologic signs in the primary aminoacidurias. Ann. Radiol., *10*:317, 1967.
41. Starer, F., and Couch, R.: Clinical atrophy in hyperammonemia. Clin. Radiol., *14*:353, 1963.
42. Malmquist, J., Jagenburg, R., and Lindstedt, G.: Familial protein intolerance. N. Engl. J. Med., *284*:997, 1971.
43. Morrells, C. L., Jr., Fletcher, B. D., Weilbaecher, R. G., and Dorst, J. P.: The roentgenographic features of homocystinuria. Radiology, *90*:1150, 1968.
44. Brill, P. W., Mitty, H. A., and Gaull, G. E.: Homocystinuria due to cystathionine synthase deficiency: clinical-roentgenologic correlations. Am. J. Roentgenol. Radium Ther. Nucl. Med., *121*:45, 1974.
45. Beeson, P. B., and McDermott, W.: *Textbook of Medicine.* 14th ed. Philadelphia, W. B. Saunders Co., 1975, p. 1645.
46. Conqvist, S.: Renal osteonephropathy. Acta Radiol., *55*:17, 1961.
47. Greiger, H.: Roentgen findings in cystinosis. Fortschr. Roentgenstr., *113*:711, 1970.
48. Becker, M. H., and Wallin, J. K.: Congenital hyperuricosuria. Radiol. Clin. North Am., *6*:239, 1968.
49. Nyhan, W. L.: Clinical features of the Lesch-Nyhan syndrome. Arch. Intern. Med., *130*:186, 1972.

DISEASES OF THE ENDOCRINE SYSTEM

THE ANTERIOR PITUITARY

Hypopituitarism

Hypopituitarism may be idiopathic, or may be secondary to a pituitary or suprasellar tumor. Rarer causes include basal meningitis and a deficient sellar diaphragm. There are positive skull findings in about one fifth of cases. In adults there may be evidence of an intrasellar lesion, usually a chromophobe adenoma. In children there may be an extrasellar lesion such as a cyst or craniopharyngioma.

Hypopituitarism in a prepubertal child results in a Lorain dwarfism, in which the body proportions are normal though the bones appear slender. Bone age is retarded, and the appearance of epiphyseal centers is delayed. Absence of marginal epiphyses in the vertebrae can result in a relative platyspondylia. The epiphyses may remain open well into adult life, sometimes up to the fifth decade. The sella is usually normal or small unless a suprasellar lesion is present.

Radiography is helpful in distinguishing pituitary dwarfism from other types of dwarfism. In many of the latter, including dwarfism from rickets, Turner's syndrome, chondrodystrophy, and Hurler's syndrome, there are characteristic bone alterations, and the appearance of the epiphyses is usually not delayed.[1-4]

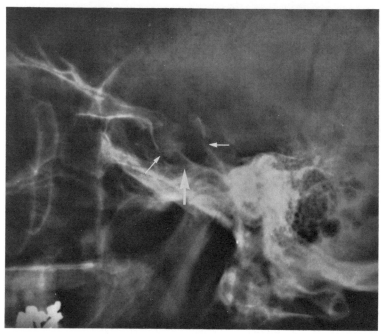

Figure 16–1 **Hypopituitarism: Chromophobe Adenoma.** In a 40 year old woman, the sella turcica is ballooned and there is downward displacement of the floor *(large arrow)* into the posterior portion of the sphenoid sinus. The floor is thinned and eroded *(small arrows)*, and the normally dense cortical line of the floor of the sella is absent — an important radiographic sign of an intrasellar mass. The anterior clinoids and dorsum sellae of this patient are intact, but the dorsum is often thinned and eroded by an intrasellar tumor. The anterior clinoids are lateral to the sella and consequently are not involved by a tumor confined to the sella. Chromophobe adenoma is the most common cause of hypopituitarism in association with sellar changes.

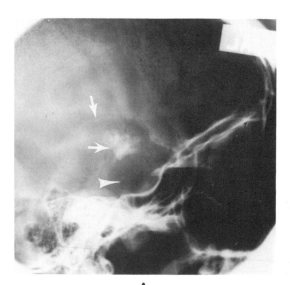

A

Figure 16–2 **Hypopituitarism and Dwarfism in 19 Year Old Male: Craniopharyngioma.**

A, Lateral skull film shows linear and amorphous calcifications *(arrows)* in the suprasellar area, associated with almost complete disappearance of the dorsum sella *(arrowhead)*. These findings are characteristic of a craniopharyngioma.

B, Ununited epiphyses in the hand and wrist are evidence of the hypogonadism secondary to the hypopituitarism.

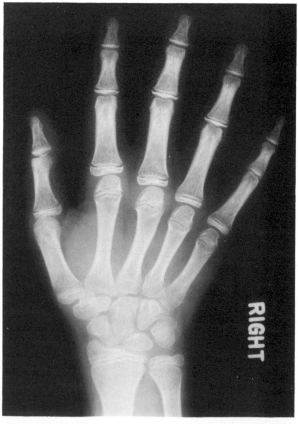

B

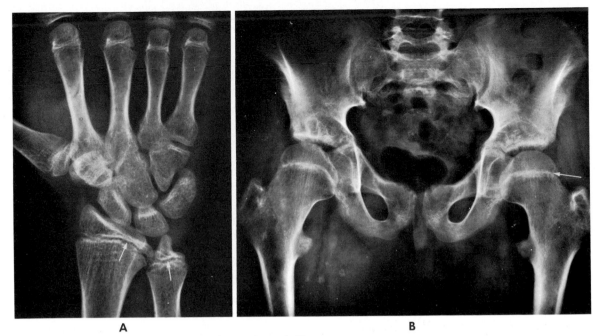

Figure 16–3 **Pituitary Dwarf: Delayed Epiphyseal Closure.**

A, In a 38 year old pituitary dwarf the bones are small but otherwise appear normal. The epiphyses of the ulna and radius are still open *(arrows)*.

B, The epiphyses of the femoral heads have not fused entirely *(arrow)*. Secondary hypogonadism causes the delayed closure of the epiphyses in hypopituitarism.

Hyperpituitarism: Acromegaly

An excess of growth hormone produced by an eosinophilic adenoma of the pituitary gland causes acromegaly in adults and gigantism in younger individuals whose epiphyses are not closed. The most frequent and significant radiographic finding is increased size and alteration of contour of the sella turcica (see *Pituitary Adenomas*, p. 346). These sellar changes occur in over 80 per cent of cases.

Overgrowth of all tissues is the basic pathologic alteration in acromegaly. This is seen most often in the soft tissues and cartilages. Increased thickness (over 23 mm.) of the soft tissue heel pad is a frequent and helpful sign. Periarticular soft tissue thickening in the small joints of the hand is also common. Cartilaginous hypertrophy causes increased width of the intervertebral disc spaces and widened spaces in many peripheral joints.

Bone changes are variable and of limited diagnostic value. In the skull the frontal sinuses are enlarged in about three fourths of cases, but prognathism due to an elongated and abnormally angulated mandible—a supposed hallmark of acromegaly—occurs in only a minority of cases. An enlarged occipital protuberance, a thickened inner table, and frontal hyperostosis are inconstant findings. Increased size of the phalangeal tufts occurs in well-developed cases. Flaring of the ends of the long bones and cystic changes especially in the carpal bones and femoral trochanters are nonspecific findings. Osteoarthritic changes, commonly seen in the knees, are frequent; the preservation of normal or even widened joint spaces in the presence of osteoarthritic bony overgrowth is a striking and suggestive finding. In the spine there may be enlarged vertebral bodies, with increased anteroposterior diameter and widened disc spaces. In about 30 per cent of cases, some degree of scalloping of the posterior vertebral bodies occurs, probably due to pressure of hypertrophied soft tissues. A generalized osteoporosis may occur late in the disease.

Visceral enlargement, especially of the heart and kidneys, may be striking. Cardiomegaly due to hypertension is common; the hypertension is apparently caused by increased aldosterone excretion. Cardiac decompensation eventually occurs in up to half the acromegalics.

In gigantism there will be evidence of sellar enlargement, and some of the bone and soft tissue changes of acromegaly are usually found in the abnormally large skeleton. The changes become more pronounced and classic if the hyperpituitarism is unchecked after epiphyseal closure. The bone age is normal in the pituitary giant.

Pituitary gigantism should be distinguished from the rare cerebral gigantism (Sotos' syndrome), which is characterized by a large skull, mental retardation with cerebral atrophy, and an advanced bone age.[1-3, 5-9]

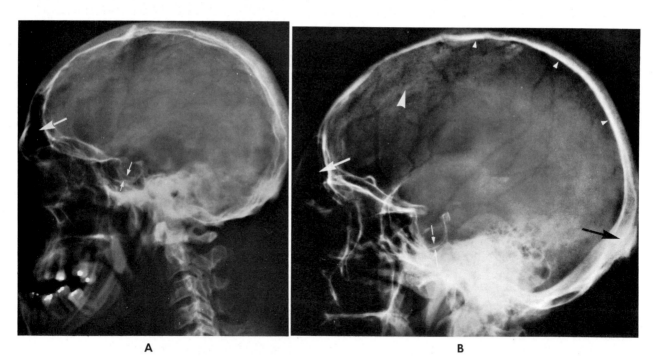

A　　　　　　　　　　　　　　　　　　　　**B**

Figure 16–4 **Acromegaly: The Skull: Two Male Patients.**

A, One side of the floor of the sella is depressed by an eosinophilic adenoma, thereby producing a double floor *(small arrows)*; otherwise, the sella appears intact. The sellar findings may vary from normal to a ballooned sella and erosion of the floor and dorsum.

The frontal sinuses are very large *(large arrow)*, and prognathism is evident. The bones of the cranial vault are somewhat thickened.

B, This skull also shows a double sellar floor *(small arrows)*. In addition there is vertical enlargement of the sella, frontal hyperostoses *(large arrowhead)*, thickening of the inner table *(small arrowheads)*, and enlargement of the external occipital protuberance (inion) *(black arrow)*. There is unrelated vascular calcification overlying the sella.

The combined findings in both skulls illustrate nearly all the roentgen features of the acromegalic skull: double sellar floor, enlargement of the sella, enlarged frontal sinuses, thickening of the vault, frontal hyperostoses (rare in normal males), prognathism, enlargement of the inion, and thickening of the inner table.

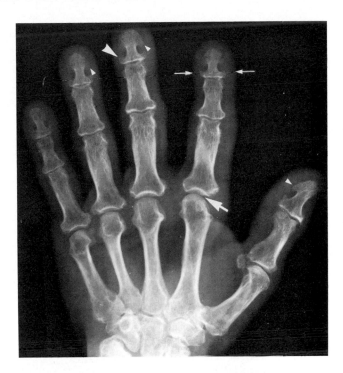

Figure 16–5 **Acromegaly: The Hand.** There is thickening of the soft tissues *(small arrows)* of the fingers. Overgrowth of the tufts of the distal phalanges *(small arrowheads)* has produced bony prominences that point proximally. Similar spurs have developed at the base of the distal phalanges *(large arrowhead).* The joint spaces of the metacarpophalangeal joints are somewhat widened *(large arrow),* but this is difficult to appreciate unless compared with a normal hand of this size.

These changes are due to bone and cartilaginous overgrowth, and are seen in long-standing cases of acromegaly.

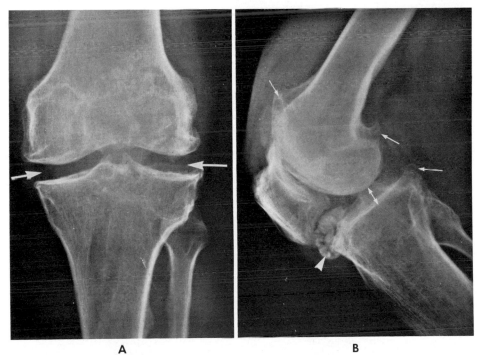

A   B

Figure 16–6 **Acromegaly: The Knee.**

A, There are hypertrophic spurs on the lateral aspect of the joint, but the cartilaginous joint spaces *(arrows)* are quite wide.

B, Extensive hypertrophic changes are seen in lateral view, with numerous spurs *(arrows)* and an osteochondroma *(arrowhead)*; the joint space remains wide *(double-headed arrow).*

Although these changes in themselves are characteristic of osteoarthritis, which often develops in acromegaly, the wide joint space is the result of enlargement of the cartilages; in osteoarthritis unassociated with acromegaly, there is cartilaginous degeneration and a narrowed joint space.

Many cartilaginous spaces, such as the intervertebral disc space and the hip joint, are unusually wide in acromegaly.

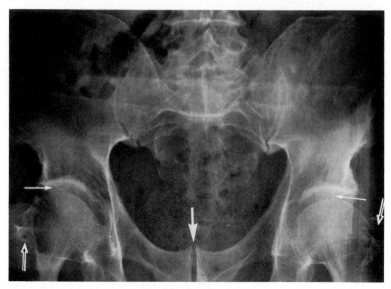

Figure 16–7 **Acromegaly: The Pelvic Bones.**   The characteristic overgrowth of bone and cartilage is well demonstrated in this 55 year old acromegalic. There is bony beaking of the symphysis *(large arrow)* and unusually wide joint spaces in the hips *(small white arrows).* Cystic changes are evident in both trochanters *(black-white arrows).*

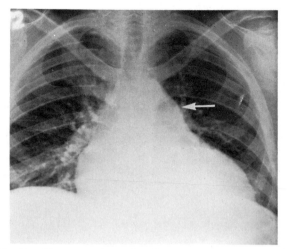

Figure 16–8 **Acromegaly: Cardiac Hypertrophy and Dilatation.**   The heart, especially the left ventricle, is greatly enlarged. The main pulmonary artery segment is dilated *(arrow),* and there is moderate vascular engorgement.

Cardiopathy occurs in over half the patients and may be associated with hypertension; decompensation often follows.

POSTERIOR PITUITARY

Diabetes Insipidus

Of the numerous causes of diabetes insipidus, only brain tumor and xanthomatosis (histiocytosis) are associated with significant roentgenologic findings. Craniopharyngioma is the most common tumor. Usually there is suprasellar calcification and pressure on the sella. Chromophobe adenoma can also cause diabetes insipidus, either as an early symptom or concomitantly with hypopituitarism.

The xanthomatous lesions of eosinophilic granuloma or Hand-Schüller-Christian disease (histiocytosis X) often give rise to punched-out lesions in the skull bones, but the lesions of the hypothalamus that cause diabetes insipidus may occur without associated bone involvement. In diabetes insipidus caused by histiocytosis in which there are no bone lesions, a honeycomb lung may be the only radiographic clue (see p. 1192).

In severe untreated diabetes insipidus there may be massive dilatation of the renal pelves, calices, and ureters, probably a compensatory alteration to accommodate the huge volume of excreted urine.[10-13]

THE PINEAL

Pinealoma

This uncommon tumor usually occurs in males under 25 years of age. The majority are teratomas, but other histologic types can occur. From 15 to 30 per cent of these tumors are associated with precocious puberty, most often when the tumor actually destroys the pineal gland. Some investigators believe that hypothalamic involvement is responsible for the endocrinopathy.

Plain skull films may be negative, but usually the pineal is calcified, occasionally with unusual circular or small linear streaks. Pineal calcification in a young child is unusual and should suggest the possibility of pinealoma.

On the CT scan, a pinealoma may appear as an abnormal mass density anterior to the quadrigeminal cistern, sometimes compressing or displacing this structure. Dilatation of the lateral and third ventricles is often apparent. Unusual and extensive pineal calcification may be seen even when the tumor itself cannot be clearly identified on the scan. Occasionally, dilatation of the lateral and third ventricles is the only finding. Contrast material administered intravenously may enhance and identify the tumor.

Ventriculography may show dilatation of the lateral ventricles and of the anterior portion of the third ventricle if the aqueduct is compressed. The definitive finding is a midline filling defect located in the posterior part of the third ventricle projecting into the air-filled portion of the ventricle.

Angiography usually reveals nonspecific findings of internal hydrocephalus, with a stretched anterior cerebral artery and a more obtuse curve to the thalamostriate vein on frontal projection.[14-19]

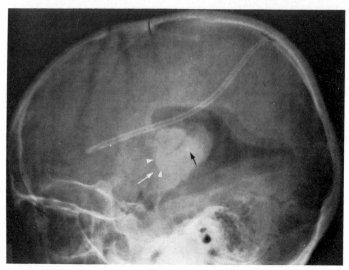

Figure 16–9 **Pinealoma: Precocious Puberty.** Pneumogram of a 7 year old boy with marked precocious puberty reveals the anterior border of a large mass *(arrowheads)* projecting into the anterior portion of the third ventricle *(white arrow)* and extending upward and posteriorly into the lateral ventricles. The pinealoma completely obliterates the posterior portion of the third ventricle. The pineal gland *(black arrow)* is calcified, always a suspicious finding in a child of this age.

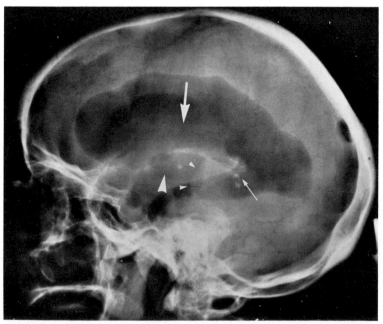

Figure 16–10 **Pinealoma: Ventriculogram.** The lateral ventricle *(large arrow)* and the third ventricle *(large arrowhead)* are dilated because of a pinealoma whose curved anterior margin projects into the third ventricle *(small arrowheads)*. Ordinarily, the air in the third ventricle extends posteriorly to the pineal. A number of discrete calcifications are in the posterior portion of the tumor *(small arrow)*, at the usual site of a normal pineal. The posterior clinoids have been eroded by pressure from the enlarged third ventricle. The tumor was not associated with precocious puberty.

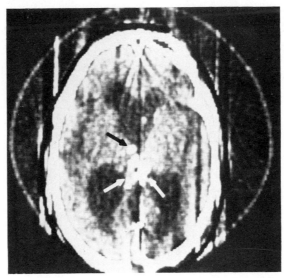

Figure 16–11 **Pinealoma: CT Scan.**   A collection of densities which have a scan μ value of calcium is seen in the midline *(arrows)*. These densities were calcifications within a pinealoma. The dilatation of the lateral ventricles indicates that the tumor is causing some obstruction of the aqueduct.

The CT scan will often demonstrate tumorous enlargement of the pineal gland, even when calcifications are absent, or will reveal calcifications that are too faint to be seen on conventional films.

THE THYROID

Hyperthyroidism (Thyrotoxicosis)

The increased circulatory flow in hyperthyroidism often leads to some cardiac enlargement, a prominent main pulmonary artery segment, and a slight increase in the caliber of the pulmonary vessels (high output heart). These changes are relatively slight and therefore easily overlooked; it may be necessary to compare films taken during the course of disease with those made before onset or after successful treatment.

The skeletal system may undergo a mild osteoporosis or osteomalacia; this too is difficult to recognize without carefully exposed comparative films. In neonates, an accelerated bone age is usually seen. A rare and late manifestation of hyperthyroidism is thyroid acropachy, which may occur even after the thyrotoxicosis has disappeared. This is characterized by swelling and clubbing of the fingers or toes and by a distinctively spiculated periosteal new bone formation in the phalanges and metacarpals. These changes may be mistaken radiographically for hypertrophic pulmonary osteoarthropathy or pachydermoperiostitis (see p. 1367). Exophthalmos, whether unilateral or bilateral, can be readily demonstrated on CT scan.[1, 20–23]

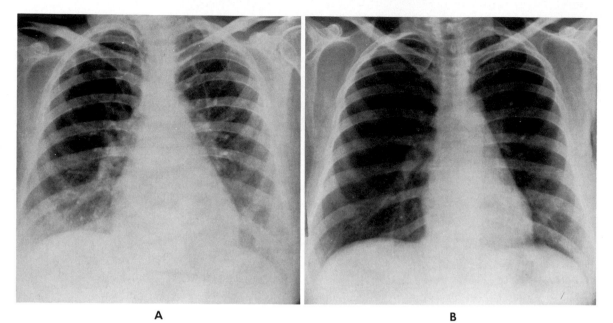

A   **B**

Figure 16–12 **The Heart in Thyrotoxicosis.**

A, The cardiac silhouette is moderately enlarged; the straight left border is due to fullness of the main pulmonary artery segment: The perihilar and basal vasculature is accentuated. This is the high output heart.

B, The heart size and vasculature have returned to normal following therapy, but the main pulmonary artery segment is still prominent.

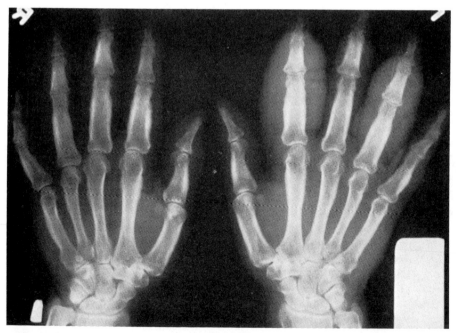

Figure 16–13 **Thyroid Acropachy.** There is characteristically spiculated periosteal new bone formation in the metacarpal and phalanges. Notice the marked soft tissue swelling. (Courtesy Dr. F. Wietersen, Wayne State University School of Medicine, Detroit, Michigan.)

Hypothyroidism

In cretinism and juvenile hypothyroidism the most common and most characteristic skeletal finding is delay in the appearance and subsequent growth of the ossification centers. Epiphyseal closure is also delayed, often well into adult life. A dysgenesis of the epiphyses characterized by fragmented epiphyses that contain multiple ossification foci (stippled epiphyses) is also frequent and highly characteristic. Skull changes are common in younger cretins and include widened sutures, widened fontanelles with late closure, delayed dentition, and delay or failure of pneumatization of the paranasal sinuses and mastoids. The interorbital space may be increased. Later, the bones of the cranial vault may become abnormally dense.

Other less specific skeletal changes include wedging of one or more dorsolumbar bodies, dense vertebral margins, metaphyseal irregularities, hip deformities, and hypoplasia of the phalanges of the fifth finger. Bone demineralization is sometimes seen, especially in longstanding cases. Vascular calcification from premature atherosclerosis is often found.

In adult cretins, bone abnormalities are less common. These include thickening of the cranial vault, vertebral wedging, and coxa vara with flattened femoral head.

There are no skeletal changes in hypothyroidism that begins in adulthood.

An enlarged cardiac silhouette may appear in adult myxedema. This is apparently due mainly to pericardial effusion, although chamber dilatation and myxedematous tissue deposits may contribute to the enlargement. Occasionally, ascites and pleural effusion are associated with the pericardial effusion. In uncomplicated hypothyroidism, the heart size returns to normal after thyroid therapy.[24-28]

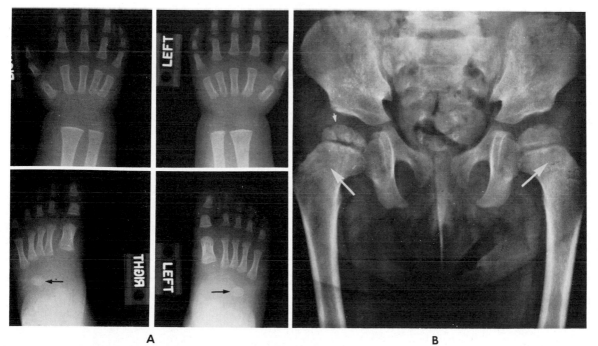

A   B

Figure 16–14 **Cretin: Bone Changes in a 3 Year Old Child.**

A, There are no ossification centers in the wrist and there is only one in the tarsal area *(arrows),* in contrast to the three to five ossification centers normally present in these regions. A delay in the appearance of ossification centers occurs in all cases of untreated cretinism. The distal two phalanges of the fifth fingers are somewhat hypoplastic, a common finding.

B, Multiple ossification centers *(small arrow)* give the right femoral head a fragmented appearance (epiphyseal dysgenesis). The femoral necks are abnormally broad *(large arrows).*

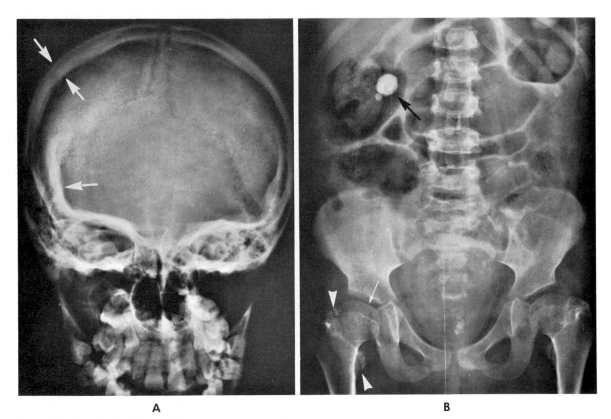

A   B

Figure 16–15   **Cretin: Bone Changes.**

A, In a 38 year old cretin, there is a marked increase in the thickness of the bones of the vault *(arrows).* The frontal sinuses are undeveloped, and the interorbital distance is widened.

B, The femoral heads are flattened *(white arrow),* the necks are broadened, and the trochanteric epiphyses are fragmented *(arrowheads).* The two calculi in the right kidney *(black arrow)* are probably unrelated to the cretinism.

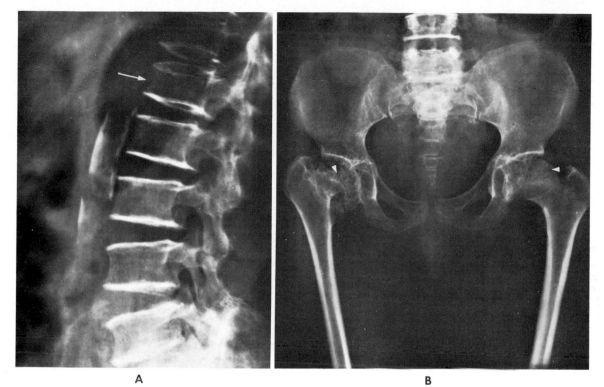

A   **B**

Figure 16–16   **Adult Cretin: Spine and Hip Changes.**

   A, The lower dorsal and lumbar bodies, especially LI *(arrow),* are slightly wedged. This juvenile ap-pearance is probably due to faulty vertebral epiphyseal development and fusion.

   There is extensive calcification of the abdominal aorta; premature arteriosclerosis is frequently seen in cretins.

   Demineralization of the vertebrae and increased density of the cortices are nonspecific findings but are often seen in older cretins.

   B, The epiphyses of the femoral head are still ununited *(arrowheads),* the femoral heads are flattened, and the necks are broadened. Severe bilateral coxa vara is apparent. There is marked demineralization of all the bones.

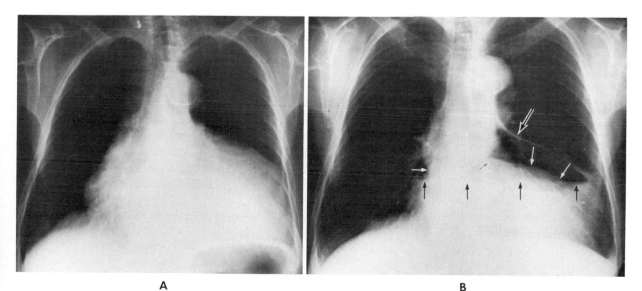

A   **B**

Figure 16–17   **Myxedema: Pericardial Effusion.**

   A, The cardiac silhouette is greatly enlarged. The pulmonary vasculature is normal.

   B, Following pericardiocentesis and air instillation, the borders of a normal-sized heart *(white arrows)* can be seen. The residual pericardial fluid forms an air-fluid level *(black arrows).* The pericardium is not thickened *(black-white arrow).*

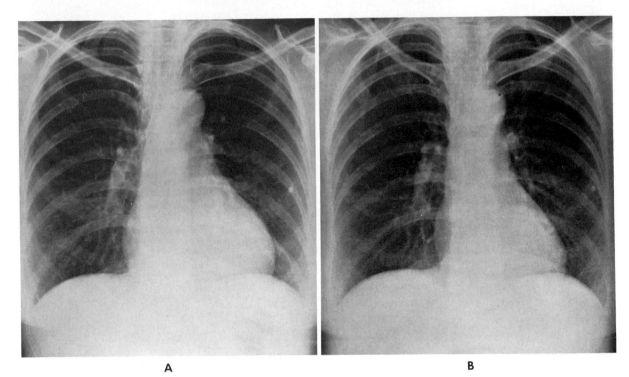

A   B

Figure 16–18 **Postoperative Myxedema: Cardiopathy.**

A, Ten days after thyroid ablation the heart is moderately enlarged, but there is no alteration in the vasculature.

B, With prolonged thyroid therapy, the heart has returned to normal size. (Courtesy Dr. F. G. Hoffmann, Louisville, Kentucky.)

Goiter: Thyroid Adenomas

An enlarged thyroid gland in the neck can usually be recognized radiographically by the deviation or indentation of the trachea. Even diffuse enlargement is rarely entirely symmetric, and tracheal deviation or compression can often be demonstrated before enlargement can be palpated. The gland itself is rarely visible radiographically, but sometimes a soft tissue mass is seen anterior to the trachea on lateral films. Adenomas may often be recognized because of local calcifications within the mass. Diffuse calcification may sometimes occur in a long-standing benign goiter.

Substernal extension of an enlarged thyroid usually produces bilateral but asymmetric widening of the superior mediastinum with sharply defined curved lateral margins. Tracheal and esophageal deviation adjacent to the substernal mass almost invariably is present. Atypical or unilateral substernal extension may simulate a mediastinal tumor. Associated tracheal deviation in the neck is a helpful finding for identifying a substernal thyroid.

The size, location, and functional activity of the thyroid gland or adenoma are most accurately shown by radioactive isotope scan of the neck.[1, 20, 29]

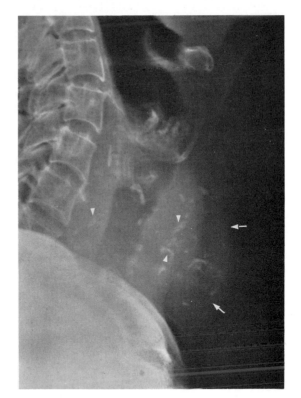

Figure 16–19 **Longstanding Goiter with Calcification.** Lateral view demonstrates a bulging soft tissue mass *(arrows),* anterior to the trachea, with irregular calification *(arrowheads)* scattered throughout. The goiter also extends posteriorly behind the trachea. The retrotracheal space is abnormally full and contains some calcifications.

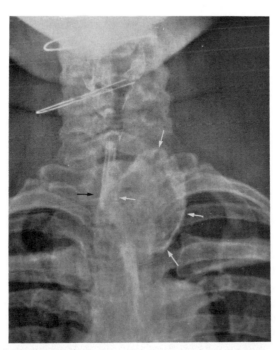

Figure 16–20 **Large Calcified Thyroid Adenoma.** A large ovoid mass having a calcified rim *(white arrows)* and containing mottled calcifications extends to the upper sternal level and causes deviation of the esophagus and trachea *(black arrow)* to the right. Most thyroid adenomas are smaller than the one above; calcifications are more frequent in longstanding cases.

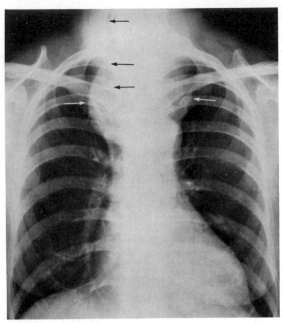

Figure 16–21 **Substernal Extension of Enlarged Thyroid.** Smooth round densities *(white arrows)* are producing bilateral but asymmetric widening of the superior mediastinum. The trachea *(black arrows)* is deviated to the right, both in the neck *(upper arrows)* and in the upper mediastinal area; the esophagus, which is not opacified in this film, was also displaced to the right. The picture suggests substernal thyroid, and if the mass extends into the neck the diagnosis is almost certain. Fluoroscopic examination with a swallow of barium often demonstrates deviation of the esophagus and upward movement of the mass on deglutition. Most other superior mediastinal tumors do not move during deglutition.

Malignant Disease of the Thyroid

Malignant nodules or tumors of the thyroid may produce a nonspecific enlargement of the gland, evidenced radiographically only by deviation of the trachea. Occasionally fine hazy calcifications arising in psammoma bodies may be seen in papillary carcinoma.

The most common metastases from thyroid carcinoma are to regional nodes, lungs, and bone.

Papillary carcinoma is most frequent in children and metastasizes mainly to the lungs. These metastases often merely cause deceptive thickening of the bronchovascular markings, but may also appear as miliary and nodular densities, most abundant in the lower lobes.

The follicular adenocarcinoma of adults most often involves bone, especially of the skull, pelvis, and upper extremities. These metastases are medullary, expansile, usually oval, and entirely lytic, eventually destroying the cortex and extending into the soft tissues. There is little or no periosteal reaction. Frequently the first symptoms of an unsuspected thyroid carcinoma arise from a bone metastasis.

Medullary carcinoma is the least frequent thyroid malignancy, and appears to have some familial tendency. It often originates in both lobes, and about one third exhibit characteristic dense calcifications. This carcinoma may be associated with pheochromocytoma and sometimes with parathyroid adenoma or hyperplasia—Sipple's syndrome.[29–31]

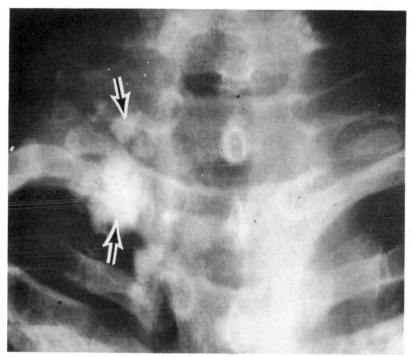

Figure 16–22 **Medullary Carcinoma of Thyroid: Characteristic Calcifications.** The collections of amorphous dense calcifications *(arrows)* in the right paratracheal area are within a medullary carcinoma of the thyroid. This type of calcification in the thyroid gland is quite characteristic of medullary thyroid carcinoma, in contrast to the psammomatous calcifications of papillary thyroid carcinoma.

Medullary carcinoma of the thyroid is often associated with Sipple's syndrome (see Fig. 16–24).

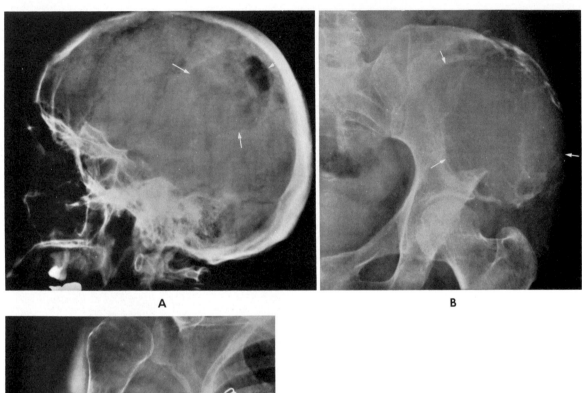

A

B

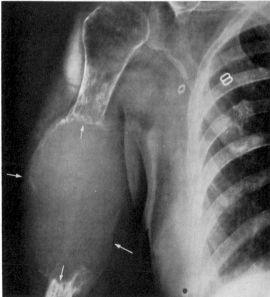

C

Figure 16–23 **Bone Metastases in Follicular Carcinoma of Thyroid.** *(A)* There are circumscribed lytic lesions of the skull *(arrows)*, *(B)* a huge expanding lytic lesion of the ilium *(arrows)*, and *(C)* expansile destruction of most of the humeral shaft *(arrows)*. The tumor has extended into the soft tissues.

Multiple Endocrine Neoplasia (Sipple's Syndrome)

This familial syndrome comprises medullary carcinoma of the thyroid and adrenal pheochromocytoma. Parathyroid hyperplasia or adenoma is often associated. Both lobes of the thyroid are usually involved by tumor, and the pheochromocytomas, usually bilateral, are found in about 50 per cent of cases. Elevated serum calcium and calcitonin levels are often encountered.

Radiographically, characteristic dense calcifications (in contrast to fine psammomatous calcifications of papillary carcinoma) are seen in the thyroid tumor in about one third of cases. This calcification may also appear in metastatic nodes. Pulmonary metastases are peculiarly reticulonodular; bone metastases are always lytic.

The pheochromocytomas only rarely can be identified by egg-shell calcification. Angiographic studies are generally necessary for identification.

The hyperparathyroidism is usually mild and without any bony changes. Renal calculi are more commonly encountered.

Characteristic dense calcification in the thyroid should suggest medullary carcinoma and initiate a search for other features of Sipple's syndrome.[31]

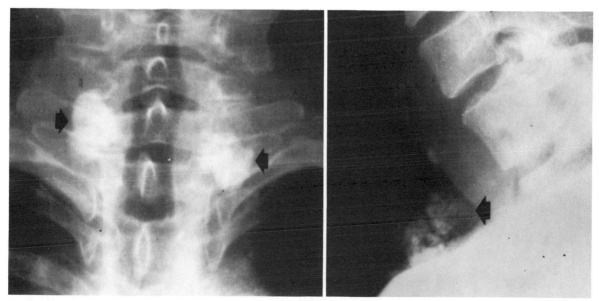

Figure 16–24 **Sipple's Syndrome.** There are dense amorphous calcifications (*arrows*) in both lobes of the thyroid. These were within bilateral medullary carcinomas (multicentric origin?).

A parathyroid adenoma was also present, but no pheochromocytomas were uncovered. The latter tumor, usually bilateral, occurs in about 50 per cent of patients with Sipple's syndrome. (Courtesy Dr. H. R. Keiser, National Institutes of Health, Washington, D. C.)

ADRENAL CORTEX

Adrenocortical Insufficiency

In infants, acute adrenal insufficiency can result from bilateral adrenal hemorrhage. Unilateral hemorrhage does not produce adrenal insufficiency. A picture of paralytic ileus may be present during the acute episode, and because of associated vomiting a high small bowel obstruction is sometimes suspected. Intravenous pyelogram may show depression of one or both kidneys by the hemorrhagic masses, which are slowly resorbed if the infant survives. The adrenal glands may subsequently calcify.

In chronic adrenocortical insufficiency (Addison's disease) there are no characteristic radiographic findings. One or both adrenals are calcified in about 25 per cent of cases, but asymptomatic adrenal calcification is also seen in normal individuals. Frequently, the heart shadow is small but will increase in size after successful therapy.

Tuberculosis of the adrenal glands was once considered to be the most common single cause of Addison's disease. Most current cases, however, result from idiopathic atrophy. Nevertheless, there may be evidence of chronic or healed pulmonary tuberculosis and, more rarely, of renal or bone tuberculosis. Other infrequent radiographic findings include an enlarged spleen (10 per cent of cases) and calcification of the pinnae of the ear.[32-37]

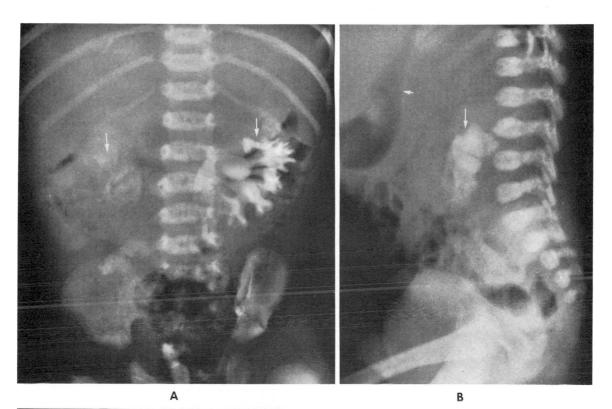

A   B

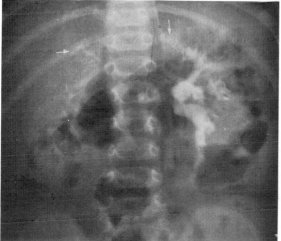

C

Figure 16–25 **Bilateral Massive Adrenal Hemorrhage in Newborn: Recovery and Calcification.**

A, Both kidneys are displaced downward and rotated outward *(arrows)* by large adrenal masses due to hemorrhage. An unrelated congenital ureteral pelvic narrowing on the left has produced dilatation of the pelvis and calices.

B, Lateral view demonstrates depression of the kidney *(large arrow)* and forward displacement of the air-filled stomach *(small arrow)* by the left adrenal mass.

C, Intravenous pyelogram seven months later shows mottled calcification *(arrows)* in both adrenal areas. Both kidneys are in normal position, and angulation is normal. There is still evidence of ureteropelvic obstruction on the left.

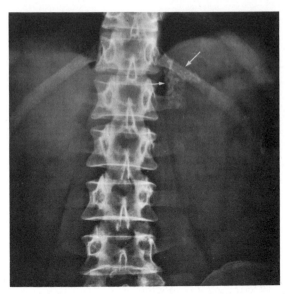

Figure 16–26 **Unilateral Adrenal Calcification in an Adult.** There are mottled calcifications throughout the left adrenal area *(arrows)* corresponding to the size and shape of an adrenal gland. The patient was asymptomatic. The calcifications might be the consequence of adrenal hemorrhage during infancy.

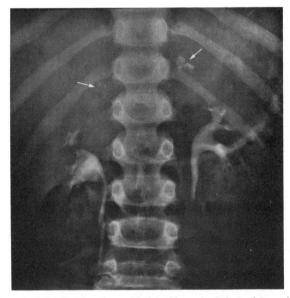

Figure 16–27 **Bilateral Adrenal Calcification in a Child: Chronic Adrenal Insufficiency.** The urogram was normal; there was clinical and biochemical evidence of mild chronic adrenal insufficiency. Both adrenals are calcified *(arrows)*. Although unilateral and bilateral adrenal calcification may be late consequences of neonatal adrenal hemorrhage, adrenal insufficiency rarely results.

     Other causes of adrenal calcification include tuberculosis, xanthomatosis (Wolman's disease), and malignant tumors.

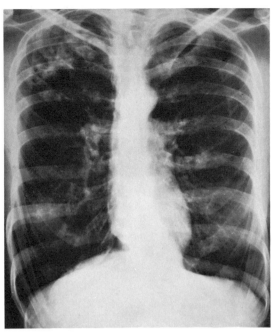

Figure 16-28 **Addison's Disease: Tuberculosis: Small Heart.** The heart is unusually small; this is common in Addison's disease but is also occasionally seen in normal persons. There is fibroid tuberculosis of the right upper lobe. Addison's disease in this instance was due to tuberculous destruction of the adrenals. Although tuberculosis is the cause of many cases of Addison's disease, roentgenologic evidence of pulmonary tuberculosis is often lacking.

An extremely small heart shadow is a nonspecific finding usually without significance, but it should suggest the possibility of Addison's disease.

Cushing's Syndrome

Skeletal changes consist of osteoporosis, pathologic fractures, abnormal callus formation, and aseptic necrosis.

The most frequent radiographic finding is osteoporosis. The spine, pelvis, ribs, and skull are most often affected; osteoporosis of the extremities is less common.

Fractures of the osteoporotic bones, especially the vertebrae and ribs, are frequent; pain is often mild or absent. Excess callus formation is characteristic of Cushing's disease and leads to cortical condensation in the margins of the vertebrae, a finding rarely present in vertebral fractures from osteoporosis due to other causes. The marginal condensation regresses with successful therapy. Rib fractures with excess callus formation have an irregular beaded appearance after healing.

The osteoporotic skull exhibits diffuse stippled demineralization. The dorsum sellae is usually demineralized with a washed out appearance.

In children, delayed skeletal maturation and osteoporosis are common. Infrequently, aseptic necrosis occurs, especially around the hip and shoulder.

Nephrocalcinosis or renal calculi develop in up to 20 per cent of cases, probably related to the hypercalcinuria.

In advanced cases, cardiomegaly may appear as a result of hypertension or myocardiopathy. Decreased cardiac size usually follows successful therapy.

Widening of the mediastinum due to mediastinal lipomatosis is an infrequent finding. It occurs more often in iatrogenic Cushing's syndrome resulting from administration of steroids.

Adrenal adenoma or carcinoma, or bilateral cortical hyperplasia is the cause of the syndrome in most cases. Only a large tumor can be demonstrated by abdominal or pyelographic films. Nephrotomography is especially useful in Cushing's disease because the increased amounts of perirenal fat may permit visualization of masses as small as 2 cm. Retroperitoneal pneumography, arteriography, and suprarenal venography, either alone or in combination, are generally necessary to demonstrate adrenal pathology.

Sellar enlargement or erosion from pituitary tumor is seen in less than 15 per cent of cases. After adrenal surgery a pituitary adenoma will develop in some patients, producing progressive sellar enlargement (Nelson's syndrome). Periodic skull films would seem to be indicated after definitive adrenal surgery.

A Cushing-like syndrome, with the attendant skeletal changes, can occur after prolonged administration of steroids.

Cushing's syndrome may be associated with neoplasia of nonendocrine origin. In these cases it is most frequently associated with tumors of the lung (especially oat cell carcinoma), of the thymus, thyroid, or of the pancreas. However, the roentgen findings of Cushing's disease are rarely seen because of the rapid course of the primary malignancy.[35, 36, 38–40]

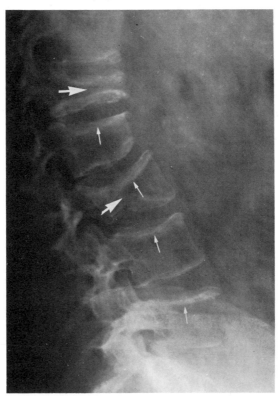

Figure 16–29 **Cushing's Syndrome: Lumbar Spine: Marginal Condensation.** Pronounced osteoporosis is associated with biconcave compression fractures *(large arrows)*. The marginal bone condensation, especially of the upper vertebral margins *(small arrows)*, is pathognomonic, occurring in about half the cases of Cushing's syndrome and in 90 per cent of cases of Cushing's syndrome associated with vertebral fractures. The marginal condensation may be indicative of the tendency toward excess callus formation that is characteristic of Cushing's syndrome, and it may be helpful in differentiating spinal osteoporosis due to Cushing's disease from osteoporosis due to other causes.

A

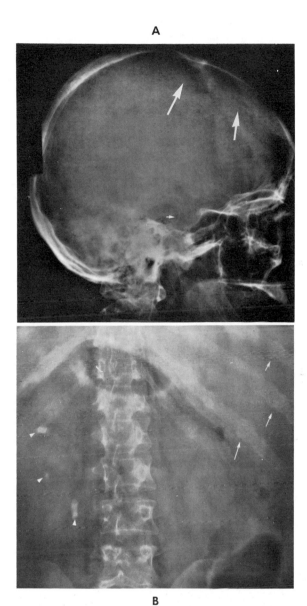

B

Figure 16–30 **Cushing's Syndrome: The Skull, Ribs, and Abdomen.**

A, Mottled areas of osteoporosis are most apparent in the frontal and parietal areas *(large arrows).* The dorsum sellae is demineralized and only faintly visualized *(small arrow).* No enlargement or erosion of the sella has occurred in this case. Sellar changes occur in only a small percentage of cases and are due to a primary or secondary pituitary adenoma.

B, The lower ribs are osteoporotic and have numerous bulbous irregularities *(arrows)* as a result of old fractures that have healed with excess callus and bone formation. Excess callus formation is characteristic of Cushing's syndrome, and often the fractures are painless. There are three calculi *(arrowheads)* in the left kidney. Calculi and nephrocalcinosis are not uncommon as a result of the excessive calcium excretion.

The lumbar bodies are osteoporotic but without compression fractures.

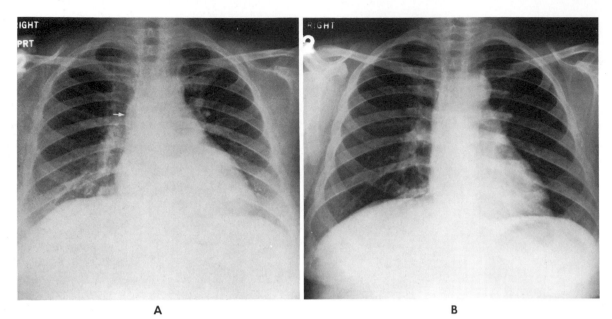

Figure 16-31 **Cushing's Syndrome: Myocardiopathy and Recovery.**

A, The heart, especially the left ventricle, is enlarged, the ascending aorta is widened (*arrow*) and prominent, and the pulmonary vasculature appears normal.

B, After removal of an adrenal adenoma, the heart size has decreased and the ascending aorta is no longer prominent.

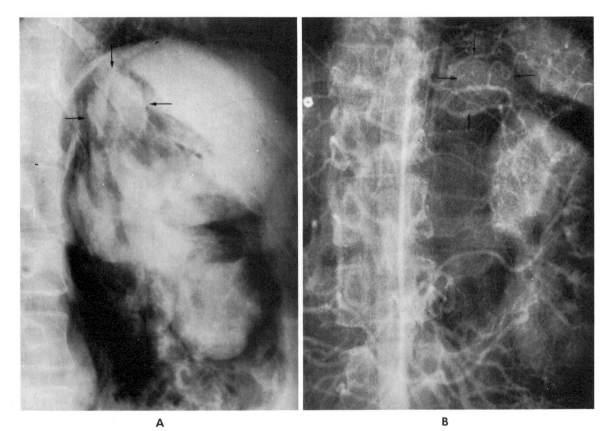

Figure 16-32 **Cushing's Syndrome: Adrenal Adenoma.**

A, Retroperitoneal air study shows enlargement of the left adrenal (*arrows*).

B, In the capillary phase of an arteriogram, a homogeneous opacification outlines the adrenocortical adenoma and encircling vessels (*arrows*).

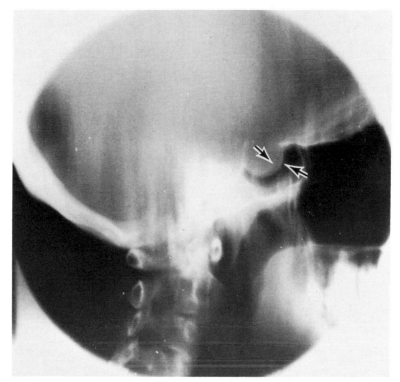

Figure 16-33 **Sellar Enlargement (Pituitary Adenoma) Following Adrenalectomy for Cushing's Disease (Nelson's Syndrome).** Laminogram of the sella turcica made about one year after bilateral cortical adrenalectomy for Cushing's disease shows a deepened, slightly expanded sella with a double floor *(arrows)*. The sella had been normal before the adrenalectomy.

The sellar enlargement is due to a growing pituitary adenoma. Some investigators report that this postadrenalectomy adenoma is usually a chromophobe lesion, but others believe it to be a pre-existing basophilic adenoma that has been stimulated to rapid growth and loss of basophilic pigment by expiration of the adrenal cortical tissue and its hormones.

Primary Hyperaldosteronism

Approximately three quarters of the patients with primary aldosteronism have an adrenocortical adenoma; the remainder have a nodular hyperplasia. Malignancy is rare, and demonstration of adrenal calcification is infrequent. Primary aldosteronism is unusual in children; if present it may lead to premature skeletal maturation and subsequent growth retardation.

Adrenal venography is the method of choice for localization and demonstration of adrenocortical hyperfunction. It also allows for selective biochemical assays of each adrenal vein. Hyperplasia can usually be distinguished from tumor. The venous pattern of the normal adrenal consists of one or two central veins running along the long axis of the gland, usually near the center. Short branching parenchymal veins, which progressively decrease in size toward the periphery of the gland, drain into these central veins. With cortical hyperplasia, the glands become large and ovoid, with spreading, somewhat dilated branches but with a normal branching pattern. If an adenoma is present the parenchymal and capsular veins are distended and spread around the tumor.

In secondary aldosteronism, which can result from renal artery stenosis or from malignant nephrosclerosis, there may also be compensatory bilateral adrenocortical hyperplasia.[35, 41, 42]

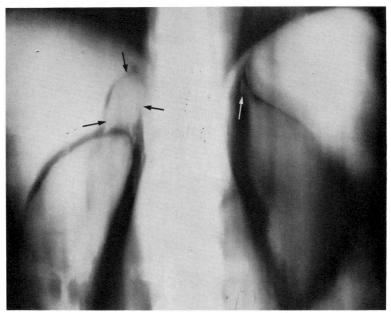

Figure 16–34 **Primary Hyperaldosteronism: Planigram: Retroperitoneal Air Study.** Air in the retro-peritoneal and perirenal spaces clearly outlines both kidneys and demonstrates enlargement of the right adrenal *(black arrows).* This was a functioning adenoma that secreted aldosterone. The left adrenal is very small *(white arrow).* Hyperfunctioning of one adrenal causes hypoplasia of the opposite one. Similar roentgeno-logic findings may be demonstrated in Cushing's disease and in the adrenogenital syndrome. (Courtesy Dr. J. W. Laws, London, England.)

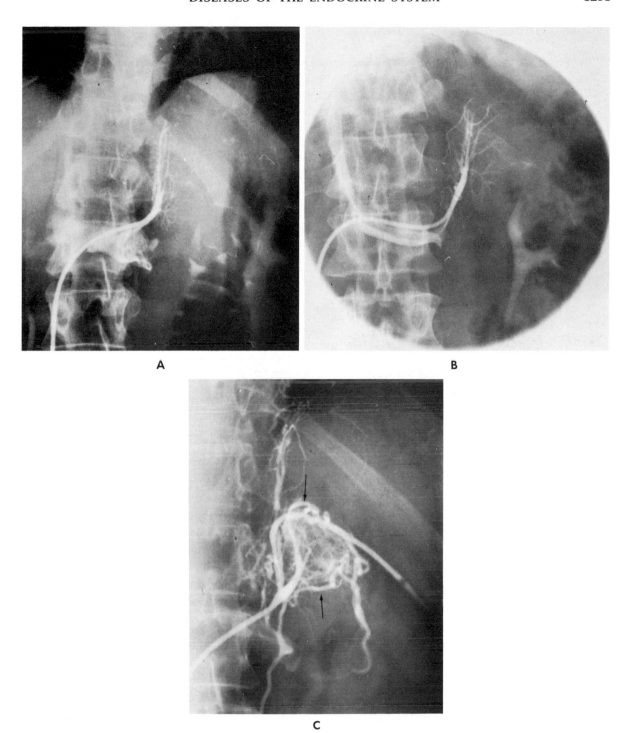

Figure 16–35 **Adrenal Venogram of a Normal Patient and of Two Patients with Hyperaldosteronism.**

A, Normal left adrenal venogram: The two central veins run along the longitudinal axis of the adrenal. Numerous short branching parenchymal veins drain into the central veins.

B, Hyperaldosteronism with adrenal hyperplasia: The adrenal is enlarged and ovoid. The veins are spread apart and slightly dilated, but they show normal branching.

C, Hyperaldosteronism with adenoma: The capsular veins *(arrows)* are enlarged and encircle the adenoma in the inferior portion of the gland. The veins within the adenoma show an irregular haphazard pattern. The adrenal veins above and medial to the adenoma are normal. (Courtesy Dr. Joseph J. Bookstein.)

Adrenogenital Syndrome

This syndrome is caused by androgenically active substances from the adrenal gland. In the congenital form there is usually adrenocortical hyperplasia; in the acquired type, an adrenal adenoma or carcinoma is usually responsible.

In the congenital form, excess androgens prevent normal development of the urogenital sinus in the female, so that a separate urethra and vagina do not develop (pseudohermaphrodism). This can be demonstrated by direct injection of contrast material into the urogenital sinus.

Skeletal maturation is accelerated, with premature epiphyseal fusion leading to dwarfism.

A large adrenal tumor may be apparent on abdominal or pyelographic films, but smaller lesions require retroperitoneal gas studies, adrenal arteriography, or adrenal venography.

The Stein-Leventhal syndrome may clinically simulate a masculinizing adrenogenital syndrome. In the former, gynecography will disclose enlarged ovaries.[35, 43]

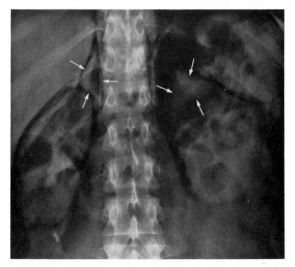

Figure 16–36 **Adrenogenital Syndrome: Adrenal Cortical Hyperplasia.** A 28 year old woman had amenorrhea and hypertrichosis and was unable to become pregnant. Retrococcygeal air study discloses enlarged adrenals bilaterally *(arrows),* particularly the left. Similar findings are often seen in full-blown Cushing's syndrome.

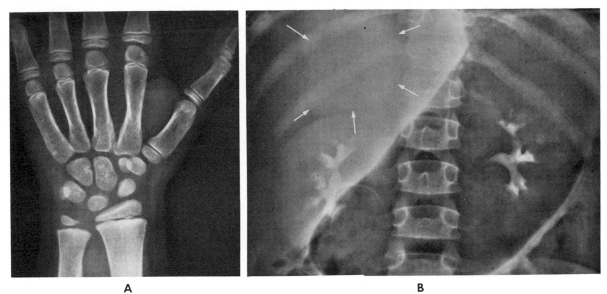

A   B

Figure 16–37 **Cortical Hyperadrenalism in a Child: Functioning Adrenal Adenoma.**

A, A 3½ year old child had clinical signs of precocious sexual development. All eight carpal bones are ossified, which does not normally occur until age 7 to 9 years.

B, Intravenous pyelography demonstrates a faint but definite rounded mass *(arrows)* above the right kidney. Both kidneys are normal. The stomach has been deliberately distended with gas by having the child ingest a carbonated drink. This procedure displaces confusing intestinal gas shadows from the kidney areas.

The mass was a functioning adrenal cortical adenoma. The excess secretion of androgens caused virilization, precocious sexuality, and advanced bone age.

Large adrenal tumors can produce a soft tissue shadow on abdominal films; retroperitoneal pneumography or adrenal arteriography is needed to identify smaller tumors or hyperplasia.

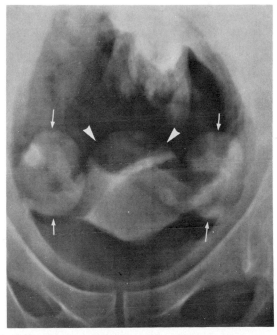

Figure 16–38 **Stein-Leventhal Syndrome: Gynecogram.** The ovaries are symmetrically enlarged *(small arrows).* The uterus *(arrowheads)* is abnormally small, being only slightly larger than the ovaries. The clinical picture is quite similar to that of the adrenogenital syndrome; gynecography may be helpful in making the distinction because in the adrenogenital syndrome the ovaries are of normal size.

Adrenal Carcinoma

Only a minority of adrenal carcinomas are associated with Cushing's syndrome; the majority produce no endocrine disturbance. Although a relatively uncommon tumor, adrenal carcinoma occurs about as frequently as pheochromocytoma.

In most cases there is radiographic evidence of a mass, best seen on the excretory urogram. The mass may become quite large and often will displace the kidney, generally without invasion. Scattered calcifications are occasionally seen.

Angiographically the lesion is usually quite vascular and will stretch the inferior adrenal artery, which is its major vascular supply. Arteriovenous lakes, abnormal vessels, and early venous filling are commonly seen, but the angiographic appearance is often quite similar to a vascular pheochromocytoma. Distinction is usually made by the elevation of blood pressure that occurs during arteriography of a pheochromocytoma (see p. 1292). Hepatic angiography should be done to uncover any liver metastasis.[44-46]

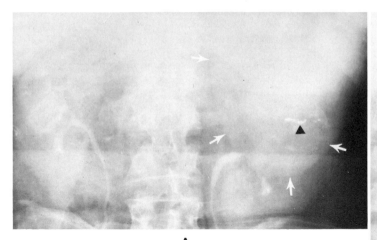

A

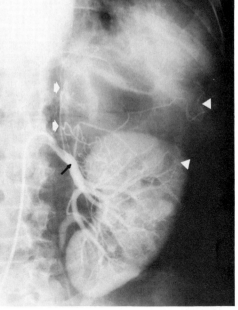

B

Figure 16–39 **Large Nonendocrine Adrenal Carcinoma.**

A, Intravenous urogram shows a huge soft tissue mass *(white arrows)* in the left upper quadrant. It is partially overlying the left kidney, whose caliceal system, although not well opacified, was not distorted. The density in the mass *(black arrowhead)* was an artifact.

B, Selective left renal arteriogram discloses a normal renal artery *(black arrow)* and renal arterial tree. The nephrogram shows that the kidney is displaced downward and its upper pole rotated laterally by the mass. No renal invasion is apparent.

The inferior adrenal artery *(wide arrows),* which arises from the renal artery, is greatly elongated and stretched around the tumor. The mass is only moderately vascularized, but abnormal vessels with small shunt densities are seen *(white arrowheads).*

Angiographically, the carcinoma simulates a pheochromocytoma.

GONADS

Hypogonadism

Long slender bones in the hands and feet owing to delayed epiphyseal closure and prolonged growth are frequently seen in eunuchoid males, and in tall thin normal males as well. In Klinefelter's syndrome, skeletal maturation and bone density are normal, although occasionally a short fourth or fifth metacarpal bone is found. In hypogonadism secondary to hypopituitarism there may be roentgenologic evidence of a pituitary or suprasellar tumor.[27]

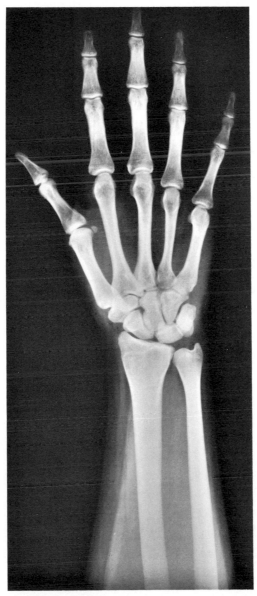

Figure 16–40 **Eunuchoid Male.**   The patient was 26 years of age. The bones of the hand and forearm are long and slender.

Gonadal Dysgenesis (Turner's Syndrome)

In this condition, the clinical features of sexual infantilism, short stature, and webbed neck are associated with numerous and varied skeletal and visceral anomalies.

The most constant and specific radiographic skeletal features are the metacarpal sign and changes in the knee. The former, found in over three fourths of cases, consists of an abnormally short fourth metacarpal and sometimes also a shortened fifth metacarpal. These changes are often bilateral, and frequently there are similar changes in the metatarsals. In the knee, the medial femoral condyle is larger and extends lower than the lateral condyle, a virtual pathognomonic finding.

Other common but less specific radiographic features are cubitus valgus, and osteoporosis especially of the spine. The osteoporosis is apparently due to gonadal hormone deficiency and appears during or after the second decade. Less frequent skeletal changes include deformed angulated epiphyses, deformities of the pelvis, ribs, and clavicles, vertebral osteochondrosis, and some delay in epiphyseal closure.

Renal anomalies, particularly malrotation of the kidneys, are quite common. Coarctation of the aorta is not rare, and its appearance in a female should suggest gonadal dysgenesis, since coarctation is predominantly a male anomaly.

Abnormalities of the lymphatic system, including intestinal lymphangiectasia and lymphedema, are often seen.

On the gynecogram (pelvic pneumogram) the infantile uterus and hypoplastic ovaries may be too small to be identified. These findings often eliminate the necessity of direct surgical visualization. After hormone therapy a striking increase in uterine size is apparent.

Although the syndrome has a wide and varied spectrum, gonadal dysgenesis without associated skeletal or visceral anomalies is very rare.[47-51]

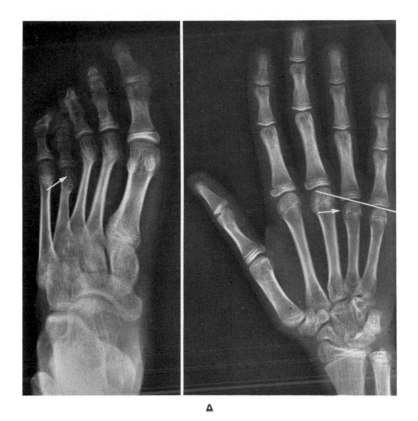

A

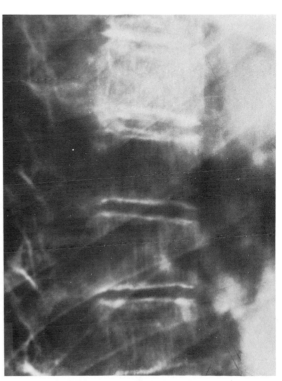

B

Figure 16–41 **Gonadal Dysgenesis: Skeletal Anomalies.**

A, The fourth metacarpal and fourth metatarsal bones are very much shortened *(arrows)*. A line drawn from the distal edges of the fourth and fifth metacarpals passes through the head of the third metacarpal; in the normal hand this line is distal to the third metacarpal. (Courtesy Dr. Bertram Levin, Chicago, Illinois.)

B, The dorsal bodies are severely osteoporotic. All the patient's bones were osteoporotic, but deformities were minimal. This type of osteoporosis develops during late adolescence in many patients with Turner's syndrome. (Courtesy Dr. Bertram Levin, Chicago, Illinois.)

Illustration continued on following page.

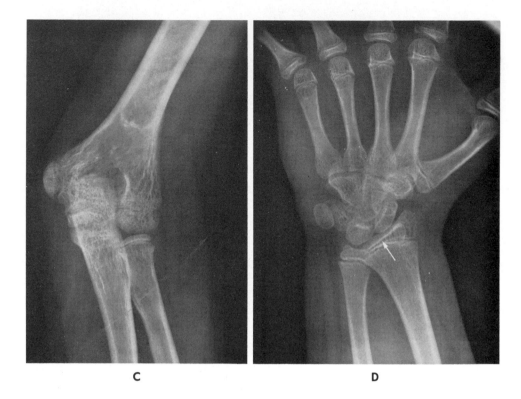

C

D

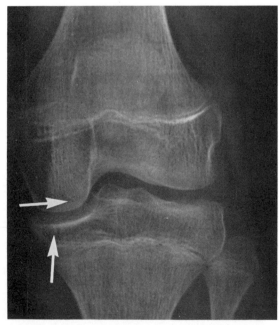

E

Figure 16–41 (Continued)

    C, A third patient had cubitus valgus.

    D, In the same patient, the radial epiphysis is abnormally angled and of irregular width *(arrow).* The third and fourth metacarpals are short. The epiphyses are ununited in this adult; this is characteristic of hypogonadism that continues into adult life.

    E, In the same patient, the medial portion of the tibial epiphysis is narrow *(lower arrow),* so that there is a lower medial tibial plateau with a consequent deeper femoral condyle *(upper arrow).* This is a frequent and characteristic finding. (Courtesy A. Lunderquist, Angelholm, Sweden.)

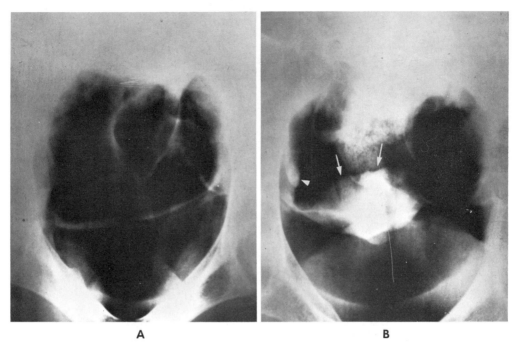

A   B

Figure 16–42   **Gonadal Dysgenesis: Gynecogram.**

A, Before therapy, the gynecogram fails to disclose uterine or ovarian shadows.

B, Following five months of hormonal therapy, the gynecogram demonstrates a definite uterine shadow *(arrows)* and a small right ovary *(arrowhead)*. (Courtesy A. Lunderquist, Angelholm, Sweden.)

Klinefelter's Syndrome

In this hypogonadal condition of males, the skeletal changes are minimal and far less frequent than in Turner's syndrome, its female counterpart. There is no osteoporosis, and a short fourth metacarpal is seen in only about 15 per cent of cases. In about half the cases, the fifth middle phalanx is short or curved (clinodactyly).[52]

Menopause

In some menopausal women, a moderate to severe osteoporosis of the axial skeleton develops; the extremities are rarely affected.

The roentgen appearance is indistinguishable from that of senile osteoporosis. In the demineralized vertebral bodies, the vertical trabeculae and cortices appear prominent. Compression fractures are frequent complications.

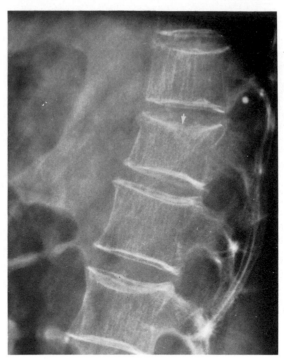

Figure 16–43 **Postmenopausal Osteoporosis.**   The patient was a 52 year old woman. All the vertebrae are demineralized, lending prominence to the cortical margins. Coarse vertical trabeculae are evident in each body. There is a concave compression fracture of the superior surface of T12 *(arrow).*

Infertility: Hysterosalpingography

Hysterosalpingography is the principal radiographic procedure employed for investigation of infertility. Although gross tubal patency may be determined by a Rubin test, hysterosalpingography yields more precise and meaningful information such as patency or obstruction of one or of both fallopian tubes, their anatomic configuration, the location of tubal obstruction, and tubal spasm. The procedure may also disclose uterine abnormalities that contribute to infertility; these include congenital and acquired malformations, severe uterine flexion or retroversion, intrauterine fibroids, polyps, and even carcinoma.

Pelvic pneumography (gynecography) is less frequently employed, but it can disclose hypoplasia, aplasia or atrophy of the uterus or ovaries, bilateral enlargement of the ovaries (Stein-Leventhal syndrome), pelvic masses from endometriosis, inflammatory disease, and ovarian tumors.[53]

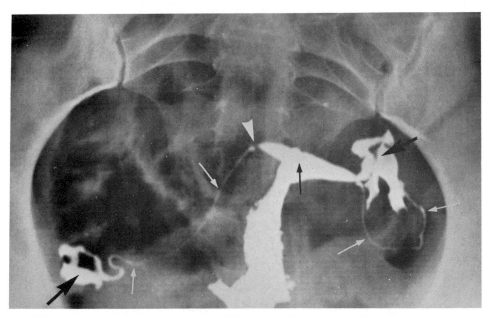

Figure 16–44 **Bilateral Patent Fallopian Tubes: Hysterosalpingogram.** The uterine cavity is somewhat small *(small black arrow)* and anteflexed, but within normal limits for a nullipara. Both tubes are filled *(white arrows)* and are normal in caliber. Patency is indicated by the presence of free contrast medium *(large black arrows)* beyond the outer end of each tube. A film made after the uterus and tubes have been allowed to empty would show the contrast medium scattered throughout the pelvis, thereby confirming patency.

The short unfilled segment at the uterine end of the right fallopian tube *(white arrowhead)* probably represents constriction of the circular muscle (sphincter?). Sometimes both tubal "sphincters" are contracted and the tubes are not opacified until constant injection pressure overcomes the spasm. Some investigators believe that tubal spasm may be a functional cause of infertility.

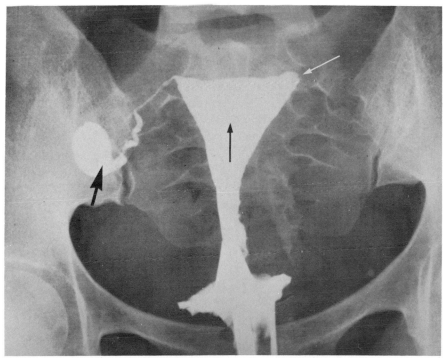

Figure 16–45 **Bilateral Occluded Fallopian Tubes: Hysterosalpingogram.** The uterine cavity is somewhat enlarged *(small black arrow)*, but is smooth and regular in outline. The right fallopian tube is opacified, but its outer end is dilated, coiled, and occluded *(large black arrow)*; no contrast medium entered the peritoneal cavity. The left tube is occluded at its cornual end *(white arrow)*.

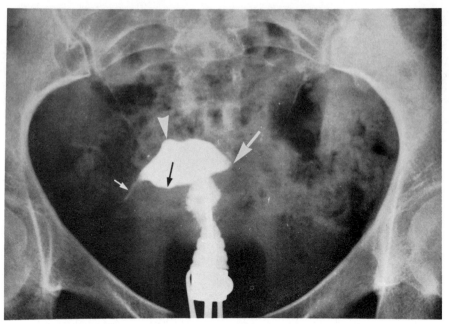

Figure 16–46 **Bilateral Occluded Fallopian Tubes: Hysterosalpingogram.**   The uterus is markedly ante-flexed, so that the fundus *(black arrow)* appears to be lower than the miduterus. Only a short segment of the right tube could be opacified *(small white arrow)*; the left tube is completely occluded at its cornual end *(large white arrow)*. The bulge in the uterine cavity *(white arrowhead)* is caused by the tip of the cannula.

Infertility: Pelvic Masses

In addition to narrowed or occluded fallopian tubes, infertility may be due to intra- and extrauterine masses that interfere with entrance of the ovum into the fallopian tube or with proper nidation of the fertilized ovum.

Fibroids are the most common uterine tumors and can reach huge proportions. They are often multiple. Radiographically they may appear as a soft tissue pelvic mass, often lobulated and usually compressing the bladder. The longstanding fibroid frequently shows characteristic and easily recognized calcifications.

Ovarian cysts may also reach tremendous proportions and present as a soft tissue mass; calcification is rare.

Dermoid cysts of the ovary are not uncommon, and they may be bilateral. The tumor may contain sufficient fatty tissue to give it a radiolucent appearance. The presence of one or more rudimentary teeth within the cyst is a pathognomonic roentgen finding.

Endometrial carcinoma may lead to enlargement of the uterine shadow. The findings in endometriosis involving the colon are discussed on page 1071.

THE ADRENAL MEDULLA AND SYMPATHETIC NERVOUS SYSTEM

Pheochromocytoma

Although pheochromocytomas are usually located in the adrenal medulla, 5 to 10 per cent may be found in the para-aortic region or in the pelvis. Rarely, multiple tumors are present. A minority of pheochromocytomas are malignant. Pheochromocytoma is occasionally associated with neurofibroma and also with such other tumors as bronchogenic carcinoma and medullary carcinoma of the thyroid (Sipple's syndrome).

The pheochromocytoma is often difficult to demonstrate on routine film studies unless it is quite large and produces a soft tissue shadow. Curvilinear or egg-shell calcification in the adrenal gland is a suggestive but unusual finding.

Pyelography will be normal unless the tumor is large enough to displace or rotate the kidneys; the caliceal system remains normal. Nephrotomography will often delineate the mass above the kidney. Occasionally, the triangular cap of residual adrenal cortex is seen above the medullary mass, the so-called apex sign.

Presacral pneumography will disclose the adrenal mass provided the tumor is in its usual adrenal location.

Definitive diagnosis of pheochromocytoma can generally be made by renal and adrenal arteriography and venography. The enlarged adrenal arteries feed a network of finely reticulated small vessels that outline the mass. A tumor stain or blush usually occurs in the highly vascular tumors. Marked elevation in blood pressure after injection of contrast material is characteristic. Adrenal venography may identify very small avascular tumors by displaced veins.

Pheochromocytoma arising from the lumbar sympathetics can sometimes be identified by angiography.

Occasionally, a large active pheochromocytoma can secrete sufficient catecholamines to produce a clinical and radiographic paralytic ileus. A higher than normal incidence of cholelithiasis is associated with this condition.[46, 54-58]

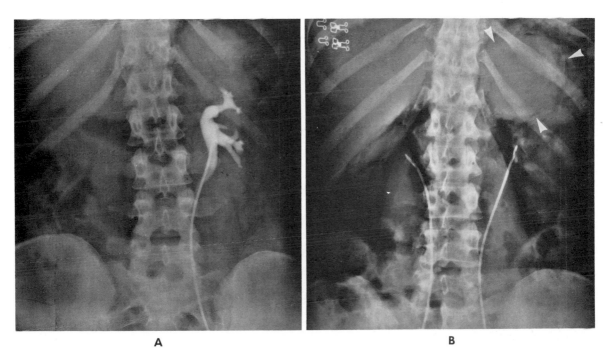

A   B

Figure 16–47 **Pheochromocytoma.**

A, In a 38 year old woman, a left retrograde pyelogram demonstrates a normal collecting system with no evidence of displacement of the kidney or pressure on the collecting system. A vague soft tissue density above the kidney is suggestive of a mass.

B, Retroperitoneal-pneumogram discloses a large soft tissue mass (*arrowheads*) outlined by the injected gas. This proved to be a pheochromocytoma.

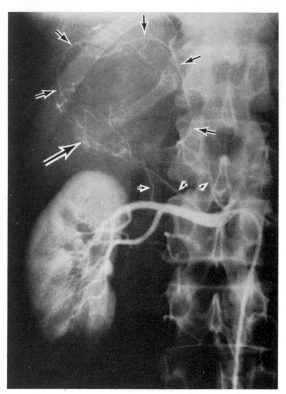

Figure 16–48 **Pheochromocytoma: Angiographic Demonstration.** An angiographic study was made because of paroxysmal hypertension in a 53 year old man; abdominal films and excretory urography were negative.

The adrenal arteries *(small arrows)* form a network of vessels that is stretched and draped *(middle-sized arrows)* around a mass above the completely normal right kidney. Abnormal vessels and a tumor stain *(large arrow)* are visible on the inferior aspect of the mass. The angiographic findings were characteristic of an adrenal tumor, probably pheochromocytoma. This was verified surgically.

Carotid Body Tumors

Tumors arising from the carotid body at the bifurcation of the carotid artery are usually chromaffin paragangliomas (chemodectoma or pheochromocytoma). Less than 10 per cent will metastasize. About 5 per cent are bilateral.

The majority are asymptomatic, but occasionally cough, dysphagia, and hoarseness occur; rarely a carotid sinus syndrome develops.

Carotid arteriography reveals a network of small vessels in a highly vascular mass at or near the bifurcation of the common carotid artery. In large lesions the internal and external carotid arteries may be displaced and separated. Contralateral angiography to rule out bilaterality is indicated.[59, 60]

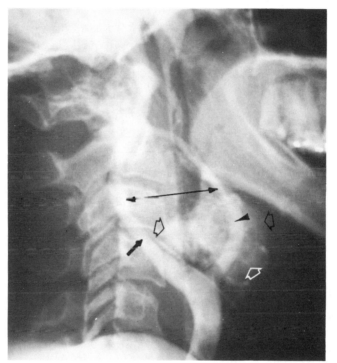

Figure 16–49 **Carotid Body Tumor.**   Arteriogram shows a large mass with homogeneous vascular blush *(open arrows)* at the bifurcation of the common carotid artery. There is marked separation and bowing *(double-headed arrow)* of the external *(arrowhead)* and internal *(black arrow)* carotid arteries.

This mass, with vascular blush at the carotid bifurcation, and separation of the arteries are virtually pathognomonic findings of carotid body tumor.

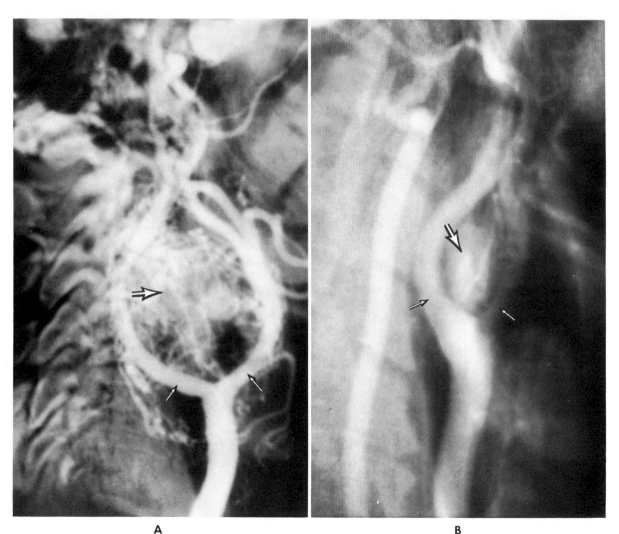

A   B

Figure 16–50   **Carotid Body Tumor: Bilateral Chemodectomas: Angiogram.**

A, On the left side, the bifurcation *(small arrows)* of the common carotid artery is greatly widened by a highly vascular tumor *(large arrow)* lying between the internal and external carotid arteries.

B, On the right side, also at the bifurcation *(small arrows)*, a smaller tumor, with intense tumor blush *(large arrow)* is present.

The location, vascularity, and widening of the carotid bifurcations are highly characteristic of carotid body tumors. Bilaterality is unusual.

(Courtesy Dr. D. W. Laster, Staten Island, New York.)

Ganglioneuroma

This benign tumor occurring in both children and adults may arise in any part of the sympathetic nervous system or in the adrenal medulla. It is found most often in the posterior mediastinum. The adrenal area is the second most frequent site. Roentgenologically it appears as a mass close to the spine. It can become huge and will displace adjacent structures. The tumor mass is sharply circumscribed and of homogeneous density. Calcification is uncommon.[61, 62]

Neuroblastoma (Sympathicoblastoma)

This is one of the most common malignant tumors in children. It arises in the adrenal gland in about three fourths of patients; the chest is the usual site in the remaining cases. Occasionally it can arise in the abdomen from a para-aortic sympathetic ganglion. The majority occur before the child reaches 5 years of age.

On plain films of the abdomen a retroperitoneal mass may be seen displacing adjacent organs. There may be local destruction of the lateral or posterior aspect of the pedicle of a vertebral body. Variably patterned calcifications are seen in two thirds of these tumors.

Pyelography usually demonstrates downward and lateral displacement of the kidney by a mass. Evidence of renal infiltration with disturbance of the caliceal system is unusual.

Abdominal angiography may prove useful, especially for planning therapy.

The neuroblastoma metastasizes early, and the metastases are often multiple and fairly symmetric. Bone metastases are frequent, generally in or near a metaphysis, and cause lysis of the medullary cavity, cortical erosion, and, often, periosteal reaction. The epiphysis is usually not involved. Skull metastases are frequent and produce a characteristic soft tissue mass with radial periosteal reaction. There may be lytic lesions and osteoporosis of the tables. Intracranial metastases may also result in wide separation of the sutures. Pulmonary metastases are rare. In some cases the paravertebral soft tissue stripe is widened from local extension or from metastases to the spine. Liver metastases may calcify.

Neuroblastoma arising in the chest presents as a mass in the posterior mediastinum; in about half of these there is calcification. Metastatic mediastinal nodes are frequently seen.[32, 61, 63, 64]

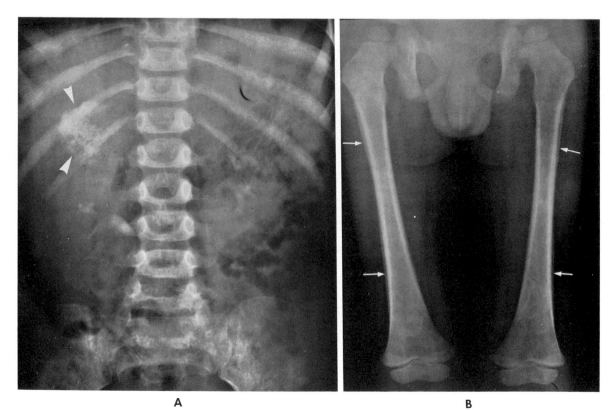

A   **B**

Figure 16–51   **Neuroblastoma of Adrenal Gland: Bone Metastases.**

A, On intravenous pyelogram there is an area of stippled calcification *(arrowheads)* above the right kidney. This kidney is displaced caudad but the pelvis and calices are normal, indicating that the kidney has not been invaded.

B, There is thin, regular, linear periosteal reaction along the outer edges of both femora *(arrows)* from metastatic involvement. Generally, cortical or medullary lysis is associated with periosteal reaction of metastatic neuroblastoma.

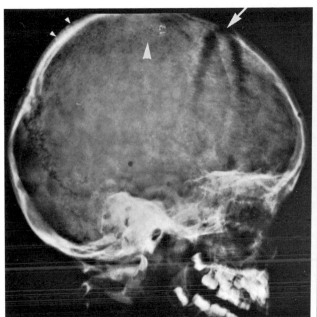

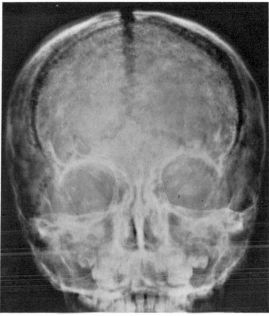

A

B

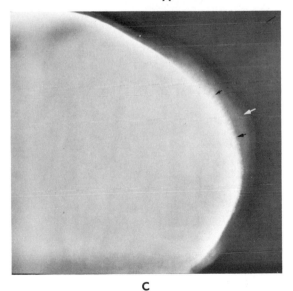

C

Figure 16–52 **Neuroblastoma of Adrenal: Metastases to Skull and Cerebrum.**

A, Lateral skull film discloses separation of the coronal suture (*arrow*). Diffuse osteoporosis has caused the granular appearance (*large arrowhead*). Some portions of the outer table (*small arrowheads*) have a brush-like appearance.

B, Separation of the sagittal suture, and the granular osteoporosis are clearly demonstrated on the posteroanterior film.

C, Soft tissue aspect of the posterior skull illustrates vertical spiculations of the outer table (*black arrows*) and thickened overlying soft tissues (*white arrow*).

The tendency of metastatic lesions from neuroblastoma to develop as plaques on the brain surface is responsible for the osteoporosis and vertical spiculation of the tables; these plaques also cause separation of the sutures. These skull changes are unique, and are virtually pathognomonic of metastatic neuroblastoma.

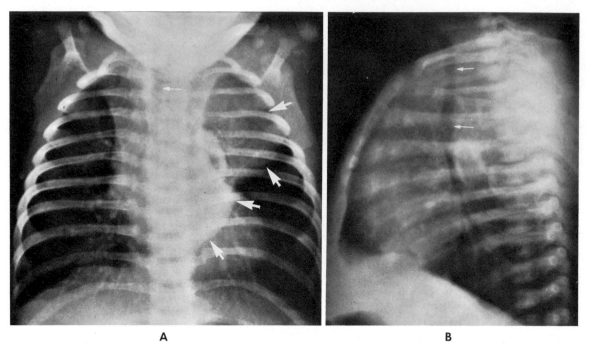

A   B

Figure 16–53 **Neuroblastoma of Mediastinum in an Infant.**

A, Posteroanterior view demonstrates a large lobulated density *(large arrows)* extending from the mediastinum to the lateral wall of the left upper chest. No calcification is evident. The trachea *(small arrow)* is displaced to the right. The esophagus (not opacified on this film) is also displaced to the right.

B, In lateral view it is difficult to identify the mass. Anterior displacement and bowing of the trachea *(arrows)* indicate that the mass is posterior to the trachea.

In infants or children, tumors of the posterior mediastinum are usually either neurogenic tumors or neuroblastoma.

THE CARCINOID SYNDROME

Malignant Carcinoid Syndrome

Serotonin-secreting malignant carcinoids occur most often in the gastrointestinal tract, especially in the ileum, but may occasionally be found in other tissues or organs. The ileal lesions are frequently multiple, small intraluminal masses. The lesions may extend through the small bowel wall into the mesentery, producing kinked and distorted loops and occasionally leading to obstruction. The radiographic picture may resemble that of regional enteritis; mesenteric angiography may be helpful in making a distinction.

In the colon, stomach, or duodenum the tumor appears as a nonspecific polypoid intraluminal mass. Metastases to the regional nodes or liver are usually present when the clinical syndrome is manifested. Hepatomegaly, however, is a late finding.

Arthralgia, especially of the hands, is a frequent symptom; occasionally there may be periarticular osteoporosis without soft tissue swelling, and small articular erosions in the interphalangeal joints.

Late in the disease, endocardial fibrosis occurs in about half the cases and can produce tricuspid insufficiency and pulmonary valvular stenosis. Alterations of the cardiac silhouette may occur.

Nonsecreting benign small carcinoid tumors are not uncommon and most frequently occur in the appendix and distal ileum. Although carcinoids are the most common small bowel lesion encountered at autopsy, because of their small size and submucosal location, the majority are not uncovered radiographically.

Benign bronchial carcinoids constitute the vast majority of bronchial adenomas. They occur intrabronchially, closer to the hilum than the periphery (see pp. 529–530). Rarely, a bronchial carcinoid can produce the carcinoid syndrome. Osteoblastic or osteolytic bone metastases occasionally occur.

A careful radiographic search of the gastrointestinal tract, especially of the small bowel, is clearly indicated in any patient with a clinically suspected carcinoid syndrome.[65–72]

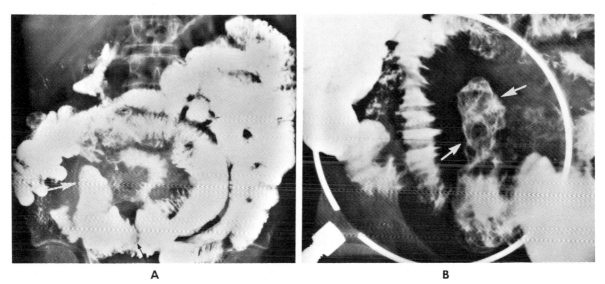

A   B

Figure 16–54 **Malignant Carcinoid Syndrome: Multiple Carcinoids of Ileum.**

A, In a 68 year old man, small bowel progress study discloses two polypoid defects in different portions of the ileum (*arrowhead and black arrow*). There is a fixed distal ileal loop (*large white arrow*) with some dilatation of most of the proximal small bowel.

B, Compression spot film of the fixed loop demonstrates multiple filling defects (*arrows*). These carcinoid tumors had invaded the mesentery.

Figure 16–55 **Carcinoid of Duodenum.** A large sausage-shaped mass (*arrowheads*) has caused distention of the third portion of the duodenum but has produced no obstruction. There were no metastases or evidence of the carcinoid syndrome. Primary carcinoids rarely attain this size.

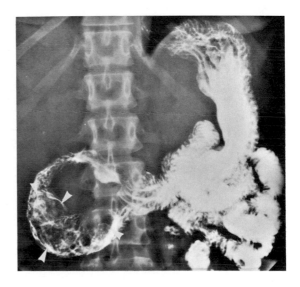

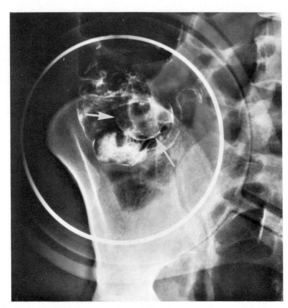

Figure 16–56 **Malignant Carcinoid Syndrome: Cecal Lesion.**   View of the cecal area following air-contrast study discloses a large sharply marginated tumor mass *(arrows)* projecting into the air-filled cecum. There were metastatic lesions in the liver.

Most colonic carcinoids are found close to the ileocecal valve, and the majority do not metastasize or cause the carcinoid syndrome.

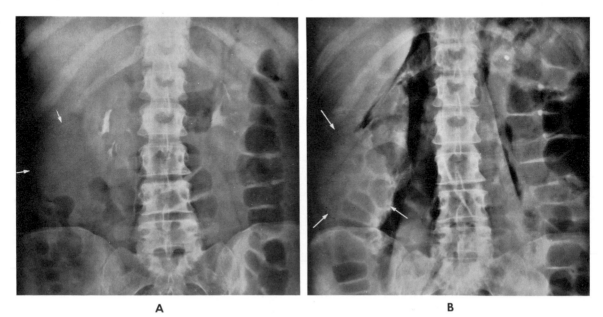

A   B

Figure 16–57 **Malignant Carcinoid Syndrome: Retroperitoneal Carcinoid.**

A, Urogram following normal gastrointestinal survey demonstrates normal kidneys, but there is a vague density *(arrows)* lateral to the right lower kidney.

B, Following retroperitoneal gas injection, a large circumscribed retroperitoneal mass is outlined *(arrows).* The mass was a huge carcinoid adherent to the right kidney. Clinical symptoms caused by secretion of serotonin cleared entirely following surgical removal of the carcinoid.

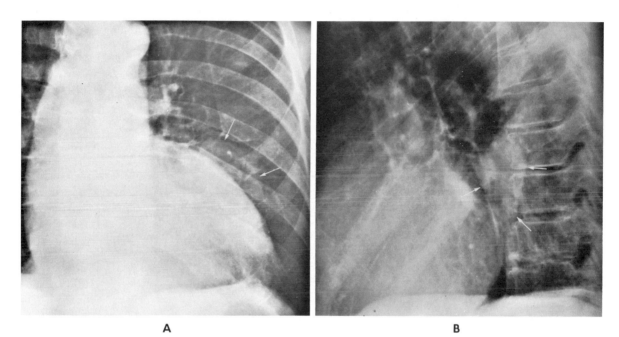

A   B

Figure 16–58   **Carcinoid of Lung.**

A, There is a faint density with distinct borders in the left lung adjacent to the heart *(arrows).*

B, In lateral view the density is more clearly defined *(arrows).* It appears to extend downward into an area of infiltration that is poorly defined *(lower arrow).*

The patient had a bronchial carcinoid; much of the density was due to associated focal atelectasis. Carcinoids of the lung usually arise in the bronchus and are difficult to detect until focal atelectasis appears. In this case, carcinoid syndrome of moderate degree was present; however, most bronchial carcinoids do not secrete enough serotonin to produce clinical effects.

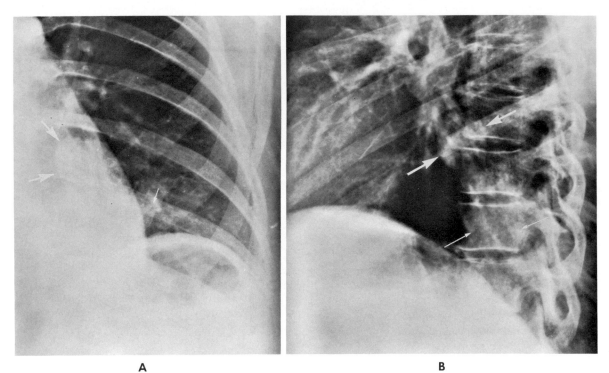

A   B

Figure 16–59 **Carcinoid of Lung.**

A, In posteroanterior view of a 36 year old woman who had had cough, hemoptysis, and fever for several weeks, a vague area of infiltration *(small arrow)* is evident at the left lung base. The inner aspect of the diaphragm is obscured. A mass with distinct borders *(large arrows)* is barely visible through the heart shadow.

B, Lateral view demonstrates the mass in the posterior lung *(large arrows).* A larger triangular density *(small arrows)* extends from the mass into the posterior lower lung field.

The mass proved to be a bronchial adenoma (carcinoid), and the basal density was an area of focal atelectasis caused by obstruction of the segmental bronchus by the carcinoid.

Ninety per cent of bronchial adenomas are carcinoids. A focal area of atelectasis is usually the earliest and sometimes the only radiographic finding on conventional films. The adenoma itself is usually not visualized until it enlarges beyond the site of origin. Planigraphy and bronchography may be aids in earlier recognition. (See also Figure 9–105.)

PARATHYROID

Hyperparathyroidism (Primary and Secondary)

Bone changes do not occur early in primary hyperparathyroidism. They are always associated with an elevated alkaline phosphatase level.

The earliest bone change is subperiosteal bone resorption. Later, trabecular resorption occurs, producing demineralization. Brown tumors, representing localized areas of extensive bone resorption, are a late development.

Small cortical erosions beginning on the radial side of the middle phalanges are among the earliest roentgenologic changes. Erosions of the distal cortex of the phalangeal tufts, resorption of the outer and, less often, inner ends of the clavicles, and disappearance of the lamina dura of the teeth are early and striking findings.

Grainy demineralization of the skull with a thinned and indistinct outer table is characteristic.

Progressive subperiosteal resorption involves other smaller and larger long bones, often producing a lacy cortical pattern. Skeletal demineralization is spotty but can become generalized. In a small percentage of cases, osteosclerosis rather than osteoporosis appears, especially in the vertebra; the mechanism is unclear.

Localized lytic areas, the brown tumors, can appear in any bone, but the jaw and facial bones are favored sites. Brown tumors can become large, sharply marginated, and expansile. In severe untreated cases these cyst-like lesions may become widespread and produce the picture of von Recklinghausen's disease (*Osteitis Fibrosa Cystica*, see p. 1328). Multiple recurring pathologic fractures can severely deform the skeleton.

Removal of the parathyroid adenoma is followed by regression of the bone lesions.

Urinary calculi apparently due to hypercalcemia and hypercalcinuria are demonstrable in a high percentage of cases. Diffuse nephrocalcinosis occurs less often.

Metastatic calcification occasionally occurs in the soft tissues, particularly around joints and in articular cartilages (chondrocalcinosis). There is an increased incidence of pancreatic calculi and pancreatitis; renal calculi in association with pancreatic calculi are a suggestive finding.

A high incidence of peptic ulcer and gallstones has been reported.

Radiologic demonstration of the parathyroid adenoma is infrequent. The adenoma rarely may be large enough to deviate the trachea, but this deviation is more often due to unrelated thyroid enlargement. In suspected but nonpalpable parathyroid adenoma, subclavian arteriography or selective opacification of the thyrocervical trunk may sometimes show tumor stain and localizing distortion or displacement of the loops of the opacified inferior thyroid artery. However, this procedure is not too reliable and is not often employed.

Secondary hyperparathyroidism due to chronic renal failure is more frequently encountered than the primary disease, probably because of the prolongation of survival, by means of dialysis, of patients with chronic renal failure. Roentgenologic changes are found in almost 80 per cent of patients on a chronic dialysis program, compared to less than 20 per cent prior to the advent of dialysis. These changes are similar to those of primary hyperparathyroidism, but there are quantitative differences. Subperiosteal resorption and grain-like osteoporosis of the skull are frequent findings in both forms, but demineralization of the spine is a more common finding in secondary hyperparathyroidism. This may be related to vitamin D resistance, which occurs in virtually every case of chronic renal failure. Resorption of the outer and sometimes inner ends of the clavicles, osteosclerosis especially in the spine and metaphyseal areas, and metastatic calcifications in periarticular soft tissues and in blood vessels are seen more frequently in secondary hyperparathyroidism, while bone cysts (brown tumors) are much less common. The mechanism of the osteosclerosis (which occurs in up to 20 per cent of cases) is unclear. (See also *Renal Osteodystrophy*, p. 780.)[73-80]

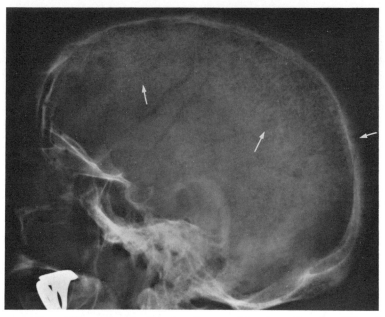

Figure 16–60 **Hyperparathyroidism: The Skull.** Small areas of demineralization diffusely scattered throughout the bones of the vault (*arrows*) combine with islands of uninvolved bone to produce the characteristic grains-of-sand appearance. The outer table (*arrow*) is considerably thinned.

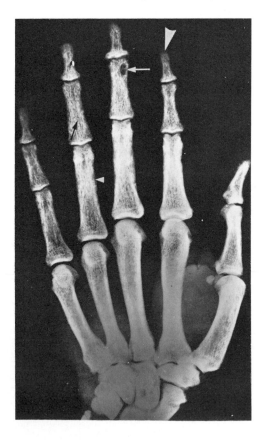

Figure 16–61 **Hyperparathyroidism: Advanced Bone Changes in Phalanges.** There is extensive subperiosteal bone resorption producing a lace-like cortical pattern and extensive cortical erosions, most prominent on the radial side of the phalanges (*small arrowhead*). The medullary cavities are demineralized with prominent spaces between trabeculae (*black arrow*). There is slight erosion of the tufts (*large arrowhead*). A sharply marginated lytic area (*white arrow*) is a small brown tumor.

Cortical, subperiosteal, and trabecular bone resorption form the basic roentgenologic picture of hyperparathyroidism.

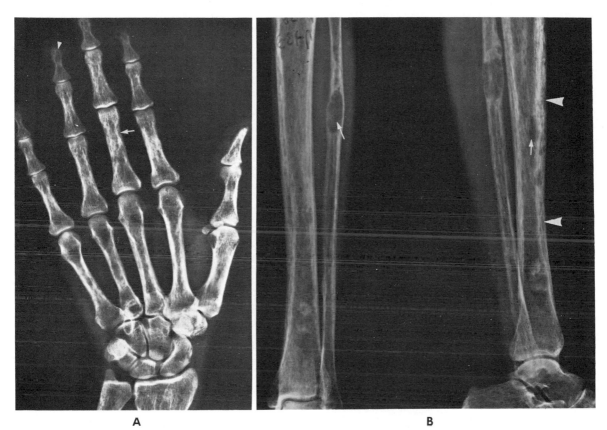

A   **B**

Figure 16–62   **Hyperparathyroidism: Extensive Changes in Long Bones.**

A, Widespread demineralization of the bones of the hand and wrist accentuates the density of the cortical bone. Extensive subperiosteal bone resorption has occurred in all the phalanges and in the fourth and fifth metacarpals (radial side). There is pronounced cortical erosion on the radial aspect of the proximal phalanx of the middle finger (*arrow*), and the digital tufts show some resorption (*arrowhead*).

B, Extensive subperiosteal resorption has also occurred in the bones of the leg (*arrowheads*), and has produced the characteristic lacy appearance. There is extensive demineralization. A number of medullary cyst-like areas (*arrows*) are seen, one of which is causing expansion of the fibula; these are brown tumors.

The characteristic roentgenologic features of bone changes in hyperparathyroidism, including cortical erosion, subperiosteal bone resorption, demineralization, and cyst-like areas, are illustrated by the above patient.

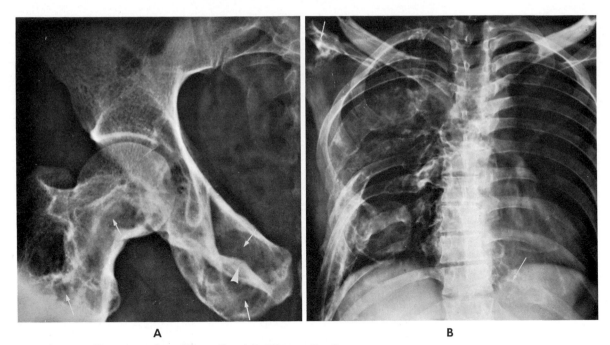

A   B

Figure 16–63 **Hyperparathyroidism: Osteitis Fibrosa Cystica.**

A, There are multiple cyst-like areas in the right femur, ischium, and pubic bones (*arrows*). There is also cortical expansion (*arrowhead*). The absence of cortical thinning and generalized demineralization makes it difficult to distinguish these findings from those of fibrocystic disease (fibrous dysplasia) unassociated with hyperparathyroidism.

B, Similar cyst-like lesions have caused expansile deformities of many ribs on the right side. The deformities are similar roentgenologically to those of fibrous dysplasia.

The eleventh left rib and the right scapula are also involved (*arrows*). Demineralization is not apparent in the uninvolved bones.

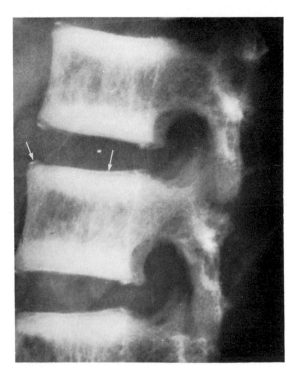

Figure 16–64 **Hyperparathyroidism: Parathyroid Adenoma: Osteosclerosis.** The patient was a 14 year old girl. There are broad bands of homogeneous density in the upper and lower margins of the vertebral bodies. The epiphyseal plates and marginal epiphyses are not fused (*urrows*). The central portions of the vertebral bodies and most of the other bones are demineralized.

Sclerotic changes are more common in hyperparathyroidism secondary to renal failure than they are in the primary forms. These changes are more apt to affect the ends of the growing bones, as in the case illustrated here. This appearance of the vertebral bodies is called the Rugger-Jersey spine. (Courtesy Dr. B. P. Vaughn, Royal Perth Hospital, Australia.)

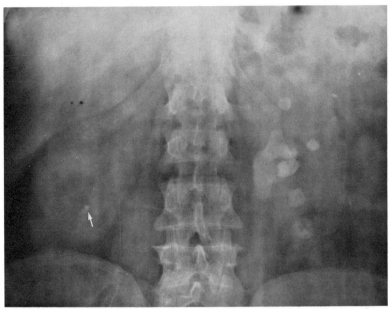

Figure 16–65 **Hyperparathyroidism: Renal Calculi.** There is a dendritic (stag-horn) calculus in the left renal pelvis, large calculi in the calices, and smaller calcifications in the lower pole of the right kidney (*arrow*). The bones are moderately demineralized. Renal calculi and parenchymal calcification (nephrocalcinosis) develop in 75 per cent of hyperparathyroid patients at some time during the disease. Occasionally, symptoms of a urinary calculus may be the first clinical manifestation of hyperparathyroidism.

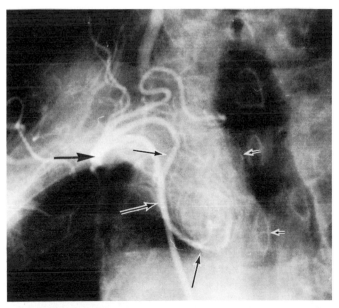

Figure 16–66 **Mediastinal Parathyroid Adenoma: Arteriogram.** Selective opacification of the right thyrocervical trunk (*black arrow*) reveals caudal displacement of an unusually large inferior thyroid artery (*large black-white arrows*), which conforms to the contours of a mass in the upper mediastinum. There are abnormal tangles of vessels within the mass. The medial border of the adenoma indents the trachea (*small black-white arrows*).

Displacement or distortion of the caudal loop of the inferior thyroid artery by a vascular mass is a characteristic angiographic finding in parathyroid adenoma. (Courtesy Dr. K. Kuroda, Philadelphia, Pennsylvania.)

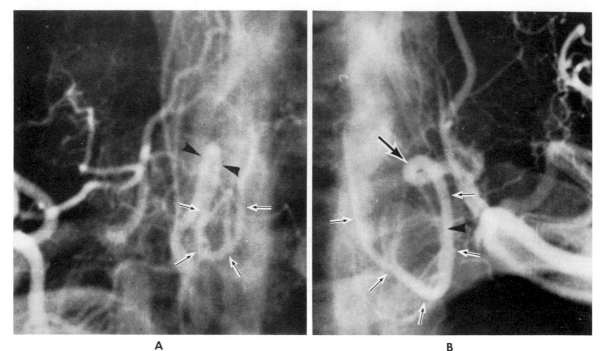

A   B

Figure 16–67 **Parathyroid Adenoma: Thyrocervical Trunk Angiogram.**

A, On the right side, the caudal (*arrows*) and cephalic (*arrowheads*) loops of the inferior thyroid artery are normal.

B, On the left side, the caudal loop is considerably widened (*small arrows*), and the cephalic loop is reversed (*large arrow*) due to lateral displacement of the proximal limb of the artery (*arrowhead*) by a parathyroid adenoma. No tumor blush was seen.

Hypoparathyroidism

In acquired or postsurgical hypoparathyroidism there are no significant radiographic findings.

In idiopathic or primary hypoparathyroidism, discrete intracranial calcifications are found in about one third to one half of cases. These calcifications are usually in the region of the basal ganglia or choroid plexus. They are apparently not related to the biochemical disturbances of hypoparathyroidism, and only rarely occur in the acquired form. Increased density in the long bones, usually localized to the metaphyseal areas, may occur in up to one fourth of cases. Rarely, osteoporosis secondary to prolonged steatorrhea can become evident.

Other infrequent radiographic findings include hip joint deformity, ligamentous and subcutaneous calcifications, and dental abnormalities. Steatorrhea, a frequent clinical symptom, may be associated with a mild malabsorption pattern or merely with hypomotility of the small bowel.

The basal ganglia calcifications that occur in idiopathic hypoparathyroidism and pseudohypoparathyroidism are often similar to those found in toxoplasmosis, in tuberous sclerosis, or familially in totally asymptomatic individuals.[78, 81-83]

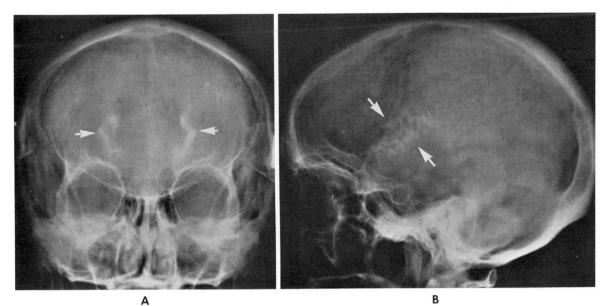

A	B

Figure 16–68   **Idiopathic Hypoparathyroidism: Calcification of Basal Ganglia.**

A, Bilateral coalescent calcifications (*arrows*) are symmetrically located in the region of the basal ganglia adjacent to the lateral ventricles.

B, In lateral view these calcifications (*arrows*) are shown superimposed and situated anteriorly.

Calcification of basal ganglia in idiopathic hypoparathyroidism probably is not related to the endocrine abnormality but is more likely a manifestation of the genetic disorder responsible for the parathyroid deficiency.

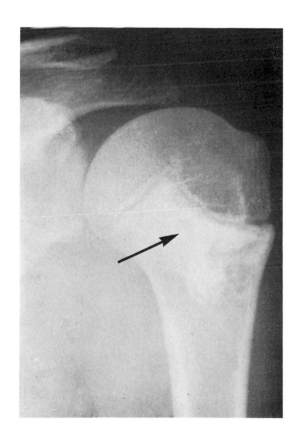

Figure 16–69   **Idiopathic Hypoparathyroidism: Sclerosis of Bone.**   In an 11 year old girl there is a wide irregular density (*arrow*) with an ill-defined lower border in the metaphyseal area of the humerus. Similar areas of metaphyseal sclerosis were found in the tibiae and femora. There was no calcification of the basal ganglia.

Sclerosis of bone is a relatively rare finding in hypoparathyroidism. (Courtesy Dr. H. Taybi, Indianapolis, Indiana.)

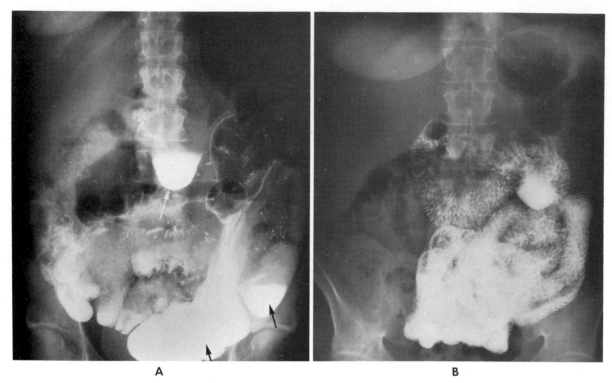

A   B

Figure 16–70   **Hypoparathyroidism: The Small Bowel.**

A, The patient was a woman with symptoms of hypoparathyroidism, severe hypocalcemia, and steatorrhea; there was no clinical malabsorption. A five-hour film of a small bowel study discloses considerable gastric retention (*white arrow*) and atonic, dilated small bowel loops (*black arrows*) in which no mucosal pattern is evident. There are areas of flocculation, and movement of the barium meal was greatly diminished. Radiographically, the picture resembles sprue, but there was no biochemical evidence of malabsorption.

B, In a small bowel study made a few months after calcium and vitamin D therapy, the small bowel appears normal; the stomach is almost emptied in 15 minutes.

Presumably, the sprue-like picture resulted from the hypocalcemia and other biochemical disturbances of untreated hypoparathyroidism. Although steatorrhea, small bowel changes, and hypoparathyroidism constitute a recognized, although uncommon, syndrome, their pathophysiological relationship is not well understood.

Pseudohypoparathyroidism and Pseudopseudohypoparathyroidism

In pseudohypoparathyroidism, multiple skeletal anomalies are associated with the biochemical changes of hypoparathyroidism (hypocalcemia and hyperphosphatemia). The parathyroid glands function normally, but there is a tissue insensitivity to the hormone. In some cases there is an excess of thyrocalcitonin (a thyroid hormone that lowers serum calcium). The most frequent findings are one or more short metacarpals or metatarsals, and soft tissue calcification. Frequently there is calcification of the basal ganglia, as in idiopathic hypoparathyroidism.

Similar skeletal anomalies can appear in other members of the patient's family in the absence of biochemical disturbances (pseudopseudohypoparathyroidism). Conversely, pseudohypoparathyroidism can exist clinically without obvious skeletal anomalies. Pseudohypoparathyroidism is further complicated by the rare development of hyperparathyroidism secondary to phosphate retention (pseudohypohyperparathyroidism).[84–87]

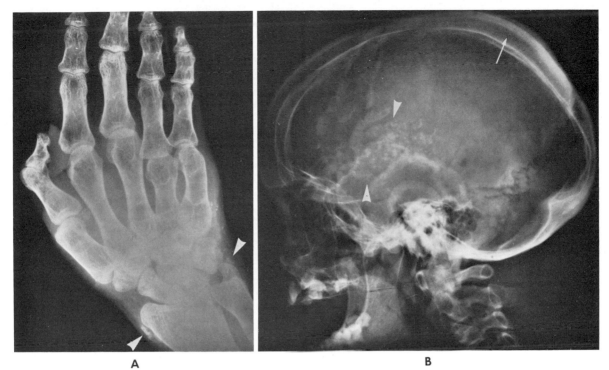

Figure 16–71 **Pseudohypoparathyroidism.**

A, The patient was a 21 year old man. The bones of the hand are short and wide; the fourth metacarpal is greatly shortened. Soft tissue calcifications (*arrows*) are seen in the wrist.

B, Symmetric, bilateral calcifications of the basal ganglia are superimposed in lateral view (*arrowheads*). The calvarium is thickened, and the diploetic space is increased (*arrow*). (Courtesy Dr. G. M. Ashurst, Lincolnshire, England.)

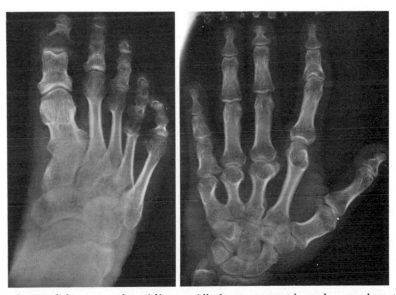

Figure 16–72 **Pseudopseudohypoparathyroidism.** All the metacarpals and several metatarsals are short and moderately deformed. Subcutaneous calcification and ossification were found in other soft tissues. The serum calcium level was normal. (Courtesy Dr. M. LeMay, Boston, Massachusetts.)

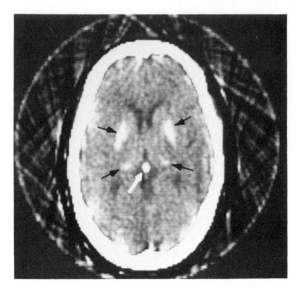

Figure 16–73 **Basal Ganglia Calcification: CT scan.** Characteristic symmetric densities of calcific μ value (*black arrows*) are in the basal ganglia. These are not as dense as the pineal calcification (*white arrow*). The cause of these calcifications was unknown; the ventricular system and the other scan findings were normal.

Basal ganglia calcifications may be a surprising finding on a CT scan, since sometimes they are not apparent on conventional films.

POLYADENOMATOSIS OF THE ENDOCRINE GLANDS (WERMER'S SYNDROME)

In this familial syndrome there are signs and symptoms of endocrinopathy due to tumors or hyperplasia of two or more endocrine glands. Most cases are associated with severe gastrointestinal symptoms from intractable peptic ulcerations. In the Zollinger-Ellison syndrome (p. 955), in which there are similar gastrointestinal symptoms and findings, only the pancreas is involved (non-beta cell tumor), and there is usually no familial history. Some investigators consider it a *forme fruste* of polyadenomatosis.

In polyadenomatosis, the parathyroids, anterior pituitary, and pancreas are most frequently involved. The adrenal cortex and, least frequently, the thyroid may also be affected. The pituitary lesions are adenomas of various types: eosinophilic, basophilic, or chromophobic. In the parathyroids, pancreas, or adrenal cortex there may be hyperplasia, single or multiple adenomas, or carcinoma, occurring either alone or in combination. The radiographic features of these various lesions are discussed elsewhere.

The radiographic findings in the upper gastrointestinal tract consist of peptic ulcerations, gastric hypersecretion, and thickened and coarsened folds in the stomach, duodenum, and jejunum. Megaduodenum is a frequent finding. The walls of the duodenum and jejunum may appear stiffened. Severe small bowel involvement may be associated with a watery diarrhea and hypokalemia. The peptic ulcers are identical in appearance to ordinary nonendocrine ulcers but often are larger, multiple, and may be in unusual locations: the postbulbar area, the distal duodenum, or the jejunum. These ulcers frequently perforate or bleed and are relatively intractable to medical management. Recurrence after surgery is common.

A higher than normal incidence of soft tissue lipomas, villous adenomas of the colon, and serotonin-secreting bronchial carcinoids are found in polyadenomatosis.

Peptic ulcerations, especially if postbulbar, in a patient with polyendocrine symptoms should suggest the possibility of polyadenomatosis of the endocrine glands.[88-90]

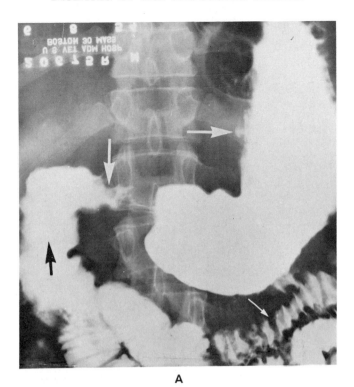

A

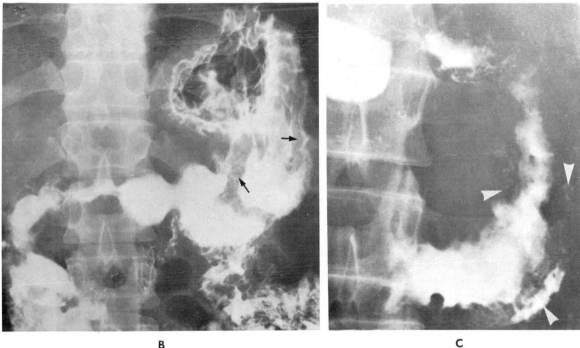

B   C

Figure 16–74 **Polyadenomatosis of Endocrine Glands.**

A, In a 35 year old man, the duodenal bulb is deformed, and there is a gastric ulcer of the lesser curvature (*large white arrows*). The descending duodenal loop is dilated (*black arrow*) and the mucosal folds are coarsened; the appearance of the jejunum is similar (*small arrow*).

B, A few months later the gastric folds (*arrows*) appear greatly enlarged, resembling Menetrier's disease.

C, Film of the duodenal loop demonstrates the large folds and submucosal sinuses containing barium (*arrowheads*) many of which proved to be ulcers.

At autopsy, islet cell carcinoma was found in the head and tail of the pancreas, as well as chromophobe adenoma of the pituitary gland and adrenal cortical hyperplasia. (Courtesy Dr. Ralph Schlaeger, New York, New York.)

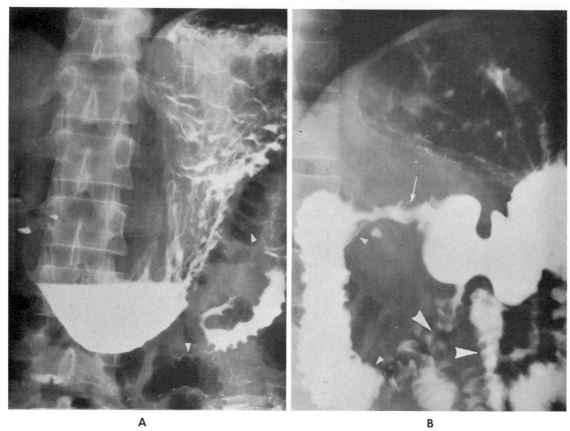

A   B

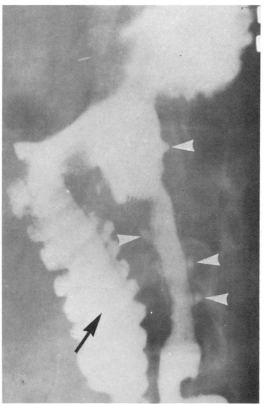

Figure 16–75 **Polyadenomatosis of Parathyroid Glands and Islet Cells.**

A, The patient was a 43 year old man. In the stomach heavy gastric folds and hypersecretion are demonstrated. The rigid edematous jejunal loops are filled with air (*arrowheads*) and barium. The jejunal folds are greatly thickened.

B, The duodenal bulb is greatly deformed (*arrow*), the duodenal loop is dilated (*small arrowheads*), and the jejunal loops are greatly thickened (*large arrowheads*) and rigid.

C, Following total gastrectomy, the afferent loop is dilated (*black arrow*), and the efferent loop is narrow and rigid, with multiple ulcerations (*arrowheads*). The ulcers and edematous folds were intractable to anti-ulcer therapy in this and the preceding patient. (Courtesy Dr. Ralph Schlaeger, New York, New York.)

C

REFERENCES

1. Spence, A. W.: The radiology of endocrine disorders. A symposium. The diagnostic value of radiology in endocrine disorders. Br. J. Radiol., 31:341, 1958.
2. Pribram, H. F. W., and Swann, G. F.: Radiologic changes and clinical evidence of endocrine effects in sellar and parasellar tumors. Radiology, 75:877, 1960.
3. Lemay, M.: The radiologic diagnosis of pituitary disease. Radiol. Clin. North Am., 5:303, 1967.
4. Mortara, R., and Norrell, H.: Consequences of deficient sellar diaphragm. J. Neurosurg., 32:565, 1970.
5. Lang, E. K., and Bessler, W. T.: Roentgen features of acromegaly. Am. J. Roentgenol. Radium Ther. Nucl. Med., 86:321, 1961.
6. Glancy, J. J.: Some radiologic aspects of acromegaly. Aust. Radiol., 11:226, 1967.
7. Posnanski, A. K., and Stephenson, J. M.: Radiographic findings in hypothalamic acceleration of growth associated with cerebral atrophy and mental retardation (cerebral gigantism). Radiology, 88:446, 1967.
8. Stuber, J. L., and Palacios, E.: Vertebral scalloping in acromegaly. Am. J. Roentgenol. Radium Ther. Nucl. Med., 112:397, 1971.
9. Strauch, G., Vallotton, M. B., et al.: The renin-angiotensin-aldosterone system in normotensive and hypertensive patients with acromegaly. Arch. Intern. Med., 130:720, 1972.
10. Freed, W. J.: Diabetes insipidus and pulmonary fibrosis. Arch. Intern. Med., 95:823, 1955.
11. Grant, L. J., and Ginsburg, J.: Eosinophilic granuloma with diabetes insipidus. Lancet, 2:529, 1955.
12. Wheeler, J. S., and Adelson, W. J.: Pituitary diabetes insipidus associated with progressive urinary tract dilatation. J. Urol., 92:64, 1964.
13. Yalowitz, P. A., Randall, R. V., and Greene, L. P.: Dilatation of the urinary tract associated with pituitary and nephrogenic diabetes insipidus. J. Urol., 103:327, 1970.
14. Cummins, F. L., et al.: Treatment of gliomas of third ventricle and pinealomas. Neurology, 10:1031, 1960.
15. Maier, J. G., and De Jung, D.: Pineal body tumors. Am. J. Roentgenol. Radium Ther. Nucl. Med., 99:826, 1967.
16. Cole, H.: Tumors in the region of the pineal. Clin. Radiol., 22:110, 1971.
17. Tod, P. A., Porter, A. J., and Jamieson, K. G.: Pineal tumors. Am. J. Roentgenol. Radium Ther. Nucl. Med., 120:19, 1974.
18. New, P. F. J., Scott, W. R., et al.: Computerized axial tomography with the EMI scanner. Radiology, 110:109, 1974.
19. Hahnemann Medical College and Hospital—Department of Diagnostic Radiology: First Conference on Computerized Axial Tomography. November, 1974.
20. Wietersen, F. K., and Balow, R. M.: Radiologic aspects of thyroid disease. Radiol. Clin. North Am., 5:255, 1967.
21. Dixon, D. W., and Samuels, E.: Acral changes associated with thyroid disease. J.A.M.A., 212:1175, 1970.
22. Moulc, B., Grant, M. C., et al.: Thyroid acropathy. Clin. Radiol., 21:329, 1970.
23. Bonakdarpour, A., Kirkpatrick, J. A., et al.: Skeletal changes in neonatal thyrotoxicosis. Radiology, 102:149, 1972.
24. Astley, R.: Radiology of endocrine disorders. A symposium. Hypothyroidism in children. Br. J. Radiol., 31:346, 1958.
25. Middlemass, I. B.: Bone changes in adult cretins. Br. J. Radiol., 32:685, 1959.
26. Kittrcdge, R. D., et al.: The role of angiocardiography in myxedema heart disease. Radiology, 80:430, 1963.
27. Williams, F. G.: Myxedema cardiopathy. Am. Heart J., 57:463, 1959.
28. Rybak, M.: Skeletal dysplasia and bony maturation in hypothyroidism of children. Ann. Radiol., 13:243, 1970.
29. Margolin, F. P., Winfield, J., and Steinbach, H. L.: Patterns of thyroid calcification. Invest. Radiol., 2:208, 1967.
30. Gombert, H. J., and Klappe, W.: Diagnosis of metastasizing thyroid adenoma. Fortsch. Roentgenstr., 86:567, 1957.
31. Pearson, K. D., Wells, S. A., and Keiser, H. R.: Familial medullary carcinoma of the thyroid, adrenal pheochromocytoma and parathyroid hyperplasia. Radiology, 107:249, 1973.
32. McAllister, W. H., and Kochler, R. P.: Diseases of the adrenal. Radiol. Clin. North Am., 5:205, 1967.
33. Brown, B. St. J., et al.: Acute massive adrenal hemorrhage in newborn. J. Can. Assoc. Radiol., 13:100, 1962.
34. Gabriele, O. T., and Sheehan, W. E.: Bilateral neonatal adrenal hemorrhage. Am. J. Roentgenol. Radium Ther. Nucl. Med., 91:656, 1964.
35. Laws, J. W.: Radiology of endocrine disorders. A symposium. Radiology of the suprarenal glands. Br. J. Radiol., 31:352, 1958.
36. Howland, W. L., et al.: Roentgenographic changes of skeletal system in Cushing's syndrome. Radiology, 71:69, 1958.
37. Kuhn, J., Jewett, T., and Munschauer, R.: The clinical and radiographic features of neonatal adrenal hemorrhage. Radiology, 99:647, 1971.

38. Janower, M. L., et al.: The radiologist in diagnosis of nonendocrine endocrinology. Radiology, 86:746, 1966.
39. Santini, L. C., and Williams, J. L.: Mediastinal widening (lipomatosis) in Cushing's syndrome. N. Engl. J. Med., 284:1357, 1971.
40. Darling, D. B., Loridan, L., and Senior, B.: The roentgenographic manifestations of Cushing's syndrome in infants. Radiology, 96:503, 1970.
41. Reuter, S. R., et al.: Adrenal venography. Radiology, 89:805, 1967.
42. Kahn, P. C., et al.: Adrenal arteriography and venography in primary aldosteronism. Radiology, 101:71, 1971.
43. Kahn, R. C.: The radiologic identification of functioning adrenal tumors. Radiol. Clin. North Am., 5:221, 1967.
44. Alfidi, R. J., Gill, W. M., and Klein, H. J.: Arteriography of adrenal neoplasms. Am. J. Roentgenol. Radium Ther. Nucl. Med., 106:635, 1969.
45. Reuter, S. R.: Arteriography vs. phlebography in the evaluation of adrenal disease. J. Belg. Radiol., 54:575, 1971.
46. Colapinto, R. F., and Steed, B. L.: Arteriography of adrenal tumors. Radiology, 100:343, 1971.
47. Levin, B.: Gonadal dysgenesis. Am. J. Roentgenol. Radium Ther. Nucl. Med., 87:1116, 1962.
48. Leszczynski, S.: Turner syndrome: report of 32 cases. Fortschr. Roentgenstr., 97:200, 1962.
49. Hung, W., and LoPresti, J. M.: Urinary tract anomalies in gonadal dysgenesis. Am. J. Roentgenol. Radium Ther. Nucl. Med., 95:439, 1965.
50. Reveno, J. S., and Palubinskas, A. J.: Congenital renal abnormalities in gonadal dysgenesis. Radiology, 86:49, 1966.
51. Altemus, R., Charles, D., and Stock, R.: Pelvic pneumography in adult gonadal dysgenesis. Surg. Gynecol. Obstet., 134:751, 1972.
52. Ohsawa, T., Furuse, M., et al.: Manifestations of Klinefelter's syndrome. Am. J. Roentgenol. Radium Ther. Nucl. Med., 112:178, 1971.
53. Yune, H. Y., Klatte, E. C., et al.: Hysterosalpingography in infertility. Am. J. Roentgenol. Radium Ther. Nucl. Med., 121:642, 1974.
54. Pendergrass, H., et al.: Pheochromocytoma. Radiology, 78:725, 1962.
55. Fry, I. K., Kerr, I. H., Thomas, M. L., and Starer, F.: Value of aortography in the diagnosis of pheochromocytoma. Clin. Radiol., 18:276, 1967.
56. Cornell, S. H.: Pheochromocytoma of lumbar sympathetic chain demonstrated by angiography. Am. J. Roentgenol. Radium Ther. Nucl. Med., 115:175, 1972.
57. Reuter, S. R.: Arteriography versus phlebography in evaluation of adrenal disease. J. Belg. Radiol., 54:575, 1971.
58. Cruz, S. R., and Colwell, J. A.: Pheochromocytoma and ileus. J.A.M.A., 219:1050, 1972.
59. Gehweiler, J. A., and Bender, W. R.: Carotid arteriography in the diagnosis and management of tumors of the carotid body. Am. J. Roentgenol. Radium Ther. Nucl. Med., 104:893, 1968.
60. Laster, D. W., Citrin, C. M., and Thyng, F. J.: Bilateral carotid body tumors. Am. J. Roentgenol. Radium Ther. Nucl. Med., 115:143, 1973.
61. Barrett, A. F.: Sympathicoblastoma (neuroblastoma). Clin. Radiol., 14:34, 1963.
62. Theros, E. G.: Radiologic-pathologic case of the mouth: mediastinal ganglioneuroma. Radiology, 93:677, 1969.
63. Burgener, F., et al.: Angiographic diagnosis of abdominal neuroblastoma. Fortschr. Roentgenstr., 114:752, 1971.
64. Young, L. W., Rubin, P., and Hanson, R. E.: The extra-adrenal neuroblastoma. Am. J. Roentgenol. Radium Ther. Nucl. Med., 108:75, 1970.
65. Bluth, I.: Gastrointestinal carcinoid tumors. Radiology, 74:573, 1960.
66. Toomey, F. B., and Felson, B.: Gastrointestinal and bronchial carcinoid tumors with osteoblastic bone metastases. Am. J. Roentgenol. Radium Ther. Nucl. Med., 83:709, 1960.
67. Castleman, B., et al.: Case reports of Massachusetts General Hospital. N. Engl. J. Med., 288:36, 1973.
68. Schulman, H., and Giustra, P.: Carcinoids of the colon. Radiology, 98:139, 1971.
69. Peavy, P. W., Rogers, J. V., et al.: Unusual osteoblastic metastases from carcinoid tumors. Radiology, 107:327, 1973.
70. Ureles, A. L.: Diagnosis and treatment of malignant carcinoid syndrome. J.A.M.A., 229:1346, 1974.
71. Plonk, J. W., and Feldman, J. M.: Carcinoid arthropathy. Arch. Intern. Med., 134:651, 1974.
72. Bancks, N. H., Goldstein, H. M., and Dodd, G. D.: The roentgenologic spectrum of small intestinal carcinoid tumors. Am. J. Roentgenol. Radium Ther. Nucl. Med., 123:274, 1975.
73. Steinbach, H. L., et al.: Primary hyperparathyroidism: correlation of roentgen, clinical and pathologic features. Am. J. Roentgenol. Radium Ther. Nucl. Med., 86:329, 1961.
74. Teng, C. T., and Nathan, M. H.: Primary hyperparathyroidism. Am. J. Roentgenol. Radium Ther. Nucl. Med., 83:716, 1960.
75. Zimmerman, H. B.: Osteosclerosis in secondary hyperparathyroidism in chronic renal disease. Am. J. Roentgenol. Radium Ther. Nucl. Med., 88:1152, 1962.
76. Newton, T. H., and Eisenberg, E.: Angiography of parathyroid adenoma. Radiology, 86:843, 1966.
77. Kleemann, C. R., et al.: The problem and unanswered questions. Renal osteodystrophy, soft tissue calcification, and disturbed divalent ion metabolism in chronic renal failure. Arch. Intern. Med., 124:262, 1969.

78. Taybi, H., and Keele, D.: Hypoparathyroidism; a review of the literature and report of 2 cases in sisters. Am. J. Roentgenol. Radium Ther. Nucl. Med., 88:432, 1962.
79. Selle, J. G., Altmeier, W. A., et al.: Cholelithiasis in hyperparathyroidism. Arch. Surg., 105:369, 1972.
80. Kuntz, C. H., and Goldsmith, R. E.: Selective arteriography of parathyroid adenomas. Radiology, 102:21, 1972.
81. Snodgrass, R. W., and Mellinkoff, S. M.: Idiopathic hypoparathyroidism with small bowel features of sprue without steatorrhea. Am. J. Dig. Dis., 7:273, 1962.
82. Bennett, J. C., Maffly, R. H., and Steinbach, H. L.: Significance of bilateral basal ganglia calcification. Radiology, 72:368, 1959.
83. Moskowitz, M. A., Winickoff, R. N., and Heinz, E. R.: Familial calcification of basal gaaglia. N. Engl. J. Med., 285:72, 1971.
84. Howatt, T. W., and Ashurst, G. M.: Pseudohypoparathyroidism. J. Bone Joint Surg., 39B:39, 1957.
85. McNeely, W. F., et al.: Dyschondroplasia with soft tissue calcification and ossification and normal parathyroid function (pseudo-pseuodhypoparathyroidism). Am. J. Med., 21:649, 1956.
86. Todd, J., III, et al.: Hereditary multiple exostoses: pseudo-pseudohypoparathyroidism. Am. J. Med., 30:289, 1961.
87. Greenberg, S. R., Karabell, S., et al.: Pseudohypoparathyroidism. Arch. Intern. Med., 129:633, 1972.
88. Schlaeger, R., et al.: Gastrointestinal tract alterations in adenomatosis of endocrine glands. Radiology, 75:517, 1960.
89. Wermer, P.: Diagnosis of polyadenomatosis of the endocrine glands. Radiol. Clin. North Am., 5:349, 1967.
90. Craven, D. E., Goodman, A. D., and Carter, J. H.: Familial multiple endocrine adenomatosis. Arch. Intern. Med., 129:567, 1972.

DISEASES OF BONE

The Osteoporoses

Osteoporosis is caused by a deficiency of organic bone matrix; in the past this has been attributed to deficient bone formation with normal bone resorption, but later studies indicate that it may be caused by a disproportion between osteoblastic bone deposition and osteoclastic bone resorption (remodeling rate). The end result is reduction in bone mass. There must be a calcium loss of from 25 to 30 per cent before osteoporosis can be detected by routine roentgenograms. In acquired or adult forms the overall size of the bone remains unchanged; in congenital forms the bones may be smaller than normal.

The serum calcium, phosphorus, and alkaline phosphatase are frequently normal.

Among the common causes of generalized osteoporosis are senility, Cushing's syndrome, prolonged cortisone therapy, postmenopausal metabolic changes, nutritional (especially protein) deficiencies, hyperparathyroidism, severe childhood anemias, osteogenesis imperfecta, and multiple myeloma. Local osteoporosis can result from disuse, neurovascular disturbances (Sudeck's atrophy), local joint disease, and so forth. In contradistinction to osteoporosis, osteomalacia is caused by deficient calcification of an otherwise normal protein bone matrix. Radiographic distinction between osteoporosis and osteomalacia is sometimes difficult or impossible, and the two disorders may coexist.

In osteoporosis there is a decrease in the number and usually in the thickness of the bony trabeculae, particularly of the secondary trabeculae. This is most apparent in cancellous bone. The trabeculae lying along the lines of stress or weight bearing or muscle contraction (primary trabeculae) are less involved and may actually show compensatory thickening, forming parallel and relatively dense coarse striations best seen in the vertebral bodies and in the neck of the femora. Later, the compact bone (the cortex) becomes thinned but appears relatively dense in contrast to the markedly decreased density of the spongiosa. In rapidly developing osteoporosis the endosteal cortex may be irregular because of the large areas of bone resorption. In severe cases, cyst-like areas of spongiosa rarefaction may simulate small lytic lesions.

Systemic osteoporosis is most marked in the spine and pelvis, where the rate of bone deposition and resorption is much greater than in the appendicular skeleton.

The vertebral bodies appear lucent with fairly dense but thin cortical plates. The prominent vertical striations are a result of preservation of the primary trabeculae along the lines of stress. Osteophytes or spurs, normally found in aging vertebral bodies, are absent or decreased in severe osteoporosis. Biconcave deformities are common and result from pressure of the nucleus pulposus on the brittle bones. There may actually be expansion of the normal intervertebral discs.

Vertebral compression fractures frequently develop; wedging of the vertebral bodies is most common in the dorsal region. Fractures of the femur are also common, especially in postmenopausal osteoporosis.

There is decreased density of the floor and dorsum of the sella turcica. Diffuse demineralization and thinning of the tables of the skull also occur.[1-4]

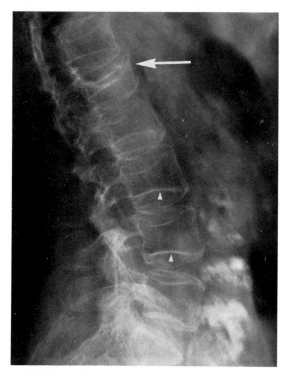

Figure 17–1 **Senile Osteoporosis of Lumbar Spine.** The pronounced lucency of the vertebral bodies is due to extensive resorption of bony trabeculae; by contrast, the cortical end plates are thinned but appear relatively dense *(arrowheads)*. There is a compression fracture of L1 *(arrow)*. The densities anterior to the spine represent residual barium from a previous contrast study.

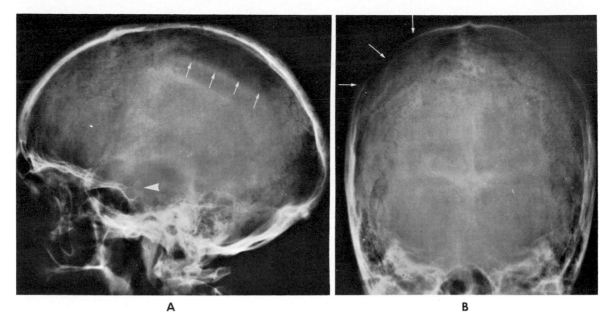

A   **B**

Figure 17-2   **Osteoporosis of Skull.**

A, Lateral view discloses spotty demineralization of the calvarium, causing a mottled appearance. The parietal bones *(arrows)* are very much thinned. The density of the dorsum sellae and posterior clinoids is decreased *(arrowhead)*.

B, In posteroanterior view the outer table of the parietal bones is virtually absent *(arrows)*, and the inner table is thinned.

Thinning of the parietal bones usually is associated with senile or postmenopausal osteoporosis. It may also occur in younger patients with hypogonadal osteoporosis. This patient manifested evidence of senile osteoporosis in other bones.

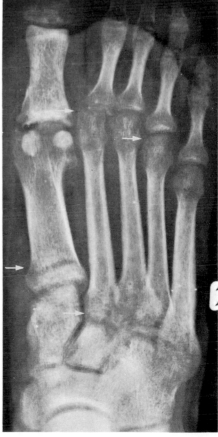

Figure 17-3   **Osteoporosis: Sudeck's Atrophy.**   Mottled patchy demineralization is greatest at the ends of the bones *(arrows)*; the shafts are nearly normal. The cortices at the bone ends are very thin but intact. Sudeck's atrophy is a severe neurovascular type of osteoporosis that usually develops following trauma.

Transient Osteoporosis of the Hip

This self-limited condition of unknown origin affects young or middle-aged adults. It is characterized by a painful hip and progressive osteoporosis of the femoral head. In more severe cases involvement spreads to the femoral neck. The joint space of the hip remains intact. Spontaneous clinical and roentgenologic recovery without residua occurs within two to four months. Rarely, there may be a second episode involving the other hip or even a shoulder, foot, or knee.

Periarticular osteoporosis is also seen in many of the infectious arthritides, but the absence of joint changes, the absence of significant demineralization of the other side of the joint (acetabulum), the minimal findings on synovial or bone biopsy, and the spontaneous recovery favor the diagnosis of transient osteoporosis syndrome.[5-8]

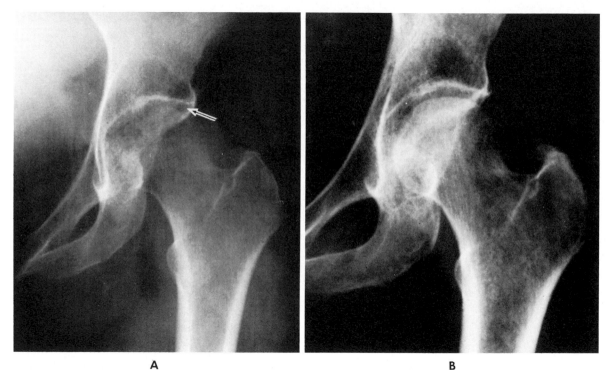

A   B

Figure 17–4 **Transient Osteoporosis of Femoral Head in a 28 Year Old Woman.**

A, Film of the left hip, made after three months of severe left hip pain, reveals marked demineralization of the femoral head. The proximal portion and articular margin of the head are virtually invisible, and the joint space is recognizable only in its extreme lateral aspect *(arrow)*. Note that the articular margin of the acetabulum is practically unaffected. The right hip was completely normal.

B, Six weeks later there was complete clinical and roentgenologic recovery without specific therapy. The femoral head is completely remineralized, and the joint space is entirely normal. (Courtesy Dr. R. A. Rosen, Bronx, New York.)

Osteomalacia

Failure of calcium and phosphorus deposition in bone matrix is usually attributable to inadequate concentration of these substances in the body fluids. The bone matrix itself is not abnormal (as in osteoporosis). Osteomalacia can result from decreased intestinal absorption of vitamin D, calcium, or phosphorus, which occurs in malabsorption, or from inadequate intake of these substances. Non-nutritional metabolic causes of osteomalacia include the various renal tubular dystrophies, chronic renal failure, hypophosphatasia, and hypercalcinuria.

Pseudofractures are pathognomonic. These bands of uncalcified osteoid tissue appear as lines of decreased density perpendicular to the cortex and extend partially across the bone. They are often bilateral, frequently symmetric, and tend to occur where arteries enter into bones. The usual sites of pseudofractures are the neck of the femur, the pubic bone, and the lateral border of the scapula. The fractures may ultimately undergo marginal sclerosis. Full healing is slow.

Continuing osteomalacia leads to demineralization of both the cortex and the spongiosa of the axial and peripheral skeleton. The texture of the bones may be coarse as a result of total demineralization of many secondary trabeculae. In advanced cases, true fractures may occur in any bone, and the vertebral bodies may show biconcave deformities and compression fractures.

In the growing skeleton the picture is that of rickets. (See p. 1129).

Radiographic distinction of osteomalacia from osteoporosis is often difficult. Frequently the two conditions coexist. Osteomalacia secondary to malabsorption or chronic renal failure is frequently associated with secondary hyperparathyroidism and its attendant roentgenologic changes. (See p. 1304).[2, 4, 9, 10]

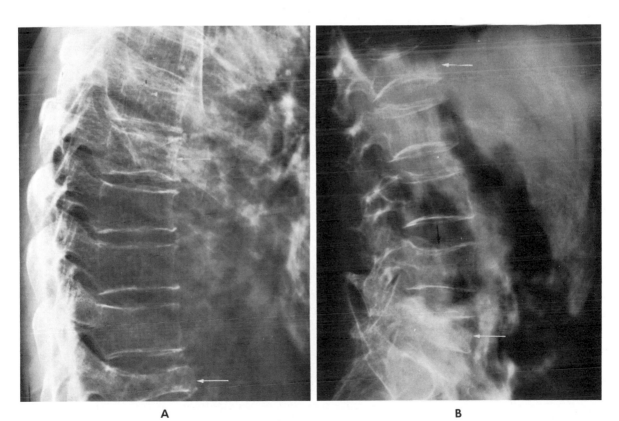

A   B

Figure 17–5 **Osteomalacia of Spine Secondary to Malabsorption.**

A, There is generalized demineralization of the spine. Compression fractures of two dorsal bodies are evident *(arrows).* The coarse striations *(arrowhead)* represent thickening of the primary trabeculae. Almost all the secondary trabeculae are completely decalcified.

B, Lateral view of the lumbar spine demonstrates two compression fractures *(white arrows).* Concavity of the vertebral margins *(black arrow)* is a result of pressure from the nuclei pulposi on the soft and brittle bodies. A virtually identical appearance is seen in osteoporosis.

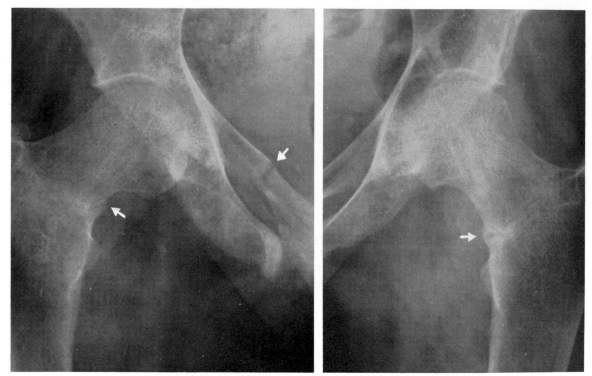

Figure 17–6 **Osteomalacia: Pseudofractures.** Bilateral horizontal lucencies in the medial aspect of the femoral necks *(lower two arrows)* represent pseudofractures. There is another pseudofracture on the superior ramus of the right symphysis pubis *(upper arrow)*. The bones are diffusely demineralized. Pseudofractures are pathognomonic of osteomalacia but may occasionally be seen in Paget's disease and fragilitas ossium. In these conditions there are other characteristic changes in the bones. (Courtesy Dr. P. G. Powell, Indiana University Medical Center, Bloomington, Indiana.)

Hypophosphatasia

In this familial condition there is a lack of alkaline phosphatase in the cells, resulting in defective mineralization of bone.

The disorder may be discovered in utero (about one fifth of cases) and usually affects the entire skeleton. Many bones are uncalcified; others are short, thin, and coarsely trabeculated, with defective metaphyseal growth. Metaphyseal factures with formation of irregular callus occur frequently and lead to marked deformity. These changes can often be demonstrated on prenatal films. As a rule, the infants are stillborn.

In infancy, the roentgenologic features of hypophosphatasia resemble those of rickets. Demineralization in the submetaphyseal area and irregular metaphyseal zones are the usual findings. Bowing deformities are common. In the skull there are unossified areas usually adjacent to the sutures and at the base, simulating greatly widened sutures. Premature closure of the sutures occurs in surviving infants, leading to craniostenosis. The skull changes will help differentiate radiographically hypophosphatasia from rickets.

In childhood the epiphyseal line is widened and irregular. Metaphyseal defects persist in less severely affected children who reach adulthood (about 40 per cent).[11, 12]

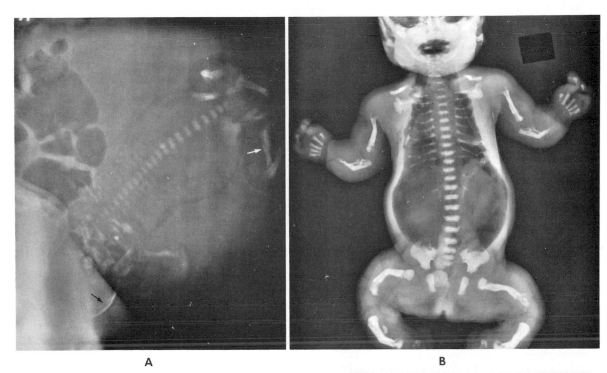

A   B

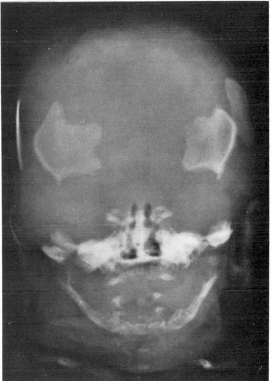

Figure 17–7 **Hypophosphatasia in Utero and Postpartum.**

A, Lateral view late in pregnancy discloses fetal bone abnormalities. Only a small segment of skull is calcified *(black arrow)*. The ribs are only partially ossified; the long bones are short and thin. These changes are virtually diagnostic of hypophosphatasia. There is intrauterine fracture of the femur *(white arrow)*.

B, Postpartum film made after evisceration of stillborn reveals that the ribs are incompletely ossified. The long bones are short and deformed by bowing or by fracture, especially at the metaphyseal end. Many bones are entirely uncalcified.

C, The skull and facial bones are almost entirely unossified. (Courtesy Dr. R. Todd, Liverpool, England.)

C

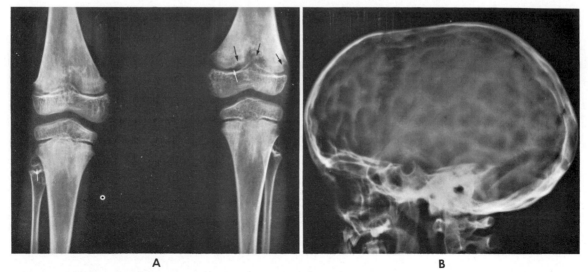

A   B

Figure 17–8 **Hypophosphatasia: Late Changes.**

A, The patient was 10 years old; rachitic changes developed when he was 6. The epiphyses show very coarse trabeculations. The metaphyseal ends are somewhat irregular, and some areas are demineralized (*black arrows*). The epiphyseal line is widened (*white arrows*), and there is evidence of demineralization in all bones.

B, The anteroposterior diameter of the skull is increased, and there are prominent digital markings; these changes were due to premature suture closure (craniostenosis). (Courtesy Drs. W. Dickson and R. Horrocks, Bolton, England.)

Renal Osteodystrophy

See page 780.

Osteitis Fibrosa Cystica

This extensive bone disease is characterized by severe demineralization of the skeleton and deformities of the bones due to bowing, expansile cystic tumors, and fractures. The condition may be produced whenever there is a rapid bone turnover. It is usually associated with severe longstanding hyperparathyroidism, usually primary. Less commonly it is associated with rickets or osteomalacia, with hyperthyroidism, and locally with rapidly developing Paget's disease. The serum alkaline phosphatase is invariably elevated.

When due to hyperparathyroidism, subperiosteal resorption progresses to generalized skeletal rarefaction and to fairly well-demarcated cystic areas of bone destruction (brown tumors) throughout the skeleton. These may cause expansion of bones. The cysts may be solitary, or multiple and contiguous, producing multilocular expansion. Such resorption and overgrowth of fibrous tissue may lead to deformity, bowing, and pathologic fracture. The mandible, pelvis, ribs, and femur are the most common sites of brown tumors.

The fundamental roentgenologic features of hyperparathyroidism — lace-like subperiosteal resorption especially in the middle phalanges, loss of the dental lamina dura, grainy demineralization of the skull, and generalized demineralization in which the trabeculae become indistinct and the cortices thinned — help distinguish osteitis fibrosa cystica from similar diseases, especially fibrous dysplasia.

If the primary cause of osteitis fibrosa cystica can be corrected (as in parathyroid adenoma), the bones usually return to normal, although the more severe bowing and shortening deformities may persist. Mineralization of the pseudocysts may make them denser than the surrounding bone, but true cysts do not disappear. (See also *Hyperparathyroidism*, p. 1304 and *Renal Osteodystrophy*, p. 780.)[13, 14]

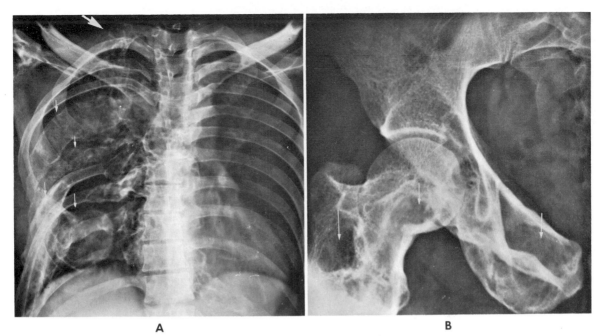

A   B

Figure 17–9   **Osteitis Fibrosa Cystica in Hyperparathyroidism.**

A, Posteroanterior view discloses great expansion and distortion of multiple ribs on the right *(arrows)*. There is cortical thinning and loss of trabeculae. The first rib has a multicystic appearance *(large arrow)*.

B, Enlarged view of the right hip area demonstrates multiple cystic lucent areas—so-called brown tumors *(arrows)*. There is resorption of bony trabeculae as well as cortical thinning and expansion.

The appearance closely resembles that of advanced fibrous dysplasia. Brown tumors may be single, or multiple and diffuse as in the present case. The serum alkaline phosphatase level is invariably elevated.

BONE INTOXICATIONS

Fluorosis

Fluorosis is characterized by generalized increased density of the skeleton associated with spicular bone deposits at the sites of muscle and ligamentous attachment. The bone sclerosis appears earliest and is most prominent in the vertebrae and pelvis. It is less marked in the peripheral skeleton.

In advanced cases the vertebrae, the pelvic bones, and occasionally the ribs become chalky white, obscuring individual trabeculae. Calcification of a portion of the sacrospinous or sacrotuberous ligaments occurs in a high proportion of cases. Sclerosis of the bones of the extremities is much less common, but periosteal roughening of the long bones at the sites of muscle and ligamentous attachment is frequent and characteristic.

Denseness of the axial skeleton associated with calcification of the sacrospinous or sacrotuberous ligaments and with periosteal exostoses and roughening of some of the long bones may help differentiate fluorosis from other conditions associated with dense bones, such as congenital osteopetrosis, sclerosing carcinomatous metastases, Paget's disease, and myelofibrosis. Calcification of pelvic ligaments, if associated with increased density of the axial skeleton, is virtually pathognomonic of fluorosis; irregular periosteal projections from the long bones to the soft tissues is another significant radiographic feature of chronic fluorosis.

Florid periostitis is characteristic of acute fluoride intoxication. In such cases the density of the bones may be either increased or decreased or a mixture of both. Calcification of ligamentous and muscular attachments is common and may be pronounced. Before the cause was established, this disorder was known as deforming periostitis of unknown origin.[15–17]

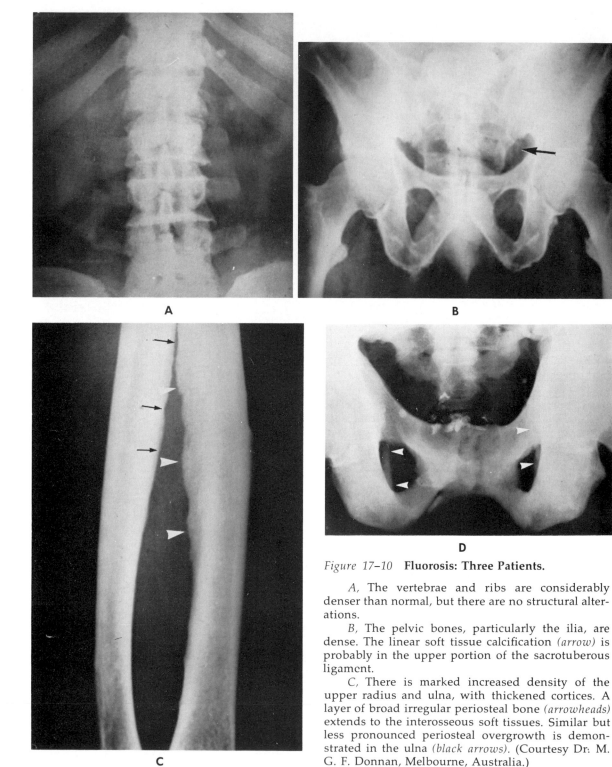

Figure 17–10 **Fluorosis: Three Patients.**

A, The vertebrae and ribs are considerably denser than normal, but there are no structural alterations.

B, The pelvic bones, particularly the ilia, are dense. The linear soft tissue calcification *(arrow)* is probably in the upper portion of the sacrotuberous ligament.

C, There is marked increased density of the upper radius and ulna, with thickened cortices. A layer of broad irregular periosteal bone *(arrowheads)* extends to the interosseous soft tissues. Similar but less pronounced periosteal overgrowth is demonstrated in the ulna *(black arrows).* (Courtesy Dr. M. G. F. Donnan, Melbourne, Australia.)

D, In another patient there is calcification of the inferior portion of both sacrotuberous ligaments *(arrowheads).* Marked osteosclerosis of the pelvic bones is evident. The patient lived in a community in which the drinking water had a high natural fluoride content. (Courtesy Dr. Clyde A. Stevenson, Spokane, Washington.)

Illustration continued on opposite page

E

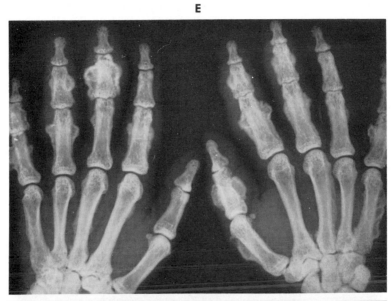

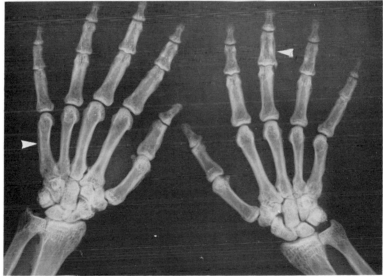

F

Figure 17–10 (Continued)

   E, In the hands of a patient who continued to drink heavily fluoridated wines there is a florid bizarre periosteal proliferation involving most of the metacarpals and phalanges. Similar changes were present in many other long bones, having developed over a period of months.

   F, Two years after the patient stopped drinking fluoridated wines, there is marked regression of the periosteal changes *(arrowheads).* (Courtesy Dr. M. Soriano, Barcelona, Spain.)

Vitamin A Intoxication (Hypervitaminosis A)

Although there are no roentgen findings in vitamin A *deficiency*, chronic *overdose* may produce significant skeletal changes.

In infants and children the most prominent feature is cortical hyperostosis, most often of the ulna and tibia. There is evidence suggesting that overdose of vitamin A may disturb bone growth, cause thinning of the epiphyseal plates, and, in severe cases, cause early closure of the epiphyses. In adults, extensive calcification may develop in the tendinous, ligamentous, pericapsular, or subperiosteal structures. These are very uncommon. Hepatic injury resulting in portal hypertension and ascites is a more frequent sequela of chronic hypervitaminosis A in adults. In both children and adults the bone and soft tissue changes usually disappear after cessation of vitamin A ingestion.[18, 19]

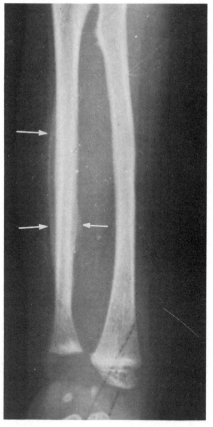

Figure 17–11   **Vitamin A Intoxication in a Child: Ulnar Hyperostosis.**   A 3 year old child was ingesting huge doses of vitamin A. There is extensive periosteal reaction *(arrows)* along the ulnar shaft. The blood level of vitamin A was 943 units (normal 30 to 60 units). (Courtesy Dr. A. Gerber, Brooklyn, New York.)

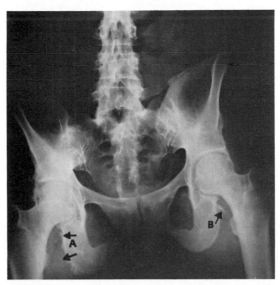

Figure 17–12 **Vitamin A Intoxication in an Adult.** A 28 year old subject had been taking large doses of vitamin A for excessive dryness of skin. There are multiple calcifications along the right ischium *(arrows at A)* and a larger area of calcification extending from the left ischium *(arrow at B).* These calcifications are in the ligamentous structures. The soft tissue calcification diminished considerably after the vitamin therapy was discontinued. (Courtesy Dr. C. N. Pease, Chicago, Illinois.)

Vitamin D Intoxication (Hypervitaminosis D)

In adults, prolonged excessive intake of vitamin D can lead to hypercalcemia and evidence of metastatic soft tissue calcification, especially around the joints and in the renal parenchyma. The calcification may diminish or disappear after discontinuation of the vitamin.

In children, hypercalcemia produces changes in the growing bones. Initially there is increased mineralization of the bony trabeculae, cortical thickening, and increased density of the zone of provisional calcification (metaphyseal line). Characteristically, the cortical end plates of the vertebrae are dense. Metastatic calcification may occur in any organ or tissue. Later, a characteristic zone of diminished density appears proximal to the metaphyseal line and gradually extends upward along the shaft. Renal damage from metastatic tubular calcification can lead to renal rickets, further complicating the roentgenologic skeletal finding. (See also *Idiopathic Hypercalcemia of Infancy,* p. 1335.)[20]

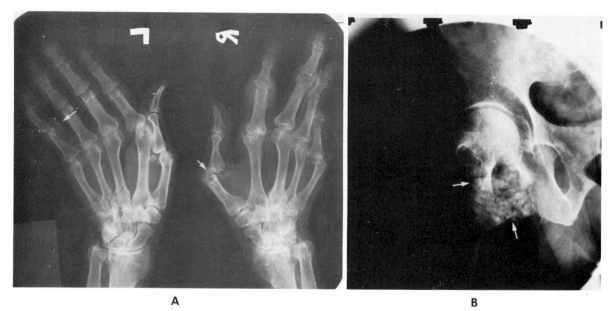

A   B

Figure 17–13   **Vitamin D Intoxication in an Adult.**

A 62 year old female with rheumatoid arthritis had been taking 200,000 units of vitamin D daily for seven years.

A, Amorphous calcification *(arrows)* developed around the finger joints in both hands. There are advanced rheumatoid changes in the joints.

B, There is an amorphous accumulation of calcium *(arrows)* in the soft tissues adjacent to the left upper femur.

The demineralization is probably due to the rheumatoid arthritis. The calcium deposits in the hands cleared when vitamin D therapy was discontinued, but those around the femur persisted and had to be removed surgically. (Courtesy Drs. C. Wilson, W. Wingfield, and E. Toone.)

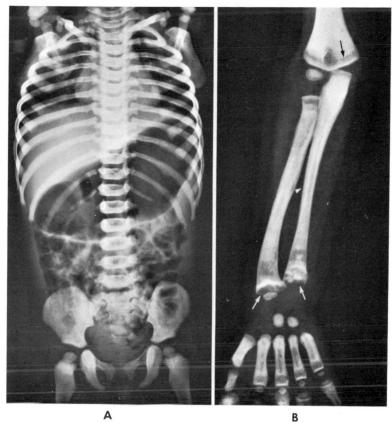

Figure 17–14 **Vitamin D Intoxication in an Infant: Renal Rickets.**

A, There is increased bone density in the ribs, spine, and pelvis.

B, The zones of provisional calcification in the bones of the elbow and hand are dense, with bands of diminished density *(black arrow)* below the metaphyseal borders; the cortices are thickened *(arrowhead),* and the bones show increased density—all characteristic changes.

Superimposed renal rickets has produced typical rachitic changes in the distal metaphyses of the radius and ulna *(white arrows).*

Idiopathic Hypercalcemia of Infancy

The condition causes changes similar to those seen in hypervitaminosis D, and may be due to hyper-reaction to this vitamin.

The bones show some increased density, due principally to trabecular, not cortical, thickening. The zone of provisional calcification is dense and broad; bands of radiolucency may appear within the metaphysis. Characteristic bands of density are seen in the acetabular roofs and in the end plates of the vertebral bodies. Islands of dense bone appear within the spongiosa.

In most patients, spontaneous resolution occurs after the age of 1 year, but nephrocalcinosis, ectopic calcification, osteoporosis, and craniostenosis may ensue in severe cases. A high incidence of supravalvular aortic stenosis is found. Other vascular anomalies include hypoplasia of the aorta, pulmonary artery stenosis, and peripheral artery stenosis. Withholding vitamin D and calcium intake may result in slow return of the bones to normal.[21, 22]

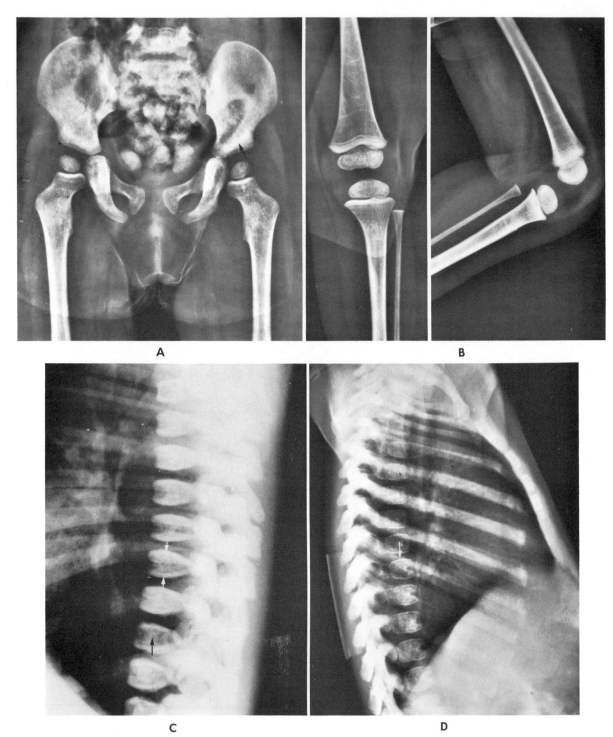

A   B

C   D

Figure 17–15 **Idiopathic Hypercalcemia in an Infant.**

    A, The characteristic wide band of increased density is demonstrated in the acetabular roof (*black arrow*). The metaphyseal lines in the upper femora are dense (*white arrow*). There are other areas of sclerosis in the pelvis and femora.

    B, The dense metaphyseal lines are demonstrated in the bones of the knee.

    C, The dorsal bodies are dense, with plates of density on the superior and inferior borders of the vertebrae (*white arrows*). There are islands of bone density (*black arrow*) in the spongiosa of almost all the bodies.

    D, Recovery is reflected in nearly normal density of the vertebrae. The vertebral plates have the normal thin lines of density (*arrow*).

OSTEOMYELITIS

Bone involvement by various microbial agents is discussed and illustrated in the section *Microbial Diseases* (see under *Staphylococcal Diseases,* tuberculosis, and specific mycotic organisms).

Bone reacts to infection in a limited number of ways, and the radiographic appearance of osteomyelitis is fashioned more by the intensity and chronicity of the infection than by the specificity of the causative organism.

Acute hematogenous osteomyelitis can be caused by any pyogenic organism; staphylococci and streptococci are the most common. The metaphysis of a long bone is the usual site, but roentgen changes in the bone may not become apparent until after 10 to 20 days. Soft tissue swelling is the earliest finding, followed by periosteal reaction and then by lytic areas of bone destruction. Later, a piece of dead bone may become detached (sequestrum) and lie within an exudate-filled lytic area. The sequestrum is of normal or increased density in contrast to the surrounding areas of bone lyses. The thickened new bone surrounding the region of the sequestrum is called the *involucrum.* In children the infection does not cross the open epiphyseal line.

In more chronic forms of osteomyelitis the cortical bone becomes thickened, and the medullary cavity develops irregular sclerosis amid the lytic areas. The bone is usually widened.

Less common forms of osteomyelitis include Brodie's abscess, which is a circumscribed lytic area surrounded by sclerotic bone, and Garré's osteomyelitis, a purely sclerotic area with a focal bulge of thickened cortex. Osteomyelitis of the skull is usually entirely lytic with little or no sclerosis or periosteal reaction.

Mycotic infections of bone are often secondary to soft tissue involvement. The cortex is then eroded or partially destroyed, and generally demarcated by surrounding sclerosis. Periosteal proliferation is often minimal or absent. Soft tissue swelling and draining sinuses are common.

In diabetics with ischemia and soft tissue infection of the feet, secondary bone involvement is marked by demineralization and irregular lysis; periosteal reaction is rare.

Ordinarily, the combined lytic and sclerotic medullary changes, together with cortical thickening, will readily identify chronic osteomyelitis radiographically. In acute or subacute osteomyelitis, however, the periosteal reaction and medullary lysis can sometimes simulate the changes of a malignant bone tumor, especially in children.

OSTEONECROSIS (AVASCULAR NECROSIS, ASEPTIC NECROSIS)

Osteonecrosis of articular bone occurs most frequently in the head of the femur; other more common sites include the bones of the knee and the head of the humerus.

The idiopathic form arises preponderantly in males (ratio of four males to one female) during adolescence or middle age. It is bilateral in about 40 per cent of cases. Other causes or associations are systemic or intra-articular corticosteroid therapy, hypothyroidism, sickle cell disease, Gaucher's disease, caisson disease, and lupus erythematosus.

There are no discernible radiographic findings during the early clinical stage. In femoral head involvement, a faint line of subchondral lucency may appear on the lateral weight-bearing side of the bone. Later, sclerotic subarticular bands or zones, often wedge-shaped, appear. Disruption of the circumference of the femoral head and mottled areas of rarefaction and condensation then develop, followed by flattening and collapse of the head. The joint space becomes irregular but remains of normal width or may even appear widened, a point of differentiation from osteoarthritis. However, eventual cartilage loss leads to joint narrowing and osteophyte formation, a picture indistinguishable from that of osteoarthritis. Similar changes are seen in osteonecrosis of other bones.

The osteonecrosis that sometimes follows administration of intra-articular steroids generally progresses much more rapidly than the other forms.[23-26]

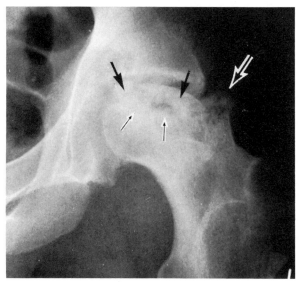

Figure 17–16 **Unilateral Osteonecrosis (Aseptic Necrosis) of Femoral Head.**   A film of the left hip of a 34 year old man shows irregular fragmentation of the articular surface of the femur (*black arrows*), with a detached lateral fragment (*large black-white arrow*). Below the fragmenting lytic areas is an irregular zone of sclerosis (*small black-white arrows*). The joint space is well preserved. The other hip was completely normal.

CONGENITAL AND/OR HEREDITARY DISORDERS INVOLVING BONE

Osteogenesis Imperfecta (Psathyrosis, Fragilitas Ossium, Lobstein's Disease)

This congenital disease is characterized by deficient formation of bone matrix and collagen, and can affect the bones, skin, sclera, and periarticular tissues.

The bone changes are due to osteoporosis and repeated fractures. The cortices are thin and sometimes do not fully extend into the metaphyses. There is a generalized osteoporosis with deficient trabecular structure. The fractures often heal with excess callus formation and in severe cases cause bizarre deformities sometimes recognizable in utero. The extreme radiolucency of the fetal skeleton in utero is virtually diagnostic. Bowing of the lower extremities is common, even without fractures.

The skull tables are thin. During infancy numerous accessory bones are found along the sutures (wormian bones), producing a mosaic appearance. The sinuses and the mastoid cells are often quite large. Basilar impression (platybasia) is frequent.

In the tardive form, clinical symptoms appear later in childhood. The long bones are slender, somewhat demineralized, and often bowed; the cortices are thin. Fractures occur after minor trauma. The pelvis is often triradiate, and biconcave deformities of the vertebrae may be found.

Mild cases may have no stigmas of the disease, and the bones appear completely normal or slightly undermineralized. Repeated fractures in later life, following inadequate trauma, may be the only clue in individuals with a genetic background of the disease.

The association of osteoporosis and bowed bones in the lower extremities is suggestive of osteogenesis imperfecta.[27-30]

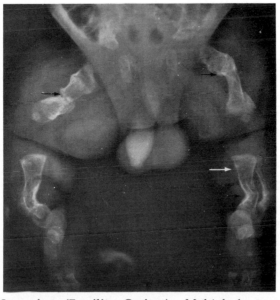

Figure 17–17 **Osteogenesis Imperfecta (Fragilitas Ossium).** Multiple fractures (*black arrows*), which were present at birth, have caused great deformity of the bones. The excess callus formation that occurred with healing has increased the deformity. Although the bones appear wide, the cortices are extremely thin and the spongiosa appears translucent, features that indicate severe osteoporosis. The cortex does not extend as far as the metaphysis (*white arrow*).

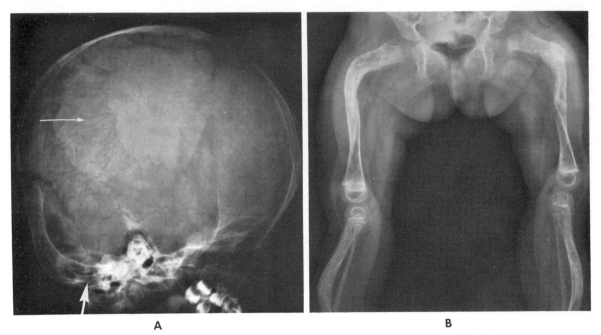

Figure 17–18 **Osteogenesis Imperfecta.**

 A, Multiple wormian bones are evident (*small arrow*). The tables are thin and demineralized, and basilar impression is demonstrated (*large arrow*). The child had blue sclera.

 B, The bones of the leg are bowed and misshapen due to multiple healed fractures. The cortices are thin. The trabeculae in the spongiosa are deficient.

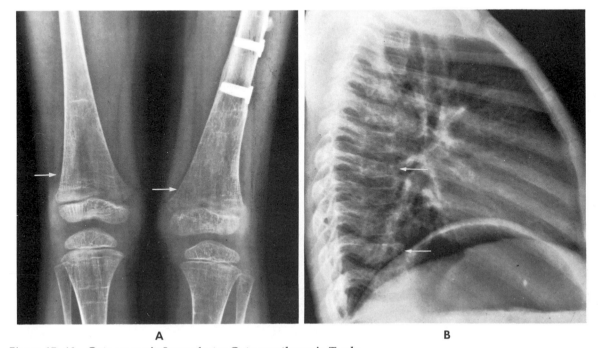

Figure 17–19 **Osteogenesis Imperfecta: Osteopsathyrosis Tarda.**

 A, The diaphyseal portions of the bones are narrow and the metaphyses appear flared (*arrows*), because of deficient modeling. The cortices are thin and the spongiosa is decreased. There are metal pins in the area of an old fracture.

 B, Osteoporosis of the dorsal bodies is evident, with multiple wedged compression fractures (*arrows*).

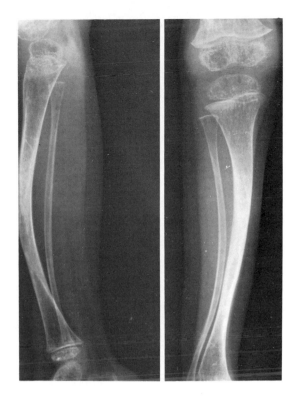

Figure 17–20 **Osteogenesis Imperfecta: Tardive Form.** The diagnosis is suggested by the thin diaphysis, flaring of the metaphysis, and bowing of the bones. The cortex is thinned, and the bones are demineralized. The area of increased density in the midshaft is secondary to an old fracture.

Osteopetrosis (Albers-Schonberg Disease, Marble Bone Disease)

In this this rare hereditary disease, failure of normal resorption of calcified chondral tissue and primitive bone leads to thickening of the cortex and narrowing of the medullary cavity.

Excessive calcified cartilaginous matrix produces a thickened cortex and a thickened, calcified spongiosa.

In severe cases, generalized increased density of *all* the bones is present at birth and even in utero. The normal architectural landmarks of cortex, spongiosa, medullary cavity, and metaphyseal zone of provisional calcification may be obliterated. Later, a layer of nonsclerotic bone may form, enclosing the original sclerotic bone and producing an outline of a bone within a bone (endobone). Normal metaphyseal constriction (modeling) fails to occur, leading to widened metaphyseal ends. Occasionally, relatively lucent bands are seen near the ends of the long bones; these probably represent periods of temporary cessation of the pathologic process. Fractures are fairly common; they are usually transverse and heal rapidly with abundant callus.

In the skull the sclerotic changes are most marked at the base; the mastoid cells, the paranasal sinuses, and even the foramina at the base may be obliterated. Cranial nerve disorders, especially blindness and deafness, may ensue.

Crowding of the bone marrow results in myelophthisic anemia; extramedullary hematopoiesis develops, enlarging the liver and spleen.

In less severe forms of this disease the onset may be later in infancy or childhood, and not all the skeletal bones are involved with osteopetrosis; involvement is usually symmetric. The pelvic bones and vertebrae are affected in almost every case. Some bones, especially those of the extremities, may show various patterns of sclerosis, including discrete areas, linear streaks, concentric layers, or diffuse involvement with thickened cortices. The varying patterns of density appear principally in the growing ends of the bones.

Somewhat similar sclerotic bone changes can occur in hypervitaminosis D, pycnodysostosis, and in fibrous dysplasia of the skull and facial bones.[31, 32]

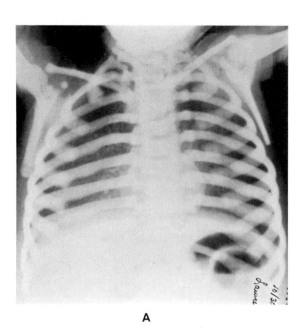

A

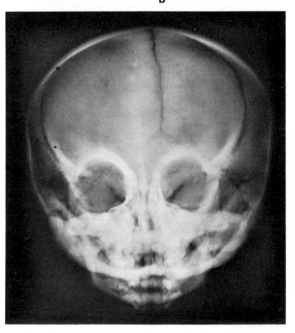

B

Figure 17–21 **Congenital Osteopetrosis (Osteosclerosis).**

A, The ribs, clavicles, scapulae, and humeri are uniformly dense; cortical-medullary distinction is obscured.

B, All the vertebrae are chalky white. The pelvic bones (seen on end) are also very dense. The overexposed film of the femur demonstrates marked cortical thickening and narrowing of the medullary cavity.

C, The orbits and facial bones are extremely sclerotic; the bones of the vault appear uninvolved. The paranasal sinuses are obliterated.

C

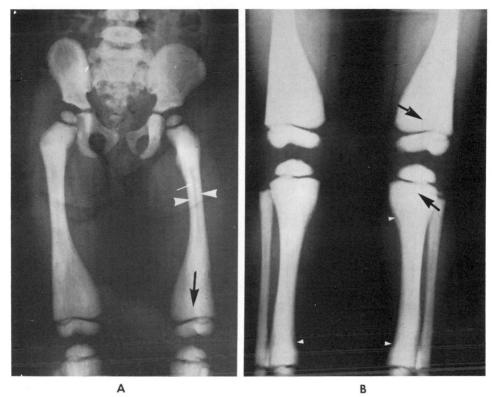

A   B

Figure 17–22   **Congenital Osteopetrosis: The Long Bones.**

A, The spine, pelvis, and femora have greatly increased density. The cortices of the femora are thickened *(arrowheads),* and the medullary cavity is markedly narrowed *(white arrow).* The metaphyseal ends of the lower femora *(black arrow)* and upper tibiae are widened, producing a flask-like appearance. This is caused by failure of normal tubulation and is characteristic of congenital osteopetrosis.

B, There is markedly increased density of the bones of the legs, with flask-like widening of the metaphyseal ends *(arrows).* A few areas of normal cortical density *(arrowheads)* have developed during periods of normal bone formation. Sometimes the entire sclerotic bone becomes surrounded by new bone of normal density, producing the bone-within-a-bone appearance.

Achondroplasia

This hereditary condition resulting in dwarfism is characterized by abnormal bone configuration due to diminished cartilaginous growth and decreased enchondral bone formation. Ossification and maturation of epiphyses, articular cartilage, and membranous bone formation are not affected.

The most constant and characteristic bone changes are in the upper extremities and lumbar spine. The humeri are disproportionately short compared to the bones of the forearm (rhizomelia). Similar but less marked shortening of the femora is usual. All extremities are disproportionately short in relation to the trunk. In the lumbar spine the interpediculate distances progressively diminish from L1 to L5, a direct reversal of normal. The pedicles also have a shortened anteroposterior diameter. Neurologic symptoms may occur as a result of the narrowed spinal canal.

Less constant changes in the spine are hypoplastic bullet- or wedge-shaped lumbar bodies, similar to the changes in Hurler's disease. A localized kyphos (gibbus) may be seen. The posterior margins of the bodies may be concave and the intervertebral foramina widened.

Numerous other bone changes are generally present. Most of the long bones of the extremities are shortened, widened, and flattened. The broad short tubular bones of the hand may be of the same length—the trident hand. The distal ends of long bones around the knees and ankles are often widened and flared; in children the metaphyses may be cupped around the epiphyses—the ball-in-socket epiphyses.

The pelvis is short and broad, with squared ilia and decreased acetabular angles. The skull is relatively large.

The typical achondroplastic dwarf is readily recognized clinically. The characteristic radiographic changes are confirmatory and may serve to distinguish achondroplasia from osteogenesis imperfecta, in which the extremities are shortened by multiple fractures, and from other forms of dwarfism.

Thanatrophic dwarfism is a lethal form of achondroplasia in which there is also a narrow thorax, generalized diminished vertebral height, and often a "cloverleaf" skull, with a large vault and short base.[33-36]

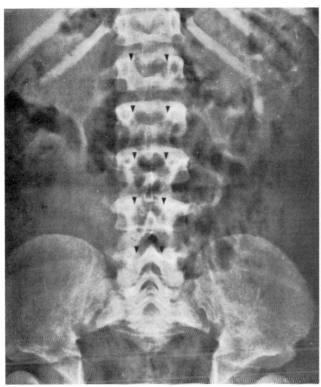
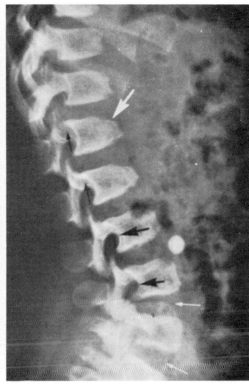

A

B

Figure 17–23 **Achondroplasia.**

A, In anteroposterior view there is a progressive decrease in the interpedicular distances *(black arrowheads)* from L1 to L5, the reverse of normal. The acetabular roof is rather flat, and the ilia are somewhat squared. The joint space of the hip is widened due to excess cartilage formation.

B, In lateral view the dorsal borders of the vertebral bodies are concave *(large black arrows),* and the pedicles are shortened *(small black arrows).* There is flattening of the anterior superior aspect of the bodies of the upper lumbar vertebrae *(large white arrow),* and the intervertebral spaces are widened *(small white arrows)* because of excess cartilage.

C, View of the extremities discloses the ball-in-socket epiphysis *(arrows)* which is characteristic of achondroplasia. The metaphyses are flared *(arrowhead),* and the bones are short and wide.

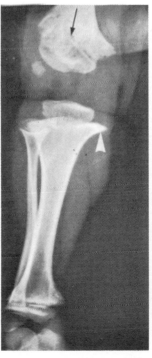
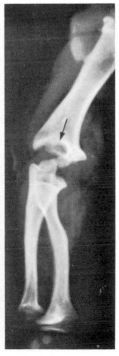

C

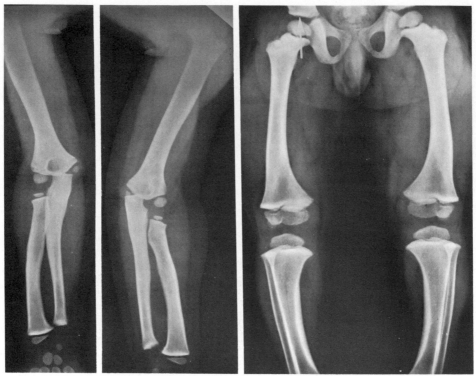

Figure 17–24 **Achondroplasia: Long Bones of Extremities in a Child.** The long bones of the upper and lower extremities are shortened and appear relatively wide, although their width is about normal for the child's age. The cortices appear somewhat thickened, and there is moderate flaring of the metaphyseal ends.

The angle of the acetabular roof is decreased *(arrow)*.

Hereditary Deforming Chondrodysplasia (Hereditary Multiple Exostosis, Skeletal Osteochondromatosis)

In this hereditary and familial condition there are multiple osteochondromas arising from any portion of the skeleton that was preformed in cartilage. The osteochondromas usually occur near the ends of long bones. They begin in childhood and continue to grow until general skeletal growth ceases.

The exostoses usually project away from the adjacent joint. The lesions extend from the cortex as spurs (exostoses) or knob-like masses (osteochondromas) and vary greatly in size. They contain both cortical and cancellous bone and merge smoothly and continuously into the normal bone. The shaft may be widened in this vicinity. The cartilaginous cap may calcify irregularly.

Alterations of long bone growth, deformities, and loss of tubulation are frequent. A shortened, deformed radius and ulna are commonly encountered.

Similar lesions can occur also in portions of flat bones that are preformed in cartilage. Occasionally, osteochondromas in the spine may produce neurologic symptoms by compression of cord or roots.

Occasionally, one of the lesions may undergo malignant degeneration.[37, 38]

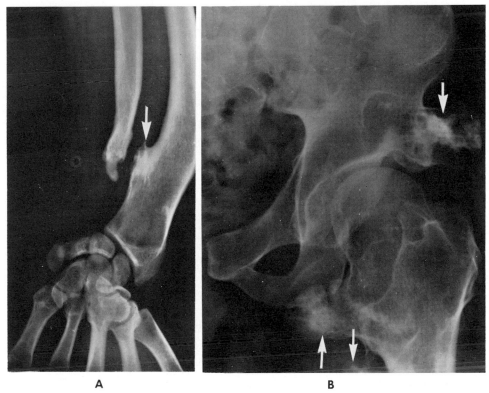

A   B

Figure 17–25 **Hereditary Deforming Chondrodysplasia.**

A, The bones of the forearm exhibit characteristic deformities: the ulna is shortened and the radius is widened and curved at the site of an exostosis *(arrow).*

B, Numerous exostoses with calcified cartilaginous caps arise in the femoral neck and ilium *(arrows),* and these bones are deformed. The cartilaginous mass may not completely calcify, so that the full extent of the exostosis may not be appreciated.

Ollier's Dyschondroplasia (Multiple Enchondromatosis)

Ollier's disease, or multiple enchondromatosis, is characterized by proliferation of cartilaginous masses within the shafts of the bone. These appear as intramedullary radiolucent areas often separated by bony septa, and sometimes as linear lucent streaks of cartilage paralleling the long axis of the bone. In the hands these lesions are ovoid or round, and usually devoid of septation. Stippled or mottled calcification within the lesion is frequent. Enchondromas may expand, erode, and destroy the cortex.

Deformities and disturbances of growth are commonly associated with the bone lesions. Involvement is frequently but not necessarily unilateral. Asymmetric shortening of the extremities is almost always present. The hands and feet are the most common sites of involvement. Cartilaginous malignancy (chondrosarcoma) may develop in a small percentage of patients with Ollier's disease, but almost never from lesions in the hands or feet.[39]

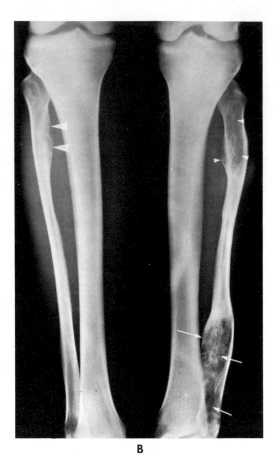

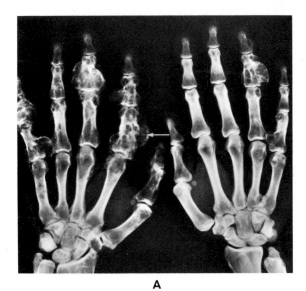

A   B

Figure 17–26 **Ollier's Dyschondroplasia: Hands and Legs.**

A, There are cystic expansile lesions in the phalanges, with thinning of the cortex and gross deformities of many of the bones. Stippled calcifications are seen within several of the lesions *(arrow)*. Involvement is considerably more extensive in the left hand *(left side of illustration)*.

B, A long expanding lesion containing calcifications is seen in the left lower fibula *(arrows)*. The cortex is expanded and thinned. A less extensive lesion is found in the upper left fibula *(small arrowheads)*. The linear band of lucency paralleling the long axis of the bone, seen in the right fibula *(large arrowheads)*, is a frequent finding and represents proliferation of cartilaginous masses.

Although bilateral involvement is present, the lesions were much more extensive unilaterally, a frequent characteristic of Ollier's disease.

Miscellaneous Congenital and/or Hereditary Disorders

A very large number of syndromes and conditions with dysplastic bone formation have been reported. A great many of these syndromes are exceedingly rare, and many have complex clinical and confusing radiographic abnormalities—the domain of the geneticist.

The conditions discussed in this section have bone changes sufficiently characteristic or unique to permit a radiographic diagnosis.

Acro-Osteolysis

This condition is a congenital osseous dysplasia, with an onset usually in the second decade. It may be idiopathic or familial.

Shortened and clubbed fingers, often painful and sometimes associated with overlying skin ulcerations, are the principal findings. Other frequent clinical features include kyphoscoliosis, progressive decrease in height, atrophy of the mandible or the maxilla with an edentulous state, and a protuberant occiput.

The striking radiographic feature is lytic destruction and resorption of the tufts of the distal phalanges of the hands and feet without reactive bone changes (acro-osteolysis). Other findings may include resorption of the alveolar processes of the maxilla and mandible, premature closure of the skull sutures, basilar impression of the skull, and demineralization of the spine with loss of vertebral stature.

Other conditions in which resorptive changes appear in the distal phalanges include Raynaud's disease or phenomenon, leprosy, exposure to vinyl chloride, and progeria. However, clinical considerations and associated skeletal changes simplify the differential diagnosis.[40]

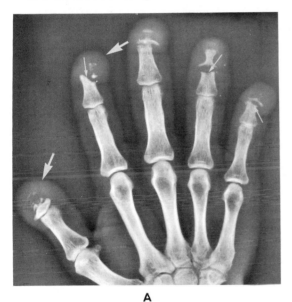 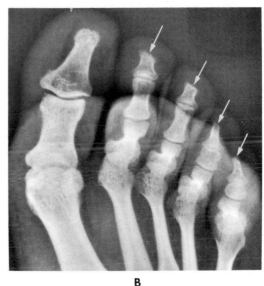

A   **B**

Figure 17–27 **Familial Acro-Osteolysis.**

This 35 year old man had a long history of back pain and had become shorter in stature. The lumbar bodies were demineralized and showed biconcave narrowing.

A, Film of the hand reveals clubbing of the distal soft tissues (*large arrows*), resorption of the tufts and portions of the distal phalanges, and sharply marginated resorption of the distal ends of the middle phalanges (*small arrows*). The index finger showed the most severe changes.

B, In the foot the phalangeal tufts have been resorbed (*arrows*); only the big toe is intact. (Courtesy Dr. W. D. Cheney, Lansing, Michigan.)

Melorheostosis

This rare disorder of unknown origin can occur at any age. It exhibits a slow chronic course in adults but progresses rapidly in children. Soft tissue contractures and deformities of the hands and feet are common, often preceding the bone changes.

The peculiar bone sclerosis or hyperostosis is usually confined to one side of a bone. Multiple long bones of the extremities are usually affected. Involvement is often predominantly or entirely unilateral.

Radiographically, irregular linear bone sclerosis of the inner cortex projects into the medullary cavity. The appearance is characteristic; the resemblance to wax drippings is responsible for the term *melorheostosis.*

In membranous bone there may be small, dense, irregular sclerotic deposits resembling osteopoikilosis.[41, 42]

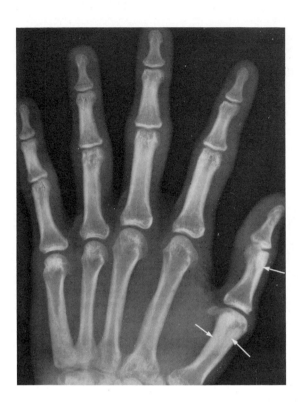

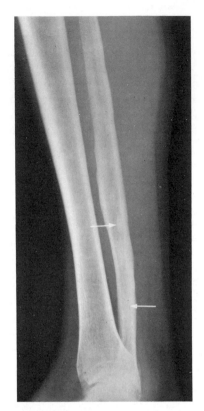

Figure 17–28 **Melorheostosis in Young Adult.** Irregular and patchy cortical thickening is seen in several bones of the hand, ulna, and fibula *(arrows).* Note the usual confinement to one side of a bone and the projection of the thickened cortex into the medullary cavity. Involvement was bilateral but considerably more marked in the left upper extremity and the right lower extremity. Pain in the hand was the only symptom.

This roentgen picture is characteristic and diagnostic.

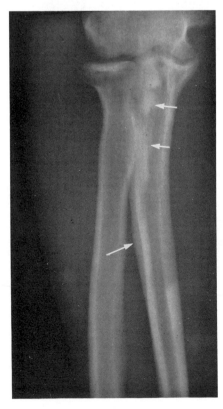

Osteopoikilosis

In this asymptomatic hereditary and familial condition, small foci of bone sclerosis are found most often in the pelvis, tarsal and carpal bones, and the epiphyses and metaphyses of the long bones. The sclerotic lesions are round or oval and vary from a few millimeters to several centimers in diameter. The involved bones have a characteristic speckled appearance.

The condition is not progressive. Although it is asymptomatic, osteopoikilosis may be associated with cutaneous abnormalities.[43]

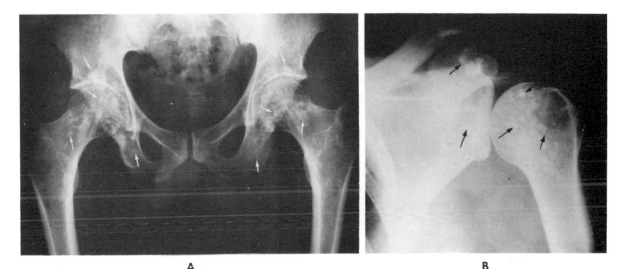

A   B

Figure 17–29   **Osteopoikilosis.**

A, Numerous round and ovoid islands of bone density are seen in both femoral heads and necks, and to a lesser extent in the pelvic bones *(arrows).*

B, Similar bone islands are present in the humeral heads and articular ends of the scapulae *(arrows).*

Pycnodysostosis

This syndrome consists of short stature, dysplasia of the skull and clavicles, and aplasia or dysplasia of the distal phalanges and tufts. The most constant and characteristic finding is increased density of all the bones. The dense long bones have a narrowed but discernible medullary cavity. Distinction from osteopetrosis may be difficult when based on the bone appearance alone.

The base of the skull is thickened, and widened sutures and wormian bones are frequent.[44, 45]

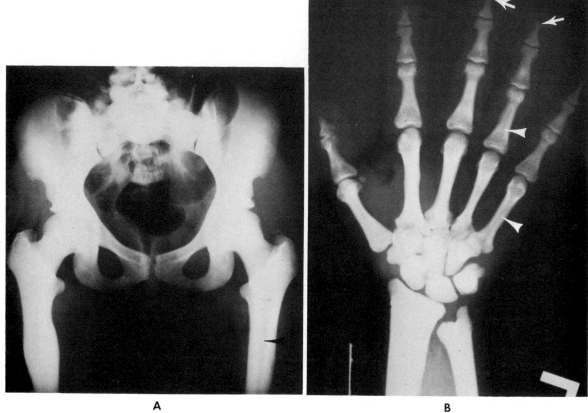

A   **B**

Figure 17–30   **Pycnodysostosis in 15 Year Old Girl.**

    A and *B,* All the bones are extremely dense. The medullary cavities of the long bones *(arrowheads)* are greatly narrowed by the thickened cortices but are not completely obliterated as in osteopetrosis. Tapering of the distal phalanges and absent tufts *(arrows)* are characteristic of pycnodysostosis.

Metaphyseal Dysplasia (Pyle's Disease)

    In this disturbance there are flask-like widenings of the metaphyses and adjacent diaphyses of the long bones. Medullary widening and diminished bone density are usually associated. Hyperostosis of the craniofacial bones and genu valgum are commonly seen.[46, 47]

Cleidocranial Dysostosis

    This hereditary defect is characterized by aplasia of the clavicles, delayed closure of skull sutures, wormian skull bones, and often defective ossification of the pubic and ischial bones. Other associated skeletal abnormalities often encountered include hemivertebrae, spondylosis, lateral notching of the femoral head epiphysis, and pointed terminal tufts in the hands.

    Both clavicles are totally or partially absent, a virtually pathognomonic finding. The thorax is almost always bell-shaped. The associated skull dysplasia and defective ossification of the symphysis pubis are found in most cases.[48, 49]

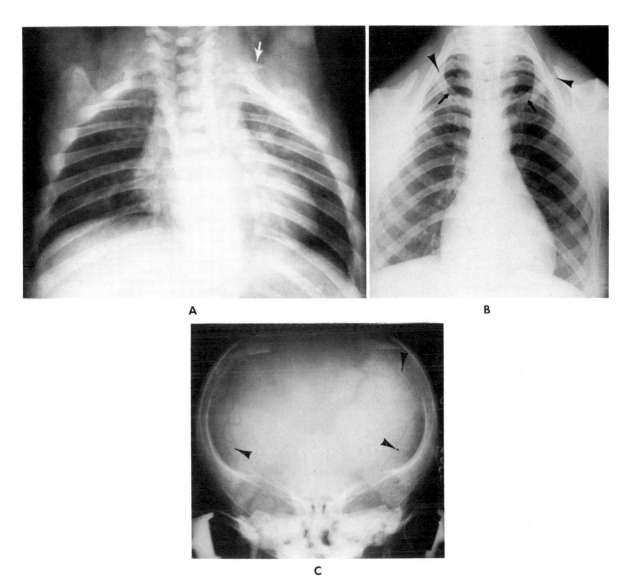

A

B

C

Figure 17–31 **Cleidocranial Dysostosis in Father and Child.**

A, Except for a rudimentary fragment on the left *(arrow)*, both clavicles are absent in the infant.

B, Both clavicles of the father are short and rudimentary *(black arrows),* and their lateral ends *(arrowheads)* do not reach the acromion processes of the scapulae. The upper thorax is tapered and narrow; both scapulae are more medial than normal.

C, Multiple irregular sutures of wormian bones *(arrowheads)* are seen through the infant's skull.

Progressive Diaphyseal Dysplasia (Engelmann's Disease)

A wide-based waddle gait and inability to gain weight during infancy are the salient features of this disease. Crippling bone deformities sometimes occur.

The diaphyses of the long bones reveal symmetric endosteal and periosteal cortical thickening, leading to progressive broadening of the shafts. Involvement extends from midshaft toward the bone ends, but the metaphyses and epiphyses usually remain unaffected. The hands, feet, ribs, and scapulae are not involved. The clavicles, cervical vertebrae, and calvarium are occasionally affected.[50, 51]

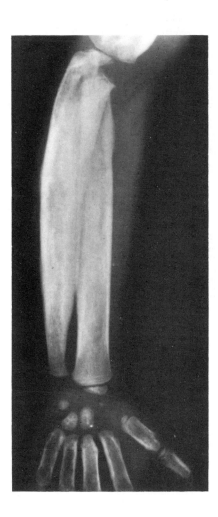

Figure 17–32 **Progressive Diaphyseal Dysplasia (Engelmann's Disease).** The shafts of the radius and ulna are widened and fusiform owing to endosteal and periosteal new bone formation. The medullary cavity of the ulna is irregularly narrowed. The metaphyses and epiphyses are not involved. (Courtesy Dr. E. B. D. Neuhauser, Children's Hospital Medical Center, Boston, Massachusetts. *In* Aegerter, E., and Kirkpatrick, J. A.: *Orthopedic Diseases.* 4th ed. Philadelphia, W. B. Saunders Co., 1975.)

Osteo-Onychodysostosis (Nail-Patella Syndrome, Fong's Disease)

This disorder is characterized by hypoplastic or absent patellae, dysplastic nails, elbow deformities, and posterior iliac horns. The latter are seen in 80 per cent of cases and are diagnostic, since they apparently do not occur in any other condition. The horns are asymptomatic bilateral bony outgrowths, occasionally capped by an epiphysis. The iliac crests are often flared, with prominent anterior superior spines.

The elbow deformity is due to hypoplasia of the radial head and capitellum. Other skeletal anomalies may be present.

Renal failure may occur in later life.[52, 53]

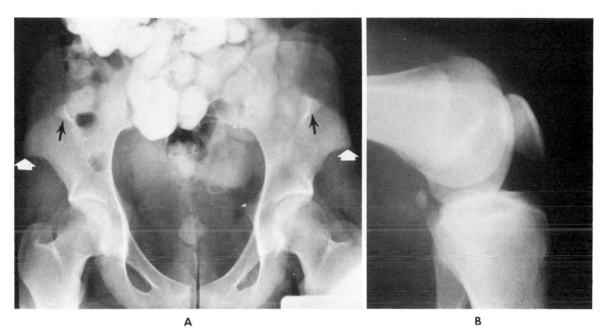

A   B

Figure 17–33   **Osteo-Onychodysostosis (Fong's Disease).**

A, There are characteristic bony "horns" (*black arrows*) arising from the posterior ilia. The pelvis is abnormally flared, and the anterior superior spines (*white arrows*) are unusually prominent.

B, The patella is hypoplastic and small for a 19 year old girl.

Chondroectodermal Dysplasia (Ellis-van Creveld Syndrome)

This condition is characterized clinically by shortening of the tubular bones, ectodermal dysplasia, polydactyly, and, frequently, congenital heart disease. It may be mistaken for achondroplasia because of the shortness of the extremities.

The most constant findings are shortening and deformities of the tubular bones of the extremities, polydactyly, and fusion of the carpal bones, although a variety of other malformations in the metaphyseal-epiphyseal area may result. Hypoplasia of dental structures is a fairly common finding. The spine is usually normal.

Generally, the thorax is elongated but otherwise normal. Sometimes, however, the thorax is narrow and immobile, indistinguishable from the changes in asphyxiating thoracic dystrophy.[54, 55]

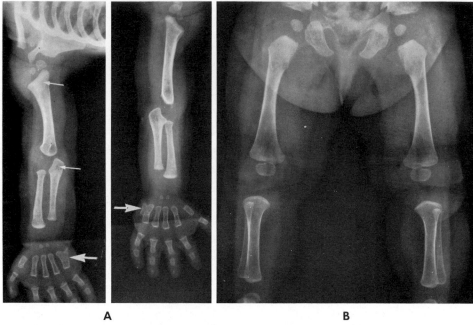

A   **B**

Figure 17–34   **Chondroectodermal Dysplasia (Ellis-van Creveld Syndrome).**

A, In a 9 month old infant, both radii and ulnae are short and consequently appear rather wide, the humeri are abnormally short, and the proximal ends of the humeri and ulnae are widened (*small arrows*). There is fusion of the fifth and a supernumerary sixth metacarpal in each hand (*large arrows*); the sixth finger on each hand had been amputated earlier. Two tiny carpal centers are demonstrated in each wrist; the extensive fusion of the carpal bones occurs after complete carpal ossification.

B, Both tibiae and fibulae are short and therefore appear to be wide. The femora are also shortened.

In achondroplasia, which resembles the Ellis–van Creveld syndrome clinically and radiographically, the humeri and femora are more shortened than the bones of the leg or forearm; whereas in chondroectodermal dysplasia the opposite occurs, and the distal long bones of the extremities are more shortened than the humeri and femora.

Familial Pachydermoperiostosis (Touraine-Solente-Golé Syndrome, Familial Hypertrophic Osteoarthropathy)

A familial form of osteoarthropathy, pachydermoperiostosis (Touraine-Solente-Golé syndrome) affects mainly male adolescents. Irregular subperiosteal ossification begins most often in distal ends of long bones, more marked in the vicinity of tendon and ligament insertions. The bones become progressively widened and irregular as the periosteal new bone merges with the cortex. Clubbing of the fingers and thickening of the facial skin are usually associated. The paranasal sinuses are often enlarged. The condition becomes stationary after several years and is not associated with neoplastic disease.

A forme fruste has been encountered in which the clinical features of pachydermoperiostosis are seen, but with little or no periosteal overgrowth.[56-59]

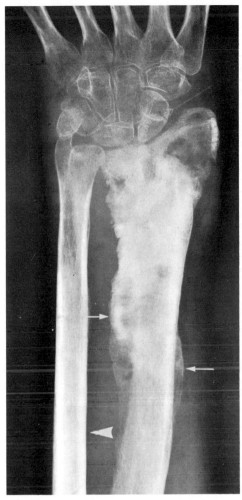

Figure 17–35 **Pachydermoperiostosis (Touraine-Solente-Golé Syndrome).** The overall density of the distal radius is increased as a result of multiple layering of the periosteum. The outer aspect of the periosteal new bone has a lacy irregularity (*arrows*); involvement is much less pronounced in the ulna (*arrowhead*).

Hyperphosphatasia

In this rare childhood condition, a high alkaline phosphatase may be associated with thickened cortices in long bones and skull thickening resembling Paget's disease. Occasionally, many of the vertebral bodies are flattened (vertebra plana).

Some authors believe this condition to be juvenile Paget's disease.[60]

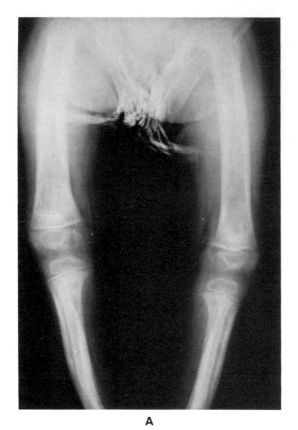

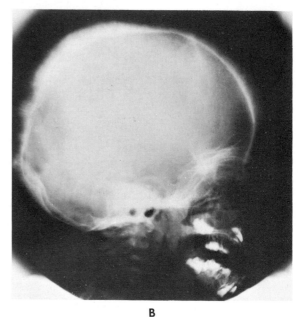

A   B

Figure 17–36 **Hyperphosphatasia.**

A, The medullary cavities are widened and the femoral cortices are thickened and dense.
B, The skull tables are thickened with scattered irregular areas of sclerosis, resembling Paget's disease. Some believe hyperphosphatasia represents juvenile Paget's disease.
(Courtesy Dr. L. Verano, Hershey Medical Center, Hershey, Pennsylvania. *In* Aegerter, E., and Kirkpatrick, J. A.: *Orthopedic Diseases.* 4th ed. Philadelphia, W. B. Saunders Co., 1975.)

OTHER BONE DISTURBANCES

Osteitis Deformans (Paget's Disease)

This common chronic disease of the adult skeleton is characterized both by loss of bone substance and by increased bone formation and repair, leading to enlargement and deformity. Both phases usually coexist, but the sclerotic changes most often predominate. Onset is usually in the fifth or sixth decade, and males are more frequently affected. Progression is slow and multiple bones are usually involved, particularly the pelvis, proximal femora, skull, tibia, and vertebrae. Infrequently, a solitary bone is involved (monostotic form).

Radiographically, early Paget's disease may be osteoporotic or sclerotic, but the fully developed form is predominantly sclerotic. The rarer osteoporotic form occurs most often in the skull, producing a sharply demarcated zone of decreased density with loss of bone detail (osteoporosis circumscripta cranii). The anterior portion of the skull is usually affected. When the osteoporotic form occurs in long bones, the area frequently terminates in a point or V.

In the more common sclerotic form the trabeculae are thickened and dense. The cortex is also thickened, a highly characteristic finding. Cyst-like areas can appear between the thickened trabeculae. Despite the increased radiographic density, the bones are soft and may become deformed or bowed. Pseudofractures occasionally occur, usually on the convex side of a bowed bone. The combination of cortical thickening and coarse dense trabeculation interspersed with lucent areas is diagnostic.

The pelvis is the most common and often the initial site of the disease. Cortical thickening adjacent to the pelvic inlet may be the earliest finding. In advanced disease the cortical thickening will distinguish Paget's disease from osteoblastic metastases to the pelvis. Vertebral involvement leads to a dense, somewhat expanded body. If vertebral involvement is solitary, the marginal thickening will distinguish Paget's disease from the dense vertebra of Hodgkin's disease, lymphosarcoma, hemangioma, or osteoblastic metastases. Pathologic vertebral fractures can occur but are relatively rare.

A serious but fortunately infrequent complication is sarcomatous degeneration, most often a chondrosarcoma but occasionally a fibrosarcoma or an osteogenic sarcoma. Another complication in far-advanced Paget's disease is cardiac enlargement and vascular engorgement (high output heart) due to widespread arteriovenous shunts in the diseased bones.

Central nervous system symptoms occasionally occur and are due to root compression by expanded vertebrae or from the basilar impression that is often encountered in advanced disease of the skull.[61-63]

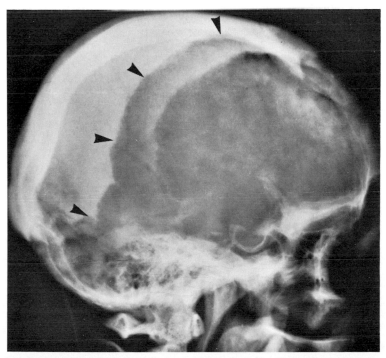

Figure 17–37   **Osteitis Deformans (Paget's Disease): Osteoporosis Circumscripta Cranii.**   In lateral view there is a sharply demarcated area of lucency of the anterior two thirds of the skull *(arrowheads)*. Bony details are lacking in this region. The picture is typical of the osteoporotic phase of Paget's disease. Eventually the more characteristic bone changes of Paget's disease develop.

DISEASES OF BONE

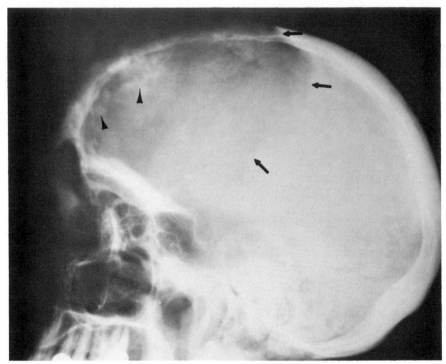

Figure 17–38 **Osteitis Deformans: Mixed Osteoporotic and Productive Stage.** In addition to a sharply marginated osteoporosis circumscripta of the anterior skull *(arrows),* there are characteristic "cotton wool" sclerotic densities *(arrowheads).*

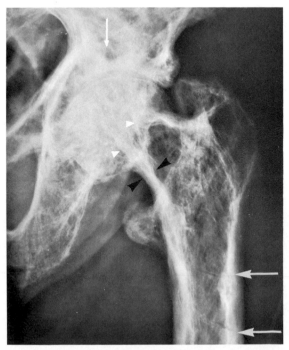

Figure 17–39 **Osteitis Deformans: Femur and Pelvis: Pseudofractures.** There is marked cortical thickening *(black arrowheads)* with dense coarse trabeculae *(white arrowheads)* interspersed with lucencies—all characteristics of Paget's disease. In the pelvis there is sclerosis of bone, cortical thickening, and medullary lucencies *(small arrow).* There are several pseudofractures in the femur *(large arrows);* when associated with the typical appearance of Paget's disease they can be differentiated from the pseudofractures of osteomalacia.

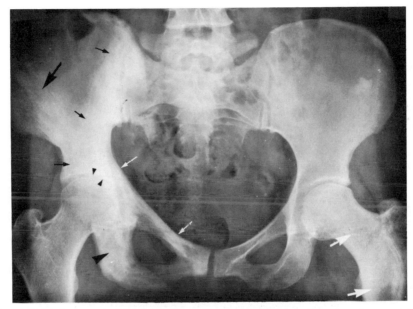

Figure 17-40 **Osteitis Deformans of Pelvis: Characteristic Findings.** The involvement is predominantly right-sided.

The inner aspects of the innominate and pubic bones show thickened cortex *(small white arrows)*; this portion of the bony pelvic inlet has become flattened, making the inlet asymmetric.

The ischial bone contains thick sclerotic trabeculae, and the entire bone is widened *(large black arrowhead)*. Sclerotic changes in the ilium extend down the medial side *(small black arrows)* to the hip joint. The expansion of bone has somewhat narrowed the joint space of the hip *(small black arrowheads)*. The wing of the ilium also contains coarsened trabeculae *(large black arrow)*.

These bony changes in the right pelvis are most apparent when compared to the left side. Incidentally, the left femoral neck and shaft are involved *(large white arrows)*.

The pelvis is the most common and often the earliest site of Paget's disease. The characteristic features of cortical thickening, trabecular coarsening and sclerosis, and widening of the affected bone are illustrated by the above patient.

The cortical thickening associated with Paget's disease will help differentiate it from osteoblastic metastasis.

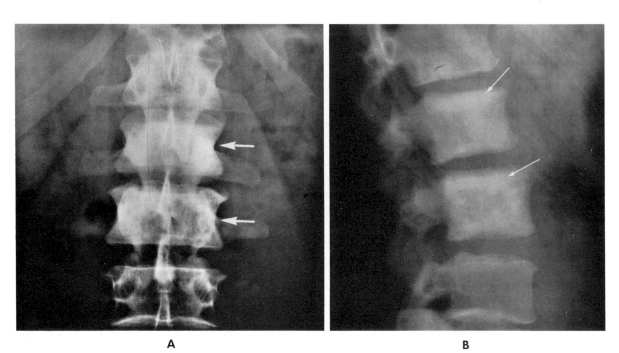

A   B

Figure 17–41 **Osteitis Deformans: Involvement Confined to Two Vertebrae.**   Anteroposterior and lateral views of the upper lumbar spine disclose increased density of L2 and L3 *(arrows)*. The posterior elements are not involved. On lateral view, it is apparent that the cortical margins are the principal sites of the sclerosis *(arrows)*. Complete skeletal survey disclosed no other osseous involvement.

In vertebral involvement with Paget's disease, the dimensions of the vertebral body frequently increase as the cortical sclerosis and thickening progresses. The cortical sclerosis and increase in dimension will aid in distinguishing a solitary dense vertebra of Paget's disease from a solitary dense vertebra due to lymphosarcoma, Hodgkin's disease, or osteoblastic metastatic disease. In the latter group, there is no cortical thickening, there is usually no increase in vertebral size, and the sclerosis is almost always medullary.

Pathologic fracture of a Paget's vertebra can occur, but is uncommon.

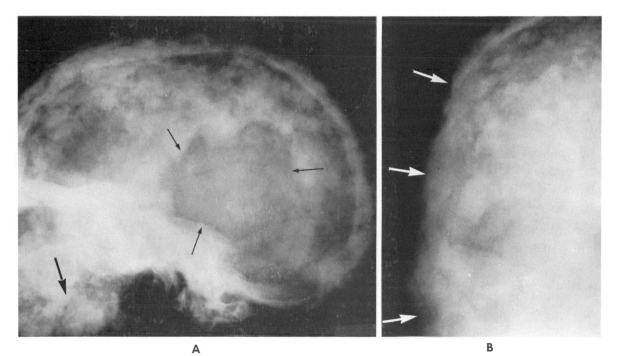

A   B

Figure 17–42 **Advanced Osteitis Deformans of Skull with Secondary Osteochondrosarcoma.**

A, There are characteristic sclerotic patches and thickening of the tables indicative of Paget's disease. Even the mandible *(large arrow)* is extensively involved. A large irregular defect *(small arrow)* is seen in the posterior parietal area, the site of a soft tissue tumor.

B, On anteroposterior view there is irregular destruction of both skull tables in the right parietal area *(arrows).* A soft tissue mass was present. This was a huge osteochondrosarcoma.

The rare complication of malignant "degeneration" is most often seen in well-advanced Paget's disease, and almost never in mild or minimal cases.

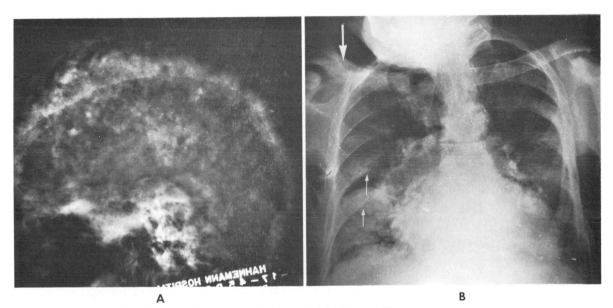

A   B

Figure 17–43 **Osteitis Deformans: Skull and Chest: High Output Heart.**

A, There is great thickening of the calvarium, particularly in the outer tables. Fragments of sclerotic bone are interspersed throughout areas of osteoporosis—the "cotton wool" appearance, which is characteristic of osteitis deformans.

B, Chest film discloses marked widening of the clavicle *(large arrow),* the acromial process, and the ribs *(small arrows).* The heart is greatly dilated because of high output failure. This is a very rare complication of Paget's disease and occurs only in far-advanced cases.

Fibrous Dysplasia of Bone

This condition is rare in infants. It begins in childhood and generally progresses until growth ceases. The serum calcium and phosphorus are normal; the alkaline phosphatase is sometimes elevated. The architecture of involved bones is distorted by replacement of the medullary bone by fibrous tissue, cysts, cartilage and osseous tissue.

Fibrous dysplasia may involve a single bone (monostotic) or multiple bones (polyostotic). When associated with pigmentary disorders and precocious puberty in females, it is called *Albright's syndrome.*

The monostotic form generally involves a femur, a tibia, a rib, or one of the facial bones, whereas the polyostotic form involves multiple bones with a tendency toward unilateral predominance.

The roentgenologic picture varies considerably. The medullary portions of the long bones usually have a homogeneous ground-glass appearance that blends with cortical bone without sharply demarcated edges. The medullary trabeculae are frequently obliterated, and the endosteal cortex is thinned and scalloped. Areas or bands of endosteal sclerosis may produce a multilocular appearance. The diaphysis may be expanded or widened. The expanding lesions are always covered by a thin shell of bone, a significant roentgen feature. Deformity of bone is common. Coxa vara — the shepherd's crook — is sometimes seen. Occasionally the sclerotic changes dominate the picture. Although the diaphyseal and metaphyseal areas are most often involved, lesions may extend into the epiphysis in children.

In the skull there may be lucent lesions or sclerotic lesions, or both. The lucent or cystic lesion is usually found in the calvarium and may be surrounded by a sclerotic zone. The diploë is widened and the outer tables bulge, but there is little or no inner table involvement. The sclerotic lesion usually involves the base of the skull, the sphenoid ridges, and the facial bones and is considered to be a form of leontiasis ossea (see p. 1366).[64-66]

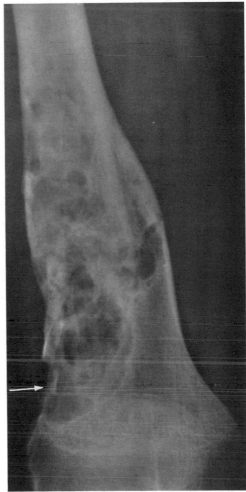

Figure 17–44 **Monostotic Fibrous Dysplasia of Femur.**
The distal femur is widened, and the cortex is thinned.
Numerous irregular bands of sclerosis traverse cyst-like
areas. The borders of the lesion are distinct. A pathologic
fracture has occurred *(arrow)*.

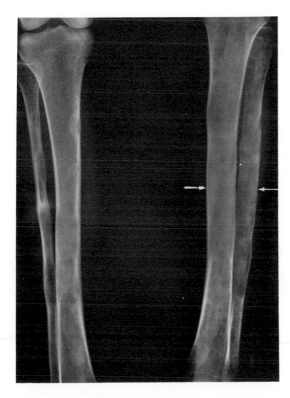

Figure 17–45 **Fibrous Dysplasia of Tibia and Fibula.**
The left side is involved to a greater degree than the
right. The diaphysis is widened *(arrows)*, the cortex is
thinned, and the bones have a homogeneous ground-
glass appearance.

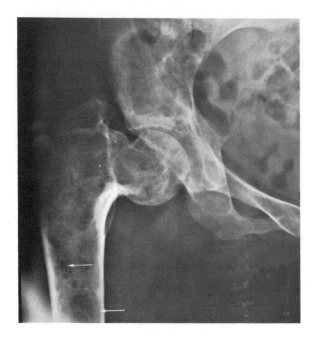

Figure 17–46 **Fibrous Dysplasia: Shepherd's Crook Deformity.** All the characteristics of fibrous dysplasia are demonstrated: pronounced bowing of the femoral neck, which has caused shortening of the leg, and multiple cystic areas of homogeneous lucency in the femur *(arrows).*

Leontiasis Ossea

This slowly progressive but benign facial deformity is usually due to fibrous dysplasia, although occasionally Paget's disease, osteopetrosis, or cranial metaphyseal dysplasia may be the cause. Marked thickening and sclerosis of the facial bones in some cases cause partial obliteration of the sinuses and orbits.

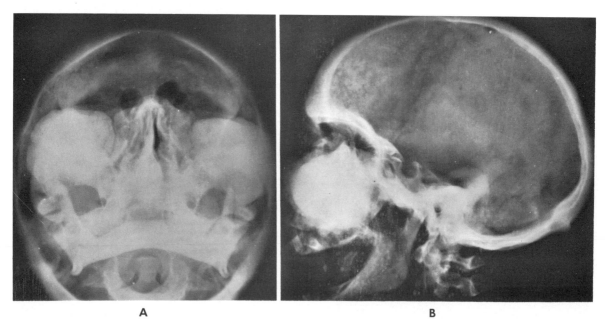

A   B

Figure 17–47 **Leontiasis Ossea.**

A, Anteroposterior view discloses homogeneously dense expansile lesions in both maxillary antra.

B, Lateral view demonstrates large sclerotic densities in the maxillary sinus and similar but less extensive sclerosis in the sphenoid ridges, frontal bones, and base of the skull.

Leontiasis ossea can sometimes occur without other skeletal lesions.

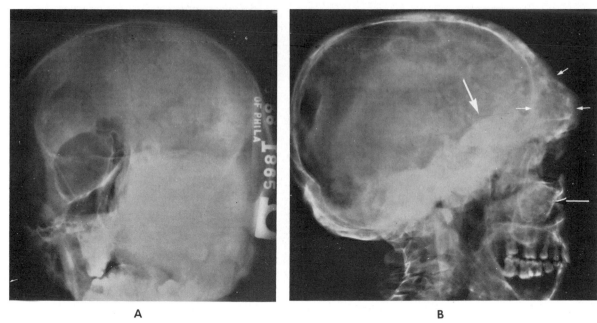

A   B

Figure 17–48   **Leontiasis Ossea in Fibrous Dysplasia: Unilateral Involvement of Skull and Facial Bones.**

A, Posteroanterior view discloses a sharply demarcated, homogeneous, dense, expansile lesion that has obliterated the left orbit and maxillary sinus.

B, Lateral view demonstrates sclerotic densities of the sphenoid wings *(large white arrow)*, maxilla *(black-white arrow)*, and base of the skull. There is mixed sclerosis and lucency in the skull tables, and expansion of the outer table in the frontal region *(small white arrows)*. The findings are characteristic of fibrous dysplasia. (Courtesy Dr. Arlyne Shockman, Veterans Administration Hospital, Philadelphia, Pennsylvania.)

Hypertrophic Osteoarthropathy

Pulmonary hypertrophic osteoarthropathy (Marie-Bamberger syndrome) is an infrequent acquired disorder characterized by periosteal bone formation secondary to primary and metastatic pulmonary malignancies, mesothelioma, mediastinal tumors, and chronic pulmonary disease. The majority of cases are seen in patients with carcinoma of the lung; osteoarthropathy may be the first roentgenologic clue to an unsuspected pulmonary neoplasm. Osteoarthropathy also occurs in a high proportion of cases of benign mesothelioma of the pleura and diaphragmatic neurolemmoma—both rare tumors. Other causes include diffuse chronic pulmonary diseases, especially cystic fibrosis; rarely, primary neoplasms of the upper gastrointestinal tract or portal cirrhosis are causative. The pathophysiologic mechanism of hypertrophic osteoarthropathy is not understood.

Radiographically, multiple layers of thin subperiosteal new bone appear along the shafts of long bones; the outer layers may be irregular. Symmetric involvement of the bones of the distal forearm and legs is the most frequent finding. Soft tissue clubbing of the digits may be associated, but without bone changes in the underlying distal phalanges. The periosteal changes of osteoarthropathy often disappear after removal of the associated neoplasm.[67, 68]

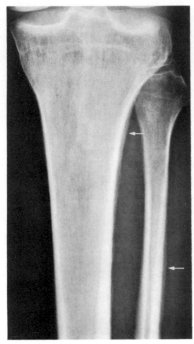 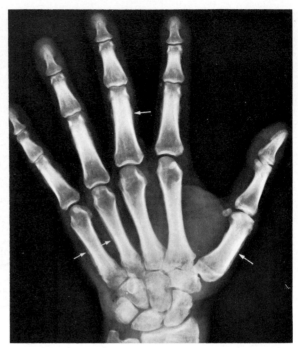

Figure 17–49 **Hypertrophic Osteoarthropathy with Bronchogenic Carcinoma.**   Layers of periosteal new bone (periostosis) have been deposited somewhat irregularly along the shafts of the tibia, fibula, metacarpals, and phalanges *(arrows)*. This patient had a bronchogenic carcinoma.

The periosteal reaction in hypertrophic osteoarthropathy occurs most often in the long bones distal to the knees and elbows. The lesions usually disappear after removal of the pulmonary neoplasm.

Hyperostosis Frontalis Interna

Thickening of the inner table of the frontal bone, occurring in about 15 per cent of normal women and in 3 per cent of normal men, is most common after the age of 40. It usually has no clinical significance, although there is a significantly higher prevalence in male patients with myotonia atrophica and in patients with the multiple nevoid basal cell carcinoma syndrome.

Skull radiograms demonstrate the smooth, symmetric, nodular bony plaques on the inner table of the frontal bone. On anteroposterior views these densities are seen on both sides of the midline. The midline groove, where the floor of the superior sagittal sinus is located, is unaffected. These hyperostoses usually have sharp margins. Extremely variable degrees of involvement are encountered.[69, 70]

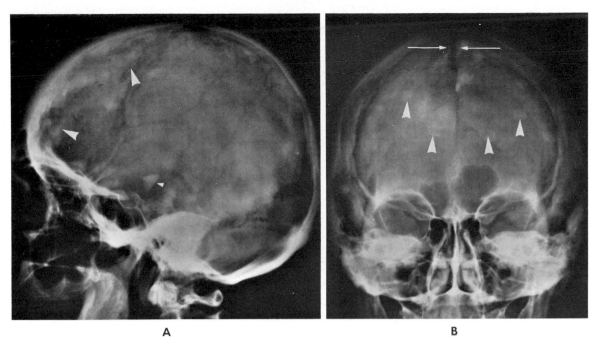

A   B

Figure 17–50 **Hyperostosis Frontalis Interna.**

A, Lateral view demonstrates nodular calcific densities in the inner table of the frontal bone *(large arrowheads)*. There is unrelated calcification of a dural plaque *(small arrowhead)*.

B, Frontal view discloses nodular densities *(arrowheads)* on both sides of the midline *(arrows)*.

TUMORS OF BONE

Radiologic evaluation of a solitary bone lesion can often determine whether the lesion is a tumor and, more important, whether it is benign or malignant. Occasionally the radiologist can suggest the specific histopathologic type, but more often he can merely narrow the diagnosis to a few likely possibilities. For accurate evaluation, both clinical and radiographic parameters must be utilized. These include age of the patient, clinical symptoms, location and extent of the lesion, sharpness of margination, condensation at margins, internal architecture, degree and type of periosteal reaction, presence and type of calcification or ossification, and presence or absence of soft tissue mass.

In general, a malignant bone tumor produces pain, is poorly and irregularly marginated, extends along the medullary cavity or subperiosteally, can break through the cortex to form a soft tissue mass, has a mottled destructive internal architecture, often contains irregular periosteal layering or spiculation at the tumor margins, and, if calcified, may show irregular deposits of density. A benign bone tumor is usually sharply marginated, often with sclerotic edges. It may thin and expand the cortex, without destruction. Periosteal reaction and soft tissue mass are usually absent. However, occasionally the radiographic appearance may suggest malignancy, particularly if pathologic fracture has occurred with reparative periosteal reaction.

In some benign and malignant primary bone tumors the radiographic features are sufficiently characteristic to suggest the correct histologic diagnosis. However, a metastatic lesion to bone is the most commonly encountered malignant bone lesion, and radiographically it can simulate almost any primary malignant tumor of bone. Lesions of the flat bones present the greatest difficulty in diagnosis, especially in the pelvis, where periosteal reaction and soft tissue mass are often difficult to recognize.

Benign Tumors

Osteochondroma (Osteocartilaginous Exostosis)

Osteochondroma is a common benign lesion that contains both bone and cartilage; the latter may frequently be calcified. It arises in childhood and continues to grow until general body growth ceases. Any juxta-epiphyseal area in a long bone may be affected, but the distal femur and proximal and distal tibia are the most frequent sites; the pelvis and scapula are also frequently involved. As a rule these lesions are asymptomatic unless they enlarge sufficiently to cause pressure symptoms or to interfere with function, or are subject to repeated trauma.

The solitary osteochondroma of a long bone has a true bony stalk, continuous with the adjacent cortex and growing away from the adjacent joint, and a bulbous irregular distal end resembling a cauliflower. The irregular cap consists of cartilage, some of which is usually calcified. Often, however, a considerable area beyond the calcification is noncalcified tumor; hence the lesion is frequently larger than it appears to be on the radiogram. The cartilaginous cap is potentially malignant, but this is a rare complication. In adults the cartilaginous portion tends to involute; growth or soft tissue calcification beyond the lesion may indicate beginning malignant change.

In the pelvis the osteochondroma appears as an irregular ball of calcification resembling a calcified uterine fibroid. Its stalk often cannot be identified.

Multiple osteochondromas are found in hereditary deforming chondrodysplasia (see p. 1346).[37, 71, 72]

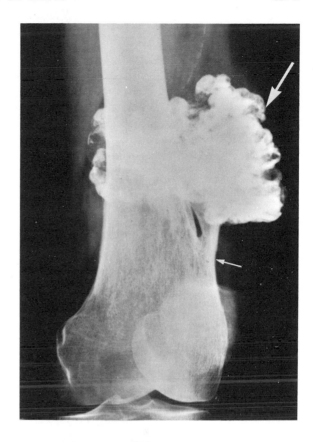

Figure 17–51 **Solitary Large Osteochondroma of Femur.** The stalk of the tumor *(small arrow)* contains normal appearing cortical and medullary bone. It is growing away from the joint, a characteristic of most osteochondromas in long bones. The bulk of the tumor is the irregularly calcified cartilaginous cap *(large arrow)*.

In long bones, an osteochondroma arises from the metaphyseal area and grows away from the joint, and its cartilaginous cap shows varying degrees of calcification. Growth ceases with skeletal maturation. Most osteochondromas are smaller and less densely calcified than the one shown here.

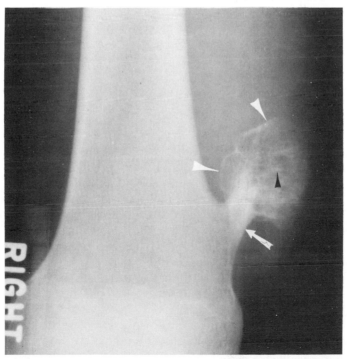

Figure 17–52 **Osteochondroma of Femur.** The stalk *(white arrow)*, which contains cortical and medullary bone, typically extends away from the knee joint. The bulbous portion contains bony trabeculae *(black arrowhead)* and a thin cortex *(white arrowheads)*. The latter is entirely covered with noncalcified and nonvisualized cartilage, in contrast to the heavily calcified cartilage of the osteochondroma of Figure 17–51.

Osteoma

Osteoma arises from membranous bone, contains no cartilage, and is considerably less common than osteochondroma. It is usually found in the skull, most often within a frontal or ethmoid sinus, or the orbit. Growth ceases after complete skeletal maturation. Radiographically the osteoma appears as a mass of dense bone with sharp borders; occasionally it becomes large and lobulated and may rarely erode the dura. Distinction from a calcified meningioma is sometimes difficult. Osteomas may be associated with colonic polyposis in Gardner's syndrome (see p. 1415).[37, 71, 73]

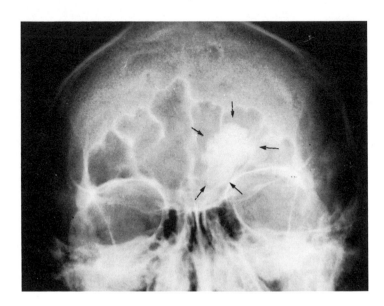

Figure 17–53 **Osteoma in Frontal Sinus.** A large, irregularly lobulated but sharply marginated mass of bony density *(arrows)* is seen within the left frontal sinus.

Osteoid Osteoma

The benign osteoid osteoma generally develops between the ages of 10 and 30, and is more frequent in males. The tibia or femur is the usual site, although any bone except the calvarium may be involved. Pain at night, generally relieved by aspirin, point tenderness, and occasionally limping are common symptoms. Vertebral lesions may cause back pain and scoliosis. Symptoms may be present for months before changes appear on roentgenograms.

There is usually a round or oval relatively radiolucent area generally less than 1 cm. in diameter located in or just beneath the cortex. This radiolucent nidus is usually surrounded by an area of reactive thickened bone that gives rise to a localized and circumscribed area of increased bone density. The lucent nidus may be obscured by the encasing sclerosis, and planigraphic studies may be needed for its demonstration. Surgical removal of the nidus is necessary for cure. The roentgenologic picture is generally characteristic and usually diagnostic. A localized chronic osteomyelitis, however, may sometimes present an identical appearance.

The rarer intramedullary osteoid osteoma may have little or no periosteal reaction, and roentgen identification of a small nidus in cancellous bone may be difficult or impossible.[74-76]

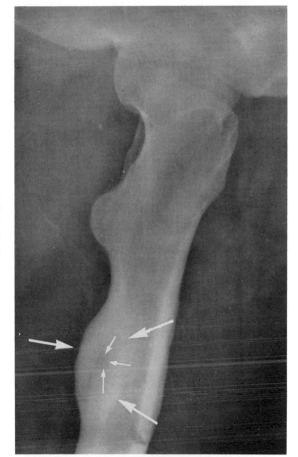

Figure 17–54 **Osteoid Osteoma.** A small area of relative lucency *(small arrows)* represents the nidus. There is marked reactive bone production in this area, producing increased density and thickening of the cortex and surrounding bone *(large arrows)*. The radiographic appearance is characteristic.

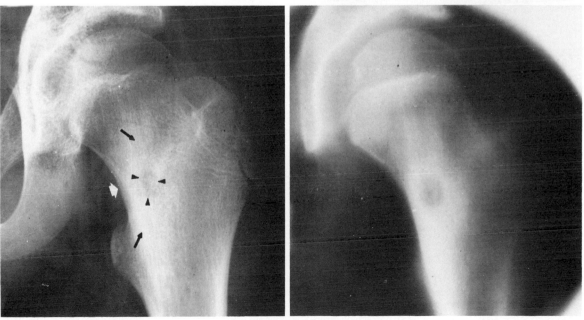

A   B

Figure 17–55 **Osteoid Osteoma: 13 Year Old Boy With Pain Around Hip.**

A, There is an ill-defined lucency *(black arrowheads)* within an area of sclerosis *(black arrows)*. Some periosteal new bone is apparent *(white arrow)*.

B, The tomogram more clearly depicts the sclerosis and its lucent nidus.

A small nidus of an osteoid osteoma within a dense sclerotic area can sometimes be identified only by tomography.

Benign Osteoblastoma

The majority (75 per cent) of these rare tumors occur between the ages of 10 and 20. Over half are found in the vertebral column, where they tend to be eccentric and to involve the neural arch or pedicle. Tubular bone involvement may be diaphyseal or metaphyseal, but the epiphysis is not involved. Local pain, tenderness, and soft tissue swelling are the most common symptoms. Nerve root or spinal cord symptoms sometimes occur.

Radiographically, the lesion is rather sharply demarcated. Although these tumors are predominantly lytic, there is usually some internal calcification, or even new bone formation. Rapid growth and cortical expansion are characteristic. Cortical erosion and soft tissue mass can occur; the latter is usually surrounded by a calcific shell, a somewhat unique appearance. Reactive sclerosis often occurs at the tumor border. At times the bizarre internal structure may simulate a malignant lesion. In the spine, if the lesion is expansile and entirely lytic it may closely resemble an aneurysmal bone cyst. In long bones the rare osteoblastoma is often mistaken for more common lesions such as giant cell tumor, osteogenic sarcoma, or chondrosarcoma.

Some pathologists consider the osteoblastoma to be a giant form of osteoid osteoma, but there are no significant radiographic similarities.[75, 77-79]

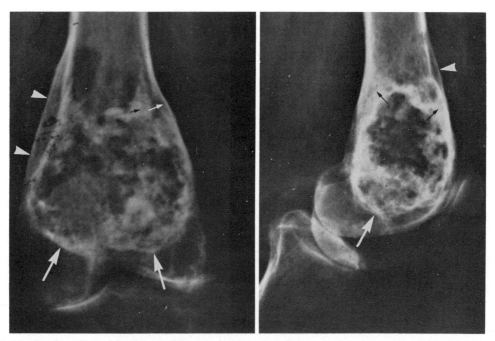

Figure 17–56   **Benign Osteoblastoma of Femur in Young Adult.**   Anteroposterior and lateral views of the lower femur disclose a large expanding lesion with a sharply demarcated and sclerotic lower border (*large arrows*). It contains numerous irregular areas of calcification of varying sizes. The surrounding bone shows some sclerosis (*black arrows*). The cortex adjacent to the upper portion of the tumor is expanded and thinned (*small white arrow*). The lesion has extended beyond the bone, and this soft tissue portion is bordered by a calcified shell (*arrowheads*) that simulates periosteal reaction.

An osteoblastoma in the epiphyseal area is virtually indistinguishable from a chondroblastoma. A chondrosarcoma may also produce a similar appearance.

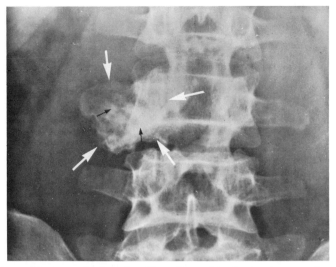

Figure 17–57 **Benign Osteoblastoma in Lumbar Vertebra.** The lesion has produced smooth expansion of the transverse process *(large arrows).* Irregular areas of calcification and sclerosis *(small arrows)* within the lesion suggest the diagnosis.

A purely lytic osteoblastoma may resemble an aneurysmal bone cyst. (Courtesy Dr. J. R. Stewart, Rochester, Minnesota.)

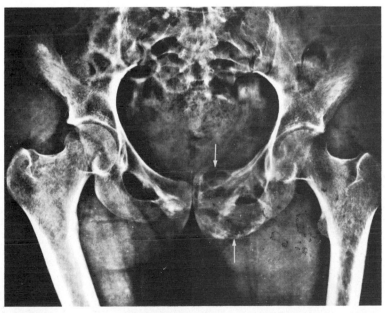

Figure 17–58 **Benign Osteoblastoma of Pubic Bone.** There is a large, sharply circumscribed cystic lesion causing expansion of the upper and lower borders of the left pubic bone *(arrows).* No calcification is evident within the lesion. The appearance is nonspecific, and the lesion cannot be distinguished from other cystic expansile lytic lesions.

Giant-Cell Tumor

Giant-cell tumor is a distinct clinical and pathologic entity. Although generally benign, it may be malignant. The vast majority are encountered in young adults after the epiphyses have closed. Over half the lesions occur around the knee; other frequent locations are the ulna, radius, and humerus. Pain and a palpable mass may develop. The pelvis and sacrum are the most common flat bones involved. Vertebral lesions have been reported and are difficult to distinguish from aneurysmal bone cyst.

Radiographically there is usually a completely lytic lesion in the epiphyseal area of a tubular bone; the epiphysis is invariably closed. The lesion is often eccentric and the cortex becomes expanded and thinned, but no periosteal new bone formation is seen unless a fracture occurs. Bony condensation at the margins is absent, making the border somewhat indistinct, although the transition from tumor to normal bone is abrupt. The lesion may extend to the articular margin, but it never invades the joint. Pathologic fracture of the thinned cortex is fairly common.

Roentgenologic distinction from benign chondroblastoma, and rarely aneurysmal bone cyst and fibrosarcoma, all of which also can involve the epiphyseal area, is sometimes difficult.

The infrequent giant-cell tumor in a flat bone produces a nonspecific, fairly sharply marginated lytic area; cortical expansion occurs in the larger lesions.

The roentgen appearance of malignant giant-cell tumor can be quite similar to benign giant-cell tumor, but the tumor's extension through the cortex to produce a soft tissue mass is highly suggestive of its malignant nature. Eventually, irregular bone destruction and some periosteal reaction may develop.[80, 81]

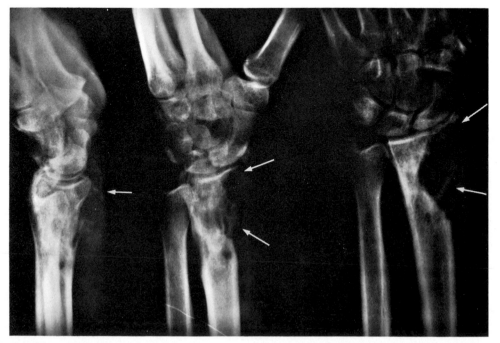

Figure 17–59 **Giant-Cell Tumor.** An eccentric lytic lesion of the epiphyseal end of the radius has caused expansion and destruction of the cortex *(arrows)*. The inner border is clearly demarcated. The location and appearance of the lesion are typical; sclerotic areas are from an old healed fracture. Giant-cell lesions rarely occur in persons under 20 years of age.

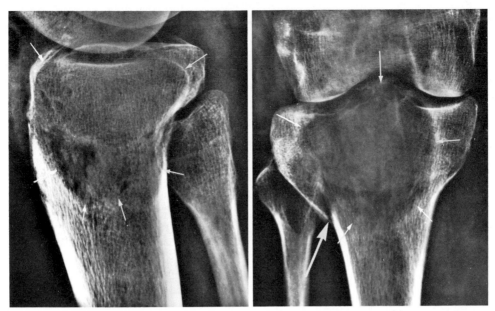

Figure 17–60 **Large Giant-Cell Tumor of Proximal Tibia.** A large, sharply demarcated area of lysis at the epiphyseal end of the tibia extends as far as the subarticular bone *(small arrows)*. The lytic lesion contains no trabeculation, and the cortex is thinned. Anteroposterior view discloses a pathologic cortical fracture *(large arrow).*

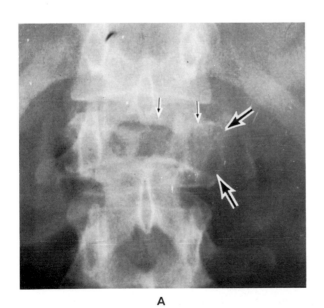

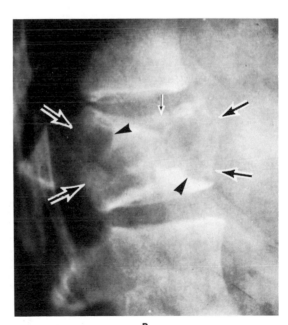

A   B

Figure 17–61 **Giant-Cell Tumor of First Lumbar Body.**

A 43 year old woman had been complaining of lumbar pain for five months.

A, Anteroposterior view shows compression of the left superior margin of the first lumbar body *(small arrows)* and a lytic expansion of its left lateral border *(large arrows)*. No paravertebral soft tissue mass was seen.

B, In lateral view there is lytic expansion of the anterior and posterior margins *(large arrows)*. The lytic areas are sharply marginated *(arrowheads)*. A pathologic compression fracture has depressed and thickened the superior margin *(small arrow)*.

Radiologically the lesion resembled an aneurysmal bone cyst; metastatic malignancy was also considered. A simple giant-cell tumor was found at surgery.

Enchondroma

These benign, slow-growing cartilaginous tumors occur most frequently in children and young adults. The bones of the hands and feet, especially the phalanges of the hand, are the most common sites. The lesions are often multiple. In other long bones, solitary lesions are the rule.

Usually these tumors are intramedullary and originate in the metaphyseal area. The central round or oval lucent area is sharply circumscribed and often contains flocculent calcification. The cortex may be expanded and thinned, and the endosteal cortex may become scalloped. This may deform the bone. Pathologic fracture may further alter the bone contour.

In larger bones the lesion may sometimes appear as spotty amorphous intramedullary calcification without bone lysis; radiographically, this resembles a calcified bone infarct.

Multiple enchondromas affecting multiple long bones occur in *Ollier's dyschondroplasia* (p. 1347) and in *Maffucci's syndrome* (see below).[37, 82]

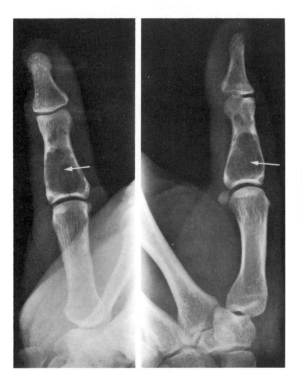

Figure 17–62 **Enchondroma of Thumb.** There is a lytic, expanded, sharply circumscribed lesion in the proximal phalanx *(arrows)*. The cortex is thinned but intact. No calcification is present. The appearance is fairly characteristic.

Maffucci's Syndrome

Enchondromatosis with soft tissue hemangiomatosis represents a distinct entity, although the association of these two conditions may be coincidental. The hemangiomas and phlebectasia may occur anywhere in the subcutaneous tissues or soft tissues, and appear unrelated to the location of the bony lesions.

In addition to the radiographic findings of Ollier's disease, multiple rounded calcific phleboliths are usually seen in the soft tissue hemangiomas, and the combination identifies the syndrome. Secondary chondrosarcoma or angiosarcoma may develop in about 15 per cent of cases.[83-85]

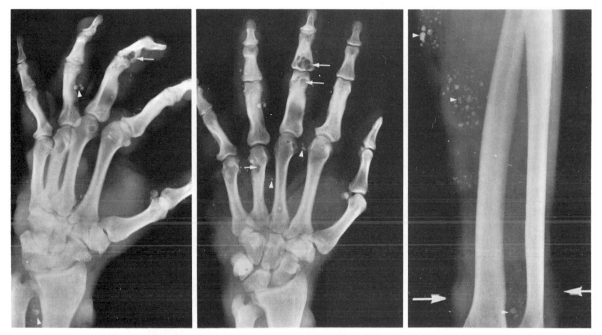

Figure 17–63 **Maffucci's Syndrome.** There are several enchondromas *(small arrows)* in the bones of the hand, and numerous phleboliths within multiple hemangiomas in the subcutaneous tissues of the fingers and forearm *(arrowheads)*. Hemangiomas have caused irregularity and swelling of the subcutaneous tissue *(large arrows)*.

Chondroblastoma

Chondroblastoma is a rare benign tumor of cartilaginous origin that occurs predominantly in adolescent males. It is found in the epiphyseal centers of the femur, tibia, or humerus. The greater tuberosity of the humerus and the greater trochanter of the femur are among the favorite sites. Pain, local swelling, and limitation of motion are the usual initial symptoms. It appears as a well-demarcated round or oval area of relative lucency in the epiphysis, most often with mottled areas of calcification. A thin sclerotic border usually surrounds the lesion. Periosteal reaction is rare. Pathologic fracture almost never occurs.

Giant-cell tumor and occasionally chondrosarcoma can resemble the chondroblastoma. In a flat bone, chondroblastoma is rare and difficult to diagnose.[86-88]

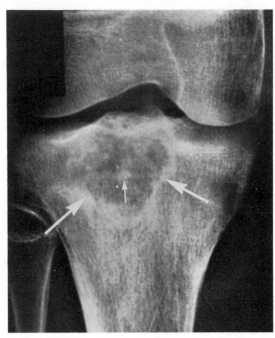

Figure 17–64 **Chondroblastoma in Adolescent Male.** A radiolucent lesion in the epiphyseal end of the tibia has a thin margin of sclerosis *(large arrows)* and numerous small areas of internal calcification *(small arrow).* The age of the patient, the location of the tumor, and the calcification are characteristic of chondroblastoma, but it cannot be radiographically distinguished from an osteoblastoma.

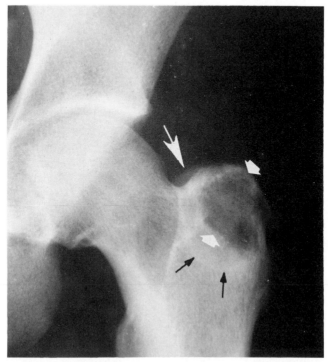

Figure 17–65 **Chondroblastoma of Femur in 17 Year Old Boy.** The somewhat mottled, well-circum-scribed lytic lesion in the greater trochanter has a sclerotic border *(short white arrows).* The posterior portion of the lesion is more expansile *(large white arrow),* producing a second medial sclerotic rim *(black arrows).*

An epiphyseal lytic lesion with sclerotic borders and possibly areas of calcification, if occurring in an adolescent male, should suggest chondroblastoma.

Chondromyxoid Fibroma

This benign tumor most frequently occurs in individuals under 30 years of age; there is no significant sex predominance. In descending order of frequency, the bones affected are the tibia, the femur, the pelvis, and the long bones of the upper extremities. Pain is the most constant symptom.

Chondromyxoid fibroma usually appears as a well-defined, eccentric, ovoid lucency generally originating in the metaphyseal area but may extend into the epiphyseal area after closure. The center appears rarefied, and the overlying cortex is thinned and bulges. Actual cortical destruction may occur without producing periosteal reaction. The border of the lesion is usually sclerotic and may be scalloped. Trabeculation is often seen, but calcification is surprisingly rare in the cartilaginous matrix. The rarer cortical chondromyxoid fibroma may present as a lytic lesion within an area of cortical thickening in a diaphysis.

In the radiographic differential diagnosis, giant cell tumor, aneurysmal bone cyst, benign chondroblastoma, simple bone cyst, and nonossifying fibroma must be considered.[41, 89, 90]

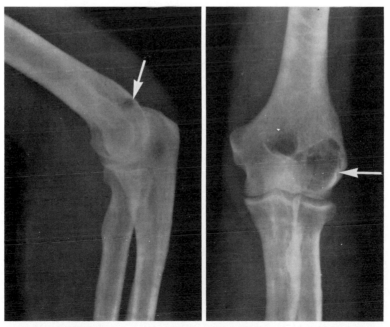

Figure 17-66 **Chondromyxoid Fibroma.** There is an eccentric, sharply demarcated lucency with a sclerotic margin in the metaphyseal and epiphyseal aspect of the distal femur *(arrows)*. Some expansion of bone has occurred, and there are a few trabeculae in the lesion.

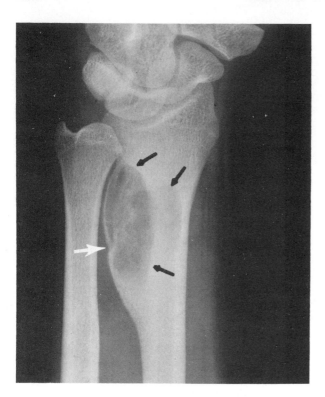

Figure 17–67 **Chondromyxoid Fibroma.** The circumscribed lytic lesion in the metaphysis of the radius shows characteristic eccentricity, marked cortical expansion with a break in the cortex *(white arrow)*, no periosteal reaction, and internal trabeculation. The lateral border is scalloped and mildly sclerotic *(black arrows)*.

The location and radiographic appearance are quite characteristic.

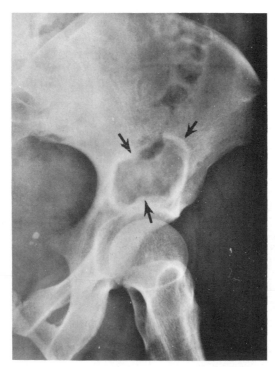

Figure 17–68 **Chondromyxoid Fibroma.** The large lytic lesion above the acetabulum is scalloped with a thick sclerotic border *(arrows)*. Some areas of density are present within the lesion.

Scalloping and a sclerotic border are characteristic of a chondromyxoid fibroma in a flat bone.

Nonossifying Fibroma

Nonossifying fibroma is a benign localized defect in enchondral bone growth, and is generally found in older children and young adults. The lower femur and upper or lower tibia or fibula are favored sites.

The lesion appears as a radiolucent defect, eccentrically placed in the metaphyses, close to the cortex and surrounded by a thin, even sclerotic layer. The defect may be round or oval or scalloped, with its long axis paralleling the long axis of the shaft. Although it is usually small, it may enlarge sufficiently to cause expansion of the adjacent cortex. Occasionally it may appear multiloculated. In thinner bones the entire width of the shaft may be involved. The radiographic appearance is usually characteristic.

Benign cortical defects have an identical roentgen appearance, but are usually smaller and less scalloped than the nonosteogenic fibroma. They arise from the inner cortex in the metaphyses of children, usually near the knee. These generally disappear before adolescence.[41, 91]

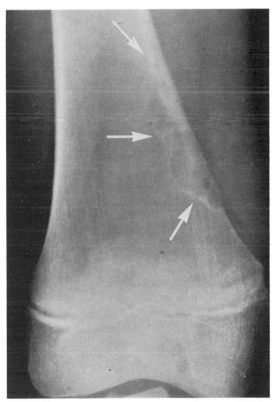

Figure 17–69 **Nonossifying Fibroma.** An eccentric proximal metaphyseal lesion has a sclerotic scalloped inner border *(arrows)*, a thin cortex, and a multilocular appearance. The long axis of the lesion corresponds to the long axis of the bone. The appearance is characteristic of a nonosteogenic fibroma.

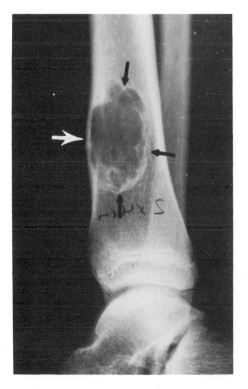

Figure 17–70 **Large Nonossifying Fibroma.** The lytic lesion in the lower tibia of a 13 year old girl is noncalcified, has a markedly scalloped and sclerotic border *(black arrows)*, is eccentrically located, and is slightly expanding the bone *(white arrow)*.

These are characteristic roentgen findings of a nonossifying fibroma.

Hemangioma of Bone

This benign tumor generally grows slowly. More than half are found in the skull and the spine; other less frequent sites are the ribs, long bones, and mandible. The lesion is usually solitary, but there may be multiple lesions scattered throughout the skeleton. Rarely, diffuse skeletal involvement is encountered.

In the skull the lesion appears as a round or oval rarefaction with fine bony striations producing a honeycomb appearance. There is a sharp, somewhat sclerotic outer margin. If the striations are coarse, the so-called sunburst pattern is seen. Expansion of the outer tables may occur.

In the vertebrae the hemangioma is usually solitary. It produces characteristic parallel vertical trabecular lines in the vertebral body. The cortex may be somewhat fuzzy but remains intact. The overall density of the body may be increased.

In the other bones the appearance is rather nonspecific and may resemble that of other benign or malignant lesions, including aneurysmal bone cyst, giant cell tumor, and osteogenic sarcoma. The lesions are primarily lytic and may involve any part of a long bone, most commonly the diaphysis. Usually the lesion is corticoperiosteal and tends to displace the cortex toward the medulla. Soft tissue hemangioma may secondarily involve bone, giving rise to smooth indentations or cortical erosions. Phleboliths in soft tissue masses strongly suggest hemangioma. In diffuse angiomatosis, the bone lesions resemble many other more common conditions such as myeloma, histiocytosis, or metastatic disease, but systemic symptoms are minimal or absent.[92, 93]

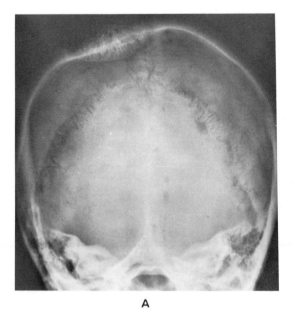 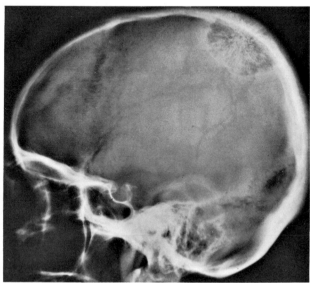

A   B

Figure 17–71 **Hemangioma of Skull.**

A, Occipital view demonstrates a round lucent area with coarse radiating striations in the parietal region. There is expansion of the outer table.

B, Lateral view discloses the lucency and the coarse sunburst pattern of the trabeculae.

The appearance is fairly characteristic.

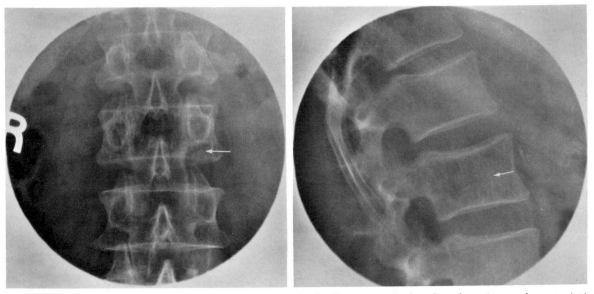

Figure 17–72 **Hemangioma of Vertebral Body.** Multiple, linear, vertical trabeculae give a characteristic appearance to this demineralized vertebral body *(arrows).* The cortex is of normal thickness and is intact. The pedicles, laminae, and spinous and transverse processes are normal. The appearance is typical of vertebral hemangioma.

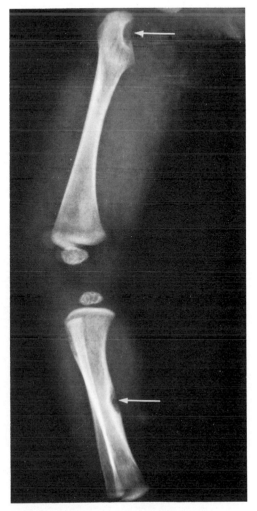

Figure 17–73 **Multiple Hemangiomas of Bone.** The subcortical defect of the femoral neck *(upper arrow)* has smooth borders; there is a similar lesion in the midtibia *(lower arrow).* The cortex around the tibial lesion is thickened.

The appearance of hemangiomas of the long bones is varied and nonspecific.

Neurofibroma

A neurofibroma usually does not arise from bone, but it may produce changes in an adjacent bone by direct pressure. Rarely, growth of the tumor into a bone produces a lytic cyst-like intraosseous defect. Neurofibromatosis of von Recklinghausen is a generalized disease and is discussed on page 1411.[94]

Massive Osteolysis (Disappearing Bones, Gorham's Disease)

This extremely rare disease usually has its onset in childhood or early adulthood and is characterized by a gradual and progressive regional loss of bone. It is apparently caused by a diffuse angiomatosis or lymphangiomatosis of bone. An entire bone or a group of bones may disappear. The shoulder girdle or pelvis is most often affected. Spontaneous arrest may occur, but without recalcification of the destroyed bones. Occasionally the angiomatous mass will invade the surrounding soft tissues. Associated chylous pleural effusion is a suggestive finding. There is usually no evidence of systemic disease or alterations of blood chemistry.

There is progressive loss of bone trabeculae and cortex in a number of contiguous bones, with eventual disappearance of these structures. The bone at the edge of the lesion may taper down to a cone-like spicule, a suggestive finding.

Lymphography may show stasis and partial obstruction of lymphatics in the involved area, with later contrast filling of the soft tissue masses and bone.[95-97]

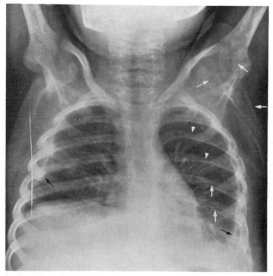

Figure 17–74 **Massive Osteolysis in a Child.** There is considerable loss of bone trabeculae in the left humerus, scapula, and a few ribs on the left *(white arrows)*. The upper borders of portions of the fourth and fifth ribs have been resorbed *(arrowheads)*. Diffuse angiomatosis (Gorham's disease) was the underlying disorder. The pelural reaction in the left chest *(black arrow)* is apparently due to involvement of the pleura; the cause of the right pleural thickening *(black arrow)* is uncertain.

Simple Bone Cyst (Unicameral Bone Cyst)

This benign lesion usually occurs in a metaphysis, most often in the proximal humerus or femur of the growing skeleton. It may be asymptomatic unless a pathologic fracture occurs. The lesion does not grow after general skeletal growth ceases.

Radiographically the lesion is a sharply demarcated, uniformly radiolucent defect. The cortex may be expanded and thinned, but it remains intact unless pathologic fracture supervenes. The lesion rarely becomes wider than the epiphyseal plate, but it can disturb the normal modeling of the bone. However, as the cyst becomes progressively more diaphyseal with skeletal growth, the modeling deformity is corrected.

Occasionally the cyst has scalloped borders and incomplete septa, giving it a somewhat multilocular appearance. Frequently, the cyst is wider at its metaphyseal end, and the length of the cyst is often greater than its width.

Periosteal reaction does not occur except as a reparative reaction to fracture. Some cysts will calcify and disappear after fracture.

The roentgen appearance is characteristic in long bones, but in a flat bone definitive diagnosis is difficult.[98, 99]

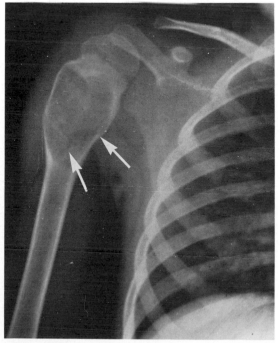

Figure 17–75 **Simple Bone Cyst.** A central lucent lesion in the metaphyseal area has distinct borders (*arrows*); the cortex is intact and somewhat expanded. The lesion is homogeneously lucent without trabeculation. The location and appearance of the lesion are characteristic of simple cyst, although expansion of the bone is unusual. With further growth of the skeleton, the cyst will become more diaphyseal in location.

Aneurysmal Bone Cyst

This benign lesion occurs most often in children and young adults and usually involves the metaphyseal area of long bones or the vertebrae. However, any flat or small tubular bone can be affected.

In the long bones, the smaller cysts are uniformly radiolucent, while larger lesions tend to become lobulated and trabeculated. Cortical expansion is frequent, and the cyst may expand eccentrically beyond the axis of the bone. Frequently, periosteal condensation and thickening occur at the lateral margin of the lesion. The intramedullary tissues are sharply marginated but without bony condensation, a finding that distinguishes aneurysmal bone cyst from chondromyxoid fibroma. If the lesion extends into an epiphysis, it resembles a giant-cell tumor.

In the vertebra, the posterior elements are usually affected, and generally there is expansion and ballooning of the bone, resembling a giant-cell tumor. Cord compression and neurologic symptoms sometimes occur. Myelography will demonstrate the extent of the compression.[75, 100-102]

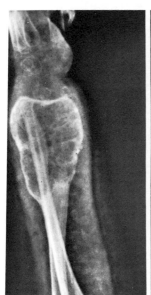
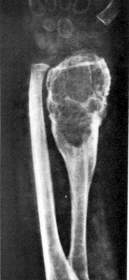

Figure 17–76 **Aneurysmal Bone Cyst.** A ballooned cyst-like lesion having coarse trabeculation has arisen in the metaphyseal region of the radius and extends to the diaphysis. The cortex is thinned.

These lesions, almost invariably metaphyseal, can extend to the diaphysis; an ununited epiphysis remains uninvolved. The coarse soap bubble appearance suggests the diagnosis, particularly in patients under the age of 17.

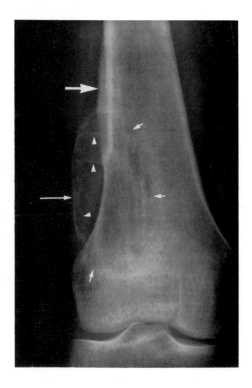

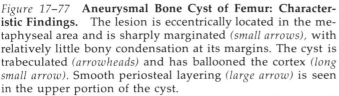

Figure 17–77 **Aneurysmal Bone Cyst of Femur: Characteristic Findings.** The lesion is eccentrically located in the metaphyseal area and is sharply marginated *(small arrows),* with relatively little bony condensation at its margins. The cyst is trabeculated *(arrowheads)* and has ballooned the cortex *(long small arrow).* Smooth periosteal layering *(large arrow)* is seen in the upper portion of the cyst.

The location, eccentric expansion, trabeculation, and smooth periosteal reaction are characteristic features of an aneurysmal bone cyst involving a tubular bone. (Courtesy Dr. J. R. Stewart, Rochester, Minnesota.)

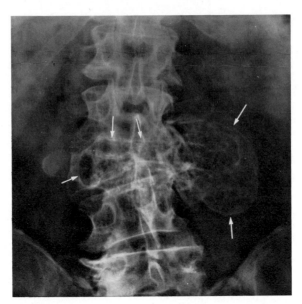

Figure 17–78 **Aneurysmal Bone Cyst of Vertebra.**   The large trabeculated cystic lesion is sharply demarcated *(arrows)*, has enormously expanded the left transverse process of L3, and involves the body almost to
its right border. The posterior elements (pedicles, lamina, and spinous process) are also involved. The
weakened body is collapsed.

In the vertebra, the aneurysmal bone cyst tends to be expansile and eccentric in location, and tends to
involve the posterior elements. (Courtesy Dr. J. R. Stewart, Rochester, Minnesota.)

Subperiosteal Desmoid (Avulsive Cortical Irregularity)

This radiographic abnormality, almost exclusively found along the posterior
aspect of the medial femoral condyle, is not a tumor but apparently a reactive bone
change due to muscular stress. It occurs most often in males between 10 and 15
years of age. It is bilateral in about one third of cases and produces few or no
symptoms.

The abnormality appears as an irregular shallow osteolytic area paralleling
the long axis of the shaft. Often there are tiny fragments in the soft tissues, and
sometimes there is a spiculated appearance. On profile view irregular cortical or
subperiosteal thickening is apparent. Occasionally, the changes may simulate a
malignant bone lesion, but its characteristic location and appearance in an asymptomatic young male should permit ready recognition. If bilateral lesions are seen,
the correct diagnosis is virtually unequivocal.[103, 104]

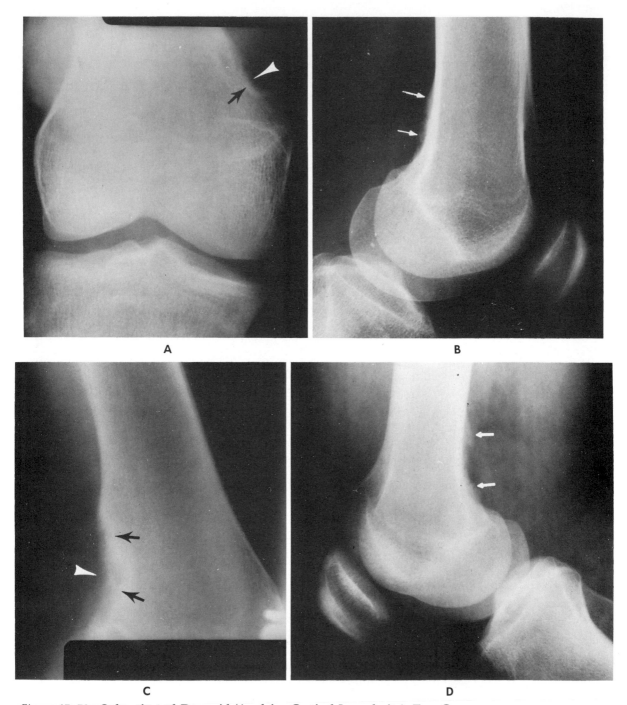

Figure 17–79 **Subperiosteal Desmoid (Avulsive Cortical Irregularity): Two Cases.**

   A and *B*, There is a marginal bone defect *(white arrowhead)* with a sclerotic base *(black arrow)* just above the medial condyle of the femur. Spiculated irregular periosteal bone reaction is best seen on the lateral film *(white arrows)*. The boy was 20 years old.
   C and *D*, In an 18 year old boy, a larger but similar defect *(white arrowhead)* on the medial side of the lower femur is seen on the tomogram *(C)*. Its base is quite sclerotic *(black arrows)*, and periosteal reaction is apparent *(white arrows)*.
   Virtually all cases have a similar appearance. Usually the changes are bilateral, although one side may be much more affected.

Intraosseous Ganglion

These benign bone lesions arise in subchondral areas close to a joint and may be single or multiple. Although they may appear as early as the second decade, most of the lesions are seen in individuals 30 years of age or older. They probably represent an intramedullary fibroplasia with secondary cystic degeneration.

The femoral neck and head and the upper and lower tibia are the common sites, but any small or large bone of the extremities can be involved. Radiographically, the lesions are juxta-articular and are always lytic and sharply circumscribed; about one half have a sclerotic margin. Occasionally, expansion, cortical thinning, and even pathologic fracture can occur.

In older patients, degenerative changes may appear in the adjacent joint, and it may be difficult to distinguish the intraosseous ganglion from cystic changes of degenerative joint disease.

In younger patients, the lesion may closely simulate chondroblastoma or giant-cell tumor.[105]

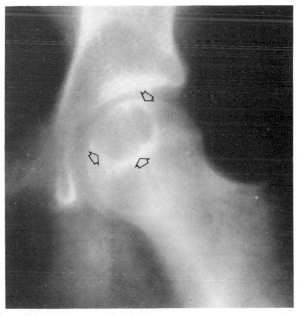

B

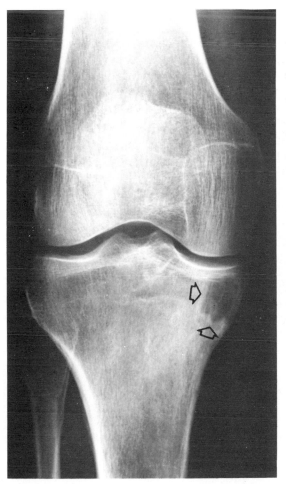

A

Figure 17–80 **Intraosseous Ganglion in Two Patients.** The cyst-like defects in the tibia and femur (tomogram, *B*) are directly subarticular; both have a slightly scalloped border and a sclerotic margin *(arrows).* The joint spaces of the knee and hip are normal. This finding helps distinguish the intraosseous ganglion from a cyst associated with degenerative joint disease in older patients. In young individuals, these lesions would be thought to be chondroblastoma radiographically. (Courtesy Dr. Frieda Feldman, New York, New York.)

Malignant Tumors

Osteogenic Sarcoma

This is the most frequent primary malignant neoplasm of bone. Males are affected almost twice as often as females. The vast majority of these tumors arise in the second and third decade and typically involve a long bone. In older individuals the tumor is usually in a flat bone and most commonly is superimposed on a pre-existing bone disturbance, particularly Paget's disease. Rarely, an osteosarcoma is a late complication of intensive radiotherapy.

The usual site is a metaphysis of a long bone, most often the lower femur or upper tibia. The upper humerus, fibula, pelvis, clavicle, ribs, and mandible are other common sites, but any bone may be involved. Rarely, lesions in several bones appear to arise simultaneously.

Clinically there is early local pain and swelling; later, fever and progressive anemia may occur. Early metastases to the lung are common.

The tumor may be entirely lytic and destructive (osteolytic form) or, more often, may also contain reactive or neoplastic new bone formation (osteolytic-sclerotic form). A completely sclerotic form is a rare occurrence. Initially there are ill-defined lucencies with trabecular destruction, usually in the metaphyseal area. Cortical involvement leads to irregular and often laminated periosteal reaction. Later, cortical destruction is followed by tumor extension into the soft tissues; often, horizontal bony spicules extend into the soft tissue mass (sunburst appearance). Elevation of the periosteum at a border of the lesion with subsequent subperiosteal calcification produces the *Codman triangle*—a significant sign of a malignant bone tumor, but not specific for osteogenic sarcoma. The bone destruction is only rarely accompanied by bone expansion.

In the more common osteolytic-sclerotic form, irregular collections of new bone appear within the lytic area; sunburst spiculation is common. Areas of calcification may appear in the soft tissue mass. The completely sclerotic lesion may appear as an innocent intramedullary density, but some periosteal reaction may suggest its neoplastic nature.

In flat bones, irregular lysis usually with some sclerotic areas is the rule; periosteal reaction may be unrecognized without special tangential views.

The classic features of a well-developed osteogenic sarcoma are irregular medullary destruction in the metaphyseal area in a young individual, irregular periosteal reaction, a sunburst spiculation, cortical destruction, a soft tissue mass, and areas of reactive bone formation. Small lytic areas with some periosteal reaction are often the earliest findings.

Radiographic distinction from Ewing's tumor is often difficult or impossible. Other bone lesions that can sometimes radiographically mimic an osteogenic sarcoma include certain forms of metastatic disease, bone lymphoma, and chondrosarcoma.[106-110]

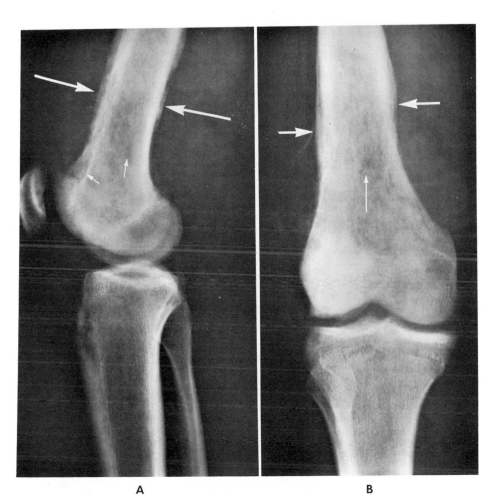

A   B

Figure 17–81   **Osteogenic Sarcoma of Femur: Mixed Form.**

    A, An irregular area of bone destruction in the distal femur involves both medulla and cortex *(small arrows).* There is irregular periosteal reaction along the lower femur with a tendency toward spicule formation *(large arrows).*

    B, There are irregular lytic areas in the medullary cavity *(small arrow),* as well as irregular periosteal layering *(large arrows).* This mixed sarcoma is predominantly lytic. There is extensive destruction of bone, yet little endosteal reactive sclerosis; however, periosteal new bone formation is a prominent feature. The findings strongly suggest the diagnosis, but Ewing's sarcoma can have a similar appearance.

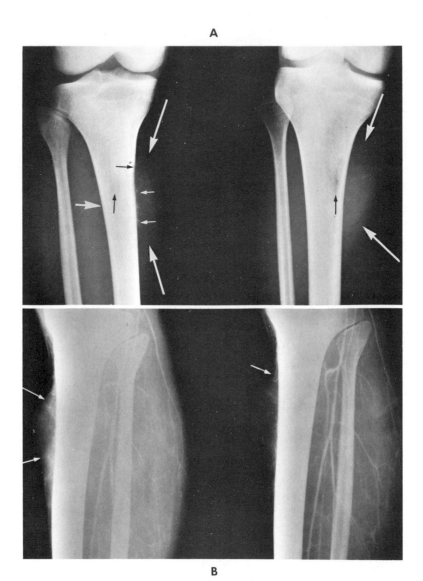

Figure 17–82   **Osteogenic Sarcoma.**

A, There is destruction of the cancellous bone and cortex *(black arrows),* a large soft tissue mass *(large arrows),* and small spicules of bone extending into the soft tissues *(small white arrows).*

B, Angiogram demonstrates diffuse tumor stains in the soft tissue due to abnormal vessels *(arrows).* The tumor is highly vascular, with an increased number of feeding arteries, abnormal vessels, and an increased number of veins.

The vessels feeding malignant tumors are frequently irregular and unusually numerous, and angiography may help distinguish benign from malignant tumors.

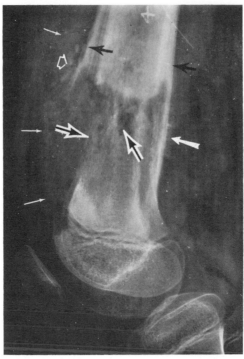

Figure 17-83 **Advanced Osteogenic Sarcoma.** Lateral knee film of a 16 year old boy reveals marked swelling of the soft tissues and an anterior soft tissue mass *(small white arrows)*. There are marked destructive changes in the metaphysis, with loss of anterior cortex *(black-white arrows)*. Spiculations into the soft tissues *(large white arrow)*, periosteal reaction *(black arrows)*, and calcifications within the tumor mass *(open white arrow)* are evident.

All the radiographic criteria of primary malignant bone tumor are present.

Parosteal Sarcoma

This rare, relatively slow-growing malignant tumor probably arises in the periosteum. It occurs in an older age group (third or fourth decade) than osteogenic sarcoma and has a far more favorable prognosis. It frequently occurs around the metaphyseal end of the long bones, most commonly in the distal or proximal femur and less commonly in the tibia or humerus.

Parosteal sarcoma appears as a juxtacortical broad-based dense area of irregular ossification. The periphery is often lobulated and less dense than the base. The lesion tends to encircle the bone, but actual bone involvement is minimal, occurring in only 10 per cent of cases. One frequently sees a linear radiolucent zone between the tumor and the bone. This rather characteristic x-ray picture usually permits accurate diagnosis.[108, 111-113]

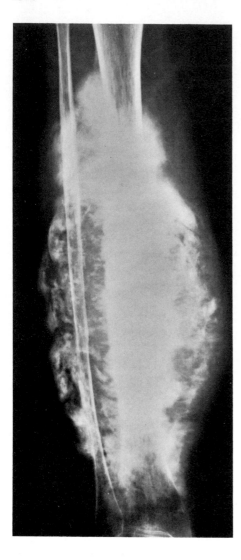

Figure 17–84 **Parosteal Sarcoma.** An extensive, dense amorphous mass along the tibial shaft essentially obscures the underlying tibia, but the bone is not involved. The density of the mass decreases toward the periphery. Multiple projections showed that the mass encircled the bone, and penetrated films revealed no significant involvement of the underlying bone.

Chondrosarcoma

This lesion is usually encountered in the later decades and may be a complication of previous bone lesions, especially enchondroma, osteochondroma, or Paget's disease. Two fairly distinct types are seen.

The central type commonly arises within a tubular bone, most often the proximal or distal femur or the proximal humerus. Radiographically it appears as a localized area of lytic bone destruction in the vicinity of the metaphysis. The margins are irregular and often ill defined. Central flocculent calcification is noted in about two thirds of these lesions. The cortex may be expanded and thinned. Periosteal reaction occasionally occurs, often as velvet-like spiculations.

The peripheral form of chondrosarcoma occurs most commonly in the ribs, scapula, or pelvis. Middle-aged males are more often affected. The tumor seems to arise from the periosteum and often is superimposed on a pre-existing exostosis. The lesion presents as a large irregular calcified mass adjacent to the bone or exostosis. The underlying bone may show some irregular areas of destruction, but these are minimal. The characteristic roentgen appearance makes diagnosis of this form of chondrosarcoma relatively easy.

Pulmonary metastases are common.[37, 108, 114–116]

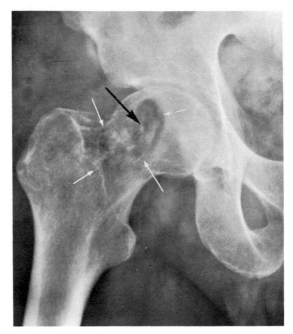

Figure 17–85 **Central Chondrosarcoma.** Irregular calcific densities *(black arrow)* are seen in a poorly demarcated area of lucency in the femoral head and neck *(white arrows).* Periosteal reaction, which is not seen in this illustration, is not uncommon in chondrosarcoma.

In cartilaginous tumors, calcium is often deposited within the cartilaginous elements. (Courtesy Dr. Arlyne Shockman, Veterans Administration Hospital, Philadelphia, Pennsylvania.)

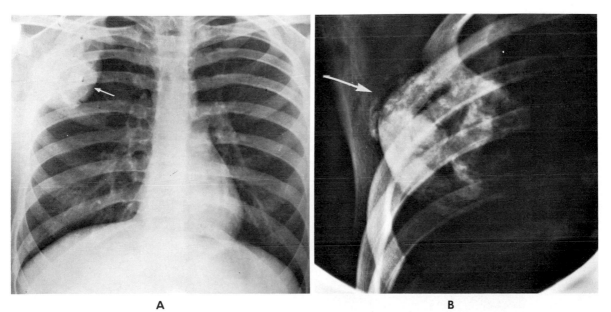

A   B

Figure 17–86 **Chondrosarcoma of Rib.**

A, Posteroanterior view discloses a dense lobulated mass in the lateral portion of the upper thorax *(arrow).*

B, Enlarged view discloses lytic areas of destruction in the rib, with marked reactive periostitis *(arrow).* There is irregular calcification throughout the lesion.

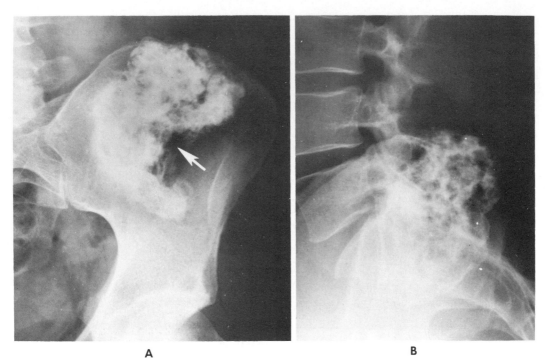

A   **B**

Figure 17–87 **Chondrosarcoma of Iliac Bone.**

A, A large collection of circumscribed amorphous calcification is associated with lytic destruction (*arrow*) of the left iliac bone.

B, Lateral view shows the cauliflower-like calcifications extending posteriorly from the iliac bone.

Without recognition of bone destruction, the radiographic appearance of the calcifications is identical to that of a cauliflower osteochondroma. Perhaps malignant degeneration of an osteochondroma occurred in this patient.

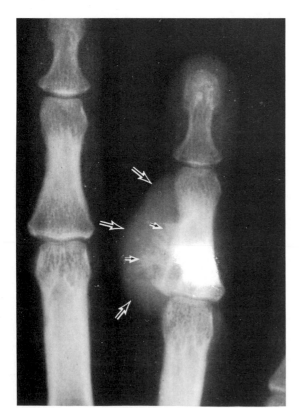

Figure 17–88 **Primary Chondrosarcoma of Phalanx.** The destructive changes on the lateral aspect of the shaft and the brush-like perpendicular bony spicules (*small arrows*) extending into a soft tissue mass (*large arrows*) are classic findings of primary osteosarcoma. The lesion in this 44 year old woman proved to be a chondrosarcoma.

Primary sarcoma of the bones of the hands or feet is extremely rare.

Ewing's Sarcoma

Ewing's sarcoma usually occurs in the first three decades with a peak incidence around 15 years of age. Males are affected twice as often as females. The femur is the most common site; it may arise in other long bones of the extremities and in the pelvis, ribs, and scapulae. The lesion has a definite tendency to metastasize to other bones.

Initially the tumor is seen as an area of medullary lysis, and it rapidly extends to involve much of the shaft of the bone. The larger lesions are usually destructive with little or no reactive changes, although occasionally there may be local areas of increased bone density. There is early cortical involvement with subsequent elevation of the periosteum. Periosteal new bone formation occurs, and the radiographic picture may simulate that of osteomyelitis. Multiple periosteal layering may occur, producing the onion skin appearance, which is suggestive of the diagnosis. Frequently, horizontal bony spicules extend into the soft tissue mass (the hair-on-end appearance). A soft tissue mass is seen in almost all cases.

The combination of ill-defined medullary lytic lesions with periosteal layering in a child strongly suggests Ewing's sarcoma, but radiographic distinction from osteogenic sarcoma or acute and subacute osteomyelitis is often difficult.

Arteriography is sometimes helpful in defining the full extent and malignant nature of the lesion, especially when it occurs in the central portion of a flat bone.[117, 118]

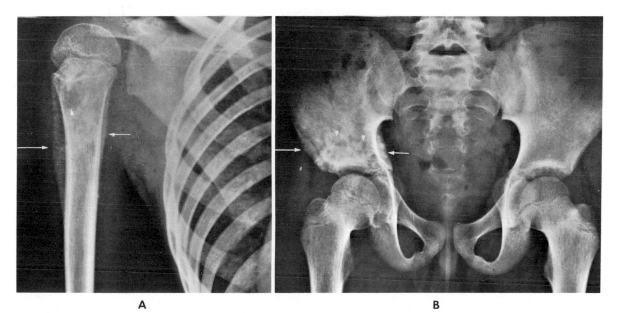

A   B

Figure 17–89 **Ewing's Sarcoma and Bone Metastases.**

A, There are diffuse osteolytic areas in the medullary cavity in the metaphysis and proximal diaphysis (*arrowhead*), and spiculated periosteal reaction (*arrows*), a combination that strongly suggests Ewing's sarcoma.

B, Bone destruction (*arrowheads*) and marked irregular spiculated periosteal new bone formation are demonstrated around the ilium (*arrows*). This was a metastatic lesion from the primary Ewing's sarcoma in the humerus.

Ewing's sarcoma is the only primary bone malignancy that often metastasizes to other bones.

Reticulum Cell Sarcoma

This primary malignant lesion of bone occurs mainly in individuals over 40 years of age and rarely is seen below the age of 20. It occurs predominantly in males, most frequently in the long tubular bones.

Reticulum cell sarcoma radiographically appears as a poorly circumscribed lytic destructive area in the medullary cavity of bone. Cortical destruction is usually present, but there is no bone expansion. Often there is amorphous and irregular periosteal new bone formation; a large soft tissue mass may ultimately develop. A Codman triangle is almost never present. Although the lesion is predominantly lytic, the endosteal bone is often thickened, producing a mixed lytic and osteoblastic picture. Reticulum cell sarcoma often resembles Ewing's sarcoma radiographically, but occurs in an older age group.[119-121]

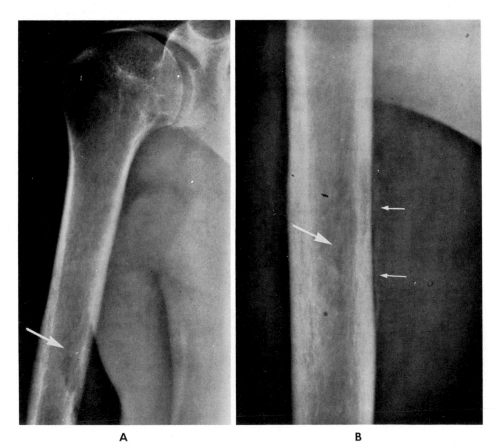

A　　　　　　　　　　　　　　　　　　　　　B

Figure 17–90 **Reticulum Cell Sarcoma of Humerus.**

A, The patient was a 50 year old man. There is an irregular area of trabecular lysis in the diaphyseal portion of the humerus *(arrow).* Cortical involvement and destruction are evident, and a large soft tissue mass is present.

B, Enlarged view of the humerus demonstrates periosteal elevation *(small arrows),* as well as destruction of bone *(large arrow).*

The appearance and location of a reticulum cell sarcoma are similar to Ewing's sarcoma, but the latter almost always occurs in children or young adults.

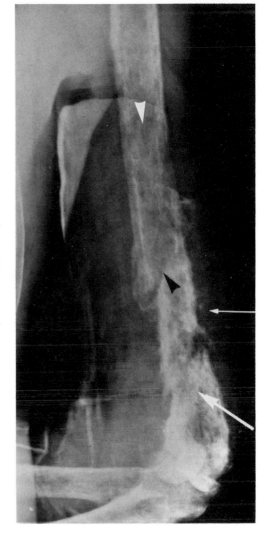

Figure 17–91 **Reticulum Cell Sarcoma.** There is extensive lysis of the medullary cavity and cortex of the lower two thirds of the humerus *(white arrowhead),* with only minimal periosteal reaction *(small arrow).* The mottled increased density in the lower humerus *(large arrow)* is due to endosteal new bone formation. A pathologic fracture has occurred *(black arrowhead).* The extensive medullary destruction in an adult is characteristic of advanced reticulum cell sarcoma.

Fibrosarcoma of Bone

This rare tumor can occur at any age, although young adults are most frequently affected. It usually appears in the metaphysis of a long bone, especially around the knee, but flat bone involvement can occur. Fibrosarcoma can be a complication of advanced Paget's disease or of an irradiated giant-cell tumor.

Radiographically, there is usually a metaphyseal area of bone destruction that is irregular and eccentric and has ill-defined margins. Endosteal erosion and scalloping are common. Larger lesions may cause cortical expansion. Periosteal reaction can occur, but without spiculation. Tumor calcifications with reactive bone formation are rare. Large lesions may invade the soft tissues.

A fibrosarcoma may extend into the epiphyseal area and resemble an aggressive giant-cell tumor, but its radiographic characteristics usually permit distinction from a benign bone lesion.[41, 122]

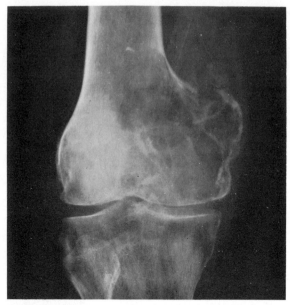

Figure 17–92 **Central Fibrosarcoma of Femur.**   The large, destructive lesion in the meta-physis of the lower femur has expanded and thinned the cortex. The cortex is broken by the perforating lesion. The lytic lesion shows no sclerosis and its margins are irregular.

Metastatic Malignancy of Bone

A metastatic lesion is the most common malignant bone tumor. Carcinomas, especially of the breast, lung, prostate, kidney, and thyroid, tend to produce distant bone metastases, while sarcomas are an infrequent cause. The bones of the axial skeleton, skull, and proximal extremities are most commonly affected; involvement of the distal extremities is uncommon.

Radiographically, most metastases appear as irregular lytic areas in medullary or endosteal bone. Eventually the cortex is destroyed, and the tumor mass may extend into the soft tissues. Pathologic fractures frequently occur, usually producing a reparative periosteal reaction. Osteoblastic metastases are less frequent and most often originate from prostatic or breast malignancies. These appear as localized areas of sclerosis, usually in the spine or pelvis; there may be diffuse increased density of one or more vertebral bodies with little or no destruction, but combined lytic-osteoblastic lesions are not uncommon. The sclerosis is due to local increased medullary bone formation, not to calcium deposits in the tumor tissue. Rarely, a metastasis primarily involves the subperiosteal area and causes a periosteal reaction, simulating a primary bone sarcoma. This type of metastatic lesion is occasionally seen in colon or thyroid carcinoma; the medulloblastoma of childhood consistently causes such metastases.

Involvement of a bone by a contiguous primary or metastatic soft tissue malignancy will cause erosion and cortical destruction; lytic extensions into the medullary cavity may occur later.

In adults, the vast majority of single or multiple destructive bone lesions are due to metastatic disease. Multiple lytic bone metastases are frequently indistinguishable from multiple myeloma.

Sizable bone metastases may be present without discernible roentgen evidence, since a significant degree of cortical or trabecular destruction is needed before radiographic changes can be perceived. (See Figs. 16–23, 16–51B, and 11–75.)

REFERENCES

1. Steinbach, H. L.: The roentgen appearance of osteoporosis. Radiol. Clin. North Am., *2*:191, 1964.
2. Rose, G. A.: The radiologic diagnosis of osteoporosis, osteomalacia, and hyperparathyroidism. Clin. Radiol., *15*:75, 1964.
3. Feist, J. H.: The biologic basis of radiologic findings in bone disease. Radiol. Clin. North Am., *8*:183, 1970.
4. Reynolds, W. A., and Karo, J. J.: Radiologic diagnosis of metabolic bone disease. Orthop. Clin. North Am., *3*:521, 1972.
5. Hunder, G. G., and Kelly, P. J.: Roentgenologic transient osteoporosis of the hip: A clinical syndrome? Ann. Intern. Med., *68*:539, 1968.
6. Rosen, R. A.: Transitory demineralization of the femoral head. Radiology, *94*:509, 1970.
7. Lequesne, M.: Transient osteoporosis of the hip. Ann. Rhem. Dis., *27*:463, 1968.
8. Longstreth, P. L., Malinak, L. R., and Hill, C. S.: Transient osteoporosis of the hip in pregnancy. Obstet. Gynecol., *41*:563, 1973.
9. Steinbach, H. L., and Noetzli, M.: Roentgen appearance of the skeleton in osteomalacia and rickets. Am. J. Roentgenol. Radium Ther. Nucl. Med., *91*:955, 1964.
10. Courey, W. R., and Pfister, R. C.: Radiographic findings in renal tubular acidosis. Radiology, *105*:497, 1972.
11. Dickson, W., and Horrocks, R. H.: Hypophosphatasia. J. Bone Joint Surg., *40*:64, 1958.
12. James, W., and Moule, B.: Hypophosphatasia. Clin. Radiol., *17*:368, 1966.
13. Steinbach, H. L., Gordon, G. S., Eisenberg, E., Crane, J. T., Silverman, S., and Goldman, L.: Primary hyperparathyroidism: a correlation of roentgen, clinical and pathological features. Am. J. Roentgenol. Radium Ther. Nucl. Med., *86*:329, 1961.
14. Czitober, H., et al.: Skeletal changes before and after operation in primary hyperparathyroidism. Fortschr. Roentgenstr., *115*:85, 1971.
15. Stevenson, C. A., and Watson, R.: Fluoride osteosclerosis. Am. J. Roentgenol. Radium Ther. Nucl. Med., *78*:13, 1957.
16. Donnan, M. G. F.: Fluorosis. Proc. Coll. Radiol. Austral., *1*:1, 1957.
17. Teotia, M., et al.: Endemic skeletal fluorosis. Arch. Dis. Child., *46*:686, 1971.
18. Pease, C. N.: Focal retardation and arrestment of growth of bones due to vitamin A intoxication. J.A.M.A., *182*:980, 1962.
19. Russell, R. M., et al.: Hepatic injury from chronic hypervitaminosis A resulting in portal hypertension and ascites. N. Engl. J. Med., *291*:435, 1974.
20. Ross, S. G.: Vitamin D intoxication in infancy. J. Pediatr., *41*:815, 1952.
21. Fraser, D.: Clinical manifestations of genetic aberrations of calcium and phosphorus metabolism. J.A.M.A., *176*:281, 1961.
22. Bliddal, J., et al.: Coarctation of the aorta with multiple artery anomalies in idiopathic hypercalcemia of infancy. Acta Pediatr. Scand., *58*:632, 1969.
23. Malka, S.: Idiopathic aseptic necrosis of the head of the femur in adults. Surg. Gynecol. Obstet., *123*:1057, 1966.
24. Patterson, R. J., Bickel, W. H., and Dahlin, D. C.: Idiopathic avascular necrosis of the head of the femur. J. Bone Joint Surg., *46*:267, 1964.
25. Miller, W. T., and Restifo, R. A.: Steroid arthropathy. Radiology, *86*:652, 1966.
26. Martell, N., and Sitterley, B. H.: Roentgenologic manifestations of osteonecrosis. Am. J. Roentgenol. Radium Ther. Nucl. Med., *106*:509, 1969.
27. Awwaad, S., and Reda, M.: Osteogenesis imperfecta: review of literature with a report of three cases. Arch. Pediatr., *77*:280, 1960.
28. Caniggia, A., Stuart, C., and Guideri, R.: Fragilitas ossium hereditaria tarda. Acta Med. Scand., supplement 340, 1958.
29. Levin, E. J.: Osteogenesis imperfecta in the adult. Am. J. Roentgenol. Radium Ther. Nucl. Med., *91*:973, 1964.
30. Navani, S. V., and Sarzin, B.: Intrauterine osteogenesis imperfecta. Br. J. Radiol., *40*:449, 1967.
31. Mosely, J. E.: *Bone Changes in Hematologic Disorders.* New York, Grune & Stratton, Inc., 1963.
32. Yu, J. S., Oates, R. K., et al.: Osteopetrosis. Arch. Dis. Child., *46*:257, 1971.
33. Caffey, J.: Achondroplasia of pelvis and lumbar spine: some roentgenographic features. Am. J. Roentgenol. Radium Ther. Nucl. Med., *80*:449, 1958.
34. Rubin, P.: Achondroplasia versus pseudoachondroplasia. Radiol. Clin. North Am., *1*:621, 1963.
35. Langer, L. O., Jr., et al.: Achondroplasia. Am. J. Roentgenol. Radium Ther. Nucl. Med., *100*:12, 1967.
36. Young, R. S., Pochazevsky, R., et al.: Thanatrophic dwarfism and cloverleaf skull. Radiology, *106*:401, 1973.
37. Levy, W. M., Aegerter, E. E. and Kirkpatrick, J. A., Jr.: The nature of cartilaginous tumors. Radiol. Clin. North Am., *2*:327, 1964.
38. Chiurco, A. A.: Multiple exostoses of bone with fatal spinal cord compression. Neurology, *20*:275, 1970.
39. Mainzer, F., Minagi, H., and Steinbach, H. L.: The variable manifestations of multiple enchondromatosis. Radiology, *99*:377, 1971.
40. Cheney, W. D.: Acro-osteolysis. Am. J. Roentgenol. Radium Ther. Nucl. Med., *94*:595, 1965.

41. Aegerter, E., and Kirkpatrick, J. A., Jr.: *Orthopedic Diseases,* 4th ed. Philadelphia, W. B. Saunders Company, 1975.
42. Campbell, C. J., Papademetriou, T., and Bonfiglio, M.: Melorheostosis. J. Bone Joint Surg., *50A*:1281, 1968.
43. Green, A. E., Ellsworth, W. H., et al.: Melorheostosis and osteopoikilosis. Am. J. Roentgenol. Radium Ther. Nucl. Med., *87*:1096, 1962.
44. Muthukrishman, N., and Shetty, M. V. K.: Pycnodysostosis. Am. J. Roentgenol. Radium Ther. Nucl. Med., *114*:247, 1972.
45. Elmore, S. M.: Pycnodysostosis: A review. J. Bone Joint Surg., *49A*:153, 1967.
46. Podlaha, M., and Kratochvil, L.: Familial metaphyseal dysplasia—Pyle's disease. Fortschr. Roentgenstr., *98*:158, 1963.
47. Fried, K., and Krause, J.: Metaphyseal dysplasia: Pyle's disease. Fortschr. Roentgenstr., *116*:224, 1972.
48. Thoms, J.: Cleido-cranial dysostosis. Acta Radiol., *50*:514, 1958.
49. Jarvis, J. L., and Keats, T. E.: Cleidocranial dysostosis. Am. J. Roentgenol. Radium Ther. Nucl. Med., *121*:5, 1974.
50. Clawson, D. K., and Loop, S. W.: Progressive diaphyseal dysplasia (Engelmann's disease). J. Bone Joint Surg., *46A*:143, 1964.
51. Mottram, M. E., and Hill, N. A.: Diaphyseal dysplasia. Am. J. Roentgenol. Radium Ther. Nucl. Med., *95*:162, 1965.
52. Williams, H. J., and Hoyer, J. R.: Radiographic diagnosis of osteo-onychodysostosis in infancy. Radiology, *109*:151, 1973.
53. Fruchter, Z.: Osteoungual dysplasia. J. Radiol., *47*:335, 1966.
54. Walls, W. L., et al.: Chondroectodermal dysplasia. Am. J. Dis. Child., *98*:242, 1959.
55. Kozlowski, K., et al.: Difficulties in differentiation between chondroectodermal dysplasia and asphyxiating thoracic dystrophy. Australas. Radiol., *16*:401, 1972.
56. Currarina, G., Neuhauser, E. B. D., Reyersbach, G. C., and Sobel, E. H.: Familial idiopathic osteoarthropathy. Am. J. Roentgenol. Radium Ther. Nucl. Med., *85*:633, 1961.
57. Rimoin, D. L.: Pachydermoperiostosis. N. Engl. J. Med., *272*:923, 1965.
58. Lazarus, J. H., and Galloway, J. K.: Pachydermoperiostosis. Am. J. Roentgenol. Radium Ther. Nucl. Med., *118*:308, 1973.
59. Harbison, J. B., and Nice, C. M., Jr.: Familial pachydermoperiostosis presenting as an acromegaly-like syndrome. Am. J. Roentgenol. Radium Ther. Nucl. Med., *112*:532, 1971.
60. Kaufmann, H. J.: *Progress in Pediatric Radiology.* Vol. 4. Basel, S. Karger, 1973.
61. Kelly, O. J., Petersson, L. F. A., Dahler, D. C., and Plum, G. E.: Osteitis deformans: morphologic study utilizing microradiography and conventional technique. Radiology, 77:368, 1961.
62. Adler, H., and Eichner, G.: Osteogenic sarcoma of the skull arising in Paget's disease. Am. J. Roentgenol. Radium Ther. Nucl. Med., *79*:648, 1958.
63. Sader, E. S., Walton, R. J., and Gossman, H. H.: Neurological dysfunction in Paget's disease of the vertebral column. J. Neurosurg., *37*:661, 1972.
64. Daves, M. L., and Yardley, J. H.: Fibrous dysplasia of bone. Am. J. Med. Sci., *234*:956, 1957.
65. Leeds, N. L., and Seaman, W. B.: Fibrous dysplasia of the skull and its differential diagnosis. Radiology, *78*:570, 1962.
66. Nixon, G. W., and Condon, V. R.: Epiphyseal involvement in polyostotic fibrous dysplasia. Radiology, *106*:167, 1973.
67. Skorneck, A. B., and Ginsberg, L. B.: Pulmonary hypertrophic osteoarthropathy. N. Engl. J. Med., *258*:1079, 1958.
68. Hallis, W. C.: Hypertrophic osteoarthropathy secondary to upper gastrointestinal neoplasm. Ann. Intern. Med., *66*:125, 1967.
69. Salmi, A., Voutilaninen, A., Holsti, L. R., and Unnerus, C. E.: Hyperostosis cranii in normal population. Am. J. Roentgenol. Radium Ther. Nucl. Med., *87*:1032, 1962.
70. McEvoy, B. F., and Gatzek, H.: Multiple nevoid basal cell carcinoma syndrome. Br. J. Radiol., *42*:24, 1969.
71. Freiberger, R. H., Loitman, B. S., Helpern, M., and Thompson, T. C.: Osteoma; eighty cases. Am. J. Roentgenol. Radium Ther. Nucl. Med., *82*:194, 1959.
72. Chrisman, O. D., and Goldenberg, R. R.: Untreated solitary osteochondroma. J. Bone Joint Surg., *50A*:508, 1968.
73. Bartlett, J. R.: Intracranial neurological complications of frontal and ethmoidal osteomas. Br. J. Surg., *58*:607, 1971.
74. Karlsberg, R. C., and Kittleson, A. C.: Osteoid osteoma. Radiol. Clin. North Am., *2*:337, 1964.
75. Stewart, J. R., Dahlin, D. C., and Pugh, D. G.: The pathology and radiology of solitary benign bone tumors. Semin. Roentgenol., *1*:268, 1961.
76. Chitale, A. R., and Kumbhani, S. J.: Osteoid osteoma. Indian J. Cancer, *8*:238, 1971.
77. Pochaczevsky, R., Ying, M. Y., and Sherman, R. S.: Roentgen appearance of benign osteoblastoma. Radiology, *75*:429, 1960.
78. Tulloh, H. P., and Harry, D.: Osteoblastoma in a rib in childhood. Clin. Radiol., *20*:337, 1969.
79. Borghi, A., and D'Ettorre, A.: The benign osteoblastoma. Riv. Radiol., *13*:47, 1973.
80. Gee, V. R., and Pugh, D. G.: Giant cell tumor of bone. Radiology, *70*:33, 1958.
81. Jacobs, P.: The diagnosis of giant-cell tumor: radiological and pathological correlation. Br. J. Radiol., *45*:121, 1972.

82. Takigawa, K.: Chondroma of the bones of the hand. J. Bone Joint Surg., *53A*:1591, 1971.
83. Marberg, K., Dalith, F., and Bank, H.: Dyschondroplasia with multiple hemangiomata (Maffucci's syndrome). Ann. Intern. Med., *49*:1216, 1958.
84. Howard, F. M., and Lee, R. E.: The hand in Maffucci syndrome. Arch. Surg., *103*:752, 1971.
85. Lewis, R. J., and Ketcham, A. S.: Maffucci's syndrome: functional and neoplastic significance. J. Bone Joint Surg., *55*:1465, 1973.
86. Plum, G. E., and Pugh, D. G.: Roentgenographic aspects of benign chondroblastoma of bone. Am. J. Roentgenol. Radium Ther. Nucl. Med., *79*:584, 1958.
87. Dahlin, D. C., and Ivins, J. C.: Benign chondroblastoma. Cancer, *30*:401, 1972.
88. Mcleod, R. A., and Beabout, J. W.: The roentgenographic features of chondroblastoma. Am. J. Roentgenol. Radium Ther. Nucl. Med., *118*:464, 1973.
89. Feldman, F., Hecht, H. L., and Johnson, A. D.: Chondromyxofibroma of bone. Radiology, *94*:249, 1970.
90. Murphy, N. B., and Price, C. H. G.: The radiological aspects of chondromyxoid fibroma of bone. Clin. Radiol., *22*:261, 1971.
91. Purcel, W. M., and Mulcahy, F.: Nonosteogenic fibroma of bone. Clin. Radiol., *11*:51, 1960.
92. Sherman, R. S., and Wilner, D.: Roentgen diagnosis of hemangioma of bone. Am. J. Roentgenol. Radium Ther. Nucl. Med., *86*:1146, 1961.
93. Brower, A. C., Culver, J. E., and Keats, T. E.: Diffuse cystic angiomatosis of bone. Am. J. Roentgenol. Radium Ther. Nucl. Med., *118*:456, 1973.
94. Hunt, J. C., and Pugh, D. G.: Skeletal lesions in neurofibromatosis. Radiology, *76*:1, 1961.
95. Johnson, P. M., and McClure, J. G.: Observations on massive osteolysis; a review of the literature and report of a case. Radiology, *71*:28, 1958.
96. Halliday, D. R., et al.: Massive osteolysis and angiomatosis. Radiology, *82*:637, 1964.
97. Winterberger, A. R.: Radiographic diagnosis of lymphangiomatosis of bone. Radiology, *102*:321, 1972.
98. Lodwick, G. S.: Juvenile unicameral bone cyst: a roentgen appraisal. Am. J. Roentgenol. Radium Ther. Nucl. Med., *80*:495, 1958.
99. Morchoisne, P., and Masse, P.: Radiological evolution of simple bone cysts. Ann. Radiol., *13*:811, 1970.
100. Donaldson, W. F., Jr.: Aneurysmal bone cyst. J. Bone Joint Surg., *44A*:25, 1962.
101. Lichtenstein, L.: Aneurysmal bone cyst; further observations. Cancer, *6*:1228, 1953.
102. Carlson, D. H., Wilkinson, R. H., and Bhakkaviziam, A.: Aneurysmal bone cysts in children. Am. J. Roentgenol. Radium Ther. Nucl. Med., *116*:644, 1972.
103. Bufkin, W. J.: The avulsive cortical irregularity. Am. J. Roentgenol. Radium Ther. Nucl. Med., *112*:487, 1971.
104. Brower, A. C., Culver, J. E., and Keats, T. E.: Histological nature of the cortical irregularity of the medial posterior distal femoral metaphysis in children. Radiology, *99*:389, 1971.
105. Feldman, F., and Johnston, A.: Intraosseous ganglion. Am. J. Roentgenol. Radium Ther. Nucl. Med., *118*:328, 1973.
106. Lindbom, A., Söderberg, G., and Spjut, H. J.: Osteosarcoma: a review of ninety-six cases. Acta Radiol., *56*:1, 1961.
107. Lagergren, C., Lindbom, A., and Söderberg, G.: The blood vessels of osteogenic sarcoma. Histologic, angiographic and microradiographic studies. Acta Radiol., *55*:161, 1961.
108. Lodwick, G. S.: Solitary malignant lesions of bone. Semin. Roentgenol., *1*:293, 1966.
109. von Ronnen, J. R.: Histological and radiographic classification of osteosarcoma in relation to therapy. J. Belge Radiol., *51*:215, 1968.
110. Finkelstein, J. B.: Osteosarcoma of the jaw bones. Radiol. Clin. North Am., *8*:425, 1970.
111. Ranninger, K., and Allner, P. C.: Parosteal osteoid sarcoma. Radiology, *86*:648, 1966.
112. Aakhus, T., and Stokke, T.: Parosteal osteogenic sarcoma. Acta Radiol., *54*:29, 1960.
113. Edeiken, J., Farrell, C., et al.: Parosteal sarcoma. Am. J. Roentgenol. Radium Ther. Nucl. Med., *111*:579, 1971.
114. Reiter, F. B., Ackerman, L. V., and Staple, T. W.: Central chondrosarcoma of the appendicular skeleton. Radiology, *105*:525, 1972.
115. Salvador, A. H., Beabout, J. W., and Dahlin, D.: Mesenchymal chondrosarcoma. Cancer, *28*:605, 1971.
116. Chavanne, G., Calle, R., and Schlienger, P.: Chondrosarcoma of bone. J. Radiol. Electrol. Med. Nucl., *52*:425, 1971.
117. Ridings, G. R.: Ewing's tumor. Radiol. Clin. North Am., *3*:315, 1964.
118. Kittredge, R. D.: Arteriography in Ewing's tumor. Radiology, *97*:609, 1970.
119. Ivins, J. C., and Dahlin, D. C.: Reticulum cell sarcoma of bone. J. Bone Joint Surg., *35A*:835, 1953.
120. Dolan, P. A.: Reticulum cell sarcoma of bone. Am. J. Roentgenol. Radium Ther. Nucl. Med., *87*:121, 1962.
121. Newall, J., Friedman, M., and de Narvaez, F.: Extra lymph node reticulum cell sarcoma. Radiology, *91*:708, 1968.
122. Greenfield, G. B.: *Radiology of Bone Diseases.* 2nd ed. Philadelphia, J. B. Lippincott Co., 1975.

18

CERTAIN CUTANEOUS DISEASES WITH SIGNIFICANT SYSTEMIC MANIFESTATIONS

Erythema Multiforme Major (Stevens-Johnson Syndrome)

Patchy pulmonary infiltrates indistinguishable from those of viral or mycoplasmal pneumonia may be seen in severe erythema multiforme.[1]

Erythema Nodosum

The inflammatory nodules in the skin and subcutaneous tissue can sometimes be seen on soft tissue films. The nodules are the result of a hypersensitivity vasculitis caused by a multiplicity of diseases and conditions.

Bilateral hilar enlargement, often associated with enlargement of the right paratracheal nodes, is found in about one fourth of cases. The adenopathy slowly resolves after clinical recovery, although a few patients develop diffuse parenchymal nodulation with small infiltrates. The roentgenologic findings are indistinguishable from those of sarcoidosis, which may be one of the underlying conditions.[2, 3]

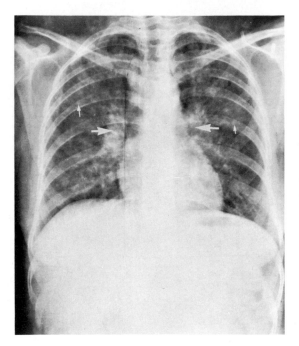

Figure 18–1 **Erythema Nodosum: Hilar Adenopathy and Pulmonary Lesions.** Chest film made during an acute phase of erythema nodosum demonstrates bilateral hilar enlargement (*large arrows*). There is also fullness of the right paratracheal area. Small nodular lesions of varying size (*small arrows*) are scattered extensively throughout both lung fields. These findings are indistinguishable from those of sarcoidosis.

Behçet's Disease

This syndrome of pyodermia and uveitis is a multisystem disease, thought to be due to vascular hypersensitivity, and analogous to a collagen disease. It chiefly affects young males in the Middle East.

In a small percentage of cases there are respiratory episodes during which there are either bronchopneumonic infiltrates or hilar adenopathy, or both, similar to the findings in some cases of erythema nodosum.

Aneurysms of large and medium-sized arteries may occur. Some patients develop a colitis indistinguishable from ulcerative colitis. Arthralgias are common but produce no radiographic changes.[4, 5]

Systemic Mastocytosis (Urticaria Pigmentosa)

Mastocytosis in adults usually affects the entire reticuloendothelial system. The childhood form is limited to the skin.

In adults the most common radiographic findings are hepatomegaly and splenomegaly. In about half the cases, osseous changes are found. Abnormalities of the gastrointestinal tract are not uncommon.

The axial skeleton is the usual site of the bone changes. Diffuse deposits of mast cells in the marrow can cause both resorption and thickening of bone trabeculae, leading to a mixed osteosclerotic-osteolytic roentgen picture. Osteosclerosis is usually predominant. Osteolytic areas are especially common in the ribs, producing a cyst-like appearance. The bone sclerosis may be diffuse or spotty, and closely resembles the changes of myelofibrosis. The diploic spaces in the skull are often obliterated by thickened sclerotic tables. Even in cases without apparent bone changes, bone marrow biopsy will usually be positive.

In the large number of patients with gastrointestinal symptoms, roentgen studies will uncover either a peptic ulcer or changes in the small bowel, or both. The small bowel may show scattered small mucosal nodules, thickened valvulae, or diffuse thickening of the bowel wall, all due to mast cell deposits. The roentgen appearance is similar to that of many of the infiltrative diseases of the small bowel, such as Whipple's disease, diffuse lymphosarcoma, collagen disease, and amyloidosis.[6-8]

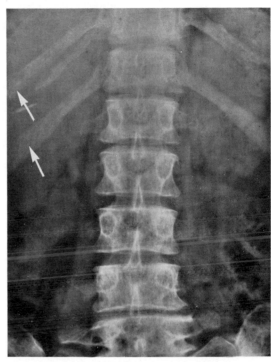

Figure 18–2 **Systemic Mastocytosis (Urticaria Pigmentosa): Bone Resorption and Trabecular Sclerosis.** There is mottled cystic osteoporosis of the ribs (*arrows*). The increased density of the lumbar bodies is due to thickening and increased density of the individual vertical bone trabeculae. Resorption between the trabeculae accentuates each of them. (Courtesy Dr. J. Snodgrass, Manhasset, New York.)

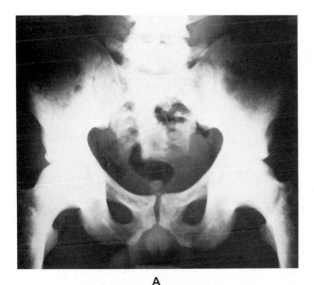

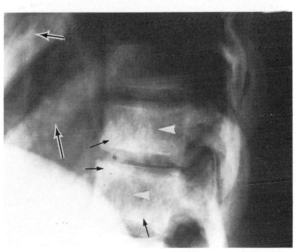

A   B

Figure 18–3 **Systemic Mastocytosis (Urticaria Pigmentosa): Spine and Pelvis.**

A, The pelvic bones, lower lumbar bodies, and upper femora are unusually dense owing to thickened sclerotic bone trabeculae.

B, The vertebrae contain areas of sclerosis (*black arrows*) and areas of osteoporosis between coarsened trabeculae (*arrowheads*). The ribs also show both osteosclerosis and osteoporosis (*black-white arrows*).

The sclerotic changes in mastocytosis are indistinguishable from the bone changes in myelofibrosis. (Courtesy Dr. D. D. Stephen, Sydney, Australia.)

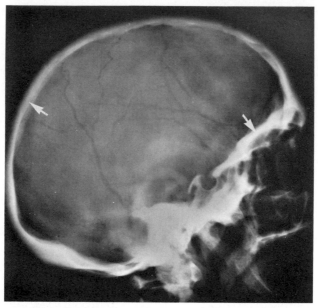

Figure 18–4 **Systemic Mastocytosis (Urticaria Pigmentosa): Skull.** The floor and tables of the anterior fossa are sclerotic *(arrows)*. The normal diploic space between the tables is obliterated.

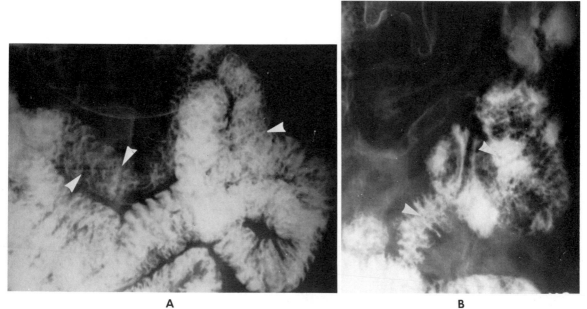

A   B

Figure 18–5 **Systemic Mastocytosis (Urticaria Pigmentosa): Jejunal Lesions in Two Patients.** Both of these middle-aged females had chronic diarrhea and other gastrointestinal symptoms. The characteristic bone changes of mastocytosis were present in only one *(B)*.

A, The nodular mucosal pattern seen throughout the upper jejunum is most apparent in the upper loops *(arrowheads)*.

B, The nodules are smaller than those in *A,* but are diffusely scattered throughout the jejunum *(arrowheads)*. (Courtesy Dr. A. R. Clemett, New York City, New York.)

Neurofibromatosis (von Recklinghausen's Disease)

Roentgenologic changes may appear in the skeletal system, the soft tissues, the central nervous system, and, least frequently, in the lungs.

Bone changes occur in about half the cases. They are usually caused either by erosions from an adjacent soft tissue neurofibroma, or by an intrinsic osseous dysplasia, or by both. Erosive deformities are most frequent in the posterior vertebral bodies and the ribs. In the latter they may simulate the rib notching from coarctation of the aorta.

The dysplastic deformities are the more common and the earlier findings. Localized scoliosis or kyphoscoliosis is the most frequent and sometimes the only osseous abnormality. Bowing of one or more long bones and absence of the posterior and superior walls of an orbit are characteristic but relatively infrequent findings. The latter abnormality is associated with pulsating exophthalmos. Scalloping of multiple vertebral bodies posteriorly can be due to neurofibromas of the posterior nerve roots but more often is due to dysplasia. Ununited fractures can lead to pseudoarthrosis. Other disorders of bone growth may be associated with minimal to massive hypertrophy of the overlying soft tissues.

Rarely, neurofibromas appear in the medullary portion of a bone, producing a cystic-appearing intramedullary lytic lesion.

Individual subcutaneous neurofibromas may produce recognizable soft tissue shadows. Massive soft tissue enlargements are usually due to both neurofibromas and soft tissue hypertrophy.

The central nervous system tumors usually arise from the spinal nerve roots and can be demonstrated by myelography. (See *Neuroma*, p. 419).

Pulmonary interstitial fibrosis is an infrequent finding in neurofibromatosis and may progress to a full-blown honeycomb lung picture.

Vascular lesions are not uncommon. Coarctation of the abdominal aorta and dysplasia of renal arteries with hypertension sometimes occur. Association of neurofibromatosis with pheochromocytoma or thyroid carcinoma has been reported.

Associated congenital anomalies are found in a small number of patients. These include spina bifida, fused vertebrae, dislocated hip, clubfoot, and meningocele.

The fairly common solitary neurofibroma in the posterior mediastinum is usually not part of a generalized neurofibromatosis.[9-11]

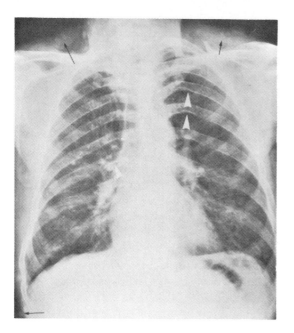

Figure 18–6 **Neurofibromatosis: Subcutaneous Nodules and Rib Notching.**   Small, discrete round or oval densities of varying sizes are present in the soft tissues of the right lower chest wall and supra-clavicular areas *(black arrows)*. There is notching of the undersurface of a number of ribs *(arrowheads)*, owing to pressure of neurofibromas of the intercostal nerves; this can simulate the notching seen in coarctation of the aorta.

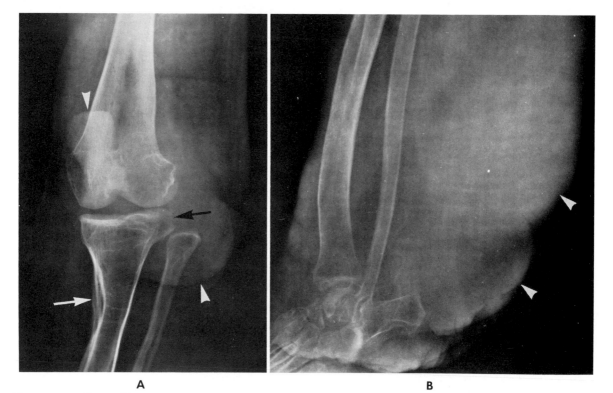

A   B

Figure 18–7   **Neurofibromatosis: Disturbance of Bone Growth, and Soft Tissue Hypertrophy.**

A, There is marked soft tissue hypertrophy around the knee and lower femur; a large neurofibroma *(arrowheads)* is outlined in the soft tissues. There is absence of modeling of the lower femur, especially on the medial side, and the upper tibia *(black arrow)* is deformed by an overgrowth of the lateral tibial condyle. Deformity of the upper tibial shaft *(white arrow)* is caused by pressure of an adjacent neurofibroma.

B, There is extreme hypertrophy of the soft tissues of the leg, in which are found lobulated neurofibromatous masses *(arrowheads)*. Marked growth disturbance is evident; the tibia is bowed, and the fibula is elongated and curved. All the bones are demineralized as a result of disuse.

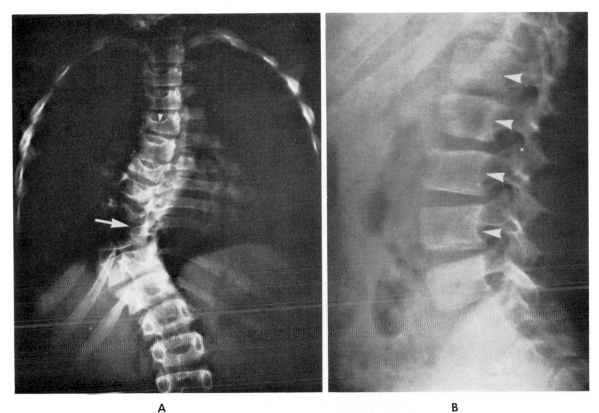

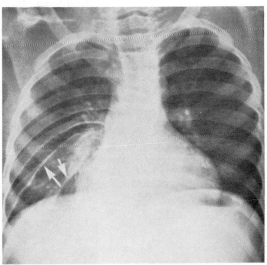

Figure 18–8 **Neurofibromatosis: Spine and Ribs.**

A, Marked scoliosis of the lower dorsal spine is due to dysplasia of the vertebrae (*arrow*). Frequently, scoliosis due to dysplasia of the vertebra without erosion may be the only roentgenographic finding in neurofibromatosis. The cervical spine is also often involved.

B, There is concave erosion of the posterior lumbar bodies (*arrowheads*) (from multiple neurofibromas arising from the spinal nerves).

C, Deformity and erosion of the proximal thirds of the eighth and ninth ribs on the right (*arrows*) are caused by neurofibromas at the site of the scoliosis. (Courtesy Dr. B. Levin, Chicago, Illinois.)

Ainhum

This is a chronic nonspecific concentric inflammation of the deep fascial layers, usually limited to the base of one or both fifth toes. Male Negroes in tropical areas are predominantly affected.

Radiographically, a sharply localized constriction of the soft tissues can be demonstrated, usually between the proximal and middle phalanges of the fifth toe. Resorption of the underlying bone depends on the duration of the disease, but eventually there is complete dissolution of the bone segment beneath the soft tissue ring without evidence of change in the adjacent bones. The appearance is quite characteristic and diagnostic.[12, 13]

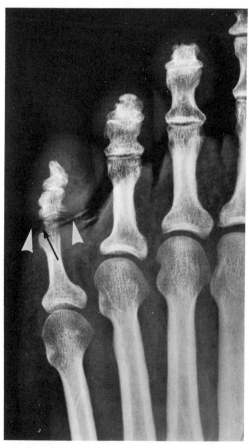

Figure 18–9 **Ainhum.** The lucent band *(arrowheads)* encircling the base of the fifth toe is due to indentation of the soft tissues. There is resorption of the lateral portion of the head of the proximal phalanx *(arrow).* (Courtesy D. Griffiths, Manchester, England.)

Gardner's Syndrome

The salient radiographic findings in this familial disease are multiple colonic polyps, multiple osteomas especially in the face and skull, and cortical thickening of the diaphyses of one or more long bones.

The colonic polyps are best demonstrated by the air-contrast barium enema. The lesions are numerous, of varying size, and tend toward malignant change. Infrequently, duodenal polyps and adenocarcinoma of the duodenum have been reported.

Lobate osteomas are most common in the maxilla and mandible but may occasionally appear in a long bone. The diaphyses of the long bones often show irregularly thickened and undulating cortices. There may also be scattered small intramedullary bone condensations, probably representing endosteal osteomas.

Dental abnormalities, including odontomas, dentigerous cysts, and supernumerary and unerupted teeth, are also frequently encountered.

The clinical soft tissue swellings are usually from underlying osteomas, but sebaceous cysts, desmoids, fibromas, and lipomas in the soft tissues are also frequent in this condition.

Recognition of the bone changes should suggest a colon study and may lead to uncovering asymptomatic but potentially malignant colonic polyps.[14-16]

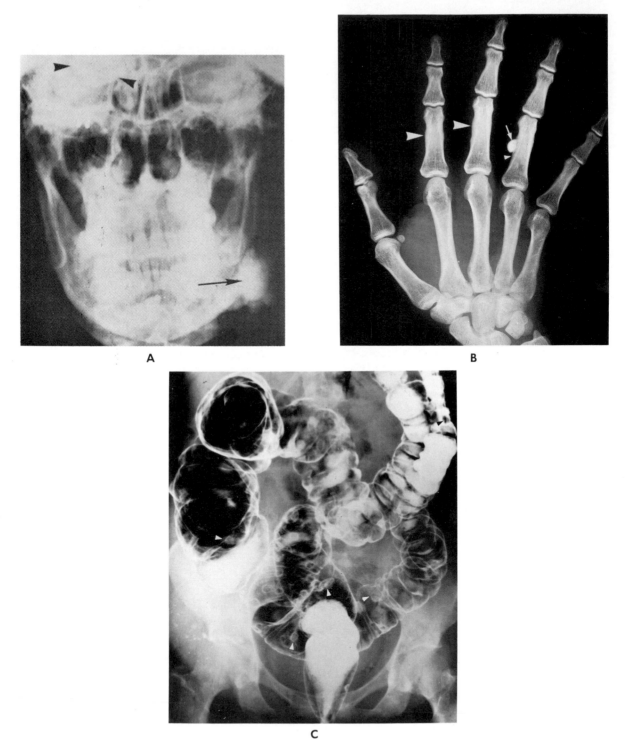

Figure 18–10 **Gardner's Syndrome.**

A, There is a multilobulated, dense osteoma at the angle of the left mandible *(arrow)* and another in the right frontal bone *(arrowheads).*

B, A dense osteoma of one phalanx *(arrow)* is associated with cortical thickening *(small arrowhead).* Other phalanges show somewhat undulating cortical thickening *(large arrowheads),* which gives these bones increased density.

C, An air-contrast enema film discloses a large number of colonic polyps of varying sizes *(arrowheads).*

The roentgenographic triad of osteomas, cortical thickening, and colonic polyps is uniquely characteristic of Gardner's syndrome. (Courtesy Dr. W. P. Cornell, Phoenix, Arizona.)

Epidermolysis Bullosa

In this rare hereditary skin disease, radiographic changes may occur in the hands or feet, and in the esophagus.

Marked webbing between the fingers is caused by epithelial bridging between opposing skin bullae. Flexion deformities of the fingers produce a claw-like hand. Soft tissue atrophy is striking. The distal phalanges may become shortened and tapered and, in advanced cases, are pointed and cone-shaped. The bone changes, apparently due to ischemia from repeated episodes of soft tissue scarring, resemble the changes of Raynaud's disease.

In patients with dysphagia, there may be strictures in any portion of the esophagus. These appear as smooth narrowings with tapering borders and are similar to the benign stenoses of peptic esophagitis.[17-19]

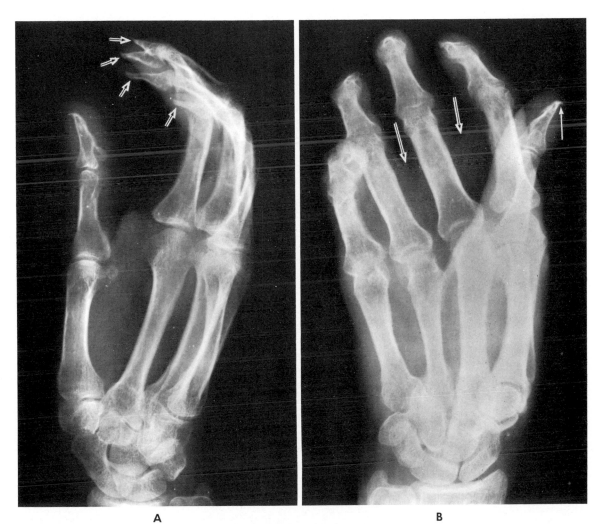

A

B

Figure 18–11 **Epidermolysis Bullosa: Characteristic Hand Changes.**

A, There is a fixed claw-like flexion of the phalanges. All the terminal phalanges taper sharply to pointed tips (*arrows*).

B, The webbing between the proximal fingers is apparent (*black-white arrows*). There is a sharp hook at the tip of the tapered distal phalanx of the thumb (*white arrow*).

The combination of flexion deformity, tapered distal phalanges, and webbing is virtually pathognomonic of epidermolysis bullosa. (Courtesy Dr. L. Brinn, Long Island, New York.)

Cronkhite-Canada Syndrome

See page 1076.

REFERENCES

1. Shapiro, H., and Lowman, R. M.: Roentgen manifestations of erythema exudativum multiforme (Stevens-Johnson syndrome). Dis. Chest, *32*:329, 1957.
2. Waisman, M., and Thomas, M. A.: Benign pulmonary hilar lymphadenopathy in erythema nodosum. Arch. Dermatol., *82*:754, 1960.
3. Wynn-Williams, N., and Edwards, G. F.: Bilateral hilar adenopathy. Lancet, *1*:278, 1954.
4. Marchi, B.: Pulmonary manifestations of Behçet's syndrome. Radiol. Med., *52*:314, 1966.
5. O'Duffy, J. D., et al.: Behçet's disease. Ann. Intern. Med., *75*:561, 1971.
6. Poppel, M., et al.: Roentgen manifestations of urticaria pigmentosa. Am. J. Roentgenol. Radium Ther. Nucl. Med., *82*:239, 1959.
7. Clemett, A. R., et al.: Gastro-intestinal lesions in mastocytosis. Am. J. Roentgenol. Radium Ther. Nucl. Med., *103*:405, 1968.
8. Robbins, A. H., Schimmel, E. M., and Krishna, C. V. G.: Mastocytosis. Am. J. Roentgenol. Radium Ther. Nucl. Med., *115*:297, 1972.
9. Levin, B.: Neurofibromatosis: clinical and roentgen manifestations. Radiology, *71*:48, 1955.
10. Hunt, J. C., and Pugh, D. G.: Skeletal lesions in neurofibromatosis. Radiology, *76*:1, 1961.
11. Smith, C. J., Hatch, F. E., et al.: Renal artery dysplasia as a cause of hypertension in neurofibromatosis. Arch. Intern. Med., *125*:1022, 1970.
12. Auckland, G., et al.: Ainhum. J. Bone Joint Surg., *39B*:513, 1957.
13. Fetterman, L. E., Hardy, R., and Lehrer, H.: The clinico-roentgenologic features of ainhum. Am. J. Roentgenol. Radium Ther. Nucl. Med., *100*:512, 1967.
14. Ziter, F. M. H., Jr.: Roentgenographic findings in Gardner's syndrome. J.A.M.A., *192*:1000, 1965.
15. Schnur, P. L., and David, E.: Adenocarcinoma of the duodenum and Gardner's syndrome. J.A.M.A., *223*:1229, 1973.
16. Dolan, K., Seibert, J., and Seibert, R. W.: Gardner's syndrome. Am. J. Roentgenol. Radium Ther. Nucl. Med., *119*:359, 1973.
17. Brinn, L. B., and Khilnani, M. T.: Epidermolysis bullosa with characteristic hand deformities. Radiology, *89*:272, 1967.
18. Alpert, M.: Roentgen manifestations of epidermolysis bullosa. Am. J. Roentgenol. Radium Ther. Nucl. Med., *78*:66, 1957.
19. Naidich, T. P., and Siegelman, S. S.: Paraarticular soft tissue changes in systemic disease. Semin. Roentgenol., *8*:101, 1973.

MISCELLANEOUS HEREDITARY DISORDERS AFFECTING MULTIPLE ORGAN SYSTEMS

Dysautonomia (Riley-Day Syndrome)

This hereditary disease of the brain stem, hypothalamus, and autonomic ganglia occurs almost exclusively in Jewish families.

Dysphagia is a constant feature from birth and may be due either to abnormal pharyngeal neuromuscular contractions or to defects in the ganglia of the esophageal wall. Radiographically, prolonged contrast filling of the pyriform sinuses is due to abnormal pharyngeal neuromuscular contractions. This finding occurs in many other brain stem lesions. Defects in the ganglia of the esophageal wall will be evidenced by a dilated and aperistaltic esophagus, an appearance quite similar to that of achalasia. In milder cases, esophageal emptying is delayed only when the patient is in the recumbent position. Recurrent episodes of bronchopneumonia due to aspiration are common.

Some teenage patients develop a neurotrophic (Charcot) joint, apparently owing to absence of pain sensitivity. Effusion, subluxation, and epiphyseal erosions are the usual findings; the knee is the most common site.[1-3]

Ehlers-Danlos Syndrome (Cutis Laxa)

In about 30 per cent of cases, multiple small, round, or oval densities with a calcified rim are found in the subcutaneous tissues of the extremities. These densities vary from 2 to 15 mm. in diameter and have a random distribution. They probably represent cystic degeneration of fatty nodules with a calcified shell. These calcified spheroids can be distinguished from phleboliths by their location and distribution. Distinction from calcified subcutaneous parasites, especially cysti-

1419

cerci, can be made by the usual alignment of the calcified cysticerci along muscular and fascial planes and by the lucent centers in the nodules of Ehlers-Danlos.

Many nonspecific musculoskeletal abnormalities are found in this syndrome and are related to tissue hyperelasticity. These include scoliosis, thoracic cage deformities, hypermobility of joints, subluxations, and osteoarthritis. Congenital anomalies are commonly associated; among them are spina bifida, spondylolisthesis, and elongation of the ulnar styloid process. A high incidence of intestinal diverticula has been observed, probably due to elasticity alterations of the intestinal walls. Vascular anomalies have been reported, including stenoses of the pulmonary arteries and tortuous systemic arteries.[4-6]

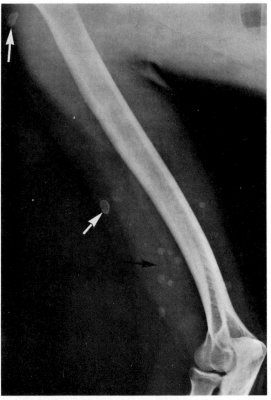

Figure 19–1   **Ehlers-Danlos Syndrome (Cutis Laxa).**   There are multiple nodules of varying sizes (*arrows*) in the soft tissues of the arm. The calcific rim is most pronounced in one of the larger nodules (*lower white arrow*). The centers of these nodules are relatively lucent because they contain fatty substance. Although the nodules are virtually indistinguishable from calcified phleboliths, the latter are rarely seen in this location; the location of these nodules, therefore, strongly suggests Ehlers-Danlos syndrome.

Familial Mediterranean Fever

Familial Mediterranean fever is a genetic disorder limited to certain ethnic groups, especially Sephardic Jews and, less commonly, Armenians and Arabs. It is characterized by multiple, self-limited, acute febrile episodes lasting from one to two days, occurring at unpredictable intervals, and accompanied by evidence of peritonitis, pleuritis, synovitis, or erysipelas-like erythema. Amyloidosis may develop in over one fourth of cases and is the usual cause of death.

Acute abdominal pain, the most common clinical manifestation, is associated with evidence of ileus, with the appearance of distended small and large bowel loops with fluid levels. Progress meal study of the small intestine reveals delayed transit time, a fragmented column, and dilated loops. Mucosal thickening is often apparent. With remission, all of these findings quickly revert to normal.

Chest films made during an attack of acute chest pain demonstrate effusion on the affected side, which disappears rapidly with clinical improvement. The rapid appearance and disappearance of effusion is a significant factor in diagnosis. During an acute attack, limited areas of basal atelectasis with little or no effusion may be demonstrated, but this is less frequent.

Joint manifestations occur in up to three fourths of the patients. The large joints are most frequently involved. Osteoporosis is common and is usually subperiosteal. During the early stages, osteoporosis may be reversible. In rare instances lytic lesions develop in bone, and there may even be destruction of the articular cartilage and subsequent formation of osteophytes. Asymptomatic changes in the sacroiliac joints sometimes occur. These changes will persist after clinical recovery.

Amyloidosis often develops after repeated acute attacks and may cause impairment of renal excretion on the intravenous pyelogram.[7-10]

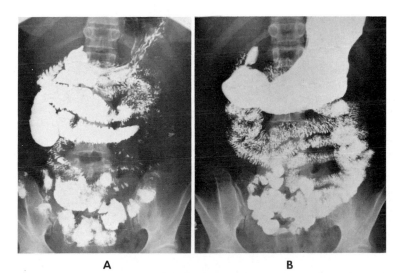

A   **B**

Figure 19–2 **Familial Mediterranean Fever: The Small Bowel During an Episode, and After Recovery.**

A, A film of the small bowel taken five hours after barium ingestion and made during an acute attack discloses discontinuous loops, dilatation of several loops, and very slow transit time.

B, During an asymptomatic period, the one and a half hour film discloses a normal small bowel. The meal has progressed in one and a half hours to a point which previously, during the attack, had required five hours. (Courtesy Dr. W. Eyler, Detroit, Michigan.)

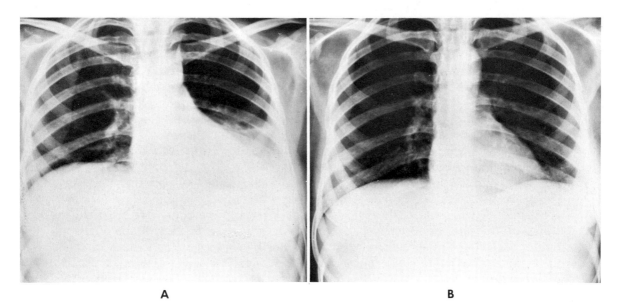

A   B

Figure 19–3 **Recurrent   Familial   Mediterranean Fever: Chest Findings.**

A, There is a left pleural effusion during an acute attack.

B, Complete clearing occurs five days later.

C, A subsequent attack of right chest pain was associated with a right pleural effusion. (Courtesy N. Shahin and F. Dalith, Tel Aviv, Israel.)

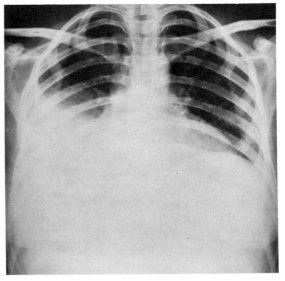

C

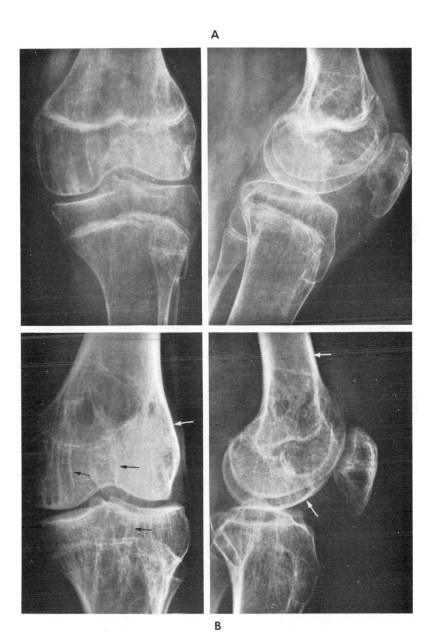

Figure 19–4 **Familial Mediterranean Fever: Changes in Joints Following Repeated Episodes.**

A, There is marked osteoporosis of the periarticular bones of the knee, with narrowing of the joint spaces. Such changes occur only following severe protracted episodes and have been misinterpreted as tuberculosis or rheumatoid arthritis.

B, Full recovery of function has occurred, although osteoporosis persists. There is increased cortical thickness *(white arrows)* and thickening of the primary weight-bearing trabeculae *(black arrows)*. (Courtesy N. Shahin and F. Dalith, Tel Aviv, Israel.)

Marfan's Syndrome (Arachnodactyly)

In this hereditary systemic disorder of connective tissue, the most frequent radiographic findings are in the cardiovascular and skeletal systems. Pulmonary changes can also occasionally occur.

Aortic involvement due to medial necrosis is present in about half the cases. Dilatation and aneurysm of the aortic sinuses and root are very common, but these changes are not seen on plain films; opacification studies are necessary. Dilatation and saccular or dissecting aneurysms of the ascending aorta are frequently encountered. (See Fig. 10–170, p. 732). Left ventricular enlargement from aortic insufficiency is also a frequent finding. Other less common anomalies include septal defects and dilatation or aneurysm of the pulmonary artery. A dilated ascending aorta and left ventricular enlargement are the most frequent findings on plain films; the other cardiovascular abnormalities of Marfan's disease usually require angiocardiographic studies.

Diffuse pulmonary emphysema or apical emphysematous bullae can occur and may lead to pneumothorax. In some cases, diffuse interstitial stranding and a honeycomb appearance are seen. In a child, these pulmonary changes are suggestive findings.

The principal skeletal change is the unusual elongation of the tubular bones, particularly in the hands and feet. The bones are long and slender, with thin cortices. The absence of osteoporosis helps differentiate Marfan's disease from homocystinuria, which it may clinically resemble. Other nonspecific skeletal anomalies that may be encountered include funnel or pigeon breast, winged scapula, and pes planus.[11-14]

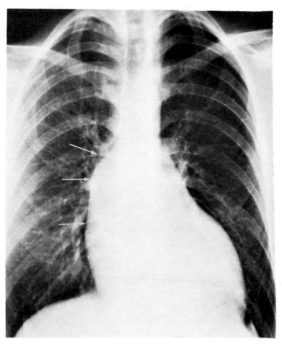

Figure 19–5 **Marfan's Syndrome: Dilated Ascending Aorta.** Cardiomegaly, left ventricular enlargement, and marked dilatation of the ascending aorta *(arrows)* are demonstrated in a young adult. The aortic knob is small.

Marked dilatation of the ascending aorta that originates at the root and that involves the aortic sinuses is characteristic of Marfan's syndrome and may result in aortic insufficiency. In aortic insufficiency due to rheumatic fever, there is generally less dilatation of the ascending aorta.

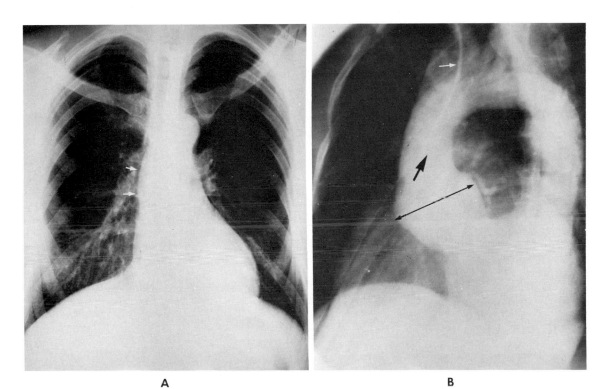

A   B

Figure 19–6 **Marfan's Syndrome: Aortic Involvement.**

A, In a 28 year old male there is slight but distinct prominence of the ascending aorta *(arrows),* a prominent aortic knob, and a cardiac configuration that suggests left ventricular enlargement.

B, Left anterior oblique view of a retrograde aortogram done by means of a brachial catheter *(white arrow)* in the ascending aorta discloses an aneurysmal dilatation of the sinuses of Valsalva *(double-headed arrow)* at the root of the aorta. Reflux of contrast material into the left ventricle (not clearly seen in film) was indicative of aortic insufficiency causing left ventricular enlargement. The proximal ascending aorta *(black arrow)* is slightly dilated.

Aneurysm or dilatation of the sinuses of Valsalva can be demonstrated only by contrast studies because the root of the aorta is intrapericardial and cannot be visualized on plain chest films.

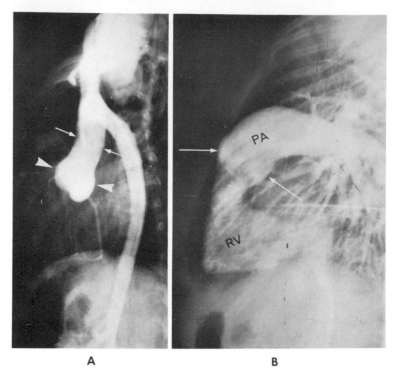

A   B

Figure 19–7 **Marfan's Syndrome: Changes in the Aorta and Pulmonary Artery.**

A, Lateral view of a retrograde aortogram in an infant with Marfan's syndrome demonstrates moderate dilatation of the sinuses of Valsalva *(arrowheads)* at the root of the aorta. The ascending aorta *(arrows)* is almost twice as wide as the descending thoracic aorta; normally it is only slightly wider.

B, Dextrophase of an angiocardiogram in another infant with Marfan's syndrome discloses dilatation of the root *(arrows)* and proximal portion of the pulmonary artery (PA). The right ventricle (RV) is opacified. There was no evidence of pulmonary stenosis either clinically or with catheterization studies.

Although dilatation of the sinuses of Valsalva and of the ascending aorta are the most common cardiovascular abnormalities in Marfan's syndrome, dilatation of the pulmonary artery is not uncommon in infants with this disease. (Courtesy Dr. A. C. Papaioannou, Athens, Greece.)

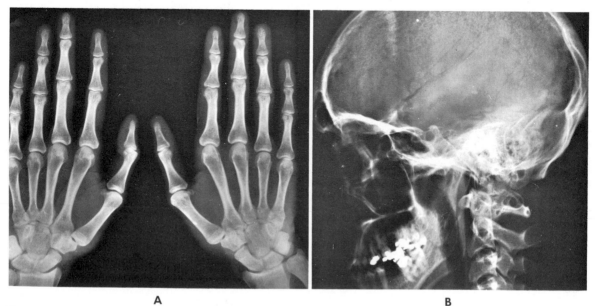

A   B

Figure 19–8 **Marfan's Syndrome: The Bones.**

A, The metacarpals and phalanges are long and slender. The cortices are somewhat thinned. This appearance is nonspecific and may occur in an otherwise normal tall asthenic individual.

B, Lateral view discloses that the distance between the brow and the tip of the mandible is abnormally long, thus accounting for the typical facies.

Hurler's Syndrome (Gargoylism)

In a fully developed case the roentgenologic skeletal findings are pathognomonic. Changes in the skull, trunk, and extremities are usual, although the bone involvement often is not uniform. The ribs and the bones of the hands and arms are most often affected; there are relatively few bony changes in the legs.

In the long bones the medullary cavity is widened, the cortex is thinned, and incomplete modeling further deforms the contour, often producing a rounded tapering at one end. This uneven increase in the bone width is the most characteristic radiographic finding. Less specific are the abnormal angles of the epiphyseal-metaphyseal margins, which are due to abnormal growth. Often the epiphyseal plates of the distal radius and ulna are tipped toward each other. The ribs are widened and have thin cortices. Coxa valga may be present.

Kyphosis in the dorsolumbar segment of the spine, resulting from underdevelopment of the superior half of one or more vertebrae, is characteristic. There is often "beaking" of the inferior border of the affected vertebral body. A somewhat similar change is seen in Morquio's disease and achondroplasia.

The skull is always abnormally large, and dolichocephaly is common, often with a prominent frontal bulge. The sella is elongated and shallow with a long anterior recess beneath the anterior clinoids; this is termed the *J-shaped sella*. Sinus and mastoid development and pneumatization are poor. Hepatosplenomegaly is fairly common.[15-17]

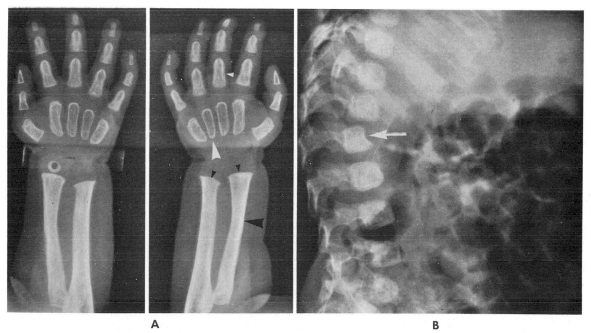

A   **B**

Figure 19–9 **Hurler's Syndrome: Extremities and Spine.**

A, The metacarpals are widened because of medullary expansion, and the cortices are thinned. Note the irregular contour of the metacarpals, especially proximally *(large white arrowhead)*, due to faulty modeling, and the irregularity in the contour of the radius *(large black arrowhead)*. The epiphyseal plates of the distal radius and ulna are abnormally angled toward each other *(small black arrowheads)*. The phalanges have the characteristic "bullet shape" as a consequence of tapering of the distal ends *(small white arrowhead)*.

B, There is localized kyphosis at L1 *(arrow),* with characteristic inferior "beaking" of the anterior aspect of L1. This is a fairly constant finding.

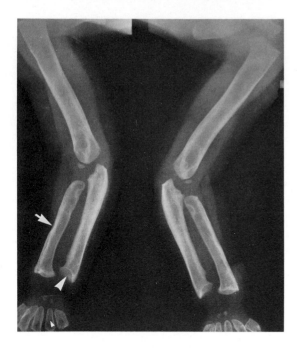

Figure 19–10 **Hurler's Syndrome: The Long Bones.** Changes in the metacarpals *(small arrowhead)* are identical with those illustrated in Figure 19–9. *A.* Irregularities in the contours of the humeri, radii *(arrow)*, and ulnae are typical of Hurler's syndrome. There is marked abnormal angulation of the distal radii and ulnae *(large arrowhead)*.

Figure 19–11 **Hurler's Syndrome: The Skull.** The skull is large and dolichocephalic, with a prominent frontal bone and small facial bones. The sella is shallow and long *(arrows)*, and there is an anterior recess under the anterior clinoids. The articular surface of the mandibular condyle is straight *(arrowheads)* instead of convex (convex is normal), and in some cases it becomes concave. These condylar changes are now considered characteristic of Hurler's syndrome. The sphenoid sinus is very small, and the other sinuses and mastoids are not pneumatized.

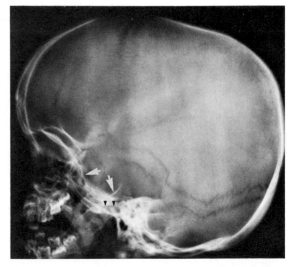

Morquio's Syndrome

This dysplasia, also called chondro-osteodystrophy, is a genetic hereditary disease involving epiphyseal cartilage; it causes dwarfism, kyphosis, and disability, but it is not associated with mental deficiency. It is somewhat akin to Hurler's syndrome, another mucopolysaccharide disturbance (see p. 1427).

Roentgen changes begin in childhood and are found in the spine, pelvis, hands, and wrist. The most constant and distinctive radiographic findings are flat, irregular vertebral bodies with a central anterior projection. Widened disc spaces, one or more wedged or oval vertebrae, and kyphosis are common. The odontoid process is either hypoplastic or absent. Atlantoaxial subluxations are very common and may cause neurologic signs. The ends of the growing long bones show irregular ossification, broadening, and irregular epiphyseal lines. The hips often Hurler's syndrome, another mucopolysaccharide disturbance (see p. 1427).

have deformed femoral heads and deep acetabula and may be subluxated. The pelvis narrows at the level of the acetabula, and the iliac wings are narrowed. The bones of the hands and feet are short and irregularly ossified. The bases of the second to fifth metacarpals are conical.

In contrast to Hurler's disease, the skull and facial bones are unaffected in Morquio's disease.[18-20]

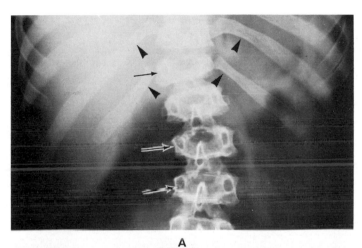

A

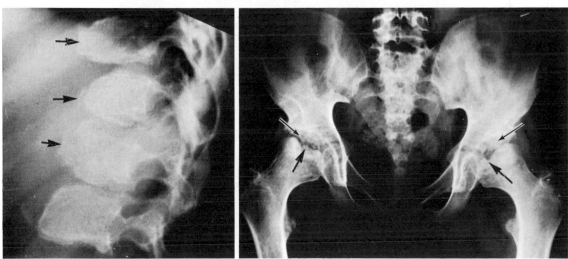

B   C

Figure 19–12 **Morquio's Syndrome in Young Adult.**

A, The dorsolumbar bodies are flat and irregular *(arrows),* and the intervertebral spaces are widened. The ribs are wider than normal but are narrowed near their proximal ends *(arrowheads).*

B, Close-up lateral view reveals irregular, deformed dorsal bodies, several of which have an oval shape. A characteristic "tongue" of bone anteriorly *(arrows)* is seen in several bodies.

C, Both femoral heads are irregularly deformed and flattened *(black arrows).* The acetabula are also irregularly ossified *(black-white arrows).* A mild bilateral coxa valga is present.

The changes in the spine, ribs, and hips are quite typical of Morquio's syndrome.

Porphyria

Repeated attacks of colicky abdominal pain and distention may suggest renal or biliary colic, appendicitis, or bowel obstruction. Chronic constipation is also common.

During an attack there may be multiple distended loops of small and large bowel. Barium transit time through the small bowel is greatly prolonged, and the dilated colon empties poorly. Sometimes gastric atony is also seen. These findings are nonspecific, but gastrointestinal studies will help exclude organic lesions.[21, 22]

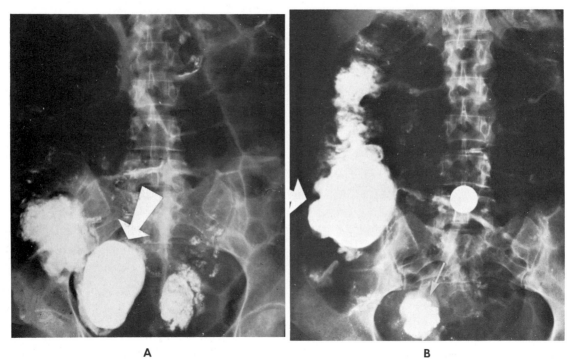

A   B

Figure 19–13   **Acute Intermittent Porphyria: Intestinal Hypomotility.**

A, A 40 year old woman experienced intermittent acute abdominal symptoms. Twenty-four hours after ingestion of barium there is an accumulation of barium in the ileum *(arrow),* which was palpable in the right lower quadrant. The colon is distended with gas. Barium is present also in the cecum and sigmoid.

B, Forty-eight hours later, some barium remains in the ileum *(small arrow),* and the remainder is in the colon. The cecum is now filled with barium *(large arrow),* and the colon remains distended with gas. (Courtesy Drs. W. Furste and P. Ayres, Columbus, Ohio.)

Pseudoxanthoma Elasticum

Roentgen findings in the soft tissues and vascular tree may be present in children and young adults. These result from degeneration of elastic tissue, the basic abnormality of this condition. Hematemesis, abdominal pain, or intermittent claudication may be the presenting symptom.

Calcifications in the soft tissues and blood vessels are the most common roentgen findings. There may be linear calcification of the dermal layer—calcinosis cutis—or extensive soft tissue or periarticular deposits. In blood vessels, either the media or intima may become calcified. Arterial opacification studies may disclose atherosclerosis-like irregularities and narrowing of the abdominal aorta or peripheral vessels.

Rarer findings include aortic dilatation, aneurysm, and hypertension with left ventricular enlargement. Miliary hemosiderin deposits may appear in a lung following pulmonary hemorrhage.

These varied roentgen findings in younger individuals are somewhat suggestive, but diagnosis can be made only by clinical and pathologic findings. A combination of angiomatous malformations and occlusive vascular changes on angiography in a young patient with recurrent abdominal pain or repeated gastrointestinal bleeding is highly suggestive.[23-26]

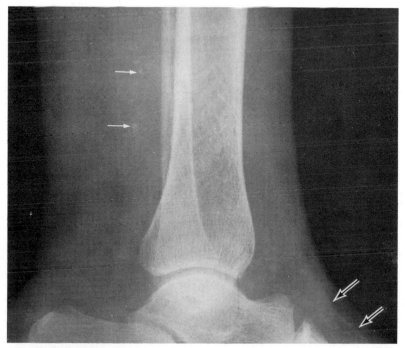

Figure 19–14 **Pseudoxanthoma Elasticum in Young Adult.**   There is linear calcification of the deep dermal layer of the dorsum of the foot *(black-white arrows)*. Vascular calcifications are seen in the soft tissues *(white arrows)*. (Courtesy Dr. A. E. James, Jr., Baltimore, Maryland.)

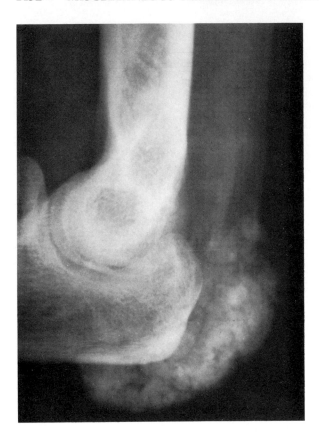

Figure 19–15 **Pseudoxanthoma Elasticum.**   An extensive collection of amorphous soft tissue calcification lies behind the elbow joint. (Courtesy Dr. A. E. James, Jr., Baltimore, Maryland.)

Figure 19–16 **Pseudoxanthoma Elasticum: Radial Artery Occlusion in Young Adult.**   The distal right artery is narrowed *(white arrow)*, and completely occluded *(black-white arrow)* proximal to the wrist joint. Tortuous collaterals *(black arrows)* from the interosseous artery supply the runoff of the distal radial artery in the hand. (Courtesy Dr. A. E. James, Jr., Baltimore, Maryland.)

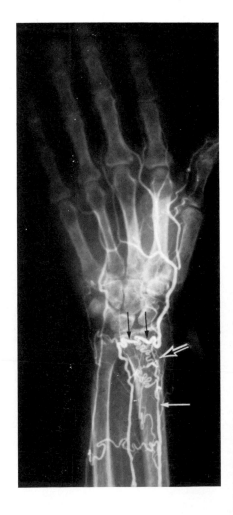

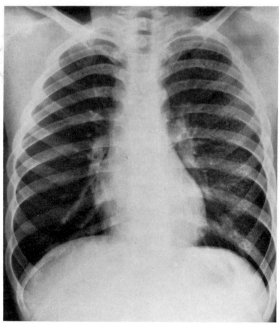

Figure 19–17 **Pseudoxanthoma Elasticum: Miliary Lung Lesions.** Discrete, moderately dense miliary lesions are scattered uniformly throughout the left lung, while the right lung is completely uninvolved. This unusual finding is probably the result of previous perivascular hemorrhage in the left lung, following which there were hemosiderin deposits limited to this side. (Courtesy L. Blair, London, England.)

Wilson's Disease (Hepatolenticular Degeneration)

In this hereditary disease characterized by excessive retention of copper, skeletal changes are found in about two thirds of the cases. Bone demineralization, evidenced by cortical thinning and coarsened trabeculations, is the most frequent finding. This may occur alone or may be associated with small subarticular cysts or small areas of periarticular bone fragmentation, most commonly in the wrists and knees. These joint changes are generally minor and asymptomatic, but occasionally a well-developed osteoarthritis may occur.

A renal tubular dysfunction of the Fanconi type can occur and may lead to renal rickets or adult osteomalacia, sometimes with pseudofractures. However, this form of renal dysfunction is seen in only a small percentage of cases. The cause of the majority of the skeletal changes is not understood.[27–29]

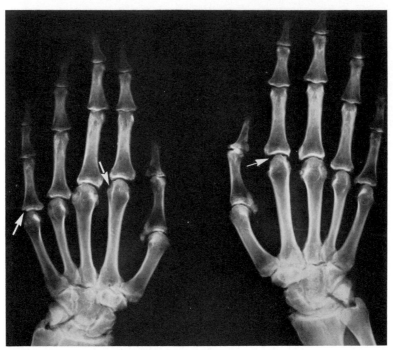

Figure 19–18 **Wilson's Disease.** A 37 year old woman had had Wilson's disease for 23 years. There is subchondral fraying and lytic areas adjacent to the metacarpophalangeal joints *(arrows)*, as well as severe osteoarthritis in both wrists, with areas of fragmentation and sclerosis. (Courtesy Drs. N. Finby and A. Bearn, New York, New York.)

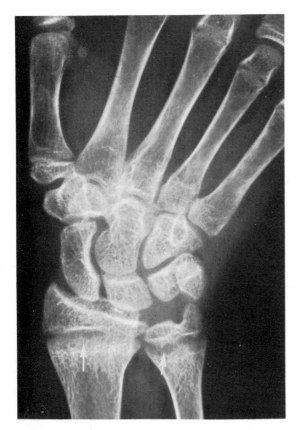

Figure 19–19 **Wilson's Disease: Rachitic Changes from Renal Tubular Dystrophy.** The patient was a 17 year old boy. There is osteomalacia, demineralization, and coarsened trabeculae. The remaining epiphyseal lines are widened, as in demonstrated in the radius and ulna *(arrows)*. The metaphyseal ends are fuzzy, and the margins are frayed. All of these changes are a result of rickets. In the adult, osteomalacia and pseudofractures would be seen. (Courtesy Drs. N. Finby and A. Bearn, New York, New York.)

Progeria (Hutchinson-Gilford Syndrome)

This rare syndrome of dwarfism with premature aging is a congenital deformity but is not hereditary. In early life it must be distinguished from other forms of hereditary or endocrine dwarfism.

The roentgen changes are generally distinctive and characteristic. Thin and often short clavicles, hypoplastic facial bones, delayed suture closure, coxa valga, and acro-osteolysis of the terminal phalanges are the most consistent and common findings. Other long bones may be strikingly slender. The bones are often diffusely osteoporotic, but epiphyseal development and bone age are generally normal. Subcutaneous fat is minimal or entirely absent. Premature atherosclerosis always occurs, and cardiomegaly, presumably from coronary artery disease, is common. Survival after age 20 is rare.

After the first few years of life, the clinical features are sufficiently unique for diagnosis. The unusual combination of roentgen findings is confirmatory.[30-32]

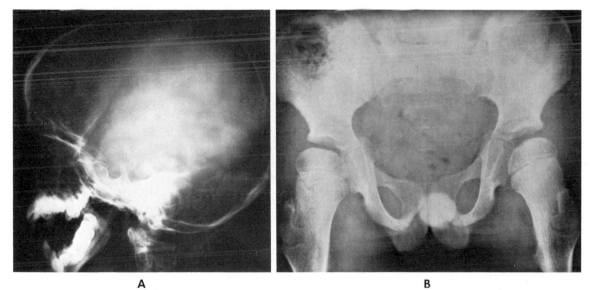

A   B

Figure 19-20 **Progeria in an 11 Year Old: Characteristic Roentgen Findings.**

A, The skull is not enlarged, but the hypoplastic mandible and facial bones are responsible for the craniofacial disproportion.

B, There is marked bilateral coxa valga.

Legend continued on next page.

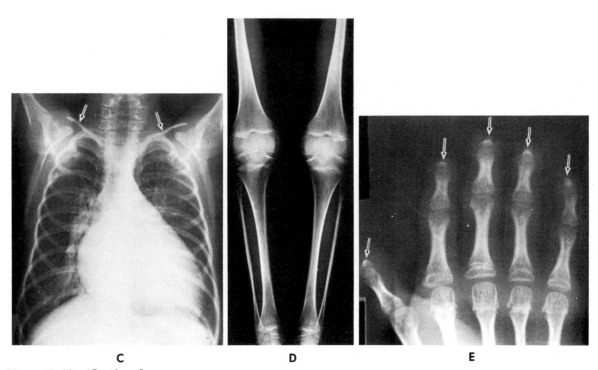

C   D   E

Figure 19–20   (Continued)

    C, The heart is greatly enlarged. The clavicles *(arrows)* are very thin and hypoplastic. Note the slender ribs.

    D, The femora, tibiae, and, especially, the fibulae are strikingly slender.

    E, Severe acro-osteolysis of the distal phalanges is evidenced by the absence of all the tufts *(arrows)*.

Pierre Robin Syndrome

The characteristic features of micrognathia and cleft palate are present at birth. The hypoplastic lower jaw crowds the tongue posteriorly and downward, causing inspiratory distress and cyanosis.

Radiographically the mandible and soft tissues of the lower jaw are extremely hypoplastic, and the tongue impinges upon the hypopharyngeal air passages. The cleft palate is recognizable on anteroposterior films. In about 10 per cent of cases, cardiac enlargement from congenital heart disease will be found.

A broad spectrum of other skeletal developmental anomalies, including limb aplasias and phalangeal abnormalities, may coexist with this syndrome.[33, 34]

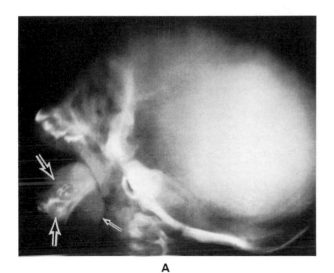
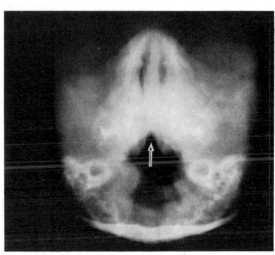

A   B

Figure 19–21   **Pierre Robin Syndrome in a Newborn.**

A, The mandible is extremely small, with poorly developed ossification *(large arrows)*. The soft tissue shadow of the tongue *(small arrow)* can be seen encroaching upon the air spaces

B, A cleft palate is apparent *(arrow)*.

Trisomy Syndromes

Among the recognized clinical conditions associated with chromosomal abnormalities are Turner's syndrome (gonadal dysgenesis), Klinefelter's syndrome (seminiferous tubule dysgenesis), and mongolism (Down's syndrome). In the latter, there is trisomy (chromosomal triplication) of chromosome 21. The radiologic features of these syndromes are discussed elsewhere.

Trisomy 13-15 and trisomy 17-18 have also been established as definite clinical syndromes. In trisomy 13-15 there are severe central nervous system defects, eye defects, harelip, cleft palate, congenital heart disease, polydactyly, and other abnormalities.

In trisomy 17-18 the anomalies are more constant, and the roentgenologic changes may suggest the diagnosis. The most constant and frequent deformities are low misshapen ears, receding chin, small mouth, a shield-like chest, hypertonia, abnormalities of the fingers and toes, and cardiac malformations, most often ventricular septal defect or patent ductus.

The most prominent radiographic findings include flexion deformities of the fingers and toes, ulnar deviation of the third, fourth, and fifth digits, defective ossification of the sternum, and an increased anteroposterior diameter of the chest.

An enlarged heart with increased pulmonary vasculature is often encountered. Many less frequent skeletal and visceral anomalies have been described, including intestinal malrotation and fused or duplicated kidneys. Affected infants rarely survive beyond a few months.[35, 36]

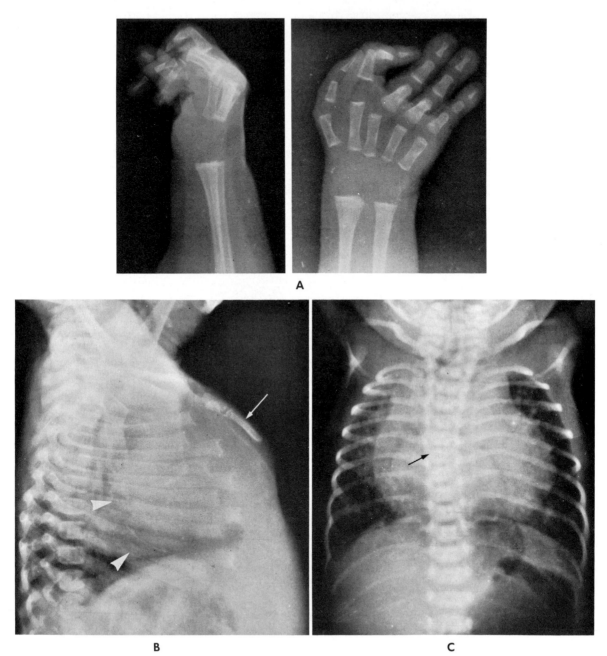

Figure 19–22   **Trisomy 17-18 Syndrome: Skeletal and Cardiac Lesions.**

A, Radiograph of the right hand, made at 13 weeks of age, shows persistent flexion of the fingers on lateral view. When the hand is straightened there is ulnar deviation of the third, fourth, and fifth fingers, and persistent flexion of the index finger (anteroposterior view).

B, Lateral film of the chest at age 6 months demonstrates a short sternum (*arrow*) and increased anteroposterior diameter of the chest. Cardiac enlargement is evident (*arrowheads*).

C, In another affected infant, a film taken at 3 weeks of age demonstrates pronounced cardiac enlargement with increased pulmonary vasculature. There is some scoliosis of the dorsal spine (*arrow*). The ribs appear thin. (Courtesy Dr. J. E. Moseley, New York, New York.)

Ring D Syndrome

A ring form of chromosome 13 in the D group is associated with this syndrome. Radiographically there are characteristic changes in the hands: the thumb is hypoplastic or absent; and there is shortening of the fifth middle phalanx and osseous synostosis between the fourth and fifth metacarpals.

Often, associated spine anomalies and dislocation of the hips are present.[37]

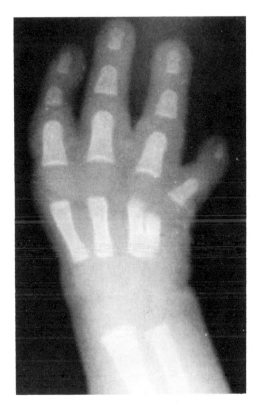

Figure 19–23 **Ring D Syndrome: Hand.** The thumb is absent, the fourth and fifth metacarpals are fused, and the middle phalanx of the fifth finger is not ossified. (From Poznanski, A. K.: *The Hand in Radiologic Diagnosis* Philadelphia, W. B. Saunders Co., 1974.)

Holt-Aram Syndrome

This familial syndrome consists of an atrial septal defect and bony deformities, most often in the wrist and thumbs. Radiographically, there is usually aplasia or hypoplasia of the thumb, inward curvature of the fifth digits, and a bifid navicular bone. Less often, there may be an absent or hypoplastic radius and various other skeletal abnormalities of the upper limbs.

Similar abnormalities of the upper limbs with or without congenital heart disease can occur in Fanconi's anemia, trisomy 18, and thalidomide phocomelia.[38]

Primary Immunodeficiency Diseases

See page 25.

Acquired Hypogammaglobulinemia

See page 28.

REFERENCES

1. McKusick, V. A., et al.: Riley-Day syndrome—observations on genetics and survivorship. Israel Med. J. Sci., 3:372, 1967.
2. Linde, L. M., and Westover, J. L.: Esophageal and gastric abnormalities in dysautonomia. Pediatrics, 29:303, 1962.
3. Gyepes, M. T., and Linde, L. M.: Familial dysautonomia; mechanism of aspiration. Radiology, 91:471, 1968.
4. Lapayowker, M. S.: Cutis hyperelastica: the Ehlers-Danlos syndrome. Am. J. Roentgenol. Radium Ther. Nucl. Med., 84:232, 1960.
5. Beighton, P., and Thomas, M. L.: Radiology of the Ehlers-Danlos syndrome. Clin. Radiol., 20:354, 1969.
6. Lee, M. H., Menashe, V. D., et al.: Ehlers-Danlos syndrome associated with multiple pulmonary stenoses and tortuous systemic arteries. J. Pediatr., 75:1031, 1969.
7. Eyler, W., et al.: Familial recurrent polyserositis. Am. J. Roentgenol. Radium Ther. Nucl. Med., 84:262, 1960.
8. Shahin, N., et al.: Roentgen findings in familial Mediterranean fever. Am. J. Roentgenol. Radium Ther. Nucl. Med., 84:269, 1960.
9. Sohar, E., et al.: Mediterranean fever. A survey of 470 cases and review of the literature. Am. J. Med., 43:227, 1967.
10. Brodey, P. A., and Wolff, S. M.: Radiographic changes in the sacroiliac joints in familial Mediterranean fever. Radiology, 114:331, 1975.
11. Papaioannou, A. C., Agustsson, M. H., and Gasul, B. M.: Early manifestations of the cardiovascular disorders in Marfan's syndrome. Pediatrics, 27:255, 1961.
12. Steinberg, I., Mangiardi, J. L., and Noble, W. J.: Aneurysmal dilatation of the aortic sinuses in Marfan's syndrome: angiocardiographic and cardiac catheterization studies in identical twins. Circulation, 16:368, 1957.
13. VanBuchem, F. S. P.: Arachnodactyly heart. Circulation, 20:88, 1959.
14. Lipton, R. A., Greenwald, R. A., and Seriff, N. S.: Pneumothorax and bilateral honeycombed lung in Marfan's syndrome. Am. Rev. Resp. Dis., 104:924, 1971.
15. Caffey, J.: *Pediatric X-ray Diagnosis.* Chicago, Year Book Medical Publishers, Inc., 6th ed., 1972.
16. Horrigan, W. D., and Baker, D. H.: Gargoylism: review of roentgen skull changes with description of a new finding. Am. J. Roentgenol. Radium Ther. Nucl. Med., 86:473, 1961.
17. Melhem, R., Dorst, J. P., et al.: Roentgen findings in mucolipidosis III (pseudo-Hurler polydystrophy). Radiology, 106:153, 1973.
18. Lomas, J. J. P., and Boyle, A. C.: Osteochondrodystrophy in three generations. Lancet, 2:430, 1959.
19. Langer, L. O., and Carey, L. S.: The roentgenographic features of the KS mucopolysaccharidosis of Morquio. Am. J. Roentgenol. Radium Ther. Nucl. Med., 97:1, 1966.
20. Blaw, M. E., and Langer, L. O.: Spinal cord compression in Morquio-Brailsford's disease. J. Pediatr., 74:593, 1969.
21. Furste, W., and Ayres, P. R.: Acute intermittent porphyria. Arch. Surg., 72:426, 1956.
22. Otte, R. C.: Gastric changes during an attack of acute intermittent porphyria. Radiology, 93:673, 1969.
23. Blair, L. G.: Disseminate lung lesions. Clin. Radiol., 6:1, 1954.
24. James, A. E., Jr., et al.: Roentgen findings in pseudoxanthoma elasticum. Am. J. Roentgenol. Radium Ther. Nucl. Med., 106:642, 1969.
25. Bardsley, J. L., and Koehler, P. R.: Pseudoxanthoma elasticum. Radiology, 93:559, 1969.
26. Altman, L. K., et al.: Pseudoxanthoma elasticum. Arch. Intern. Med., 134:1048, 1974.
27. Finby, N., and Bearn, A. G.: Skeletal system in Wilson's disease (hepatolenticular degeneration). Am. J. Roentgenol. Radium Ther. Nucl. Med., 79:603, 1958.
28. Mindelzun, R., Elkin, M., et al.: Skeletal changes in Wilson's disease. Radiology, 94:127, 1970.
29. Askoy, M., Camali, M., et al.: Osseous changes in Wilson's disease. Radiology, 102:505, 1972.
30. Margolin, F. R., and Steinbach, H. L.: Progeria. Am. J. Roentgenol. Radium Ther. Nucl. Med., 103:173, 1968.
31. Schwarz, E.: Roentgen findings in progeria. Radiology, 79:411, 1962.
32. DeBusk, F. L.: The Hutchinson-Gilford progeria syndrome. J. Pediatr., 80:697, 1972.
33. Denison, W. M.: The Pierre Robin syndrome. Pediatrics, 36:336, 1965.
34. Holthusen, W.: The Pierre Robin syndrome. Ann. Radiol., 15:253, 1972.
35. Moseley, J. E., et al.: The trisomy 17-18 syndrome. Am. J. Roentgenol. Radium Ther. Nucl. Med., 89:905, 1963.
36. James, A. E., Merz, T., et al.: Radiologic features of the most common autosomal disorders. Clin. Radiol., 22:417, 1971.
37. Juberg, R. C., et al.: Multiple congenital anomalies associated with a ring D chromosome. J. Med. Genet., 6:314, 1969.
38. Chang, C. H.: Holt-Aram syndrome. Radiology, 88:479, 1967.

SPECIAL
ROENTGENOLOGIC
PROCEDURES

This glossary contains a brief description and radiographic illustrations of many of the special roentgenologic procedures currently employed. Technical details, as well as contraindications, untoward reactions, and complications, have been omitted. The success and safety of many of these procedures require the skill and experience of specially trained radiologists or other trained physicians.

Abdominal Aortography

See *Aortography*.

Air Studies, Retroperitoneal

See *Retroperitoneal air studies*.

Angiocardiography

During contrast opacification of the cardiac chambers and the great vessels, a rapid series of films is made to follow the sequence of chamber and vessel opacification. Cine studies (*cineangiocardiography*) are often used instead of regular films; sometimes both cine and rapid film series are made. The contrast medium is injected rapidly into a peripheral vein (*intravenous angiocardiography*) or via a catheter into the vena cava (*venous angiocardiography*) or a specific cardiac chamber (*selective angiocardiography*).

Angiocardiography is the definitive procedure for roentgenologic diagnosis of congenital and acquired lesions of the heart and great vessels. Pericardial effusion or thickening can also be demonstrated.

Aortography (Abdominal Aortography, Thoracic Aortography)

Opacification of the abdominal or thoracic aorta can be achieved through retrograde insertion of a catheter into a peripheral artery (femoral or brachial). Direct insertion of the needle into the abdominal aorta through the lumbar area is sometimes employed (*translumbar aortography*).

1441

Aortography can disclose aneurysm, atherosclerosis, narrowing, occlusion, or malformations of the aorta or its branches. Deformity or insufficiency of the aortic valve can be demonstrated. The catheter tip can be directed into a specific aortic branch, allowing *selective arteriography* of this specific artery.

Normal Abdominal Aortogram

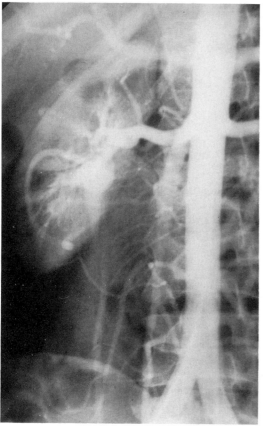

The abdominal aorta and its major branches are opacified. The common iliac arteries are also opacified.

Normal Thoracic Aortogram, Including Arch Vessels

The entire aorta, the left and right coronary arteries, and the right innominate *(small arrow),* the left common carotid *(large arrow),* and the subclavian *(arrowhead)* arteries are opacified.

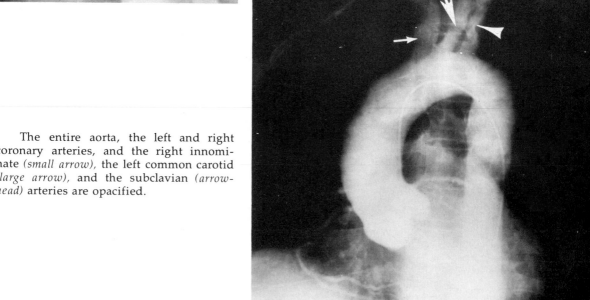

Arteriography

Direct injection of a contrast medium into an artery opacifies the vessel and its branches. Rapid film sequences are usually employed. The procedure is generally named by the artery injected (*coronary arteriography, celiac arteriography,* and so forth). Late films will usually show opacification of the venous drainage.

Arteriography permits visualization of vascular abnormalities, including atherosclerosis, stricture, occlusion, and malformation. Displacement of vessels and abnormal vasculature due to tumor or inflammatory lesions can often be recognized.

Arteriography, Celiac

Selective catheterization of the celiac axis and its branches will permit opacification of the vascular supply to the liver, spleen, stomach, and duodenum. Aneurysms, vascular abnormalities, displacements, and tumor vessels can be visualized. Temporary opacification of the liver and spleen parenchyma may be informative. Later venous filling of the splenic and portal veins can demonstrate venous occlusions and lower esophageal and gastric varices.

Displacement of pancreatic vessels can sometimes aid in diagnosis of pancreatic lesions. Occult sites of upper gastrointestinal bleeding can sometimes be demonstrated by extravasation of contrast material.

Normal Celiac Arteriogram

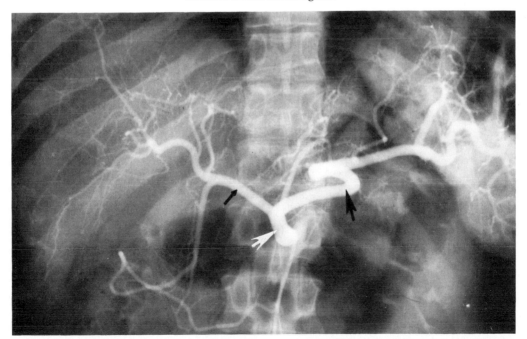

Both the splenic artery (*large black arrow*) and the main hepatic artery (*small black arrow*) arise from the common celiac trunk (*white arrow*). The intrasplenic and intrahepatic branches are well opacified. The gastroduodenal branch of the hepatic artery is filled.

Arteriography, Cerebral (Cerebral Angiography, Carotid Arteriography, Vertebral Arteriography, Brachiocephalic Arteriography)

Opacification of the arteries, arterioles, and veins of the brain can be obtained by rapid injection of contrast material into a major artery supplying the brain. Rapid sequential films are made in at least two projections to record all phases of vascular filling.

After direct injection into a carotid artery (*carotid arteriography*), the supratentorial vasculature (anterior and middle cerebral vessels) is opacified on the side of the injection. Direct injection into a vertebral artery (*vertebral arteriography*) produces opacification of the basilar artery and the infratentorial vasculature (posterior cerebral and cerebellar arteries) bilaterally. Injection into the right brachial artery (*brachiocephalic arteriography*) opacifies both the right internal carotid and the vertebral arteries and their intracranial branches, but usually less completely and less intensely than direct carotid or vertebral injection.

Currently, visualization of the carotid and vertebral arteries and their intracranial branches is obtained by opacification of the aortic arch via femoral catheterization.

Cerebral arteriography is a definitive method for disclosing vascular malformation, aneurysm, and arteriosclerotic or occlusive vascular change. Supratentorial neoplasms, subdural hematomas, and other mass lesions may be recognized and localized by arteriography. Tumor vascular stain is often produced. Infratentorial lesions frequently are best demonstrated by CT scan or pneumography, although vertebral arteriography may disclose subtle vascular changes due to small infratentorial tumors.

Normal Internal Carotid Arteriogram

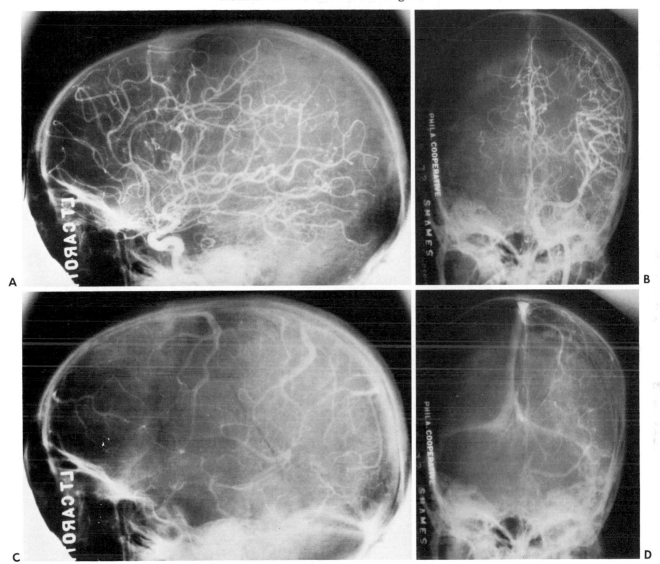

A, Arterial phase—lateral view; *B,* arterial phase—frontal view; *C,* venous phase—lateral view; *D,* venous phase—frontal view.

Arteriography, Coronary

The coronary circulation can be opacified after opaque material is instilled through a catheter into the root of the aorta. The catheter tip can usually be directed into one coronary ostium, so that a detailed outline of one coronary vessel is obtained (*selective coronary arteriography*). Rapid sequential films or cine studies may be made.

Coronary arteriography is employed to demonstrate atherosclerotic plaques, narrowing, occlusion, and malformations of the coronary circulation, and to determine patency of a bypass graft.

The Coronary Arteries: Aortogram

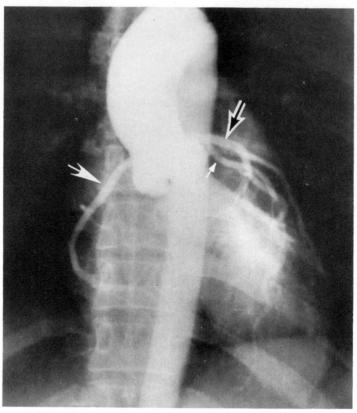

Injection of contrast material via a catheter in the root of the aorta has opacified the entire thoracic aorta and the proximal portions of the coronary arteries. The right coronary artery *(large white arrow),* the left coronary artery *(black-white arrow),* and its circumflex branch *(small white arrow)* are well opacified.

Detailed visualization of the coronary circulation requires selective coronary catheterization, oblique projections, and cineradiography.

Arteriography, Femoral

Films of the lower extremity made during and after injection of contrast medium into the femoral artery demonstrate the arterial tree of the lower extremity.

This procedure will reveal atherosclerotic plaques, stenosis, occlusion, and vascular malformations, and the collateral circulation can be estimated in the presence of arterial obstruction.

Normal Femoral Arteriogram

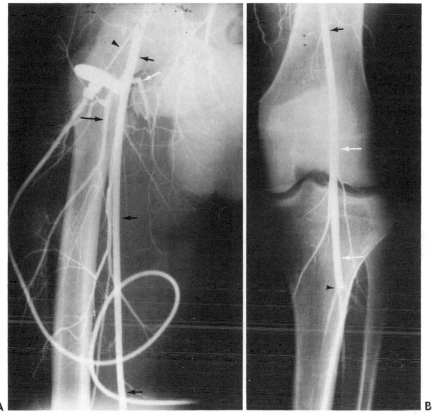

A, After injection of contrast material through a needle *(black arrowhead),* the entire femoral artery *(short black arrows),* and its profunda *(long black arrow)* and external pudendal *(white arrow)* branches are opacified.

B, The femoral artery *(black arrow)* becomes the popliteal artery *(white arrows)* and divides below the knee into the tibial and peroneal arteries *(arrowhead).*

Films taken slightly later would show opacification of the major arteries of the leg, ankle, and foot.

Arteriography, Mesenteric

Opacification of the superior or inferior mesenteric artery and its branches can be made via an aortic catheter directed into the appropriate artery.

This study may disclose narrowing, occlusion, and other abnormalities of the mesenteric artery or its major branches. Bleeding areas in the small bowel or colon can be identified by extravasated contrast material.

Normal Superior Mesenteric Arteriogram

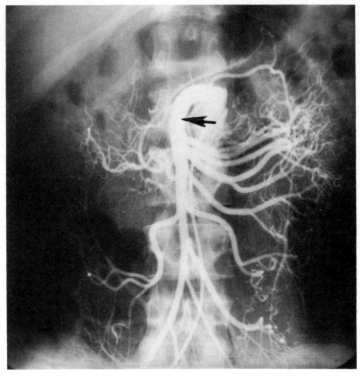

The superior mesenteric artery *(arrow)* and all its small intestinal and right colonic arterial branches are opacified.

Arteriography, Pulmonary

The pulmonary arteries and veins can be opacified most satisfactorily if the opaque material is introduced directly into the right ventricle or main pulmonary artery. This can usually be accomplished by passing a catheter into the right atrium and then through the tricuspid valve into the right ventricle and pulmonary artery.

The procedure will demonstrate congenital abnormalities of the pulmonary tree, including absence or hypoplasia of a major vessel. Pulmonary emboli can be identified and localized. Arteriovenous malformations and attenuated peripheral vessels of cor pulmonale and pulmonary hypertension can sometimes be demonstrated.

Normal Pulmonary Arteriogram

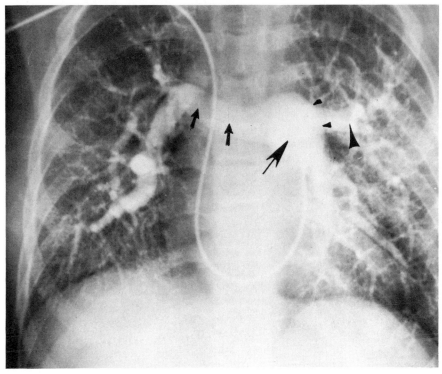

The catheter is in the main pulmonary artery *(large arrow and small arrowheads)*. The left *(large arrowhead)* and right *(small arrows)* pulmonary arteries and their peripheral branches are well opacified.

Later films would demonstrate the pulmonary veins and contrast material in the left atrium.

Arteriography, Renal

The renal arteries of both kidneys are opacified during abdominal aortography. Unilateral opacification of a renal arterial system can be obtained by selective catheterization of a renal artery *(selective renal arteriography)*.

Renal arteriography will disclose arterial abnormalities such as atherosclerosis, stricture, aneurysm, and occlusion. Arterial and arteriolar abnormalities due to tumor, degenerative diseases, or trauma can often be demonstrated. The nephrogram that develops shortly after arterial opacification is usually very dense, and small cortical lesions can appear as filling defects.

Renal arteriography is an essential study in cases of suspected renal vascular hypertension; the narrowed segment of the renal artery must be demonstrated before surgical treatment can be instituted.

Normal Midstream Renal Arteriogram

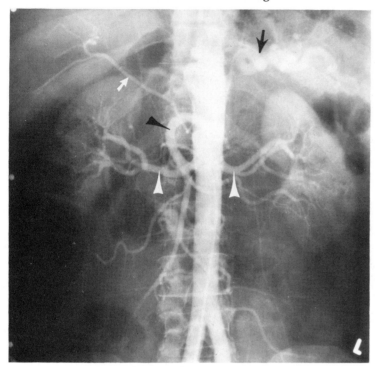

The splenic artery *(black arrow)*, the superior mesenteric artery *(black arrowhead)*, and the renal arteries *(white arrowheads)* are seen arising from the opacified aorta. A hepatic artery *(white arrow)* is arising from the superior mesenteric artery, a common variation.

Normal Nephrogram: After Midstream Renal Arteriography

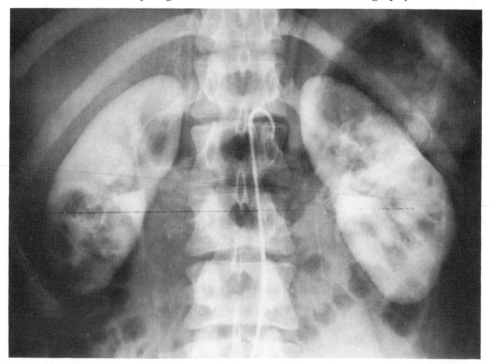

Both kidneys are diffusely opacified. The overlying gas shadows obscure portions of the nephrogram.

Arthrography

Direct injection of air or contrast medium, or both, into the synovial cavity of a joint permits visualization of enlarged joint spaces, synovial tumors or thickening, and, in the knee, cartilaginous tears or fragmentation. Arthrography is most often performed in the knee or shoulder.

Normal Arthrogram of Knee (Oblique View)

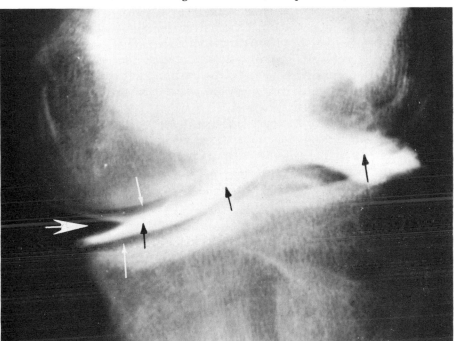

The opaque contrast material *(black arrows)* is in the synovial space and permits identification of the triangular medial meniscus *(large white arrow)* and the medial articular cartilages of the femur and tibia *(small white arrows)*. The cartilages are lucent relative to the contrast material and bones. Films are made in various projections to demonstrate the other joint structures and the various portions of the menisci.

Barium Enema Examination

Opacification of the colon by administration of an enema containing a barium sulfate suspension is the standard procedure for radiographic examination of the colon. In addition to films of the filled colon in various projections, spot films during fluoroscopy are routinely obtained. Frequently the terminal ileum is also opacified.

A postevacuation film is made for mucosal pattern visualization. If this is followed by instillation of air, double contrast opacification is obtained, which is useful for visualization of polyps, intraluminal tumors, and mucosal ulcerations.

Most colonic lesions are demonstrated by these studies; however, rectal lesions are best diagnosed by direct visualization during sigmoidoscopy, and a negative barium enema does not rule out rectal lesions.

Barium Meal Studies

These include roentgenologic and fluoroscopic examination of the esophagus, stomach, duodenum, and small intestine following ingestion of the barium sulfate suspension.

Fluoroscopy, spot films, and regular films are routinely employed. Cine studies or video tapes are sometimes made to supplement routine studies if subtle alterations of peristaltic activity are in question, especially in the esophagus or antrum. Roentgenologic examination of the esophagus, stomach, and duodenum is also termed *upper gastrointestinal series.*

In the small bowel examination, barium meal is ingested and serial films of the abdomen are taken at intervals until the barium column reaches the large bowel. Fluoroscopy and spot films are sometimes employed. This examination has been termed the *small bowel series* or *progress meal studies.* More complete small bowel opacification can be obtained by injecting the barium mixture directly into the duodenum through a gastric tube; this is a *small bowel enema,* and it produces continuous opacification of loops of small bowel.

Barium meal studies will uncover most of the significant lesions of the esophagus, stomach, and duodenum. Lesions of the small bowel are more difficult to detect, and repeat examination is frequently required.

Lesions outside the gastrointestinal tract frequently can be recognized by displacement or pressure deformities of the opacified esophagus, stomach, or small bowel.

Body Section Radiography

See *Planigraphy.*

Brachiocephalic Arteriography

See *Arteriography, cerebral.*

Bronchography

Opacification of the bronchial tree is obtained by instilling an opaque medium into the bronchi, usually through a tracheal catheter or by percutaneous transcricoid injection.

Bronchography demonstrates bronchiectasis, communicating pulmonary cavities, mucosal alterations in chronic bronchitis, bronchial obstructions, deformity or displacement from masses and bronchopleural fistula, and other disorders.

Normal Bronchogram

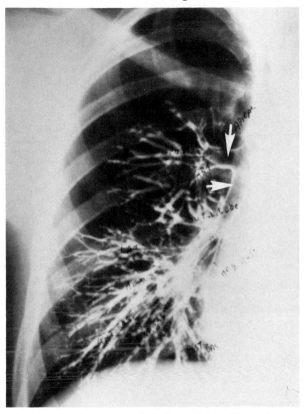

The major right bronchi (*arrows*) and their peripheral branches are opacified.

Cardiac Ventriculography

See *Ventriculography, cardiac.*

Carotid Arteriography

See *Arteriography, cerebral.*

Cavography

The inferior vena cava can be opacified by rapid injection of contrast material into the larger veins of the lower extremity, or by a catheter inserted via this route.

Rapid injection into an antecubital vein or via subclavian vein catheter opacifies the superior vena cava. The study can show narrowing, obstruction or displacement of the vena cava, and also the collateral pathways in cases of caval obstruction.

Normal Superior Vena Cavagram

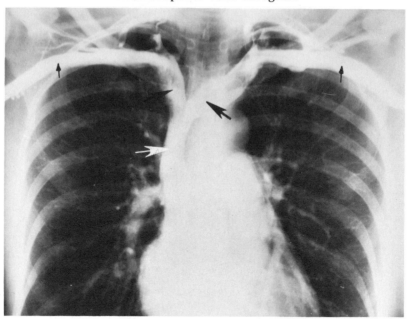

Bilateral injections of contrast material have opacified both subclavian *(small black arrows)* and both innominate veins *(large black arrows),* which join to form the superior vena cava *(white arrow).*

Normal Inferior Vena Cavagram

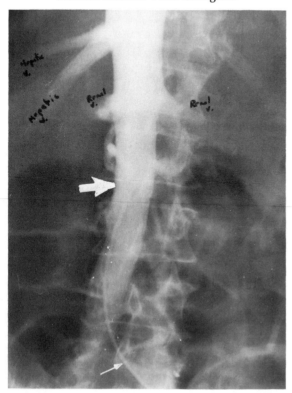

The vena cava *(large arrow)* and segments of the renal and hepatic veins *(labeled)* are opacified via a catheter *(small arrow)* introduced through the left femoral vein.

Celiac Arteriography

See *Arteriography, celiac.*

Cerebral Arteriography

See *Arteriography, cerebral.*

Cerebral Pneumoencephalography

See *Pneumoencephalography* and *Ventriculography, cerebral.*

Cerebral Sinusography

See *Sinusography, cerebral.*

Cerebral Ventriculography

See *Ventriculography, cerebral.*

Cholangiography, Intravenous

The larger hepatic ducts and the common duct are usually opacified within 10 minutes after intravenous injection of a special contrast medium (Cholografin). Frequently, planigraphy is employed to eliminate confusing gas shadows and to demonstrate more clearly a faintly opacified common duct. If the gallbladder has not been removed, it will usually be opacified within one to three hours following injection (*intravenous cholecystography*).

Intravenous cholangiography will not opacify the ducts in the presence of severe liver disease or jaundice; even in 10 to 20 per cent of normal subjects, duct opacification fails to occur after the injection, and most of the contrast material is excreted by the kidney.

The study is most commonly employed for determining the presence of common duct obstruction or calculi in a patient whose gallbladder has been removed. In the patient whose gallbladder is not visualized after oral cholecystography, the intravenous study will often produce opacification first of the common duct and subsequently of the gallbladder if the cystic duct is not obstructed.

Normal Intravenous Cholangiogram

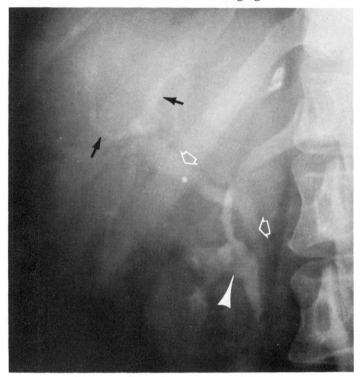

The common duct *(open white arrows)* and intrahepatic ducts *(black arrows)* are opacified. Better detail is usually obtained by tomography.

Note the opacification of the renal pelvis and calices *(white arrowhead)*, since some of the contrast material is always excreted directly by the kidneys.

Cholangiography, Transhepatic

This procedure permits opacification of the hepatic and common ducts in the presence of jaundice, when oral and intravenous cholangiography is generally useless.

A needle or catheter is introduced percutaneously into the liver substance; its entrance into the dilated bile duct can be verified by withdrawing bile. The contrast material is then injected, and opacification of the hepatic and common ducts will ensue.

The dilated biliary tree will be opacified up to the point of obstruction, usually in the common duct. The configuration at the obstructive site can often distinguish a calculus from a neoplastic or inflammatory lesion. Chronic pancreatitis may also cause a recognizable change in the common duct.

Because of the danger of bile peritonitis, transhepatic cholangiography is generally performed shortly before surgery.

The current use of a thin, flexible needle inserted deep in the direction of the porta hepatis has largely obviated the hazard of bile peritonitis or bleeding. Moreover, ductal opacification is usually successful even when the ducts are not dilated.

Cholangiography, T-Tube

The hepatic and common ducts can be opacified by injecting opaque material through the external opening of a drainage T-tube that has been placed in the common duct during surgery.

This procedure is frequently employed postoperatively in order to demonstrate any calculi or obstructive lesions in the common duct prior to removing the T-tube.

Normal T-Tube Cholangiogram

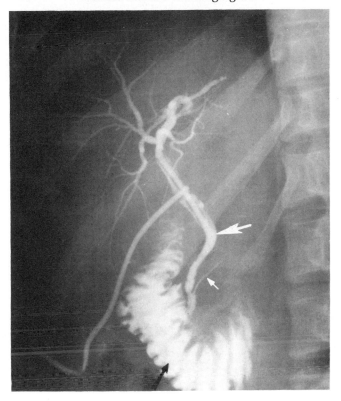

Injection of contrast material into the T-tube permits opacification of the common duct *(large white arrow)* and the intrahepatic ducts. Contrast material is seen in the duodenum *(black arrow),* indicative of patency of the duct. A small segment of the pancreatic duct *(small white arrow)* is sometimes opacified.

Cholangiopancreatography, Endoscopic Retrograde (Transduodenal Cannulation)

The ampulla of Vater can be identified visually with a flexible fiberoptic duodenoscope and cannulated. Contrast material is instilled, and the pancreatic duct or common duct or both are opacified.

Successful opacification will often permit identification of calculi, strictures, tumors or obstructions of the biliary ducts, and pancreatic carcinoma, pancreatitis, or pseudocysts.

Cholecystography, Intravenous

See *Cholangiography, intravenous.*

Cholecystography, Oral

Films of the gallbladder area are made eight to twelve hours after ingestion of an opaque medium. Erect or decubitus films are essential for exclusion of small calculi.

Nonvisualization may be due to a diseased gallbladder, impaired liver function, obstruction of the cystic duct, or intestinal malabsorption. The oral cholecystogram is useless in the presence of jaundice, since gallbladder opacification virtually never occurs.

The procedure is definitive for diagnosing gallstones, papillomas, and the cholecystoses. In the absence of liver disease, nonvisualization of the gallbladder generally indicates impaired concentrating power due to chronic cholecystitis or blockage of the cystic duct.

Cineangiocardiography

See *Angiocardiography*.

Cineradiography (Cinefluorography)

Motion pictures can be made of any radiographic procedure, utilizing an image amplifier and a specially mounted camera. Film or video tape can be used.

Cineradiography is valuable for demonstrating abnormalities of peristalsis and motility that often are not apparent on routine film studies. It is particularly useful when esophageal lesions are suspected.

Cine studies are employed in angiocardiography and coronary arteriography, either alone or in conjunction with conventional rapid sequential films. They are useful whenever a radiographic record of a functional movement is desired and are frequently employed in the study of normal and abnormal movements of joints. In some departments, video tape recording during fluoroscopy has replaced some cine studies, especially of the gastrointestinal tract.

Computerized Tomography (CT)

This study, also known as *computerized transaxial tomography (CTT)* and *computerized axial tomography (CAT),* is discussed on page 293.

Contrast Laryngography

See *Laryngography, contrast.*

Contrast Ventriculography

See *Ventriculography, cerebral.*

Coronary Arteriography

See *Arteriography, coronary.*

Cystography

The urinary bladder is readily opacified by introduction of an opaque medium through a urethral catheter. After the patient has voided, air may be introduced to obtain a double contrast study.

Cystography can disclose abnormalities in shape or position of the bladder, tumors, polyps, calculi, diverticula, and the degree of trabeculation. Vesicoureteral reflux can be readily detected, although it may occur only during voiding (see *Cysto-urethrography, voiding*).

Cystourethrography, Voiding

After contrast material has been instilled into the urinary bladder, films are made of the bladder and urethra during the act of voiding. Frequently, cine studies are made instead of serial films.

This study discloses evidence of vesicoureteral reflux, and demonstrates bladder neck obstruction, urethral stricture, and congenital urethral valves.

Normal Male Voiding Cystourethrogram

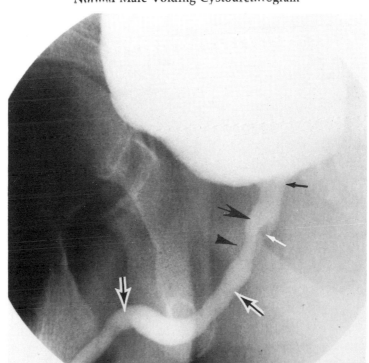

The bladder neck *(small black arrow)*, the prostatic urethra *(large black arrow)*, which contains the lucent verumontanum *(small white arrow)*, the short membranous portion of the urethra *(black arrowhead)*, and the long cavernous urethra *(black-white arrows)* are demonstrated.

Discography

This infrequently performed study consists of direct injection of a water-soluble opaque material into the nucleus pulposus of an intervertebral disc. Disintegration and herniation of the nucleus can often be demonstrated.

Drip Infusion Pyelography

See *Pyelography, intravenous.*

Duodenography, Hypotonic

The entire duodenal loop is rendered atonic and dilated by an injection of 60 mg. of Pro-Banthine (propantheline bromide). A water-barium mixture followed by air is introduced into the dilated duodenum through a previously swallowed tube. The resultant air-barium contrast visualization of the duodenum can be filmed in various projections.

Intrinsic and extrinsic lesions of the duodenum are more readily recognized on films made after this procedure. Equivocal pressure changes on the duodenal loop from pancreatic lesions may be demonstrated more conclusively.

Femoral Arteriography

See *Arteriography, femoral.*

Gastrointestinal Series

See *Barium meal studies.*

Gynecography

Nitrous oxide gas or carbon dioxide is introduced into the peritoneal cavity through an abdominal needle, with the patient in the Trendelenburg position to allow the gas to accumulate in the pelvis. The pelvic organs, including the uterus, fallopian tubes, and ovaries, are delineated by the surrounding gas. This procedure allows estimation of the size of the uterus and can usually demonstrate abnormalities of ovarian size and shape.

Hepatography

A transient opacification of the liver parenchyma (hepatogram) occurs during the capillary phase of selective celiac or hepatic arteriography. The size and shape of the liver are usually accurately delineated. Intrahepatic masses may be identified, either as a defect in the hepatogram or as an area of increased density, depending on the vascularity of the mass.

Normal Selective Hepatic Arteriogram

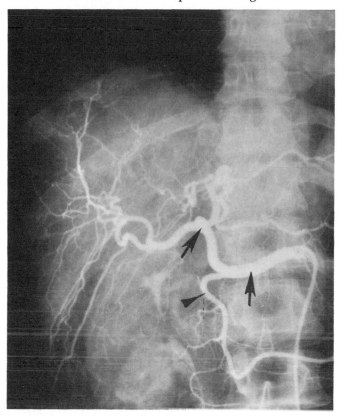

The hepatic artery *(arrows)*, its intrahepatic branches, and the gastroduodenal branch *(arrowhead)* are opacified.

Normal Hepatogram: After Celiac Arteriography

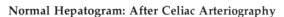

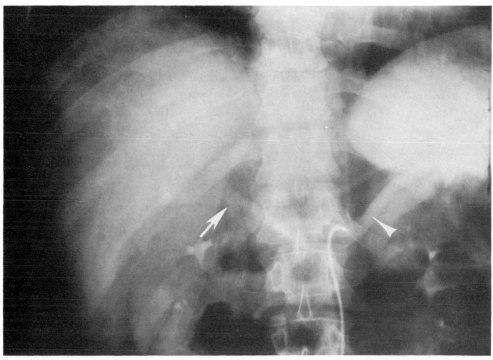

The entire liver is moderately opacified and of homogeneous density. The spleen is also opacified. The splenic vein *(arrowhead)* and portal vein *(arrow)* are easily identified.

Hepatosplenography

Satisfactory hepatograms and splenograms can be obtained during the capillary phase of selective celiac, hepatic, or splenic arteriography.

Opacification of the liver and spleen allows determination of their size, shape, and position. Tumors or other masses will appear as filling defects in the opacified liver or spleen.

Hysterosalpingography

Contrast material (usually water soluble and absorbable) is introduced into the uterus through a cannula. Injection is continued until the fallopian tubes fill and some contrast material spills into the peritoneum. Films are taken immediately.

This procedure allows estimation of the size and shape of the uterine cavity and can demonstrate intrauterine masses or tumors, and other anomalies. The size and patency of the fallopian tubes can be determined. The ovaries are not visualized. This examination is most frequently performed during investigation of infertility.

Normal Hysterosalpingogram

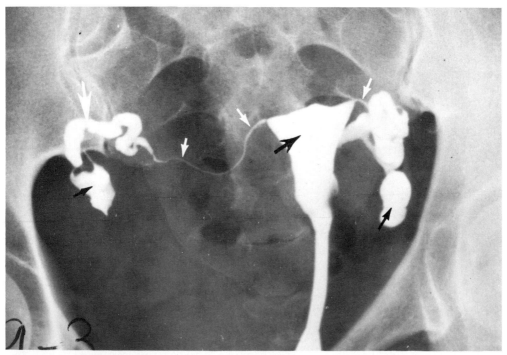

Contrast material has opacified the uterus (*large black arrow*), the fallopian tubes (*small white arrows*), and the fimbriated (outer) ends of the tubes (*large white arrow*).

Globules of contrast material (*small black arrows*) have passed through the outer ends of the tubes, indicating patency of these structures.

Intravenous Carbon Dioxide

Carbon dioxide in amounts of 50 to 100 cc. can be injected intravenously with the patient in the left decubitus position. The gas will temporarily accumulate in the right atrium. Radiograms are made with the patient in this position.

The space between the gas bubble and the right cardiac border will be increased in cases of pericardial effusion or pericardial thickening. The procedure is primarily used for pericardial measurement.

Intravenous Cholangiography

See *Cholangiography, intravenous.*

Intravenous Cholecystography

See *Cholangiography, intravenous.*

Intravenous Pyelography, Intravenous Urography

See *Pyelography, intravenous.*

Laminography

See *Planigraphy.*

Laryngography, Contrast

After administration of a topical anesthetic, an oily opaque material is dropped over the tongue during quiet inspiration. This produces an opaque coating of the laryngeal structures and effects an excellent anatomic portrayal on the radiograms.

This procedure is employed mainly to demonstrate the size and location of a laryngeal tumor, and is a supplement to direct laryngoscopy. Progress of a lesion during and after irradiation can be followed by contrast laryngography.

Normal Contrast Laryngogram: Frontal View

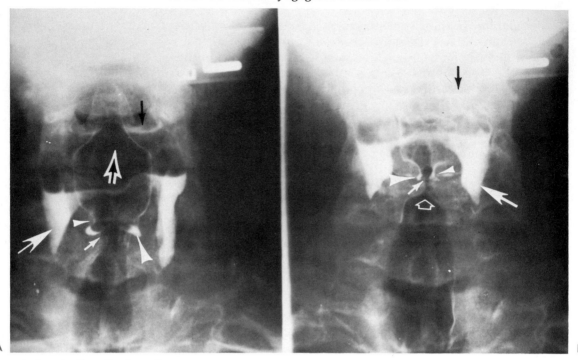

A, Inspiration; *B,* phonation.

Valleculae *(black arrows);* pyriform sinuses *(large white arrows);* true cord *(small white arrows);* false cord *(small arrowheads);* laryngeal vestibule *(black-white arrow);* subglottic angle *(open arrow);* collapsed ventricle *(large arrowheads).*

Limb Venography

See *Venography, peripheral.*

Lymphangiography and Lymphography

After direct injection of iodinated oil into a lymphatic vessel on the dorsum of the foot, there will be opacification of the lymphatic channels of the lower extremity, and of the inguinal, iliac, and retroperitoneal lymph nodes on the injected side. Larger injections produce opacification of the thoracic duct. Axillary nodes can be opacified after injection of a lymphatic vessel on the dorsum of the hand.

Lymphangiography is useful for diagnosing lymphatic channel block and diseased lymph nodes. Retroperitoneal node involvement in the lymphomatous diseases can be recognized.

Since the lymph nodes remain opacified for many months after lymphangiography, the effects of radiotherapy or chemotherapy can be evaluated by serial radiograms.

Normal Lymphangiogram

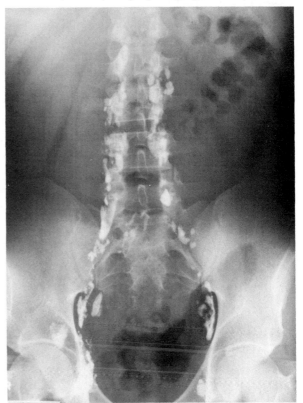

Injection of contrast material (iodinated oil) into a dorsal lymphatic vessel of each foot permits opacification of the pelvic and para-aortic lymph nodes. Earlier films would also show the lymphatic vessels.

Mesenteric Arteriography

See *Arteriography, mesenteric.*

Myelography

Opacification of the spinal subarachnoid space can be obtained by intrathecal injection of an iodinated oil. The column of oil is moved up and down the spinal canal by gravity under fluoroscopic guidance, allowing examination of any portion of the canal. This opaque oil is removed after examination.

Air can be used as a contrast medium after removal of spinal fluid, but this does not always produce satisfactory diagnostic films.

In some countries, water-soluble opaque materials are used for lumbar myelography. These produce total opacification of the canal but are irritating, even though absorbable.

Myelography is the standard procedure for demonstrating lesions of the cord and canal, for diagnosing disc herniation, and for localizing subarachnoid block.

Nephrography

See *Pyelography, intravenous,* and *Angiography, renal.*

Nephrotomography

Body section films (*planigram, tomogram*) are made of the kidneys after rapid intravenous injection of the opaque material, or during drip infusion pyelography. If properly timed after the injection, the films will opacify the renal parenchyma (*nephrogram*). Confusing shadows due to overlying gas are eliminated by the body section films.

An important use of this procedure is to demonstrate filling defects in the nephrographic density. Renal cysts can often be distinguished from tumors by the roentgenologic characteristics of the filling defect. Greatly improved detail of the pelves and calices is also obtained.

Normal Nephrotomogram

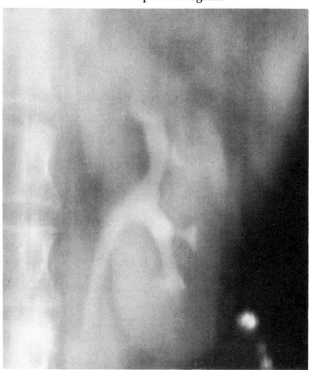

Delineation of the renal outline and collecting system and elimination of overlying bowel gas shadows can be obtained on nephrotomographic sections.

Oral Cholecystography

See *Cholecystography, oral.*

Perinephric Air Injection

See *Retroperitoneal air studies.*

Peripheral Venography

See *Venography, peripheral.*

Phlebography

See *Venography, peripheral.*

Planigraphy (Laminography, Tomography, Body Section Radiography)

Radiographic films which show the structures in a limited plane of the body by blurring out the structures above and below this level can be made with the aid of special mechanical equipment. The cassette and the x-ray tube move simultaneously in opposite directions during exposure. The stationary pivot point of this dual motion determines the level of the plane that is "in focus." Confusing shadows above and below this level are blurred out, giving a clearer view of the structures within the predetermined levels.

Planigraphy is employed to supplement any radiographic examination in which a structure is obscured by overlying gas or by other overlying or underlying structures. In pulmonary radiography it is particularly useful to demonstrate questionable cavities, masses, and calcifications, and to delineate clearly the air-filled tracheobronchial tree. Tomograms of the middle and inner ear can demonstrate anatomic detail and abnormalities that cannot be seen on conventional radiograms. Suspected fractures of the spine or facial bones can usually be readily clarified by tomographic studies.

Planigraphy is widely employed in diagnostic roentgenology to obtain better visualization of a radiographic abnormality, but it is rarely of value if employed in search of a lesion in an area that appears normal on conventional films.

Pneumoencephalography

Skull films are made using multiple projections after air has been introduced into the ventricular and subarachnoid cavities of the brain. The air is introduced into the lumbar subarachnoid space after an appropriate amount of spinal fluid has been removed. With the patient erect, the air rises into the cerebrospinal fluid spaces of the brain including the basal cisterns. The head is moved in various positions so that the air can be made to rise to any area of the ventricular and subarachnoid system.

Pneumoencephalography has been an invaluable procedure for diagnosis and localization of many neoplastic, degenerative, and congenital abnormalities of the brain. It is particularly useful for detecting infratentorial mass lesions; supratentorial lesions are usually more readily discovered and localized by carotid arteriography. However, the noninvasive CT scan is now frequently employed instead of pneumoencephalography.

Normal Pneumoencephalogram

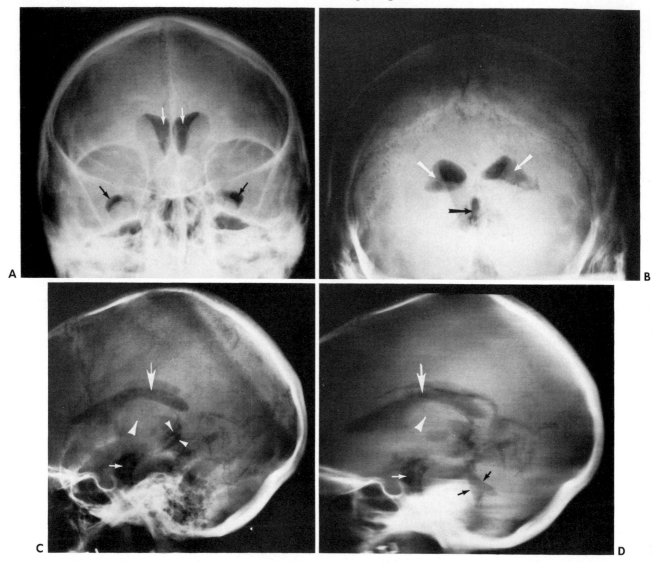

A, Frontal view; *B,* frontal view with chin flexed (occipital view).

Air is outlining the triangular frontal horns *(small white arrows),* the bodies of the lateral ventricles *(large white arrows),* the third ventricle *(large black arrow),* and a portion of the temporal horns *(small black arrows).* The cortical sulci are not well filled with air.

C, Lateral view; *D,* midline lateral tomogram.

The lateral ventricles *(large white arrows),* the ambient cisterns *(small white arrowheads),* the basal cisterns *(small white arrows),* and the fourth ventricle *(black arrows)* are filled with air. Air is also outlining the superior cerebellar sulci and cistern. The third ventricle *(large white arrowheads)* contains some air but is difficult to delineate on these films.

Pneumography, Cerebral

See *Pneumoencephalography* and *Ventriculography, cerebral.*

Pneumoperitoneum, Diagnostic

After 300 to 500 cc. of air is injected through the abdominal wall into the peritoneum, films can be made with the patient placed in various positions. The air will act as radiographic contrast to the intra-abdominal organs and the diaphragm.

The procedure is employed mainly to delineate masses in the upper abdomen, especially when the masses cannot be clearly or definitely visualized on ordinary films. The pneumoperitoneum will also aid in distinguishing a subphrenic abscess from an intrahepatic lesion and from an intrathoracic lesion that has completely obscured the diaphragm.

The pelvic organs will be outlined if the patient is placed in the Trendelenburg position (see *Gynecography*).

Pneumothorax, Diagnostic

An artificial pneumothorax can be produced by injecting air into a pleural cavity. If pleural fluid is present, it is usually withdrawn before the air is injected.

Chest radiograms made after this procedure can demonstrate adhesions between visceral and parietal pleura, can help delineate pleural masses, and will usually distinguish pleural from parenchymal lesions.

Portosplenography

See *Splenoportography.*

Progress Meal

See *Barium meal studies.*

Pulmonary Arteriography

See *Arteriography, pulmonary.*

Pyelography, Intravenous
(Intravenous Urography)

Within minutes after intravenous injection of a proper opaque medium, the collecting system (calices, pelvis, and ureter) of each kidney is progressively opacified. Films are made at intervals of five to fifteen minutes until the urinary bladder is also well opacified.

If the contrast material is rapidly injected, films made within two or three minutes will usually show opacification of the renal parenchyma (nephrogram) before the pyelogram develops.

A useful modification of conventional pyelography is the *drip infusion technique*. Four to six times the usual amount of contrast material, in diluted form, is infused. This produces far better filling and greater density in the collecting system. It is particularly useful when opacification by the conventional technique is diagnostically unsatisfactory.

Intravenous pyelography is employed for radiographic diagnosis of hydronephrosis, pyelonephritis, tumors, cysts, and many other renal and ureteral lesions. It will aid in the diagnosis of ureteral calculi, obstructive uropathy, congenital abnormalities, and so forth. The pyelogram is also a crude measure of renal function.

Certain alterations in the nephrogram and pyelogram may strongly suggest a renovascular cause of hypertension.

Pyelography, Retrograde

The pelvis, calices, and ureter of a kidney can be opacified by instilling contrast material through a catheter inserted into the ureter or up into a renal pelvis.

This procedure is currently used much less frequently than in the past. The intravenous pyelogram performed with the newer opaque media or with the drip infusion technique is usually as informative as the retrograde study; however, in a completely nonfunctioning kidney, the retrograde study often discloses the underlying disturbance. In general, the retrograde study is used when satisfactory delineation of the urinary tract cannot be obtained with intravenous techniques.

Renal Angiography

See *Angiography, renal.*

Retrococcygeal Air Studies

See *Retroperitoneal air studies.*

Retrograde Pyelography

See *Pyelography, retrograde.*

Retroperitoneal Air Studies

Air or carbon dioxide can be injected into the perirenal retroperitoneal space unilaterally by direct needle puncture of the perirenal space (*perirenal air study*).

If the gas is injected through a needle in the soft tissue plane between the rectum and coccyx, it will enter the retroperitoneal spaces bilaterally (*retrococcygeal air study*).

The gas will surround the kidney and adrenal gland, and will permit radiographic identification of these structures.

This procedure allows identification of retroperitoneal masses, abnormalities of renal outline, and tumors or hyperplasia of the adrenal gland. However, renal and adrenal arteriography and venography have largely replaced retroperitoneal air studies.

Normal Retroperitoneal Air (Carbon Dioxide) Study

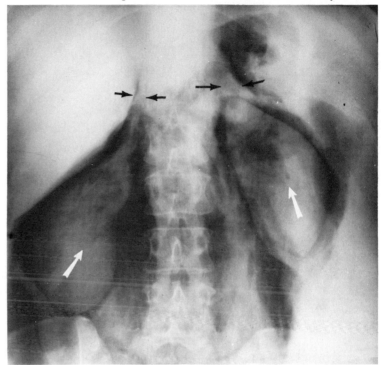

Both kidneys *(white arrows)* are clearly outlined by surrounding air. The triangle-shaped adrenal glands *(black arrows)* are fairly well delineated.

Selective Arteriography

See *Arteriography* and *Aortography*.

Sialography

The salivary ducts and glands can be opacified by injecting contrast material into the duct openings in the mouth. This is easily accomplished for parotid sialography; submaxillary opacification is more difficult. Sublingual sialography is rarely attempted, because of the multiplicity and minuteness of these ducts.

Sialography is used to demonstrate obstructive calculi in Stensen's or Wharton's duct, structural alterations of the ductile pattern in a diseased gland parenchyma, sialectasis, or neoplastic change.

Normal Sialogram: Parotid Gland

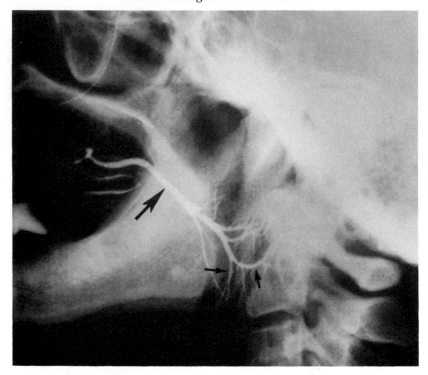

Stensen's duct *(large arrow)* and the intraparotid branch ducts *(small arrows)* are opacified.

Normal Submaxillary Sialogram

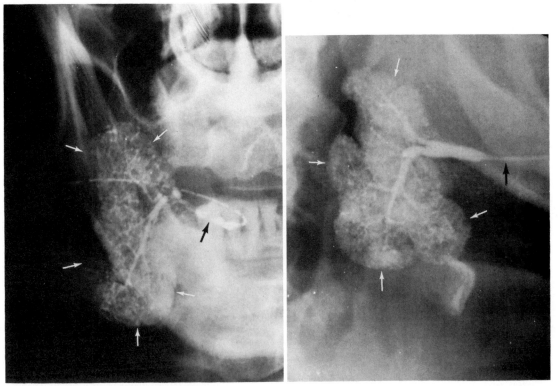

A, Anteroposterior view; *B,* lateral view.

Wharton's duct *(black arrows)* and the lobulated gland *(white arrows)* are well opacified. The submaxillary gland lies at and below the angle of the mandible.

Sinusography, Cerebral

Contrast material can be injected through a catheter into the anterior portion of the superior sagittal sinus of the skull to outline the sagittal sinus, the confluence of the sinuses, and both transverse sinuses. The other dural sinuses and veins are not opacified.

In obstruction of the superior sagittal or transverse sinuses, this study will locate the site of obstruction and will demonstrate opacification of the collateral veins.

Sinus Tract Injection

Oily or aqueous contrast material can be instilled into a sinus tract opening in the skin or mucous membrane. The tract and its origin will be opacified, and the roentgenogram will provide information about the size, shape, and origin of the tract.

Small Bowel Series

See *Barium meal studies.*

Splenoportography (Portosplenography)

If a water-soluble opaque medium is injected percutaneously directly into the spleen, it will opacify the splenic vein, and subsequently the portal vein and the portal vessels of the liver. This procedure is most frequently employed to demonstrate increased pressure of the portal circulation. In portal hypertension there will be opacification of other veins that drain into the portal circulation. These veins are not opacified in a subject with normal portal pressure. Splenoportography can also demonstrate the state of the peripheral portal vasculature, occlusion of the splenic or portal vein, and gastric or lower esophageal varices. Alteration and displacement of the intrahepatic vessels by tumor, cirrhosis, and other degenerative or inflammatory conditions can sometimes be demonstrated.

This procedure has been largely replaced by selective celiac or splenic arteriography. The venous phase will satisfactorily opacify the splenic and portal veins.

Normal Splenoportogram: After Celiac Arteriography

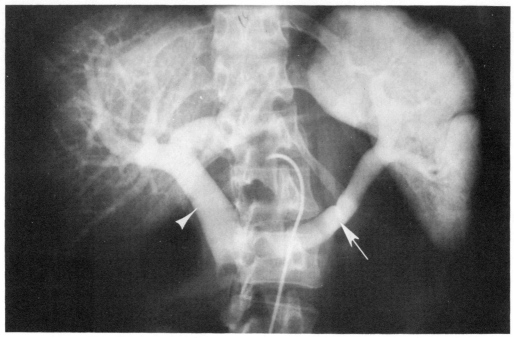

The late phase of selective celiac arteriography shows dense opacification of the spleen, the intrasplenic veins, the splenic vein *(arrow)*, the portal vein *(arrowhead)*, and the intrahepatic branches of the portal vein.

Thoracic Aortography

See *Aortography.*

Tomography

See *Planigraphy.*

Transhepatic Cholangiography

See *Cholangiography, transhepatic.*

Translumbar Aortography

See *Aortography.*

T-Tube Cholangiography

See *Cholangiography, T-tube.*

Urography, Intravenous

See *Pyelography, intravenous.*

Venography, Peripheral
(Limb Venography, Phlebography)

Opacification of the venous channels of an extremity is usually performed in the lower extremity. Contrast material is injected percutaneously into a vein on the foot or ankle. A tourniquet may be used to occlude the superficial veins so that opacification of the deep veins can be obtained in the leg and thigh.

Venography of the lower extremity is employed to determine patency of the deep veins, to demonstrate areas of deep venous thrombophlebitis or occlusion, and to demonstrate the condition of the valves.

Venography of the upper extremity is also used to demonstrate superior vena caval obstruction, particularly in superior mediastinal lesions.

Normal Venogram: Leg and Thigh

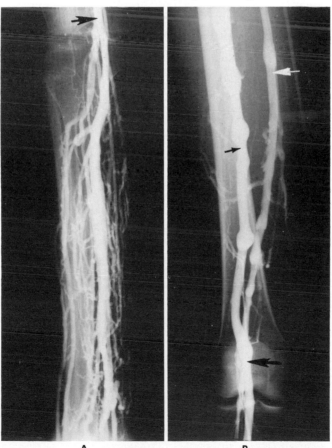

A   **B**

There is opacification of the deep and superficial veins of the leg *(A)*. The popliteal *(large black arrows),* the deep femoral *(small black arrow),* and greater saphenous *(white arrow)* veins are well opacified *(B)*.

Venography, Selective

This procedure is usually employed for opacification of a branch of the vena cava. A catheter in the vena cava is directed into the desired vein, which is then opacified. Normally, vena caval opacification alone will not produce satisfactory visualization of tributary veins because of the direction of normal blood flow.

Occlusion, compression, or displacement of a specific vein or group of veins can be ascertained. Selective renal or adrenal venography is sometimes performed to supplement arteriographic findings.

Normal Renal Venogram

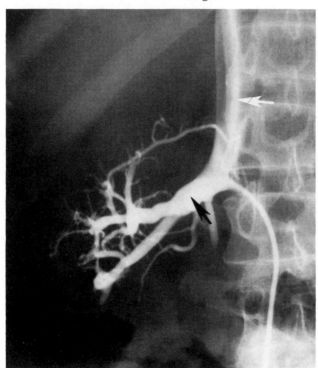

The intrarenal veins join to form the main right renal vein *(black arrow)*, which empties into the vena cava *(white arrow)*.

Ventriculography, Cardiac

Opacification of the left or right ventricle can be obtained by direct injection through a catheter into these chambers. Rapid serial films or cine studies are made after injection of contrast material. Left ventriculography is used mainly to demonstrate and quantitate mitral insufficiency. The degree and type of aortic stenosis can also be evaluated by this procedure.

Ventriculography, Cerebral

This procedure consists of direct injection of air into a lateral ventricle, usually through a burr hole in the skull. The cerebrospinal fluid is removed first; the air then enters and fills the ventricular system. Films are made in various projections. The position of the head is varied to allow the air to rise to the desired portion of the system. The basal cisterns and the subarachnoid pathways are not visualized by ventriculography.

Cerebral ventriculography is used when there is clinical evidence of increased intracranial pressure and particularly if obstructive internal hydrocephalus is suspected. In these cases there is danger of herniation of the cerebellar tonsils through the foramen magnum during pneumoencephalography.

Ventriculography is of great aid in demonstrating mass lesions of the brain and obstructive hydrocephalus. The site of obstruction can usually be determined by this study.

Sometimes opaque oil is injected into the ventricular system to produce greater contrast of the ventricles; greater diagnostic detail is usually obtained (*contrast ventriculography*).

The CT scan has decreased the use of ventriculography.

Vertebral Arteriography

See *Arteriography, cerebral.*

Voiding Cystourethrography

See *Cystourethrography, voiding.*

ROENTGEN SIGNS AND ASSOCIATED DISEASES

In this section, diseases and disorders are alphabetically listed under categories of roentgen signs or appearance. With a few exceptions, the roentgen signs are broad in scope and fairly frequently encountered. Highly specific or pathognomonic roentgen findings have been intentionally omitted.

For purposes of differential diagnosis, the list of conditions under each roentgen category is reasonably complete but not exhaustive. Disorders which are extremely infrequent or those in which the designated roentgen sign is seen only rarely may be absent from the list. Many conditions appear in several lists, which may help narrow the differential diagnostic possibilities.

ROENTGEN SIGNS OF JOINTS

ROENTGEN SIGNS OF KIDNEYS AND URINARY TRACTS

ROENTGEN SIGNS OF OSSEOUS SYSTEM

MISCELLANEOUS ROENTGEN SIGNS

I. CARDIOVASCULAR SYSTEM

ROENTGEN SIGNS OF CARDIOVASCULAR SYSTEM

(1) Increased Pulmonary Vascularity

Predominantly Venous	Predominantly Arterial
Congestive failure	Atrial septal defect
Cor triatriatum sinistrum	Congenital coronary fistula
Left atrial ball valve thrombus	Endocardial cushion defects
Left atrial myxoma	High output heart
Mitral insufficiency	Lutembacher's syndrome
Mitral stenosis	Partial anomalous venous return
Pulmonary venous obstruction by tumor, thrombus, or mediastinal fibrosis	Patent ductus arteriosus
Total anomalous venous return to below diaphragm	Pickwickian obesity
	Primary polycythemia
	Single ventricle
	Taussig-Bing complex
	Transposition of great vessels
	Truncus arteriosus
	Ventricular septal defect

(2) Pulmonary Hypertension and Cor Pulmonale

Chronic Hypoxia	Diffuse Pulmonary Arteritis
Chest deformities	Idiopathic
Chronic airway obstruction (adenoids)	Left to right shunts (Eisenmenger's physiology)
High altitude dwelling	Mitral stenosis (longstanding)
Pickwickian obesity	Schistosomiasis

Diffuse Interstitial Lung Disease	Thromboembolism
Chronic bronchitis	Recurrent pulmonary emboli
Dermatomyositis	Sickle cell anemia (pulmonary thrombi)
Emphysema	
Hamman-Rich syndrome	**Hypervolemia of Right Heart**
Idiopathic fibrosis	
Lupus erythematosus	Ventriculoatrial shunt for hydrocephalus
Lymphangitic metastases	
Mucoviscidosis	
Periarteritis nodosa	
Pneumoconioses	
Scleroderma	
Tuberculosis with extensive fibrosis	

(3) High Output Heart

Arteriovenous fistula (extrapulmonary)
Beriberi
Hypervolemia (transfusions, fluid overload)
Paget's disease
Pickwickian obesity
Pregnancy
Primary polycythemia
Pyrexia
Severe anemia
Sickle cell anemia
Thyrotoxicosis

ROENTGEN SIGNS OF CARDIOVASCULAR SYSTEM *(Continued)*

(4) Prominent or Enlarged Ascending Aorta and/or Aortic Arch

Aneurysm
Ankylosing spondylitis
Aortic insufficiency
Aortic stenosis
Atherosclerosis
Coarctation of aorta
Homocystinuria
Marfan's disease
Patent ductus arteriosus
Pseudocoarctation
Pseudoxanthoma elasticum
Syphilitic aortitis
Takayasu's arteritis
Tetralogy of Fallot
Tricuspid atresia without transposition
Truncus arteriosus (type IV)

(5) Enlarged Left Atrium

Constrictive pericarditis
Heart failure (left sided)
Left to right shunt (excluding atrial septal defect)
  Congenital coronary fistula
  Patent ductus arteriosus
  Ventricular septal defect
Mitral valvular disease
  Insufficiency
  Stenosis
Myocardiopathies
Myxoma of left atrium

(6) Pericardial Effusion

Amebic pericarditis
Congestive failure
Coxsackie pericarditis
Dissecting aneurysm with leakage
Histoplasmosis
Idiopathic
Lupus erythematosus
Mycotic infection
Myxedema
Neoplastic pericarditis
Nephrosis
Periarteritis nodosa
Postcoronary artery bypass surgery
Postmyocardial infarction syndrome
Pyogenic pericarditis
Rheumatic fever
Scleroderma
Syphilis
Toxoplasmosis
Trauma
Tuberculosis
Uremia
Viral infections

(7) Cardiac Calcifications

Aneurysm of coronary artery
Aneurysm of sinus of Valsalva
Atrial clot
Coronary atherosclerosis
Left atrium (mitral disease)
Malignant tumor of heart
Mitral annulus
Myocardial infarct
Myxoma of atrium
Pericardium
Valvular
  Aortic (aortic stenosis)
  Mitral (mitral stenosis)

Table continued on following page.

ROENTGEN SIGNS OF CARDIOVASCULAR SYSTEM *(Continued)*

(8) Vascular Calcifications

Arterial	Venous
Arteriosclerosis	Arteriovenous malformation
Homocystinuria	Hemangioma
Hyperparathyroidism	Maffucci's syndrome
Premature arteriosclerosis	Phleboliths
Familial hyperlipemias	Varicose veins
Progeria	
Secondary hyperlipemias	
Cushing's syndrome	
Diabetes	
Glycogen storage disease	
Hypothyroidism	
Lipodystrophy	
Nephrotic syndrome	
Renal homotransplantation	
Pseudoxanthoma elasticum	
Werner's syndrome	

ROENTGEN SIGNS OF CHEST

(9) Disseminated Alveolar Infiltrates

Infectious	Neoplastic	Other
Bacterial pneumonias (diffuse)	Alveolar cell carcinoma	Alveolar microlithiasis
Giant-cell pneumonia	Hodgkin's disease	Alveolar proteinosis
Mycotic infections	Leukemia	Aspiration pneumonia
Pneumocystis carinii pneumonia	Lymphoma	Blast injury
Tuberculosis		Chemical inhalation
Viral pneumonias (diffuse);		Congenital pulmonary
especially influenzal virus,		lymphangiectasis
measles, varicella		Contusion
		Desquamative interstitial
		pneumonia
		Drug hypersensitivity
		Fat emboli
		Goodpasture's syndrome
		Hemosiderosis
		Hyaline membrane
		disease
		Hydrocarbon pneumonia
		Idiopathic respiratory
		distress syndrome
		Lipoid pneumonia
		Mucoviscidosis
		Oxygen toxicity
		Pulmonary edema
		(see following table)
		Pulmonary hemorrhage
		Rheumatic fever
		pneumonia
		Riley-Day syndrome
		(aspiration)
		Sarcoidosis
		Shock lung

ROENTGEN SIGNS OF CHEST (Continued)

(10) Pulmonary Edema

Acute glomerulonephritis
Aspiration
Cardiac failure (left heart)
Chest trauma
Diffuse capillary leak syndrome
Diffuse pulmonary embolism
Drug hypersensitivity
Drug overdose (heroin)
Fluid overload
High altitude
Hypoalbuminemia
Inhalation of toxic agents
Intracranial disease
Malaria (falciparum)
Mediastinal tumor (with venous or lymphatic obstruction)
Near drowning
Oxygen toxicity
Shock lung
Uremia

(11) Disseminated Interstitial (Reticular-Reticulonodular) Infiltrates

Inflammatory	Neoplastic	Other
Diffuse mycotic infections	Hodgkin's disease	Chemical inhalation
Diffuse viral and adenoviral pneumonia	Leukemia	Dermatomyositis
Schistosomiasis	Lymphangitic metastases	Desquamative interstitial pneumonia
Tuberculosis	Lymphomas	Diffuse interstitial fibrosis (idiopathic)
		Drug hypersensitivity
		Goodpasture's syndrome
		Hamman-Rich syndrome
		Hemosiderosis
		Histiocytosis X
		Interstitial pulmonary edema
		Mucoviscidosis
		Neurofibromatosis
		Niemann-Pick disease
		Organic dust inhalation
		Oxygen toxicity
		Pneumoconioses
		Polyarteritis
		Recurrent pulmonary infarction
		Rheumatoid arthritis
		Sarcoidosis
		Scleroderma
		Tuberous sclerosis

Table continued on following page.

ROENTGEN SIGNS OF CHEST *(Continued)*

(12) Pulmonary Fibrosis (Diffuse)

Chemical inhalation (late stage)
Dermatomyositis
Desquamative pneumonia
Hamman-Rich syndrome
Histiocytosis X
Idiopathic pulmonary hemosiderosis
Mucoviscidosis
Mycotic diseases

Neurofibromatosis
Pneumoconioses (organic and inorganic)
Radiation fibrosis
Rheumatoid lung
Sarcoidosis
Scleroderma
Tuberculosis
Tuberous sclerosis

(13) Kerley B Lines

Congestive failure
Diffuse interstitial fibrosis of varied etiology
Hamman-Rich syndrome
Interstitial lower lobe pneumonia
Lipoid pneumonia
Lymphangitic metastases
Mitral stenosis
Pneumoconioses
Pulmonary alveolar proteinosis (unusual)
Sarcoidosis

(14) Miliary and Small Nodular Lesions (Disseminated)

Inflammatory	Neoplastic	Other
Cytomegalovirus pneumonia	Alveolar cell carcinoma	Amyloid disease
Dirofilariasis	Hodgkin's disease	Arteriovenous mal-
Fungal infections	Lymphosarcoma	formation
Listeriosis	Metastatic disease	Caplan's syndrome
Miliary tuberculosis		Gaucher's disease
Paragonimiasis		Hemosiderosis
Septic infarcts		Histiocytosis X
Varicella pneumonia		Niemann-Pick disease
Viral pneumonia		Pneumoconioses
		Polyarteritis and vasculitis
		Pseudoxanthoma elasticum
		Rheumatoid nodules
		Sarcoidosis
		Siderosis
		Wegener's granulomatosis

(15) Large Nodular Lesions

Inflammatory	Neoplastic	Other
Abscess (pyogenic and others)	Alveolar cell carcinoma	Amyloidosis
Dirofilariasis	Bronchogenic carcinoma	Anthracosilicosis
Mycotic infections	Hamartoma	Arteriovenous malformation
Paragonimiasis	Hodgkin's disease	Caplan's syndrome
	Lymphosarcoma	Lipoid pneumonia
	Metastases	Pulmonary hematoma
	Papilloma	Rheumatoid nodules
	Plasmacytoma	Sequestration
		Wegener's granulomatosis

ROENTGEN SIGNS OF CHEST *(Continued)*

(16) Cavitary Lesions

Inflammatory	Neoplastic	Other
Abscess (pyogenic)	Bronchogenic carcinoma	Bulla (infected)
Amebic abscess	Hodgkin's disease	Cyst
Bronchiectasis	Metastatic lesions	Infarct
Echinococcus disease	(especially squamous cell)	Polyarteritis
Gram-negative infections		Polycystic lung
B. proteus		Rheumatoid nodules
E. coli		Sequestration
Pseudomonas		Traumatic lung cyst
Klebsiella pneumonia		Wegener's granulomatosis
Melioidosis		
Mycotic infections		
Actinomycosis		
Aspergillosis		
Blastomycosis		
Coccidioidomycosis		
Cryptococcosis		
Histoplasmosis		
Mucormycosis		
Nocardiosis		
Sporotrichosis		
Paragonimiasis		
Staphylococcal pneumonia		
Tuberculosis		

(17) Atelectasis (Obstructive)

Inflammatory	Neoplastic	Other
Middle lobe syndrome	Bronchial adenoma	Agammaglobulinemia
Pertussis	Bronchogenic carcinoma	Bronchial asthma
Tuberculosis	Granular cell myoblastoma	Bulbar poliomyelitis
	Invasive mediastinal	Chondromalacia of
	malignancy	bronchus
	Metastases to bronchus	Foreign body
		Lymph node enlargement
		(peribronchial)
		Mucoviscidosis
		Papilloma of bronchus
		Peritoneal dialysis
		Postoperative mucus plug
		Primary polycythemia

Table continued on following page.

ROENTGEN SIGNS OF CHEST *(Continued)*

(18) Adenopathy—Hilar and/or Mediastinal

Infectious	Neoplastic	Other
Adenoviral infections	Bronchogenic carcinoma	Behçet's disease
Bacterial pneumonias	Extramedullary	Erythema nodosum
(children)	plasmacytoma	Sarcoidosis
Blastomycosis	Follicular lymphoma	Silicosis
Candidiasis	Hodgkin's disease	
Coccidioidomycosis	Leukemia (acute and	
Histoplasmosis	chronic)	
Infectious mononucleosis	Lymphosarcoma	
Measles	Metastatic disease	
Mycoplasma	Reticulum cell sarcoma	
Pertussis		
Plague pneumonia		
Psittacosis		
Sporotrichosis		
Tuberculosis		
Tularemia		
Varicella pneumonia		
Viral pneumonias		

(19) Mediastinal Masses and Widening

Inflammatory	Neoplastic	Other
Acute mediastinitis	Bronchogenic carcinoma	Aneurysm
Chronic mediastinitis	Extramedullary	Cushing's syndrome
Histoplasmosis	plasmacytoma	Myasthenia gravis
Lymph nodes	Follicular lymphoma	Sarcoidosis
Tuberculosis	Hodgkin's disease	Steroid lipomatosis
	Leukemia	Substernal thyroid
	Lymphosarcoma	Superior vena caval
	Metastatic disease	obstruction
	Reticulum cell sarcoma	Thymic enlargement
	Thymic tumors	
	Tumors, benign and	
	malignant	

ROENTGEN SIGNS OF CHEST *(Continued)*

(20) Pleural Fluid and/or Thickening

Inflammatory	Neoplastic	Other
Amebiasis	Bronchogenic carcinoma	Acute pancreatitis
Bacterial pneumonia	Hodgkin's disease	Asbestosis
Coccidioidomycosis	Leukemia	Cirrhosis
Coxsackie infections	Lymphosarcoma	Constrictive pericarditis
Empyema	Malignant mesothelioma	Familial Mediterranean
Hemophilus influenzae pneumonia	Metastatic disease	fever
Mycoplasma pneumonia	Primary macroglobulinemia	Heart failure
Nocardiosis	of Waldenström	Lupus erythematosus
Pneumococcal pneumonia		Meigs' syndrome
Q fever		Nephrotic syndrome
Staphylococcal pneumonia		Peritoneal dialysis
Tuberculosis		Postmyocardial infarction
Tularemia		syndrome
Viral pneumonia		Pulmonary infarction
		Rheumatoid arthritis
		Subdiaphragmatic abscess
		Superior vena caval
		obstruction
		Trauma

(21) Pneumothorax

Bronchopleural fistula
Bullous emphysema
Chemical pneumonitis
Histiocytosis X
Honeycomb lung
Ruptured esophagus
Spontaneous pneumothorax
Staphylococcal pneumonia
Trauma
Tuberculosis

ROENTGEN SIGNS OF GASTROINTESTINAL TRACT AND ABDOMEN

(22) Esophagus—Delayed Emptying and/or Dilatation

From Diffuse Peristaltic Abnormality	From Segmental Peristaltic Abnormality
Aperistalsis (achalasia)	Chalasia
Chagas' disease	Diffuse lower esophageal spasm
Dermatomyositis	Hypertrophic esophagogastric sphincter
Diabetes	Myasthenia gravis
Moniliasis	Myotonia atrophica
Riley-Day syndrome	Pseudobulbar palsy
Scleroderma	

Table continued on following page.

ROENTGEN SIGNS OF GASTROINTESTINAL TRACT AND ABDOMEN
(Continued)

From Intrinsic Obstructive Lesion	From Extrinsic Obstructive Lesion
Benign tumors	Aneurysm
Carcinoma and other malignant tumors	Cricopharyngeal muscle hypertrophy
Congenital strictures	Mediastinal tumors and masses
Duplication of esophagus	Vascular ring (aortic)
Foreign body	
Peptic or reflux esophagitis	
Peptic ulcer of esophagus	
Schatzki ring	
Sideropenic web	
Stricture (inflammatory or chemical)	
Zenker's diverticulum	

(23) Distal Esophagus — Narrowing and/or Deformity

Achalasia
Carcinoma of esophagus
Carcinoma of gastric cardia
Chagas' disease
Diffuse lower esophageal spasm
Duplication cyst
Hypertrophic esophagogastric sphincter
Leiomyoma
Peptic esophagitis
Reflux esophagitis
Stricture (chemical, inflammatory)
Trauma (intubation and instrumentation)

(24) Stomach — Dilatation

Acute hemorrhagic gastritis	Obstructive pyloroduodenal lesions
Anticholinergic drugs in gastric ulcer disease	Inflammatory
Bezoar	Neoplastic
Diabetes	Postoperative gastric dilatation
Duodenal ulcer with obstruction	Pyloric stenosis
Generalized ileus	Small bowel obstruction
Hypokalemia	Uremia and other toxic states
	Volvulus

(25) Stomach — Intraluminal Filling Defects

Aberrant pancreas	Carcinoma
Benign tumors	Duplication of stomach
Angioma	Eosinophilic granuloma
Carcinoid	Foreign body
Fibroma	Leiomyosarcoma
Leiomyoma	Lymphosarcoma
Lipoma	Polyposis (multiple)
Polyp	Varices (multiple)
Bezoar	Villous adenoma
Blood clots	

ROENTGEN SIGNS OF GASTROINTESTINAL TRACT AND ABDOMEN
(Continued)

(26) Stomach—Antropyloric Narrowing

Amyloidosis
Antral gastritis
Antral or pyloric ulcer
Carcinoma of antrum
Eosinophilic gastroenteritis
Foreign body
Granulomatous enteritis with antral involvement
Hypertrophic pyloric stenosis (infantile, adult)
Inflammatory and chemical stricture
Pancreatic tumors
Perforation and abscess
Syphilis (rare)
Tuberculosis (rare)

(27) Mesenteric Small Intestine—Mucosal Thickening Usually With Thickened Wall

Acute radiation injury
Amyloidosis
Eosinophilic gastroenteritis
Giardiasis
Hodgkin's disease
Hypoalbuminemia (bowel edema)
  Cirrhosis of liver
  Nephrotic syndrome
Intestinal lymphangiectasia

Intramural hemorrhage
  Anticoagulants
  Hemophilia
  Purpuras
Lymphosarcoma
Mastocytosis
Primary macroglobulinemia of Waldenström
Reticulum cell sarcoma
Scleroderma
Vascular occlusion
Whipple's disease

(28) Mesenteric Small Intestine—Multiple Intraluminal Defects

Carcinoids
Cronkhite-Canada syndrome
Dysgammaglobulinemia
Hodgkin's disease
Lymphosarcoma
Metastatic nodules (usually malignant melanoma)
Nodular lymphoid hyperplasia
Peutz-Jeghers syndrome
Regional enteritis
Reticulum cell sarcoma
Submucosal hemorrhages
  Anticoagulants
  Hemophilia
  Purpuras
  Vascular occlusion
Typhoid fever

Table continued on following page.

ROENTGEN SIGNS OF GASTROINTESTINAL TRACT AND ABDOMEN
(Continued)

(29) Mesenteric Small Intestine—Inflammatory-Like Appearance
(mucosal thickening or deformity, thickened walls, segmental narrowing)

Actinomycosis
Carcinoids
Enteritis necroticans
Eosinophilic gastroenteritis
Granulomatous enteritis
Hodgkin's disease
Parasitic infections
Potassium thiazide enteritis
Radiation injury
Retractile mesenteritis
Strongyloidiasis
Tuberculosis
Vascular occlusion
Zollinger-Ellison syndrome

(30) Mesenteric Small Intestine—Deficiency Pattern

Carcinoid syndrome
Celiac disease
Chronic mesenteric vascular insufficiency
Emotional states
Familial Mediterranean fever
γ-A heavy chain disease
Gastrointestinal allergy
Hyperthyroidism

Hypoparathyroidism
Kwashiorkor
Lymphosarcoma
Mucoviscidosis
Nontropical sprue
Pancreatic insufficiency
Parasitic infections
Tropical sprue

(31) Colon—Inflammatory-Like Appearance
(mucosal changes, ulcerations, irritability, segmental narrowing)

Actinomycosis
Amebiasis
Antibiotic-induced enterocolitis
Bacillary dysentery
Diverticulitis
Granulomatous colitis
Ischemic colitis

Lymphogranuloma inguinale
Lymphoma (diffuse)
Postirradiation colitis
Schistosomiasis
Trichuriasis
Tuberculosis
Ulcerative colitis

(32) Colon—Solitary Mass Defect

Adenomatous polyp
Ameboma
Benign tumors (leiomyoma, fibroma, etc.)
Carcinoid
Carcinoma
Endometrioma
Fecal impaction
Lipoma
Lymphosarcoma
Schistosomiasis
Villous adenoma

ROENTGEN SIGNS OF GASTROINTESTINAL TRACT AND ABDOMEN
(Continued)

(33) Colon—Multiple Filling Defects

Amebomas
Amyloidosis
Ischemic colitis
Lymphosarcoma
Nodular lymphoid hyperplasia
Pneumatosis cystoides intestinalis
Polyps
  Cronkhite-Canada syndrome

Familial polyposis
Gardner's syndrome
Nonfamilial polyposis
Peutz-Jeghers syndrome
Pseudopolyps in ulcerative colitis
Pseudopolyps in granulomatous colitis
Retained fecal contents

(34) Megacolon

Chagas' disease
Chronic constipation
Diabetes
Familial Mediterranean fever
Generalized peritonitis
Granulomatous colitis
Hirschsprung's disease
Lead poisoning
Low mechanical obstruction
Parkinsonism
Porphyria
Toxic ileus
Ulcerative colitis (toxic megacolon)

(35)   Intra-abdominal Calcifications

Inflammatory	Neoplastic	Other
Amebic abscess	Dermoid cyst	Adrenal
Echinococcus cyst	Hemangioma	Aneurysm
Healed splenic	Hepatoma	Arteriosclerotic vessels
histoplasmosis	Mucus-producing	Atherosclerotic aorta
Meconium peritonitis	adenocarcinoma	Epiploic appendages
Mesenteric lymph nodes	Neuroblastoma	Fecolith (appendix, colon)
Schistosomiasis	Ovarian carcinoma	Gallbladder wall
Tuberculous peritonitis	Peritoneal metastases	Gallstones
	Pheochromocytoma	Hematoma
	Renal cyst or tumor	Mesenteric cyst
	Retroperitoneal sarcoma	Milk of calcium bile
	Uterine fibroids	Nephrocalcinosis (see
		Table 44)
		Pancreatic calculi
		Phleboliths
		Prostatic calculi
		Pseudocyst of pancreas
		Renal (see Tables 42–45)
		Retroperitoneal
		hematoma
		Rib cartilage (extra-
		abdominal)
		Seminal vesicles
		Urinary tract calculi
		Vas deferens

Table continued on following page.

ROENTGEN SIGNS OF GASTROINTESTINAL TRACT AND ABDOMEN
(Continued)

(36) Splenomegaly

Inflammatory	Neoplastic	Other
Cytomegalic inclusion disease	Hodgkin's disease	Acute infarct
Echinococcus cyst	Leukemia	Adrenocortical insufficiency
Histoplasmosis	Lymphosarcoma	Amyloidosis
Infectious mononucleosis	Sarcoma	Cirrhosis of liver
Malaria		Congestive splenomegaly
Miliary tuberculosis		Cooley's anemia
Subacute bacterial endocarditis		Dysgammaglobulinemia
Viral hepatitis		Felty's syndrome
		Gaucher's disease
		Hemochromatosis
		Hemolytic anemia
		Hurler's syndrome
		Juvenile rheumatoid arthritis
		Lupus erythematosus
		Mastocytosis (urticaria pigmentosa)
		Mucoviscidosis
		Myelofibrosis
		Myelophthisic anemia
		Niemann-Pick disease
		Osteopetrosis
		Portal hypertension
		Primary polycythemia
		Sickle cell anemia (S-C)
		Splenic cyst
		Splenic rupture
		Trauma

(37) Liver Calcifications

Abscess (pyogenic or amebic)	Gumma
Alveolar hydatid disease	Hemangioma; A-V malformation
Aneurysms of hepatic artery	Hepatic duct calculi
Congenital cysts	Metastases (ovary, breast, colon, mesothelioma, neuroblastoma)
Cystic hydatid disease	Portal vein thrombus
Granulomas (tuberculosis, histoplasmosis, brucellosis)	Primary neoplasm (malignant hepatoma, cholangioma)

ROENTGEN SIGNS OF JOINTS

(38) Rheumatoid and Rheumatoid-Like Arthritis

Agammaglobulinemia arthritis
Gout
Hemochromatosis (rare)
Juvenile rheumatoid arthritis
Lupus erythematosus
Polychondritis
Psoriatic arthritis
Reiter's syndrome
Sjögren's syndrome
Ulcerative colitis arthritis

(39) Osteoarthritis—Degenerative Joint Disease

Acromegaly
Aseptic necrosis (late)
Ehlers-Danlos syndrome
Familial Mediterranean fever
Frostbite
Gout
Hemochromatosis (rare)
Hemophilia
Hepatolenticular degeneration
Late result of joint inflammation or trauma
Ochronosis
Osteoarthritis and spondylosis of aging
Trauma

(40) Neuropathic Joint (Charcot Joint)

Diabetes
Leprosy
Riley-Day syndrome
Spinal cord disease
Steroid therapy (Charcot-like)
Syphilis (tabes dorsalis)
Syringomyelia

(41) Periarticular Calcifications

Dermatomyositis
Hyperparathyroidism
Hypervitaminosis A
Myositis ossificans
Neurotrophic joint
Pseudogout
Pyogenic arthritis
Scleroderma
Synovioma
Trauma
Tuberculosis

ROENTGEN SIGNS OF KIDNEYS AND URINARY TRACTS

(42) Enlargement

Unilateral	Bilateral
Acute pyelonephritis	Acromegaly
Acute transplant rejection	Acute glomerulonephritis
Compensatory hypertrophy	Acute renal failure
Cyst and cystic disease	Amyloidosis
Duplicated kidney	Bilateral acute pyelonephritis
Echinococcus disease	Bilateral metastatic disease
Hematoma	Bilateral obstructive hydronephrosis
Multicystic kidney	Idiopathic lipoid nephrosis
Neoplastic lesions	Leukemia
(primary and secondary)	Lymphosarcoma
Obstructive hydronephrosis	Polycystic kidneys
Renal vein thrombosis	Renal cortical necrosis
	Renal vein thrombosis
	Tuberous sclerosis (bilateral angiomyolipomas)

(43) Decreased Size

Unilateral	Bilateral
Chronic pyelonephritis	Balkan nephritis
Congenital hypoplastic kidney	Bilateral renal artery stenosis
Obstructive atrophy	Chronic glomerulonephritis
Renal artery stenosis	Chronic gouty nephritis
Renal infarction (late)	Chronic interstitial nephritis
	Chronic pyelonephritis
	Diffuse fibromuscular hyperplasia
	Hereditary nephritis (Alport's disease)
	Kimmelstein-Wilson disease
	Medullary cystic disease
	Scleroderma
	Systemic lupus erythematosus

(44) Nephrocalcinosis

Intrinsic Renal Disease	Systemic Disturbance
Medullary sponge kidney	Carcinomatosis of bone
Papillary necrosis	Cortisone therapy
Renal tubular acidosis	Cretinism
Tuberculosis	Cushing's disease
	Hyperoxaluria
	Hyperparathyroidism
	Hypervitaminosis D
	Idiopathic hypercalcinuria
	Idiopathic hypercalcemia
	Milk-alkali ingestion
	Multiple myeloma
	Sarcoidosis
	Sjögren's syndrome
	Sulfonamide therapy

ROENTGEN SIGNS OF KIDNEYS AND URINARY TRACTS *(Continued)*

(45) Focal Calcifications

Abscess
Aneurysm (intrarenal artery)
Benign tumors
Chronic glomerulonephritis (cortical calcification)
Cyst
Cystinuria lithiasis
Echinococcus disease
Gouty lithiasis
Hematoma
Hydronephrotic cavity
Infarct
Lithiasis (idiopathic)
Malignant tumors
Ochronosis lithiasis
Pyonephrosis
Renal cortical necrosis (tramway calcification)
Tuberculosis and any condition causing nephrocalcinosis
   (see preceding table)
Vascular malformation

ROENTGEN SIGNS OF OSSEOUS SYSTEM

(46) Demineralization and/or Osteoporosis

Acromegaly	Hypothyroidism (cretinism)	Postmenopausal
Acro-osteolysis	Idiopathic hypercalcemia (late)	Primary macroglobulinemia
Ankylosing spondylitis	Immobilization	of Waldenström
Cooley's anemia	Iron deficiency anemia	Protein deficiency
Cortisone therapy	(severe, in children)	Renal osteodystrophy
Cushing's disease	Juvenile rheumatoid arthritis	Renal tubular acidosis
Dermatomyositis	Leukemia (acute)	Rheumatoid arthritis
Familial Mediterranean	Malabsorption	Rickets
fever	Multiple myeloma	Scurvy
Fanconi's syndrome	Muscular dystrophy	Senility
Frostbite	Niemann-Pick disease	Shoulder-hand syndrome
Gaucher's disease	Ochronosis	Sickle cell anemia
Hemochromatosis (systemic)	Osteitis fibrosa cystica	Sudeck's atrophy
Hemophilia	Osteogenesis imperfecta	Thyrotoxicosis
Hepatic rickets	Osteomalacia	Turner's syndrome
Hepatolenticular	Osteoporosis circumscripta	
degeneration	Oxalosis	
Homocystinuria	Paget's disease	
Hyperparathyroidism	Phenylketonuria	
Hyperthyroidism		
Hypoparathyroidism with		
steatorrhea		

Table continued on following page.

ROENTGEN SIGNS OF OSSEOUS SYSTEM *(Continued)*

(47) Osteosclerosis

Inflammatory (Focal)	Neoplastic (Usually Focal, Occasionally Diffuse)	Other (Usually Diffuse)
Brodie's abscess	Hodgkin's disease	*Engelmann's disease
Cytomegalic inclusion disease	Leukemia (chronic)	Fibrous dysplasia
Garre's osteomyelitis	Lymphoma	Fluorosis
Osteomyelitis (chronic and healed)	Metastatic carcinoma	Hyperparathyroidism
	Multiple myeloma (rare)	Hypoparathyroidism
		Hypothyroidism
		Idiopathic hypercalcemia
		Lipoatrophic diabetes mellitus
		Mastocytosis
		Melorheostosis
		Myeloid metaplasia
		Osteopetrosis
		Paget's disease
		Pycnodysostosis
		Renal osteodystrophy
		Tuberous sclerosis
		Vitamin D intoxication

(48) Periosteal Reaction

Caffey's disease
Congenital syphilis
Fluorosis
Hypertrophic pulmonary osteoarthropathy
Juvenile rheumatoid arthritis
Leukemia (acute)
Malignant bone tumors
Metastatic neuroblastoma
Osteoid osteoma
Osteomyelitis (acute)

Pachydermoperiostosis
Reiter's syndrome
Rickets (healing)
Scurvy
Thyroid acropachy
Trauma
Tropical ulcer
Tuberous sclerosis
Varicose ulcers
Vitamin A intoxication

(49) Rickets and Rachitic-Like Changes

Atresia of common duct (hepatic rickets)
Fanconi's syndrome
Hepatolenticular degeneration
Homocystinuria
Hypophosphatasia
Malabsorption
Oxalosis
Phenylketonuria
Renal tubular acidosis
Uremic osteodystrophy
Vitamin D deficiency

ROENTGEN SIGNS OF OSSEOUS SYSTEM *(Continued)*

(50) Rib Notching or Erosion

Aplasia of pulmonary artery
Bulbar poliomyelitis
Coarctation of aorta
Increased pulse pressure
Neurofibromatosis
Vascular malformation (intercostal artery)
Vascular obstruction (vena caval, subclavian, or
    innominate artery or vein)
Vascular surgery, for correction of tetralogy of Fallot

(51) Aseptic Necrosis

Caisson disease
Cushing's syndrome
Gaucher's disease
Hemophilia joint disease
Hypothyroidism
Idiopathic
Lupus erythematosus
Sickle cell anemia
Steroid therapy
Trauma

(52) Bone Infarcts

Arteriosclerosis
Caisson disease
Idiopathic
Pancreatitis (acute and chronic)
Sickle cell anemia

(53) Acro-osteolysis

Angiomatous malformation
Epidermolysis bullosa
Familial acro-osteolysis
Hyperparathyroidism
Occupational (vinyl chloride)
Progeria
Raynaud's phenomenon
Scleroderma

(54) Advanced Bone Age and Skeletal Maturation

Adrenogenital syndrome (adrenal hyperplasia or adenoma)
Constitutional
Exogenous obesity
Juvenile rheumatoid arthritis
Lipoatrophic diabetes mellitus
Ovarian endocrine tumors
Pinealoma
Polyostatic fibrous dysplasia (Albright's syndrome)
Primary hyperaldosteronism
Sato's syndrome (pituitary gigantism)

Table continued on following page.

VI. OSSEOUS SYSTEM

ROENTGEN SIGNS OF OSSEOUS SYSTEM *(Continued)*

(55) Retarded Bone Age and Skeletal Maturation

Congenital hyperuricosuria
Cushing's syndrome
Homocystinuria
Hypogonadism
Hypopituitarism
Hypothyroidism
Malnutrition
Phenylketonuria
Turner's syndrome

(56) Skull Tables—Thickening and/or Sclerosis

Acromegaly
Anemias of childhood (severe: Cooley's, sickle cell,
    spherocytosis, iron deficiency)
Cerebral atrophy (childhood)
Craniostenosis
Engelmann's disease
Fibrous dysplasia
Hyperostosis frontalis interna
Idiopathic
Meningioma
Microcephaly
Myotonia atrophica
Neuroblastoma (metastatic)
Osteoma
Osteopetrosis
Paget's disease

VII. MISCELLANEOUS

MISCELLANEOUS ROENTGEN SIGNS

(57) Soft Tissue Calcifications in Extremities (Excluding Focal Soft Tissue Disease)

Metabolic and Collagen	Parasitic	Vascular
Chronic renal disease (amorphous, periarticular)	Cysticercosis (oval, in muscle planes)	Atherosclerosis
Dermatomyositis (amorphous, subcutaneous sheets)	Dracunculosis (coiled, tubelike)	Medial sclerosis (Mönckeberg's)
Ehlers-Danlos syndrome (ring calcifications)	Filariasis (coiled, linear)	Phleboliths
Fluorosis (ligamentous)	Leprosy (linear, in nerve sheaths)	Venous stasis
Gout (amorphous, periarticular)		
Hyperparathyroidism, primary and secondary (amorphous, periarticular; more common in secondary disease)		
Hypervitaminosis A (ligaments)		
Hypervitaminosis D (flocculent periarticular masses)		
Hypoparathyroidism (arterial, periarticular)		
Idiopathic calcinosis (amorphous, plaques)		
Idiopathic hypercalcemia (flocculent periarticular masses)		
Milk-alkali syndrome (amorphous, periarticular)		
Ochronosis (ligaments, cartilage)		
Paraplegia (periarticular)		
Poliomyelitis (periarticular, disc cartilage)		
Progressive myositis ossificans (massive, subcutaneous, bone formation)		
Pseudogout (synovial, cartilage)		
Pseudohypoparathyroidism (small subcutaneous)		
Pseudopseudohypoparathyroidism (small subcutaneous)		
Pseudoxanthoma elasticum (faint subcutaneous sheets)		
Scleroderma (amorphous, subcutaneous sheets, periarticular in hands)		
Werner's syndrome (amorphous, vascular, ligaments, periarticular)		

VII. MISCELLANEOUS

MISCELLANEOUS ROENTGEN SIGNS (*Continued*)

(58) Cartilage Calcifications

Adrenal insufficiency (ear cartilage)
Chondrocalcinosis (joint cartilage)
Chronic respiratory poliomyelitis
Gout (joint cartilage)
Hypercalcemia (ear cartilage)
Hyperparathyroidism (joint and ear cartilage)
Ochronosis (intervertebral discs, ear cartilage)
Osteoarthritis (joint cartilage)
Physiologic (costal and laryngeal cartilage)
Polychondritis (joint, ear and other cartilage)
Senility
Tietze's syndrome (late)
Trauma
Vitamin D intoxication (joint cartilage)

(59) Intracranial Calcifications

Asymptomatic-Physiologic	Inflammatory	Neoplastic	Other
Choroid plexus	Abscess	Craniopharyngioma	Aneurysm
Dura	Cysticercosis	Gliomas	Arteriosclerotic vessels
Falx	Cytomegalic inclusion disease	Hemangioma	Arteriovenous malformation
Habenula	Paragonimiasis	Lipoma of corpus callosum	Familial cerebral calcification
Internal carotid artery (parasellar)	Torulosis (rare)	Meningioma	Hemorrhage
Petroclinoid ligament	Toxoplasmosis	Metastatic disease (rare)	Idiopathic basal ganglia calcification
Pineal	Trichinosis (rare)	Metastatic retinoblastoma	Primary hypo-parathyroidism
Tentorium	Tuberculoma	Pinealoma	Pseudohypopara-thyroidism
	Tuberculous meningitis	Pituitary adenoma (rare)	Pseudopseudo-hypopara-thyroidism
			Sturge-Weber disease
			Subdural hema-toma
			Tuberous sclerosis

INDEX

Note: Page numbers in **boldface** refer to illustrations.
"vs." denotes differential diagnosis.

INDEX v

Berylliosis, 516, **516**, **517**
Beryllium, and pneumoconiosis, 509
Bile ducts, diseases of, 1079–1103
Bilharziasis, 270, **271, 272, 273**
Biliary cirrhosis, primary, 1102, **1102**
Biliary ducts, carcinoma of, 1098, **1098, 1099, 1100**
Biliary fistula, 1086, **1087**
Biliary tree, normal, T-tube cholangiogram of, **1089**
Bladder
  anomalies of, 874
  elevation of, in prostatic enlargement, A40
  extrophy of, 874
  in pelvic lipomatosis, 1239, **1240**
  in pneumaturia, 863, **863**
  neurogenic, 372, **373**
  schistosomiasis of, 270, **273**
  tumor of, **833**
    and obstructive nephropathy, **829**
Bladder outlet, obstruction of, 827
Blast injury, 20, **20**
Blastomycosis, 229, **229**, 230, **231**
  and infectious arthritis, 54
Blebs, in anthracosilicosis, 510, **511**
Bleeding. See also *Hemorrhage.*
Bleeding diverticulum, 931, **933, 934**
Blind loop, and intestinal malabsorption, **975**
Blood cells, white, diseases of, 1162–1171
Bone. See also *Joints.*
  cyst of, aneurysmal, 1388, **1388, 1389**
    simple, 1387, **1387**
  demineralization of, diseases associated with, B19
  disappearing, 1386, **1386**
  diseases of, 1321–1405
    congenital, 1338–1358
    hereditary, 1338–1358
  fibrosarcoma of, 1401, **1402**
  fibrous dysplasia of, 1364, **1365, 1366**
    leontiasis ossea in, **1367**
  hemangioma, 1384, **1384, 1385**
  in Cushing's syndrome, 1275, **1276, 1277**
  in decompression sickness, 17, **18, 19**
  in diabetes mellitus, **1230, 1231**
  in electric injury, 15, **15, 16**
  in eosinophilic granuloma, 1191, **1192, 1193**
  in familial hyperlipemia, 1235, **1236**
  in Gaucher's disease, 1195, **1196, 1197**
  in gonadal dysgenesis, 1286, **1287, 1288**
  in Hand-Schüller-Christian disease, **1193, 1194**
  in hemophilia, 1217, **1218, 1219, 1220, 1221**
  in Hodgkin's disease, 1185, **1188**
  in homocystinuria, **1247**
  in hyperparathyroidism, 1304
  in hypogonadism, 1285, **1285**
  in hypopituitarism, 1253
  in hypothyroidism, 1263, **1264, 1265**
  in iron deficiency anemia, **1144, 1145**
  in leukemia, acute, **1163, 1164**
    chronic, 1165, **1168**
  in lymphosarcoma, 1175, **1177, 1178**
  in Marfan's syndrome, 1424, **1426**
  in multiple myeloma, 1200, **1201, 1202, 1203**
  in myelofibrosis, 1168, **1171**
  in neurofibromatosis, 1411, **1412, 1413**

Bone (*Continued*)
  in phenylketonuria, **1246**
  in radiation injury, 10
  in sickle cell disease, 1148, **1149, 1150, 1151, 1152**
  in thalassemia major, 1155, **1155, 1156, 1157**
  in trisomy 17–18, **1438**
  in tuberous sclerosis, 395, **396, 397, 398**
  infarctions of, diseases associated with, B21
  intoxications of, 1329–1336
  invasion of, from soft tissue lesion, A46
  lesions of, in decompression sickness, 17
    in echinococcosis, 274
    in pancreatitis, acute, 984, **988**
      chronic, **991**
    in sarcoidosis, 107, **111, 112**
    lytic, A46, A47, A48
    permeating, A47
    sclerotic border around, A47
  marble, 1341
  metastatic malignancy of, 1402
    in carcinoma of thyroid, **1270**
    neuroblastoma and, 1297, **1298, 1299**
  osteoblastic changes in, A45
  osteoblastic nodules of, A45
  roentgen signs of, A42–A49, B19
  sclerosis of, in hypoparathyroidism, **1311**
  skull. See *Skull.*
  tumors of, 1369–1402
    benign, 1370–1391
    malignant, 1392–1402
  wormian, A49
    in osteogenesis imperfecta, 1339, **1340**
Bone age, advanced, diseases associated with, B21
  retarded, diseases associated with, B22
Bone density, increased, in tuberous sclerosis, 395, **398**
Bone resorption, in psoriatic arthritis, 74
  subchondral, in juvenile rheumatoid arthritis, **71**
Bony ankylosis, A36
Bony nasal septum, 294
Bowel. See *Colon* and *Small intestine.*
Brachial plexus, traumatic avulsion of, **369**
Brachycephaly, 385
Brain
  arteriovenous malformation of, 306, **306, 307**
  computerized tomography of, normal findings in, **294, 295**
  infarction of, 297, **299**
  tuberculoma of, 354, **354**
  tumors of, metastatic, 350, **350, 351, 352, 353**
Brain atrophy, 377, **377, 378, 379**
  in phenylketonuria, 1245
  in Sturge-Weber disease, 394, **394**
Breast, metastatic carcinoma from, and myelophthisic anemia, **1142**
Brill-Symmers disease, 1183, **1183**
Brodie's abscess, 1337
Bronchial adenoma, 529, **530**
Bronchial papilloma, 532, **533**
Bronchiectasis, 463, **463, 464, 465, 466, 467**
  cylindrical, 463, **464, 466, 467**
  cystic, 466
  in congenital agammaglobulinemia, **26**
  saccular, 463, **465, 466**

VOLUME I–Pages 1 to 774 — VOLUME II–Pages 775 to 1478